Biomedical and Health Research Program (Biomed)

Concerted Action:
"Restoration of Muscle Activity through FES
and Associated Technology – RAFT"

Springer
Berlin
Heidelberg
New York
Barcelona
Budapest
Hong Kong
London
Milan
Paris
Santa Clara
Singapore
Tokyo

A. Pedotti, M. Ferrarin, J. Quintern, R. Riener (Eds.)

Neuroprosthetics

from Basic Research to Clinical Application

Biomedical and Health Research Program (BIOMED) of the European Union. Concerted Action: Restoration of Muscle Activity through FES and Associated Technology (RAFT)

With 275 Figures, 56 Tables, and 40 Photographs

Springer

Antonio Pedotti and Maurizio Ferrarin
Centro di Bioingegneria
Fondazione Pro Juventute
Politecnico di Milano
Via Capecelatro 66
I-20148 Milano

Jochen Quintern
Neurologische Klinik
Klinikum Großhadern
Marchioninistr. 23
D-81366 München

Robert Riener
Lehrstuhl für Steuerungs- und Regelungstechnik
Technische Universität München
Arcisstr. 21
D-80333 München

ISBN 3-540-61084-7 Springer-Verlag Berlin Heidelberg New York

Cataloging-in-Publication Data applied for
Die Deutsche Bibliotek - CIP-Einheitsaufnahme
Neuroprosthetics from basic research to clinical application: biomedical and health research program (BIOMED) of the European Union; concerted action: restoration of muscle activity through FES and associated technology (RAFT); with 56 tables / A. Pedotti ... (ed.). -Berlin; Heidelberg; New York; Barcelona; Budapest; Hong Kong; London; Mailand; Paris; Santa Clara; Singapur; Tokyo: Springer, 1996
ISBN 3-540-61084-7
NE: Pedotti, Antonio [Hrsg.]

Typesetting: Camera-ready by authors
Cover design: Lewis und Leins, Berlin
Production: PRODUserv Springer Produktions-Gesellschaft, Berlin
Printing: Hieronymus Buchreproduktions GmbH, München

SPIN: 10516469 62/3020-5 4 3 2 1 0 – Printed on acid-free paper.

Preface

There are almost 250,000 paraplegics and tetraplegics in Europe. Every year another 5,000 people have accidents that confine them to a wheelchair. Depending on the level of the lesion on the spinal cord their lower limbs (paraplegics) or their upper and lower limbs (tetraplegics) are paralysed and, if the lesion is very high (cervical), also the vital breathing function is comprised.

All these subjects still have muscles and nerves below the lesion which are in principle able to be reactivated and to produce the desired motor functions, such as standing, walking, reaching, manipulating, or breathing.

To achieve this goal we should be able to send to those nerves and muscles the same neural commands that our brain normally produces when we stand, walk, manipulate, or breath.

The idea is not new, and several results have been obtained. In general, however, they are insufficient and too critical to be really helpful for a large number of patients. Mainly because the most trivial movement is really the result of a very complex coordination, in which many muscles must be simultaneously controlled according to a sophisticated motor strategy.

Thus, a clinically viable solution must provide acceptable answers to various questions:

How is the artificial neuroprosthesis to be integrated in the general natural sensory control system?

How can optimal control strategies be designed and adapted to the individual patient in order to ensure the best functional recovery, considering also the use of mechanical devices and specific training procedures?

How should the most suitable candidate patients be selected and recruited so that the localisation of the lesion, physical conditions, as well as physiological attitudes are taken into account?

How should the interface electrode-nerve, the implantable device, and the surgical procedures be designed in order to guarantee the best results?

To answer these questions a basic understanding of natural sensorimotor integration must be combined with knowledge of neuromotor disorders, biomechanics of movement, and advanced technologies of microelectronics, sensors, mathematical modelling, and self-learning procedures. These interdisciplinary problems require the contribution of different researchers working in complementary areas, e.g., neurophysiology, neurology, rehabilitation, bioengineering, and advanced technologies of informatics.

For these reasons the European Union, in the framework of the BIOMED Programme, has chosen neuroprosthetics as one of the topics of major interest for collaborative European research and has financed the *RAFT (Restoration of muscle Activity by Functional electrical stimulation and associated Technologies)* Concerted Action. Funds were provided by the EU for relevant activities involving research collaboration and coordination among the most qualified European scientists. In this three year programme, a network of more than twenty research institutes was set up and promoted by meetings, workshops, staff exchanges, visits, ready access to relevant information, and the rapid dissemination of clinical results.

The main goal of these collaborative efforts in basic research and clinical investigation was to identify the best procedure for reactivating paralysed or poorly controlled muscle function in order to permit patients with a wide range of disabilities to perform activities of dialy life more effectively. This will in turn increase their independence and reduce the financial burden of support which such patients require from the national health services.

Efforts were particularly concentrated on restoring the ability to walk. Close contacts were maintained with other European programmes, such as the CALIES, and the ongoing activities in this field in the USA and other non-European countries. Research was also performed to identify the most suitable procedures for achieving upper limb functions and improving the restoration of autonomous respiration in tetraplegics. Five main workshops were organised in Salford (UK), Milan (I), Montpellier (F), Enschede (NL), and Grainau-Eibsee (D).

This book is derived from the contributions presented by leading scientists at these workshops. It represents an updated review of the main findings of European research and clinical developments on neuroprostheses and their applications for restoring movement.

Such fascinating topics as neural control, movement strategies, the pathophysiology of posture and gait, advancements in artificial and natural sensors, biomechanics and neural networks are presented in light of their application to the paralysed patient. Major clinical problems such as spasticity, muscle fatigue, patient training and selection, orthotics, and surgical problems are also treated.

Finally, I would like to express my gratitude to all contributors and especially to Pierre Rabischong, Herman Boom, Thomas Brandt, Thomas Sinkjaer, George Anogianakis, and John Stallard, who have fruitfully collaborated as members of the Project Management Group of the RAFT Concerted Action. A special thanks to Jack Edwards, Peter Veltink, Maurizio Ferrarin, Jochen Quintern, Robert Riener, Günther Schmidt, Carla Finocchiaro, and Matilde Cordella, who contributed to the organisation of the topical workshops that made possible the publication of the present book.

Prof. Antonio Pedotti

Project Leader
"Restoration of Muscle Activity by Functional Electrical Stimulation and Associated Technologies" Concerted Action

Table of Contents

Chapter 1: Natural control of movement and posture 1

Feedforword postural control during movement
J. Massion, S. Vernazza, A. Alexandrov 3

Is the center of gravity controlled during movement?
S. Vernazza, M. Cincera, J. Massion, A. Pedotti 11

Basic neurophysiology and FES
J. Duysens, B. M. H. Van Wezel, H. Van de Crommert 15

Correlation analysis as a tool for defining strategies of movement
G. Anogianakis, D. Koutsonicolas, E. Bela, M. Apostolakis 21

Plasticity of primary motor areas of the brain after stroke -
a motor cortex stimulation study
G. Rapisarda, E. Bastings, A. Lozza,
A. Maertens de Noordhout, P. J. Delwaide 33

Locomotor capacity of spinal cord in paraplegic patients
L. Jensen, G. Colombo, V. Dietz 41

Stretch reflex variations during gait
J. B. Andersen, T. Sinkjær 45

Modulation of the Hoffmann reflex of soleus during the walking cycle
in stroke patients and associated control of ankle joint movement
M. Garrett, B. Caulfield 51

Chapter 2: Contraction and fatigue of stimulated muscles 59

Muscle recruitment with surface and implanted electrodes
E. Rabischong 61

The effect of contractile activity on the damaged
skeletal muscle and the application on paraplegic locomotion
T. Seene, M. Umnova, P. Kaasik, J. Järva,
K. Alev, R. Puhke, A. Pehme, M. Pääsuke 67

A dynamic model of electrically stimulated
knee muscles in healthy and paraplegics
M. Ferrarin, P. Iacuone, A. Mingrino, C. Frigo, A. Pedotti 81

A model for an artificially activated musculoskeletal system
S. J. Dorgan, M. J. O´Malley 91

Physiologically based multi-input model of muscle activation
R. Riener, J. Quintern, E. Psaier, G. Schmidt 95

Novel stimulation strategies for the
recruitment of paralysed muscle
D. J. Maxwell, M. H. Granat, R. H. Baxendale 115

Towards an optimized muscle controller
J. C. Jarvis, H. Gollee, M. M. N. Kwende, S. Salmons, D. J. Murray-Smith ... 123

The function of neuromuscular junction
in upper motor neuron weakness
J. V. Trontelj, J. M. Fernandez, M. Mihelin, D. Rugelj 129

Fatigue indices in electrically stimulated
quadriceps muscle with surface electrodes
E. Rabischong, D. Guiraud 137

Muscle fatigue facing continuous and intermittent
simulation and recovery from fatigue
E. Rabischong, M. Gaviria 145

Fatigue of intermittently stimulated human quadriceps:
influence of knee angular velocity
H. M. Franken, P. H. Veltink, H. B. K. Boom 155

Chapter 3: Control strategies in FES 161

A comprehensive FES control system for mobility restoration in paraplegics
P. H. Veltink, W. de Vries, H. J. Hermens, G. Baardman,
M. Ijzerman, S. Heinze, A. V. Nene, G. Zilvold, H. B. K. Boom 163

Control of the first generation CALIES implants
J. H. Hermens, G. Baardman 171

Description of the CALIES external controller
D. Guiraud, M. Beliaeff, B. Gilbert, J. C. Repetto, E. Rabischong 179

Design of a multisensor closed-loop neurostimulator. Part A:
Communication unit with wireless data link and digital signal processor
M. Keller, P. Krauß, G. Hoch, J. Quintern 183

Design of a multisensor closed-loop neurostimulator.
Part B: Input and output stage
A.Weiß, P. Krauß, G. Hoch, J. Quintern 189

A modular system for controlled FES and therapy of paralyses
R. Rupp, A. Nützel, G. Vossius 195

Optimized experimental control of
FES-induced swing phase of paraplegic gait
H. M. Franken, P. H. Veltink, G. Baardman, H. B. K. Boom 201

Development of control strategies for
FES- supported closed-loop standing-up
S. Heinze, P. H. Veltink, P. L. Jensen, R. E. Mayagoitia,
H. J. Hermens, H. F. J. M. Koopman, P. A. Huijing 209

Unsupported standing of paraplegics by stimulation
of the plantarflexors: some results from the wobbler apparatus
N. de N. Donaldson, F. M. D. Barr, G. F. Phillips, T. A. Perkins 217

Biomechanical simulation of the lower extremity
for the development of control strategies for FES
R. Riener, J. Quintern 233

Biomechanical modelling in artificial control of FES assisted mobility
P. H. Veltink 245

Inverse models for control of movements
J. Quintern, R. Riener, S. Rupprecht, S. Volz, A. Straube 255

Neural networks for the control of posture and locomotion
W. J. Daunicht 263

Self tuning control in FES with compensation of nonlinear
recruitment characteristics by artificial neural networks
J. Schultheiss, T. Keller 275

Chapter 4: Biomechanics applied to neuroprosthetics 279

Biomechanical simulation and animation of the
lower extremity for the design of neural prostheses
R. Riener, S. Villars, J. Quintern, G. Schmidt 281

Optimal trajectory generation for a paralegic
patient raising from a chair by means of FES
F. Bahrami, R. Riener, M. Buss, G. Schmidt 285

Crutch assisted FES gait and upright stability assessment
T. Karcnik, A. Kralj, T. Bajd 293

Sensor staircase for the measurement
of ground reaction loads: preliminary results
R. Riener, J. Quintern, H. Boedrich, T. Barner, F. Freyberger, G. Schmidt ... 301

Modeling of joint-rotations during line tracking arm movements
J. Laczko, J. Quintern, S. Krafczyk 305

Chapter 5: Artificial and natural sensors 315

3D movement analysis using accelerometry - theoretical concepts
P H. Veltink, H. B. K. Boom 317

Restoration of lateral hand grasp using natural sensors
A. Lickel, M. Haugland, J. Haase, T. Sinkjær 327

Extraction of slip information from digital nerve signals in man
A. Lickel, M. Haugland 335

Characterization of the ENG activity from a digital
nerve for feedback control in grasp neuroprostheses
R. R. Riso, P. J. Slot 345

Selective intraneural sensing for neuroprosthetics
L. C. W. Rutten, H. J. Meier 359

Myoelectric signals from paretic wrist extensor
controlling electrical stimulation of the same muscle
R. Thorsen, F. Biering-Sørensen, S. D. Hansen, O. T. Andersen 373

Study of methods for decomposition of superimposed
signals with application to electromyograms
D. Zazula, D. Korze, A. Sostaric, D. Korosec 377

Chapter 6: Spasticity: pathophysiology, evaluation, and treatment 391

Which spinal cord neurophysiologic
mechanisms are responsible for spasticity?
P. J. Delwaide, G. Rapisarda, A. Lozza 393

Biomechanical and neurophysiological
implications on spasticity assessment
M. Osio, M. Ferrarin 401

A new biomechanical approach to
pendulum test for spasticity evaluation
M. Ferrarin, M. Osio, G. Abello 411

A comparison of clinical and biomechanical
assessments of spinal spasticity
R. H. Baxendale 429

Parameters controlling antispastic electical stimulation:
clinical application and theoretical considerations
G. Vossius, R. Frech 437

Clinical considerations on spasticity and FES
V. Alfieri, A. Alfieri 447

Pharmacologic management of spasticity
S. Sorbi, G. Sorrentino 461

Management of spasticity - Southport experience
B. M. Soni 469

Chapter 7: Orthotics and hybrid systems 481

Powered hip orthosis
J. Edwards, S. V. S. Rithalia 483

On the improvement provided by hip transversal rotation
on paralegic gait walking with reciprocating orthosis
M. Ferrarin, M. Rabuffetti 493

Mechanical orthoses and FES for patients with complete thoracic lesions
J. Stallard 503

Hybrid FES/reciprocating gait orthosis design
L. Yang, M. H. Granat, D. J. Maxwell,
J. P. Paul, D. N. Condie, D. I. Rowley 513

Hybrid system for upright mobility with unlockable
orthotic knee for knee bending during swing phase
J. Edwards, A. O. P. Bataweel 523

Chapter 8: Clinical application of surface FES for motor functions 531

Multichannel electrical stimulation in hemiparatic patients
S. Hesse, M. Malezic, K.-H. Mauritz 533

Multi-channel FES therapy in rehabilitation of gait in stroke patients
U. Bogotaj, N. Gros, M. Kljajic, R. Acimovic-Janezic 541

Restoration of gait by FES in stroke and spinal cord injury patients
M. Malezic, S. Hesse, K.-H. Mauritz 553

Long term electrically induced cycling in SCI. A pilot study
T. Mohr, P. Tornøe, F. Biering-Sørenson, J. Pødenphant, J. Andersen, A. Wagner, H. Galbo, M. Kjær 569

Preliminary results of muscle strength, indurance and metabolism in the wrist extensors of tetraplegics following 12 weeks of electrically induced training
A. Hartkopp, S. D. R. Harridge, M. Mizuno, A. Ratkevicius, H. Gregersen, E. Hagen, M. Kjær, B. Quistorff, F. Biering-Sørensen 579

Chapter 9: Implanted systems and neuroprosthetics for autonomic functions 591

Biomechanical basis of the choice of the stimulated muscles for CALIES program
P. Rabischong 593

Dual channel implantable stimulator system for selective stimulation of ankle dorsal flexors and evertors
M. Tomsic, U. Bogataj, U. Stanic, M. Kljajic, R. Acimovic, F. Gider 603

Lumbar anterior root stimulator for lower limb control in paraplegia
D. N. Rushton, N. de N. Donaldson, F. M. D. Barr, V. J. Harper, T. A. Perkins, P. N. Taylor, A. M. Tromans 611

Initial results with a lumbar/sacral anterior root stimulator implant
J. Perkins, N. de N. Donaldson, A. C. Worley, V. Harper, P. Taylor, D. E. Wood, D. N. Rushton 623

Augmentation of pulmonary ventilation by electrical stimulation of abdominal muscles.
U. Stanic, L. Lenart, J. Sorli, F. Kandare, R. Jaeger 635

Functional recovery of respiration: phrenic nerve stimulation
D. Caldiroli 639

Modelling and evaluation of a nerve cuff electrode
D. M. Fitzpatrick, L. M. Costa Monteiro, R. H. Baxendale 647

List of authors 653

Chapter 1

Natural Control of Movement and Posture

Feedforward Postural Control during Movement

J. Massion[1], S. Vernazza[1], A. Alexandrov[2]
[1]Laboratory of Neurobiology and Movements, C.N.R.S., Marseille, France
[2]Institute of Higher Nervous Activities, Academy of Science, Moscow, Russia

Abstract - Controlling balance while performing a movement is one of the main constraints involved in trunk and arm movements. Two questions are addressed in the present paper. First, is the Center of Gravity (CG) shift which normally occurs during upper trunk or arm movements minimized during the performance of a movement? Secondly, how is the CG control centrally organized during a movement? It was established here that an active control of the CG actually occurs during trunk bending and arm raising, which minimizes the CG shift during the movement, and that this control increases in efficiency when the equilibrium constraints increase. A single automatic control is responsible for both the movement performance and the balance control; the kinematic synergies which achieve the two goals depend both on a control signal which fixes the time course of the movement and on a second control which fixes the ratio between the angle changes on the basis of a memorized representation of the body segments'geometry and mass. This representation is updated by the sensory inputs monitoring the support conditions and the equilibrium constraints.

1 Introduction

Controlling balance is one of the main constraints involved in everyday activities. We live in a world which is subjected to the forces of gravity. In the presence of a support such as a floor, contact forces are generated, which tend to make the body collapse. Postural tone, which is mainly distributed among the extensor muscles provides muscular forces which counteract the effects of gravity and contribute to building up an erect posture such as that involved in standing. There exists however a further constraint to be dealt with, namely controlling balance. This means that under static conditions, many postures can be set up within the limits of the joint mechanics. However, with a given posture, the distribution of the body segments has to be such that the CG projection remains within the area of support. The CG projection onto the ground is tightly regulated by the CNS. During quiet stance, the CG projection does not move randomly inside the whole supporting area, but remains preferentially located within a narrow area, which is usually located 6-8 cm in front of the ankle joint axis. When a postural disturbance occurs, postural reactions can be observed which tend to restore the initial CG position (Horak and Macpherson, 1996).

Balance control is also a major issue during movement performance. Two modes of control can be identified, depending on which body segments are involved (see Massion, 1992).

The first mode of control minimizes the anteroposterior or lateral CG shift which occurs during upper trunk or arm movements. Moving these body parts will shift the CG in the direction of the movement, and thus possibly cause a state of imbalance. Opposite displacements of other body segments occur however simultaneously, which minimize the CG shift in the horizontal plane.

The second mode of control operates when the leg is engaged in a movement. This occcurs for example when a standing subject is flexing or raising a leg, or initiating a step. The leg movement is then preceded by a shift of the CG toward the supporting leg. This initial shift frees the moving leg from the part of the body weight it supports and serves to maintain the balance during the leg movement.

Two opposite modes of balance control can therefore be observed, depending on which body segments are to be moved. The one minimizes the CG shift in the horizontal plane when upper trunk or arm movements occur, and the other shifts the CG toward the supporting leg when leg movements are being performed.

The questions which will be discussed here concern two main aspects of balance control during movement.

The first relates to a debate in the literature which has not yet been definitely settled : is the center of gravity a regulated value contributing to balance during quite stance or movement?

The second question relates to balance control during upper trunk movements : how is the central control responsible for minimizing the CG shift during the movement organized?

2 Is the Center of Gravity Regulated During Movement?

Balance control is a contact force task, as recently illustrated by Macpherson (1994) in the cat. Leg muscles can be subdivided into two groups in the standing cat: those which exert vertical forces counteracting of the forces of gravity in order to support the body's weight, and those which orient the contact force vector in order to maintain balance.

Do these contact forces control the body's geometry as proposed for example by Lacquaniti (1992) and by Fung and Macpherson (1995) in the case of the leg or trunk axis, or is it the body mass and more specifically the CG position which is regulated ?

According to Lacquaniti (1992) and Fung and Macpherson (1995), the CG is not primarily regulated in the cat. It is the leg orientation with respect to the vertical or the trunk axis with respect to the ground which are actually the values regulated during stance, and the CG position is determined secondarily by the body's geometry.

Human stance, unlike that of quadrupeds, is bipedal and the supporting surface is rather narrow. Moreover, the CG position is located much higher above the ground.

Two sets of data favour the hypothesis that the CG is actually controlled during movements in humans. The first evidence was provided by experiments in which the subjects performed fast upper trunk bending. It was observed that by the end of the movement, the CG had shifted a few cm forward or backward. In a population of 5 subjects, each performing a series of 10 forward or backward movements, a mean shift ranging between - 1.7 and 2.8 cm occured with forward movements and between - 0.2 and 5.8 cm with backward movements. Upon making comparison between the theoretical CG shift liable to occur in the absence of the opposite displacements of the lower body segments (from 8 to 12 cm with forward movements and from - 3.6 to - 5.5 cm with backward movements), and the actual CG shift observed, it was noted that more than 80% of the theoretical shift was compensated for by the active control during forward and backward bending. Interestingly, the CG position at the end of the movement was not scattered over the whole supporting area, although it covered a larger area than prior to the movement (Fig.1).

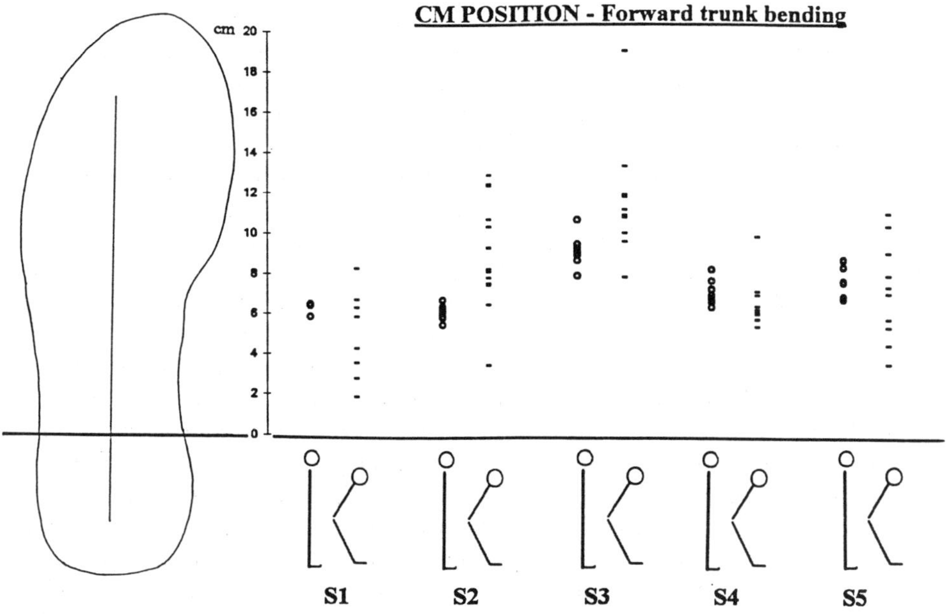

Fig. 1. Position of the center of mass before and 300ms after the end of a forward trunk movement. The subject was instructed to perform the movement as fast as possible in response to a tone. On the left, the shape of the foot. On the right, the initial and final CM projection with each of the 5 subjects. Note that the initial position was located in a narrow zone from 6 to 10 cm in front of the ankle joint axis. At the end of the movement, the positions were more widely distributed but remained inside the support area.

This finding indicates that the final CG position at the end of the movement was actually calculated and that the control of the movement was associated with the control of the CG position. It could be argued that the CG control might result from a passive interaction between segments, which actually occurs during upper trunk movements (Ramos and Stark, 1990). A Principal Component analysis of the axial synergies indicated however that in addition to the interaction between segments, there exists a neural control which actively regulates the CG position (Alexandrov et al., 1994).

The second line of evidence was provided by experiments in which the subjects performed fast upper trunk bendings with an additional 10 kg load placed on their shoulders. In this series, the CG shift at the end of the upper trunk bending was recorded when the subject was not supporting a load and was compared with that observed when he was bearing the 10 kg load. Performing the upper trunk movement with a load could be expected to result in an additional CG shift of about 4 cm forward or backward, due to the mechanical action of the load. If the CG shift turned out to be smaller, this would indicate that the additional mass was included in a representation of the body CG and that the control of the movement is associated with a feedforward control of the CG which takes the additional mass into account. In 3 subjects, the CG shift was the same both with and without a load. This resulted from a change in the kinematic synergy between the ankle, knee and hip joints which control the CG position : the ankle joint (plantar flexion) has increased. This result indicates that there exists an internal representation of the body mass which is actually involved in the feedforward control of the CG during upper trunk movements. This control of the additional mass was found to occur in 3 out of the 5 subjects

Does the control of the CG during upper trunk movements also exist with arm raising? Martin (1967) reported that this was so and published a photograh of a standing man before and after raising the arm. It could be seen that a trunk inclination did occur toward the side opposite that of the moving arm. To investigate this point, Vernazza et al. (this volume) compared the center of gravity shifts recorded when a standing subject raised an arm laterally under various standing conditions (bipodal, unipodal) and in the absence or presence of a load on the moving hand. The CG shift to be expected during arm raising is rather weak (about 1 cm without a load and 3 cm with a load) and the disturbance of equilibrium very mild in comparison with the supporting area during bipodal stance. The results indicate that a CG control does exist, that this control is subject dependent, and that only about 40% of the CG shift was compensated for by the active control 1 second after the end of the movement, based on the combined data obtained on the whole population. During unipodal stance, however where the support area is narrow, about 75% of the CG shift is compensated for both with and without load. This result suggests that the support conditions and the putative balance disturbance are taken into account by the central control mechanism which rules out both the movement and the CG control as possible contributing factors.

To conclude this part, there therefore exists evidence that in humans, during upper trunk movement and arm raising, the CG position is controlled in the anteroposterior and lateral directions and that this control takes into account the actual body mass and the support conditions. It can thus be concluded that an internal representation of the body mass does exist and that it is used to organize the CG control during movement.

3 How is the CG Regulated During Movement?

During upper trunk movement, the main control is that exerted on the amplitude and velocity of the trunk bending. An additional constraint is included however in the control, normally stabilizing the center of mass position. This is achieved by kinematic synergies which move the upper trunk and the lower body segments in opposite directions.

How are the kinematic synergies organized?

There are two schools of thoughts about the control of balance during upper trunk movement. According to the first, there exist two parallel controls, the one dealing with upper trunk bending, and the other with balance control. These two controls might be coordinated during the same motor act. According to the second hypothesis, a single control exists, which fixes the angle changes with time in such a way that both the movement time course and the CG stabilization are achieved simultaneously.

We now propose a series of data, based on kinematic, dynamic and EMG analyses, suggesting that the central nervous system uses a single, one degree of freedom, automatic control which fixes both the movement velocity and amplitude and stabilizes the CG by fixing a ratio between the joint angle changes:

1. The EMG analysis shows that an early activation of trunk, thigh and shank muscles occurs prior to the movement onset. This indicates that the central nervous system exerts a direct simultaneous command on the various segments participating in the kinematic synergy.
2. The peak velocity of the various markers occurs synchronously. This points to the existence of a timing signal which synchronizes the movement of the various segments, each having its own mass and inertia, and argues against the hypothesis that the movements might only depend on dynamic interactions between segments, although these do actually occur (Ramos and Stark, 1990).
3. The results of a principal component analysis performed by Alexandrov et al. (1994) show that there exists a fixed ratio between the hip, knee and ankle joints angle changes and thus that only one degree of freedom is controlled.

This analysis showed that the first principal component (PC1) accounts for between 96 and more than 99% of the angle joint changes in the case of both slow and fast forward and backward movements and those with low and high amplitudes.

Is the kinematic synergy defined by PC1 of central or peripheral origin?

The fact that PC1 remains stable with movements of various amplitudes and velocities argues in favour of the idea that the synergy is of central origin. The interactions between segments, which actually occur, may vary depending on the movement velocity and the ratio between the angles may change accordingly.

Another finding indicating that the kinematic synergy is of central origin was based on experiments carried out under microgravity, where the external constraints are greatly modified. In 0G, with the feet fixed to the floor, the CM is still stabilized and the multijoint kinematic synergy was still present.This indicates that the kinematic synergies are preserved although the equilibrium constraint is absent. The EMG activity was greatly modified however. This suggests that the CNS primarily controls the kinematic synergy, i.e. the ratio between the angle changes, whereas the internal muscle forces generated to perform the task adapt to the new environmental constraints.

To conclude, the upper trunk movement and the balance are simultaneously controlled and can be accounted for by the performance of a one degree of freedom multijoint movement with fixed ratios between the angle changes. This is in line with the hypothesis first forward by Bernstein (1967) that during learning, the CNS may reduce the number of degrees of freedom and that the learned control may include the anticipatory correction of the usual dynamic disturbances occurring during movement performance.

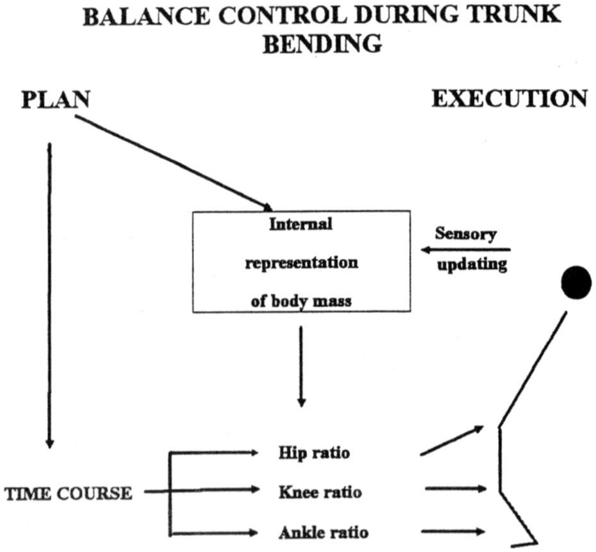

Fig. 2. Schema indicating how the balance is controlled during upper trunk movement. For explanation, see text.

4 Conclusions

During upper trunk movements in the sagittal plane or arm movements in the frontal plane, a feedforward control of balance takes place. This control minimizes the CG shift that would otherwise result from changing the position of the moving segment. The results of experiments where an external load was added to the moving segment argue in favour of the hypothesis that an internal representation of the body segments mass and inertia is built up which is used to control the CG during the movement and that this representation is under the form of a repertoire of memorized angle ratios which are appropriate for maintaining balance. For example, bending the trunk 30° forward gives rise to a CG shift which is compensated for by an ankle plantar flexion of 10° (which shifts the hip backwards). The ratio between the angle changes here is 3 to 1. Once this ratio has been fixed, a simple central signal may control the time course of the movement.

A second aspect of the control is represented by the sensory updating of the internal representation of the body mass. This occurs for example when a mass is added to the moving segment. An evaluation of the equilibrium constraints, such as the extent of the support base is also occuring (Fig. 2).

Might a simple control mechanism of this kind be a useful means of helping paraplegic patients to control their equilibrium? The question cannot be easily answered. The control exerted by electrostimulation is translated into muscle force and thus into torques, whereas the parameters controlled in the case of balance may be expressed in terms of angles. If a simple transformation of torques into angles does occur, equilibrium control might be planned by adapting the muscle control at each joint in such a way that the kinematics can be executed with an appropriate time course and angle ratio. In paraplegic patients, however where the segmental circuits do not function properly, this would not be appropriate. The control system would then have to operate on a feedback basis according to a template taking both the angle ratios and the time course into account. This would necessitate the use of sensors monitoring the trunk, thigh and shank axes.

References

Alexandrov, A., Frolov, A., and Massion, J. (1994) Voluntary forward bending movement in human : a principal component analysis of axial synergies. In : K. Taguchi, M. Igarashi and S. Mori (eds.) *Vestibular and neural front*, Elsevier Science B.V. *International Congress Series*, **1070**, pp 345-348.

Bernstein, J. (1967) The co-ordination and regulation of movements. Pergamon Press. Fung, J. and Macpherson, J.M. (1995) Determinants of postural orientation in quadrupedal stance. *J. Neuroscience*, **15**: 1121-1131.

Horak, F.B. and Macpherson J.M. Postural orientation and equilibrium. In: *Handbook of Physiology*. Neural control of movement.
Lacquaniti, F. (1992) Automatic control of limb, movement and posture. *Curr. Opin. Neurobiol.*, **2**: 807-814.
Massion, J. (1992) Movement, Posture and Equilibrium: interaction and coordination. *Progress in Neurobiol.*, **38**: 35-56.
Macpherson, J.M. (1994) Changes in a postural strategy with inter-paw distance. *J. Neurophysiol.*, 71: 931-940.
Martin, J.P. (1967) The basal ganglia and Posture, Pitman: London.
Ramos, C.F. and Stark, L.W. (1990) Simulation experiments can shed light on the functional aspects of postural adjustments related to voluntary movements. In: J.M. Winters, L.Y. Woo (eds.) *Multiple muscles systems biomechanics and movements organization*, Springer-Verlag, New York, pp. 507-517.
Vernazza, S., Cincera, M., Massion, J., and Pedotti, A. (1995) Is the center of gravity controlled during movement? (*this volume*)

Is the Center of Gravity Controlled during Movement?

S.Vernazza[1], M.Cincera[2], J.Massion[1], A.Pedotti[2]
[1]Laboratory of Neurobiology and Movement, CNRS, Marseille, France
[2]Centro di Bioingeneria, Fond. Pro Juventute Don Gnocchi, Milan, Italy

Abstract- The present study is aimed at answering two questions. First, is there during arm raising in the frontal plane a minimization of the Center of Gravity (CG) shift which results from the arm movement? Second, is the putative CG control dependent on equilibrium constraints such as the support conditions (unipodal versus bipodal) or an additional load on the moving hand? It is shown that the CG shift is actually minimized during arm raising and that this active control is markedly increased with increasing balance constraints (additional load and unipodal stance).

1 Introduction

In humans adopting a standing position, voluntary movements such as trunk bending or arm raising involve the equilibrium maintenance constraint, which means that the Center of Gravity (CG) projection has to be stabilized inside the supporting surface. Both arm and trunk movements cause the CG to shift toward the side of the movement, and are thus liable to imbalance. It has been reported that during trunk movements, a feedforward CG control occurs which minimizes the CG shift (Babinski 1899, Crenna etal 1987, Alexandrov et al. 1994).

The aim of the present study was to determine whether a CG stabilization also occurs with arm raising in the frontal plane and to check the effect of increasing the equilibrium constraints by reducing the supporting surface (unipodal versus bipodal stance) adding a load to the moving hand (3.5 Kg, approximately 5 % of the total body weight).

2 Methods

The experiments were performed on 9 adults, 5 seniors (54 to 65 years) and 4 young adults (25 to 30 years). The subjects were asked to stand on a Kistler platform with their eyes open and their arms placed along their body. They were instructed to place their left or right arm at the horizontal in response to a tone and to stabilize their final position for 3 seconds. With each arm, a total of 40 tests was performed with two stance conditions : bipodal and unipodal, and two load conditions : without any load and with a 3.5 Kg load (10 trials with each experimental condition). The order in which the tests were performed was randomized.

The kinematic analysis was performed by means of the E.L.I.T.E system (Ferrigno and Pedotti, 1985). 22 passive markers were placed along the body at specific body segments. Two cameras recorded trajectories of the markers in the frontal plane.

The CG position was calculated from the kinematic recordings, on the basis of the anthropometric model using Zatsiorsky's regression equations (Zatsiorsky et al., 1983) and the following parameters were measured:

- **actual CG shift** (dCGa) measured at the beginning of the movement and one second after the end of the movement.

The beginning and the end of the movement were the onset and the end of the change in the angular velocity curve of the arm, with a threshold corresponding to 5% of the peak velocity.

- **theoretical CG shift** (dCGt) corresponding to the mechanical effect of the arm movement on the CG position measured at the same times.
- **index of active control of CG** (IAC) corresponding to the difference between the theoretical and the actual CG shift with respect to the theoretical CG shift (see fig 1.).
- **index of active control of the load** (IACl) corresponding to the difference between the theoretical and actual CG shift due to the load with respect to the theoretical CG shift due to the load (see fig 2.).

The statistical analysis was carried out with the Mann-Whitney test. The Wilcoxon test was used in order to determine whether the active index was significantly different from zero.

3 Results

As no significant difference was found to exist between the seniors and young adults, the results analysed here are those obtained on the population of the 9 subjects.

The index of active control of CG based on the mean value of the 9 subjects indicates that a weak active control was present in bipodal stance (34.8 % without any load and 24.4 % with the load) which increased significantly in unipodal stance (65.4 % without any load and 76.8 % with the load).

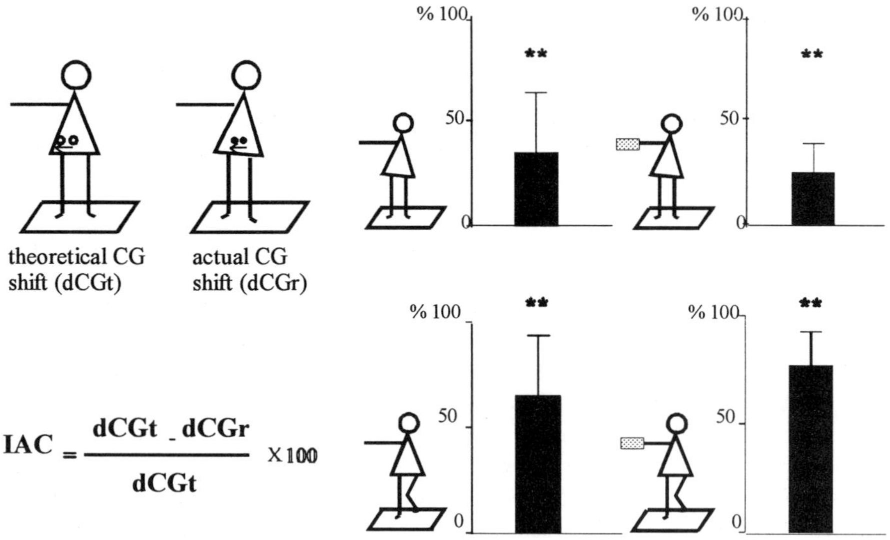

Fig. 1. Index of Active Control of CG (IAC)

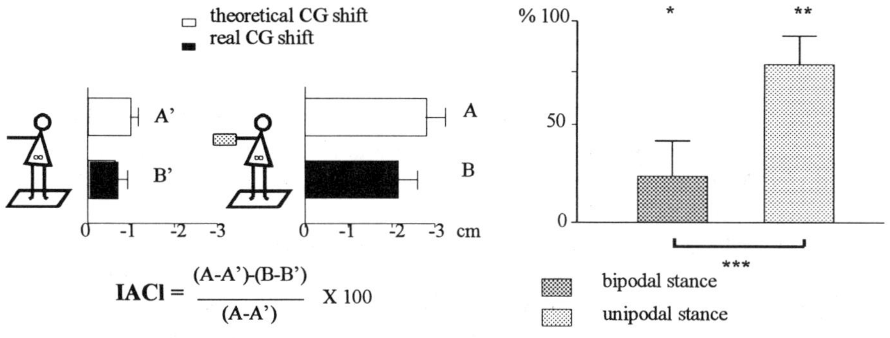

Fig. 2. Index of Active Control of the load

The index of active control of the load based on the mean value of the 9 subjects indicates that a weak active control occured in bipodal stance (23.1 %) which increased significantly in unipodal stance (78.6 %).

4 Conclusion

During arm raising in the frontal plane, an active automatic control of the CG occurs which minimizes the CG shift during the movement. This control is weakin the case of bipodal stance and large in that of unipodal stance, when the equilibrium constraints increase.

During arm raising with an additional load on the hand, the load is taken into account in stabilizing the CG during the movement. This control is weak in the case of bipodal stance and increases significantly in that of unipodal stance.

On the whole, these results indicate that a CG control exists which minimizes the CG shift during arm raising. This control increases with increasing equilibrium constraints such as those which arise when supporting an additional load on the hand and adopting unipodal stance.

During voluntary movements such as trunk bending or arm raising, equilibrium control seems to rely on two components of CG control. The first consists of a learned automatic control which fixes the ratios between joint angle changes. The axial synergies occuring during upper trunk bending are examples of this component of the control (ALEXANDROV et al 1994). The second component, which was found to exist in this study, consists of a mechanism updating this automatic control based on a sensory evaluation of the equilibrium constraints, depending on the area of the supporting surface or the weight (or inertia) of the segment performing the movement.

References

Alexandrov, A., Frolov, A., and Massion, J. (1994) Voluntary forward bending movement in human : a principal component analysis of axial synergies;

Tagushi, M., Igarashi and Mori, S. *(eds.) Vestibular and Neural front*, 345-348, Elsevier, Amsterdam.

Babinski, J. (1899) De l'asynergie cérébelleuse. *Rev Neurol* 7 : 806-816.

Crenna, P., Frigo, C., Massion, J., and Pedotti, A. (1987) A forward and backward axial synergies in man. *Exp Brain Res* 65: 538-548.

Zatsiorsky, V. and Seluyanov, V. (1983) The mass and inertia characteristics of the main segments of the human body. In : H. Matsui, K. Kobayashi (eds) *Biomechanics*, VIII-B: 1152-1159.

Basic Neurophysiology and FES

J. Duysens, B. M. H. Van Wezel, H. Van de Crommert
Dept. of Med. Physics & Biophysics, K. U. N., Nijmegen, The Netherlands.

1 Introduction

Over the years FES has become a widely accepted technique and nowadays it is common that basic scientists place their fundamental work in the context of FES (see Smits et al., 1994 for recent example). From work on cats and on humans it appears that sensory feedback during gait is very important and that a number of reflex pathways assist in adapting this automated type of movement to the environment. One of the most exciting prospects in FES research is the use of feedback either from natural sensors (Sinkjaer et al., 1994) or from artificial devices. Can we learn from basic physiological work what type of sensory feedback is necessary and how it can be incorporated in artificial "motor programs"? FES mostly relies on direct stimulation of muscles but in how far do we have to consider the secondary effects, such as the activation of muscle afferents either directly by the electrical stimulation or by the induced muscle contractions? What are the reflex consequences of this type of induced afferent input? In addition, electrical stimulation of peripheral nerves is used for FES to induce the flexor reflex for the initial part of the swing phase. Is this the only type of reflex available or are there other more subtle reflex effects which could be considered?

2 FES and Load Feedback

In some FES applications the artificial feedback about the load on the supporting limb is used to activate quadriceps FES during standing (see Stein, 1992). At first sight this type of reinforcing force feedback does not fit physiological models based on research on cats. In mammals the loading of the limb and the force of extensors is measured by Golgi Tendon Organs (GTO's) and Ib afferents which are thought to provide autogenic inhibition in the extensors producing the force (negative feedback). At present it is evident that this simple view has to be abandoned. The general idea emerging is that Ib afferent input feeds into pathways to a variety of motoneurones and that these pathways show convergence from other afferents. The gating of the activity in one pathway or the other may depend on the context of the motor task in which the animal is involved. In cats walking on a treadmill the activation of Ib afferents from extensors leads to autogenic excitation rather than to autogenic inhibition (Duysens and Pearson, 1980). More recent work has confirmed these observations and conclusions (Conway et al. 1987; Gossard et al.,1994). Conway et al.(1987) used experiments in immobilized spinal cats in which rhythmic locomotor neural activity was induced by injecting L-DOPA. Low-intensity stimulation of an extensor nerve was used to activate Ib afferents. Such stimuli increased extensor bursts and eliminated flexor bursts. From these results it appears that Ib autogenic feedback may be suppressed during gait.

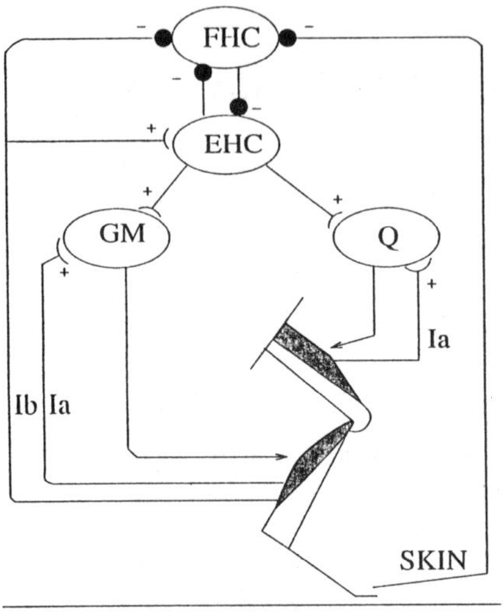

Fig. 1. Schematic representation of current hypotheses about the reflex pathways of load-detecting.afferents in cat. FHC and EHC: flexor and extensor half-centre, GM: gastrocnemius medialis, Q: quadriceps.

Instead, extensor force feedback suppresses flexor activity. The pathway for the latter effect is often only apparent in the movinganimal, since it involves motor centra which are essential for the execution of a given motor task. In the case of locomotion, the centre for the generation of flexion during swing plays a crucial role. For the cat the hypothesis was advanced that load detecting afferents, inhibit this centre during the stance phase (Fig. 1 based on Duysens and Pearson, 1980).

A second group of important afferents during locomotion are the cutaneous afferents from the foot. In humans, the activity from cutaneous afferents during movement has been recorded through microneurography (Hulliger et al., 1979). These studies have confirmed that activity from mechanoreceptors can signal changes in joint angles. However, this technique can only be used for small movements and for laboratory experiments. To record the afferent activity from the foot during gait an implanted cuff electrode has been used both in the cat (Duysens and Stein, 1978; Hoffer and Haugland, 1992) and in man (Sinkjaer et al., 1994). In the latter study the activity in the sural nerve was largest just after the foot hit the floor, although the innervation area of the nerve did not touch the ground. Moreover, a series of small bursts was seen throughout stance, coinciding with fluctuations in heel contact, as measured by separate sensors. In the cat it has been shown that induced low-threshold afferent activity from the foot can reinforce extensor activity during the stance phase of gait (Duysens and Pearson, 1976; Duysens and Stein, 1978).

3 Nerve Stimulation: Beyond the Flexor Reflex

In FES strong stimulation of the peroneal nerve is used to induce the flexor reflex. The question is whether nerve stimulation can evoke other reflexes as well (see above) and if so, whether the evoked responses can be used for FES related applications.

To answer such questions we started to investigate reflex responses in normal subjects during gait. For these experiments a bipolar stimulation electrode was positioned at the ankle over the left sural nerve (near the middle of the distance between the external malleolus and the Achilles tendon). The stimulation consisted of a train of 5 rectangular pulses of 1 ms, given over a period of 20 ms. These shocks were first applied while the subjects were standing on the treadmill to determine the perception threshold.

During the experimental runs, stimulus trains were given in some of the step cycles at a predetermined delay after footfall. Stimuli were either at 0 ("controls") or at 2 times perception threshold. The stimuli were delivered at one of a series of 16 intervals, spread evenly over the step cycle period.

To measure the reflex peaks, a fixed time window was set around the averaged rectified responses and the mean amplitude was calculated within the window. The same measurement was made on the averaged controls.

In response to sural nerve stimulation, normal subjects showed facilitatory and/or suppressive responses not only in pure flexors but also in muscles with an important extensor function (i.e. Gastrocnemii). In tibialis anterior these responses had a mean onset latency of 79 ms. It was found that the amplitude of these P2 responses to sural nerve stimulation varied as a function of the phase of stimulus application within the step cycle.

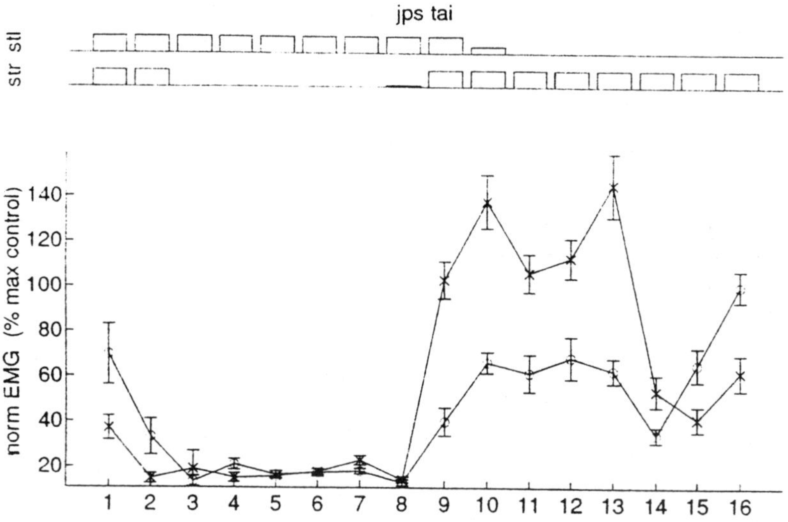

Fig. 2. Phase-dependent modulation of responses in Tibialis Anterior in a typical normal subject. At the top of each graph the stance phases are indicated for the ipsilateral (stl) and the contralateral side (str). These were obtained by sampling the signals from footswitches during the response periods. The amplitudes of the mean (N=10) responses (x symbols) are normalized with respect to the maximum (100 %) background activity in the step cycle.

The TA responses to 2xT stimulation of the sural nerve were absent during most of the stance phase but they were prominent near the transition from stance to swing. At the end of the swing phase, the response amplitude again decreased despite the high amount of background activity. Finally, a reversal from facilitatory to suppressive responses occurred. Amongst the 10 subjects investigated, 6 showed a reversal such as shown in Fig. 2, and 4 subjects showed only TA suppressive responses at all phases when TA was active.

Before being able to extend such findings to FES it is essential to investigate whether the responses are present in patients with spinal cord lesions and how strong the mechanical effects are of these evoked responses. Nevertheless, the application of this type of findings to patients has already yielded some promising results and insights in the pathophysiology of gait. For example for spastic patients Fung et al. (1990) and Yang et al. (1991) showed that there is a loss in the normal phase-dependent modulation of soleus H-reflexes during gait. In particular, Yang et al. (1991) described large Soleus H-reflexes in early stance in these patients and they proposed that this finding could explain the frequently observed clonus in this period of the step cycle. Interestingly, Fung et al. (1990) found that some improvement of gait was obtained by restoring the phase-dependent modulation of H-reflexes through conditioning by cutaneous stimuli.

Possibly the restoration of the modulation of cutaneous reflexes is also beneficial. Recently, Jones and Yang (1994) showed that reflexes elicited through stimulation of the posterior tibial nerve (containing large cutaneous and other afferents from the foot) were abnormally modulated in spinal-cord-injured patients. In particular in muscles such as Tibialis Anterior, there was no longer a phase-dependent reversal in these patients because they lacked the suppressive responses normally seen at the end of the swing phase. The ankle extensor Soleus was activated in reflexes in the swing phase. The resulting plantar flexion may have been one of the causes of their frequent falls.
It is a challenge for the future to find ways to restore normal phase-dependent modulation in such patients. However, already now it is clear that the use of peripheral nerve stimulation in FES may itself be beneficial. For example, Crone et al. (1994) recently showed that MS patients, treated with peroneal stimulation, had improved reciprocal inhibition as compared to patients without such treatment.

From work on cats it appears that the spinal cord itself can be the source of the phase-dependent modulation. Experiments with chronic spinal cats walking on a treadmill have convincingly shown that supraspinal structures are not essential to explain the phase-dependent modulation of reflexes observed in intact walking cats. Moreover, some evidence is available from experiments on fictive locomotion of spinal paralysed cats to demonstrate that part of this modulation persists in the absence of movement related feedback and thus is likely to be caused by the output of a spinal locomotor CPG (Central Pattern Generator). However, in fictive locomotion, the phase-dependent modulation is weaker, thereby indicating that under normal circumstances the afferent input may contribute significantly to the changes in reflex gain observed during locomotion.

It is worth mentioning that some data are available on humans as well. In patients with complete spinal cord transection, rhythmic locomotor-like contractions are very rare but they could indicate the existence of a CPG (Calancie et al.,1994). It has been reported that such discharges can be entrained by afferent (FRA) stimulation, indicating that cat and man may share common basic principles of afferent control of locomotor centres (Roby-Brami and Bussel, 1987).

4 Muscle Stimulation and its Afferent Consequences

In FES the direct stimulation of muscles is performed to yield a direct mechanical effect. However, such stimulation also activates muscle afferents. In the cat the stimulation of muscles yields P1 and P2 responses which are very similar to the responses evoked with cutaneous stimulation. In preliminary experiments (Van de Crommert, Van Wezel and Duysens) it was found that this also applies to humans. Stimulation of the Rectus Femoris with FES electrodes yields responses in a wide variety of ipsilateral and contralateral leg muscles, both flexors and extensors (Fig.3). The distribution and the latency of these responses is strikingly similar to those found following cutaneous stimulation of the foot.

Finally, it should be mentioned that the interaction between basic sciences and FES can go in the inverse direction as well. FES itself can be used to tackle some basic biomechanical questions about muscle functioning. For example, in our laboratory we were able to show that Medial Gastrocnemius has more of an exorotatory moment than Lateral Gastrocnemius on the basis of FES stimulation experiments (Muller and Duysens, unpublished observation).

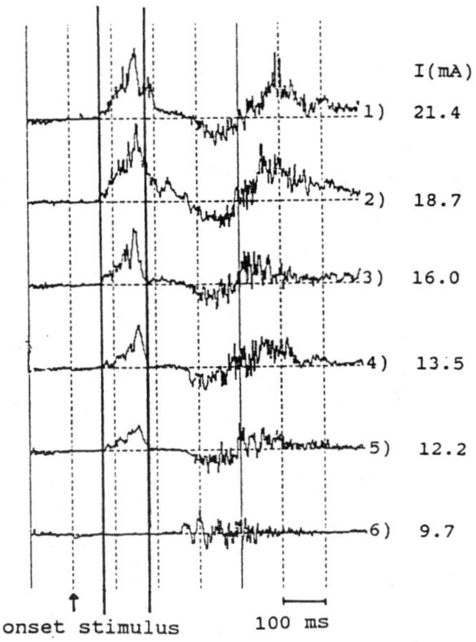

Fig. 3. Reflex responses (following subtraction of control activity) in Biceps Femoris following Quadriceps contractions elicited by electrical stimulation at various intensities in a normal subject during the early swing phase of walking on a treadmill.

References

Calancie, B., Needham-Shropshire, B., Jacobs, P., Willer, K., Zych, G., and Green, B. A. (1994) Involuntary stepping after chronic spinal cord injury. *Brain 117: 1143-1159.*

Conway, B. A., Hultborn, H., and Kiehn, O.(1987) Proprioceptive input resets central locomotor rhythm in the spinal cat. *Exp Brain Res 68: 643-656.*

Crone, C., Nielsen, J., Petersen, N., Ballegaard, M., and Hultborn, H. (1994) Disynaptic reciprocal inhibition of ankle extensors in spastic patients. *Brain 117: 1161-1168.*

Duysens, J. E. J. and Pearson, K. G. (1976) The role of cutaneous afferents from the distal hindlimb in the regulation of the step cycle of thalamic cats. *Exp Brain Res 24: 245-255.*

Duysens, J. E. J. and Pearson, K. G.(1980) Inhibition of flexor burst generation by loading ankle extensor muscles in walking cats. *Brain Res 187:321-332.*

Duysens, J. and Stein, R. B.(1978) Reflexes induced by nerve stimulation in walking cats with implanted cuff electrodes. *Exp Brain Res 32: 213-224.*

Fung, J., Blunt, R., and Barbeau, H. (1990) The soleus H-reflex modulation pattern in spastic paretic subjects during standing and walking. *In: Disorders of posture and gait 1990*, edited by Brandt T., Paulus W., Bles W., Dieterich M., Krafczyk S., Straube A. Georg Thieme Verlag Stuttgart - New York. pp. 107-110.

Gossard, J.-P., Brownstone, R. M., Barajon, I., and Hultborn, H. (1994): Transmission in a locomotor-related group Ib pathway from hindlimb extensor muscles in the cat. *Exp Brain Res 98: 213-228.*

Hoffer, J. A. and Haugland, M. K. (1992) Signals from Tactile Sensors in Glabrous Skin Suitable for Restoring Motor Functions in Paralyzed Humans. *In: Neural Prostheses*, edited by Stein R.B., Peckham P.H., Popovic. D.B. Oxford University Press - New York. pp. 99-128.

Hulliger, M., Nordh, E., Thelin, A. E., and Vallbo, A. B. (1979): The responses of afferent fibres from the glabrous skin of the hand during voluntary finger movements in man. *J Physiol (Lond) 291, 233-249.*

Johansson, R. S. (1988) Programmed and triggered actions to rapid load changes during precision grip. *Exp Brain Res 71(1): 72-86.*

Jones, C. A. and Yang, J. F. (1994) Reflex behavior during walking in incomplete spinal-cord-injured subjects. *Exp Neurol 128: 1-10.*

Roby-Brami, A. and Bussel, B. (1987) Long-latency spinal reflex in man after flexor reflex afferent stimulation. *Brain Res 110:707-725.*

Sinkjaer, T., Haugland, M., and Haase, J.(1994) Natural neural sensing and artificial muscle control in man. *Exp Brain Res 98: 542-545.*

Stein, R. B.(1992) Feedback Control of Normal and Electrically Induced Movements. *In: Neural Prostheses*, edited by Stein R.B., Peckham P.H., Popovic. D.B. Oxford University Press - New York. pp. 281-297.

Smits, E., Rose, P. K., Gordon, T., and Richmond, F. J. R. (1994) Organization of single motor units in feline sartorius. *J Neurophysiol, 72(4): 1885-1896*

Yang, J. F., Fung, J., Edamura, M., Blunt, R., Stein, R. B., and Barbeau, H. (1991) H-Reflex modulation during walking in spastic paretic subjects. *Can J Neurol Sci 18: 443-452.*

Correlation Analysis as a Tool for Defining Strategies of Movement

G. Anogianakis, D. Koutsonicolas, E. Bela, M. Apostolakis
Department of Physiology, Aristotle University of Thessaloniki, Greece

Abstract - Motor programs are defined sets of rules for executing a movement. Their definition includes the muscles involved and the timing of their actions. The combination of motor programs required to carry out a complex motor act is a motor plan. Since gait analysis provides accurate measurements of the position and velocity of defined points on the human body, this paper explores the applicability of correlation analysis in extracting, out of gait analysis data, sufficient information to permit the definition of complex motor programs and strategies of movement. Two subjects, a healthy male medical student and a female school of economics student suffering from limb girdle syndrome volunteered for providing the necessary data for testing the potential of the method. The initial results suggest that correlation analysis can be a powerful tool in identifying specific aspects of movement that can be considered both essential in describing specific movement components and, at the same time, "hidden" from common view. This permit the prediction that correlation analysis, will prove to be a valuable tool for describing the spatiotemporal evolution of the motions of the human body.

1 Introduction

Motor programs can be conceived of as defined sets of rules for executing a movement. Since the definition of a motor program must include the muscles involved (i.e. agonists, antagonists, synergists and postural fixators) as well as the timing of their actions (which must be predictably related), it is evident that, for a movement of given amplitude and speed, the rules of the program must specify the relative activity for each muscle and the exact timing between them.

Present evidence suggests that a single rapid movement at one joint is controlled by a single program. This assertion is supported by the EMG in the form of the well-known triphasic burst pattern of the agonist, antagonist and agonist muscle. More complex tasks, i.e. tasks involving a series of movements at several joints, are thought to be controlled either by a single motor program or by a number of separate programs (Benecke et al., 1986, 1987). The combination of motor programs required to carry out a complex motor act can be defined as a motor plan. The function of the motor plan would be to time the onsets of the individual programs which make up the total movement.

Humans are capable of calling up motor programs without reference to external feedback as it is evidenced by the extensive range of simple or complex motor acts that can be executed by a deafferented man (Rothwell et al., 1982). In another case it has been shown that formal aspects of motor programs are preserved in Parkinson's disease. Thus, the selection of muscles and the correct sequence of muscle activation (i.e. the invariant characteristics of a motor program) remain intact whereas the variant characteristics (speed and amplitude) are inadequately scaled. These disturbances imply a difficulty in switching from one motor program to the next or in running two motor programs at the same time.

The inability of patients to execute complex movements like walking or dressing, or the apparently abnormal slowness of their movements is of great clinical value to physicians who are interested in exploring the physiological basis of motor performance. Up to now such explorations focused on rapid simple movements. However, in most cases of clinical interest it is the performance of complex movements which is disturbed rather than single separate movements. Furthermore, in the case of rehabilitation it is the study of the strategies of movement that is important. By strategies of movement, we mean the various ways in which motor plans are altered to take into account restrictions imposed upon human motor activity either by its physiology or by its environment.

Attempts to physiologically analyze the deficits in complex movements date from 1954 when patients were asked to trace the outline of a triangle and to draw perpendicular lines with their dominant hand while repetitively squeezing the rubber bulb of a sphygmomanometer with the other hand. A little over 20 years later, studies performed on a larger spatial scale, such as kinesiologic analyses of ballistic goal- directed movements of different distances, showed that patients with Parkinson's disease perform these movements with inadequate speeds, i.e., movements of growing amplitude positively correlate with longer durations (Flowers,1976), in contrast to the behavior of normal subjects who use faster speeds for longer distances and keep movement duration relatively constant (Benecke et al., 1985).

In recent years, gait analysis has provided the means to accurately measure the position and velocity of defined points on the human body as that moves through the 3D space. This capacity opens up new vistas in the definition of complex motor programs as well as of strategies of movement. This paper represents a first attempt to explore the applicability of correlation analysis in extracting out of gait analysis data sufficient information to permit the definition of complex motor programs and strategies of movement.

2 Materials and Methods

2.1 Subjects

A healthy, 22 years old, male medical student (DA) and a 25 year old female school of economics student (AA) suffering from limb girdle syndrome volunteered for providing the necessary data for testing the potential of the method.

DA was chosen on the basis of his regular but mild involvement in physical activities in his everyday life (exercised in the university gym twice a week). In the case of AA, the limb girdle syndrome had been diagnosed through EMG 10 years ago (1984) and that diagnosis had been confirmed by biopsy in 1986. The choice of two subjects with different anatomical characteristics who had at the same time developed entirely different strategies of propulsion was dictated by the exploratory nature of the experiments reported here, i.e., it was chosen so that it maximizes the anticipated differences in the results of the correlation analysis. Indeed, the experimental paradigm and the mathematics of correlation analysis ensure that differences in anatomical characteristics play a minor role in the outcome (see discussion) in contrast to differences in the timing of the different events that are studied.

In addition in the case of AA, since she could also move without using a walking cane, it was possible to study her strategy of movement with and without such assistance.

2.2 Data Acquisition

The experimental set-up has been described in detail in the available literature (e.g. Ferrigno and Pedotti 1985), and for this reason only a brief reference will be made here.

Kinematics of the subjects propulsion movements were analyzed by a commercially available ELITE system (BTS, Milano) which has been recently installed in the Department of Physiology of the Faculty of Medicine of the University of Thessaloniki. The trajectories of eight retroreflective markers glued on the main reference points on one side of the subject were computed. The markers were placed on both subjects on the shoulder, elbow, wrist, trochanter, knee, external maleolus, heel and V metatarsal on the right side of the body. Sampling rate was 50 Hz.

The subjects were asked to walk along a prescribed, 5 meter long corridor across the room at a comfortable pace and at their normal stride. Following a few (20 - 30) trials during which they familiarized themselves with the task, 30 repetitions of the task were repeated for data acquisition purposes. During both the familiarization or the data acquisition periods the subjects were free to interrupt the routine if they felt tired and resume the process when they felt comfortable. Subject AA repeated the task both totally unassisted and using a walking cane.

The data acquired had the form of x (distance transversed from origin, i.e. from the beginning of the corridor), y (distance from the corridor), and z (height from the floor) coordinate time series for each marker, i.e. the data set for a given marker represented the x, y and z coordinates for that marker sampled every 20 milliseconds. Of these the x coordinate time series were analyzed by correlation analysis.

2.3 Analytical Methodology

The main technique used in the processing of the data was the calculation of the linear correlation coefficient (Pearson) between the x coordinate time series for every pair of markers for each subject:

$$r = \sum_t (x_t - \hat{x})(y_t - \hat{y}) \Big/ \sqrt{\sum_t (x_t - \hat{x})^2 \sum_t (y_t - \hat{y})^2} \qquad (1)$$

where x_t, y_t are the values of the two signals at time t and $\hat{x}, \hat{y}$ are the mean values of x_t, y_t accordingly.

The values of r vary between -1 and 1. Thus the value of r is near 1 when both x_t, y_t are varying in a linear fashion and both increase or decrease simultaneously. In this case we say that the two signals are positively correlated. The value 1 is independent of whether the signals increase or decrease as long they both vary in the same (positive or negative) direction.

When both x_t, y_t are varying in a linear fashion but the values of x are increasing while the values of y are decreasing or vice versa, then the value of r is -1. In this case we say that the two signals are in complete negative correlation.

A value of r that is very close to 0 indicates that the two signals are non-correlated.

The procedure for calculating the Pearson correlation coefficient r was repeated after shifting the time series of the second marker with respect to the first by a time τ

$$r_\tau = \sum_t (x_t - \hat{x})(y_{t+\tau} - \hat{y}) \Big/ \sqrt{\sum_t (x_t - \hat{x})^2 \sum_t (y_{t+\tau} - \hat{y})^2} \qquad (2)$$

where τ: -20N ... 20N msec, N: number of samples by which the second time series is shifted with respect to the first. In this way it is possible to estimate the linear dependence of the different instances of signal y on instances of signal x, i.e., it is possible to estimate whether a certain behavior of signal x has a linear effect on signal y, τ msec later. By repeating the process for increasing values of τ a sequence of r_τ is generated whose peaks identify the instances where the signals have maximum correlation. If the peak appears when $\tau > 0$ or $\tau < 0$, then the two signals have maximum correlation with a phase shift of τ msec.

The technical details of performing correlation analysis have been extensively described in the literature (e.g. Stearns, 1983). For the purposes of the present paper it must be noted that to avoid the effects of circular convolution of the x and y signals, both time series were padded with N zeroes (Stearns, 1983) before performing the necessary calculations. It must be also noted that the correlograms presented (Figs 1 to 9) represent averages of all 30 individual records obtained from each subject / condition.

3 Results

3.1 Subject DA

The main features of the correlation analysis between the shoulder marker of subject DA and the rest of the markers are shown in Fig. 1, which depicts the effects of the movement of the shoulder upon the movement of the rest of the body.

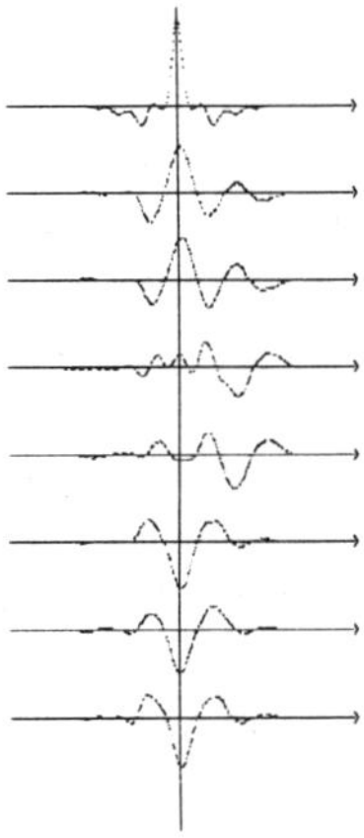

Fig. 1. Subject DA. Correlograms between the signal generated by the shoulder marker and that generated by each of the rest of the markers. The top trace represents the autocorrelation signal (i.e., the correlation of the signal generated by the shoulder marker with itself). The following traces represent the crosscorrelograms between (top to bottom of figure): shoulder and elbow, shoulder and wrist, shoulder and trochanter, shoulder and knee, shoulder and external maleolus, shoulder and heel and shoulder and V metatarsal. Total duration of signal used in calculating the correlograms was 2500 msecs.

The top most correlogram represents the autocorrelation of the signal generated by the shoulder marker. It is evident that the correlogram is absolutely symmetric about the origin (zero delay) as would be expected for the autocorrelation of a signal with itself. It is also evident that its peak at the origin falls off sharply indicating a minimal dependence of the future values of the signal upon its present values.

The second correlogram from the top represents the crosscorrelation between the signal generated by the shoulder marker and that generated by the elbow marker while the third from the top represents the crosscorrelation between the shoulder marker and the wrist. A sinusoidal dependence between the shoulder movement and the movement at the elbow and wrist is clearly evident which extends to positive as well as negative values of ô, i.e. the position of the wrist and elbow influence the evolution of the shoulder position in time and vice versa.

Further analysis of the relation between the movement of the elbow and the wrist in subject DA (Fig. 2, top two traces) shows that the two signals have almost identical characteristics allowing for the conclusion that their relative position changes very little during movement, i.e. the elbow angle changes very little during the arm swing that accompanies regular walking movement.

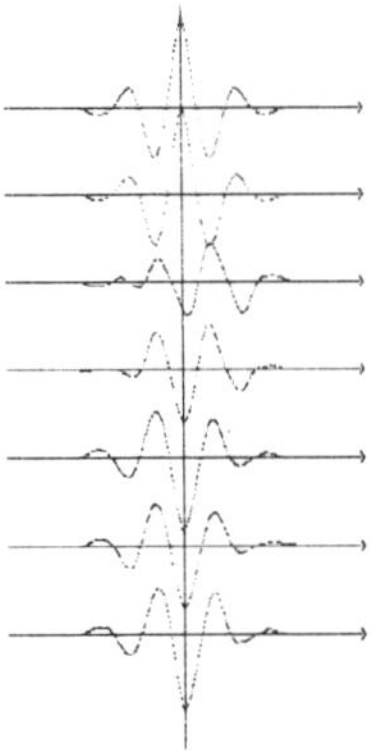

Fig. 2. Subject DA. Correlograms between the signal generated by the elbow marker and that generated by each of the rest of the markers. The top trace represents the autocorrelation signal (i.e., the correlation of the signal generated by the elbow marker with itself). The following traces represent the cross-correlograms between (top to bottom of figure): elbow and wrist, elbow and trochanter, elbow and knee, elbow and external maleolus, elbow and heel and elbow and V metatarsal. Total duration of signal used in calculating the correlograms was 2500 msecs.

The relative movement of the trochanter with respect to the rest of the body is also interesting (Fig. 1, 4th trace from the top). Thus, small sinusoidal movements of the trochanter seem to preceed the positioning of the shoulder, whose positioning in turn forces the trochanter into a large sinusoidal movement probably associated with the beginning of the next stride. This conclusion seems to be borne by the fact that the knee behaves in the same way (Fig. 1, 5th trace from the top), a reasonable expectation since the relative position of the knee to the trochanter remains constant.

Finally, there is a very interesting conclusion to be drawn from the relative movements of the external maleolus (Fig. 3, 3rd trace from the top), the heel (Fig. 3, 4th trace from the top) and the V metatarsal (Fig. 3, 5th trace from the top) with respect to the knee(Fig. 3, 2nd trace from the top) or the trochanter (Fig. 3, 1st trace from the top). Indeed the lower foot is determining the future position of the leg during stride while the reverse is not true.

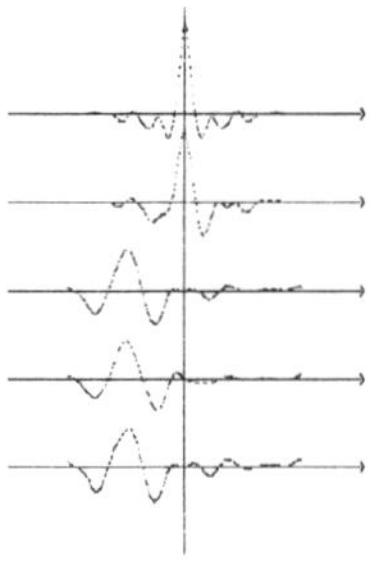

Fig. 3. Subject DA. Correlograms between the signal generated by the trochanter marker and that generated by each of the rest of the markers. The top trace represents the autocorrelation signal (i.e., the correlation of the signal generated by the trochanter marker with itself). The following traces represent the crosscorrelograms between (top to bottom of figure): trochanter and knee, trochanter and external maleolus, trochanter and heel and trochanter and V metatarsal. Total duration of signal used in calculating the correlograms was 2500 msecs.

3.2 Subject AA moving without support

The main features of the correlation analysis between the shoulder marker of subject AA and the rest of the markers are shown in Fig. 4, which depicts the effects of the movement of the shoulder upon the movement of the rest of the body.

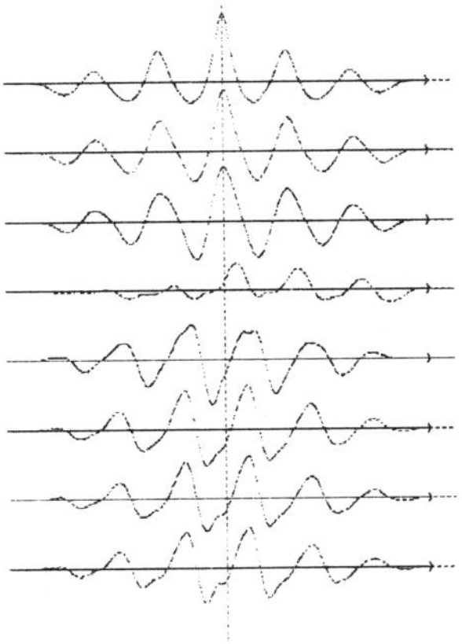

Fig. 4. Subject AA moving without support. Correlograms between the signal generated by the shoulder marker and that generated by each of the rest of the markers. The top trace represents the autocorrelation signal (i.e., the correlation of the signal generated by the shoulder marker with itself). The following traces represent the crosscorrelograms between (top to bottom of figure): shoulder and elbow, shoulder and wrist, shoulder and trochanter, shoulder and knee, shoulder and external maleolus, shoulder and heel and shoulder and V metatarsal. Total duration of signal used in calculating the correlograms was 5000 msecs.

The top most correlogram represents the autocorrelation of the signal generated by the shoulder marker. Again, as in the case of subject DA, the correlogram is absolutely symmetric about the origin (zero delay). However, in contrast to the correlogram of subject DA, the correlogram of subject AA walking without support does not show the sharp fall off about the origin indicating a great dependence of the future values of the signal upon its present values and a sinusoidal motion in space, result of the inability of subject AA to fix the position of her body in space.

As in the case of subject DA, the second correlogram from the top of Fig. 4 represents the crosscorrelation between the signal generated by the shoulder marker and that generated by the elbow marker while the third from the top represents the crosscorrelation between the shoulder marker and the wrist. Again a sinusoidal dependence between the shoulder movement and the movement at the elbow and wrist is evident, while analysis of the relation between the movement of the elbow and the wrist in subject DA (Fig. 5, top two traces) shows, just as it was evident in subject DA, that the elbow angle changes very little during the arm swing that accompanies regular walking movement.

The relative movement of the trochanter with respect to the rest of the body (Fig. 4, 4th trace from the top) indicates that, despite the inherent instability of subject AA's gate, the positioning of the shoulder forces the trochanter into a large sinusoidal movement associated with the beginning of the next stride.

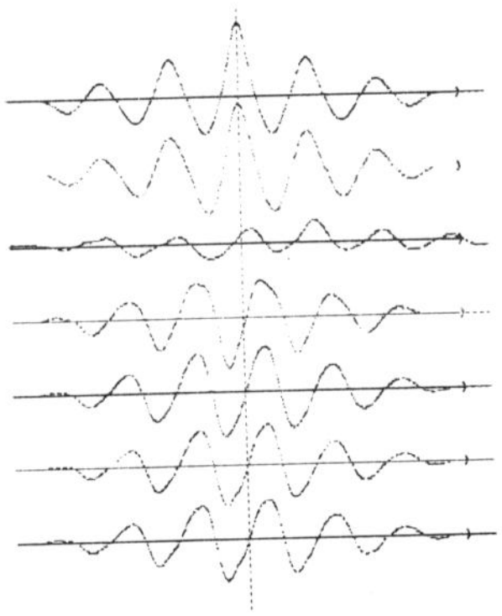

Fig. 5. Subject AA moving without support. Correlograms between the signal generated by the elbow marker and that generated by each of the rest of the markers. The top trace represents the autocorrelation signal (i.e., the correlation of the signal generated by the elbow marker with itself). The following traces represent the crosscorrelograms between (top to bottom of figure): elbow and wrist, elbow and trochanter, elbow and knee, elbow and external maleolus, elbow and heel and elbow and V metatarsal. Total duration of signal used in calculating the correlograms was 5000 msecs.

Finally, the relative movements of the external maleolus (Fig. 6, 3rd trace from the top), the heel (Fig. 6, 4th trace from the top) and the V metatarsal (Fig. 6, 5th trace from the top) with respect to the knee (Fig. 6, 2nd trace from the top) or the trochanter (Fig. 6, 1st trace from the top) indicate that in contrast to the case of subject DA the position of the lower foot is not determining the next position of the trochanter during stride. Furthermore, the movement of the knee is always in phase with that of the lower foot, indicating that during stride the whole lower limb freely swings about the hip joint.

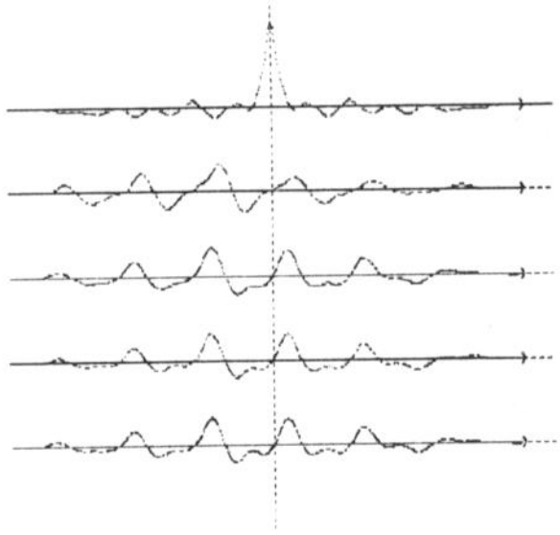

Fig. 6. Subject AA moving without support. Correlograms between the signal generated by the trochanter marker and that generated by each of the rest of the markers. The top trace represents the autocorrelation signal (i.e., the correlation of the signal generated by the trochanter marker with itself). The following traces represent the crosscorrelograms between (top to bottom of figure): trochanter and knee, trochanter and external maleolus, trochanter and heel and trochanter and V metatarsal. Total duration of signal used in calculating the correlograms was 5000 msecs.

3.3 Subject AA supported by walking cane

Correlation analysis of subject AA's walking pattern when using a walking cane shows that her strategy of movement remains amazingly unaltered with respect to her unaided gait (Figs. 7, 8 and 9). This leads to the conclusion that the strategy of movement adopted by AA does not depend on external support.

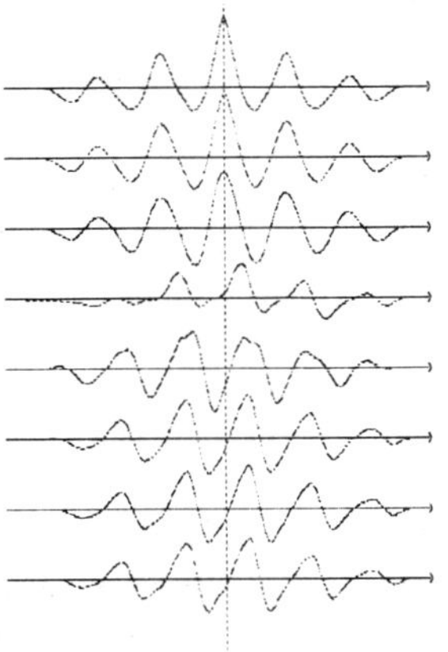

Fig. 7. Subject AA supported by walking cane. Correlograms between the signal generated by the shoulder marker and that generated by each of the rest of the markers. The top trace represents the autocorrelation signal (i.e., the correlation of the signal generated by the shoulder marker with itself). The following traces represent the crosscorrelograms between (top to bottom of figure): shoulder and elbow, shoulder and wrist, shoulder and trochanter, shoulder and knee, shoulder and external maleolus, shoulder and heel and shoulder and V metatarsal. Total duration of signal used in calculating the correlograms was 5000 msecs.

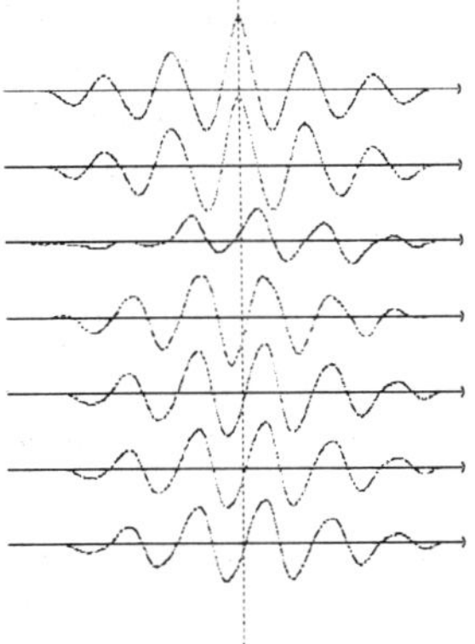

Fig. 8. Subject AA supported by walking cane. Correlograms between the signal generated by the elbow marker and that generated by each of the rest of the markers. The top trace represents the autocorrelation signal (i.e., the correlation of the signal generated by the elbow marker with itself). The following traces represent the crosscorrelograms between (top to bottom of figure): elbow and wrist, elbow and trochanter, elbow and knee, elbow and external maleolus, elbow and heel and elbow and V metatarsal. Total duration of signal used in calculating the correlograms was 5000 msecs.

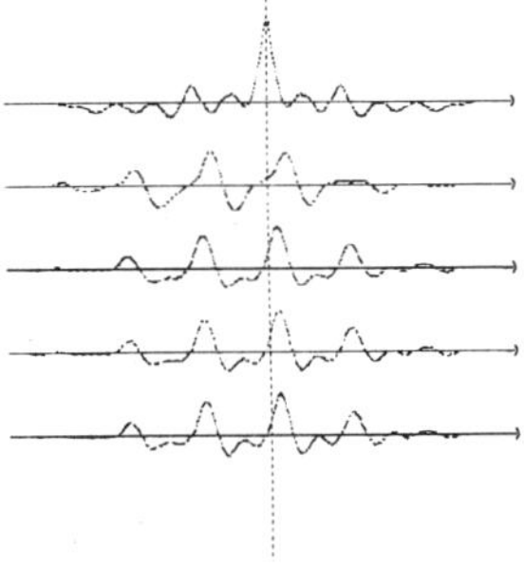

Fig. 9. Subject AA supported by walking cane. Correlograms between the signal generated by the trochanter marker and that generated by each of the rest of the markers. The top trace represents the autocorrelation signal (i.e., the correlation of the signal generated by the trochanter marker with itself). The following traces represent the crosscorrelograms between (top to bottom of figure): trochanter and knee, trochanter and external maleolus, trochanter and heel and trochanter and V metatarsal. Total duration of signal used in calculating the correlograms was 5000 msecs.

4 Discussion

Correlation analysis is an old, time tested technique in signal analysis that has been used to unravel coincidences between two signals as well as hidden periodicities that may be contained in them. It has not been used in the past for the description of spatiotemporal functions / signals mainly because the mathematics and the computational intricacies of multiple correlation analysis have been developed to a substantial degree only the last 15 years. The purpose of the present study has been to explore the potential contributions of correlation analysis in the elucidation of the strategies of movement. A simple experimental paradigm (movement alongside a straight line) was chosen in order to permit an easy assessment of the potential of this method of analysis. Two subjects with radically different movement strategies were chosen so that the method would be tested, initially, under optimal conditions and its results could be related to specific propulsion patterns. Therefore, the present report is of an exploratory nature.

The results that have been presented suggest that correlation analysis can be a powerful tool in identifying specific aspects of movement that can be considered both essential in describing specific movement components and, at the same time, "hidden" from common view. The fact, for example, that it is possible to clearly identify the absence of movement of the wrist with respect to the elbow despite the swing of the upper limb during normal walking, underscores the merits of the method and raises the hope that through correlation analysis it will be possible to consistently break up movement into simpler components, which can be identified with specific motor programmes.

The application of the method in the case of movement strategies that evolved upon a pathological substrate further elucidates this point. Indeed, the exaggerated dependence of the development of motion, in the case of subject AA, on the past positions of her body, is diametrically opposite to the strategy of movement that DA is using. Thus, while DA utilizes the thrust generated by the forward leaning of the body to initiate motion, as it is evident from Fig. 1 (where the movement of the shoulder proceeds and influences the motion of the rest of the body-points studied), AA has adopted a strategy whereby the body moves forward through the rhythmic coordination of the movement of its limbs. What is interesting about the particular strategy is the fact that it does not seem to be overtly dependent upon "breaking" mechanisms, which, had they been operational they would have tended to damp the rhythmicity of the crosscorrelations between the signals generated by the different markers.

The particular conclusions drawn above for subject AA, permit the prediction that subject AA will have substantial difficulty in terminating a sequence of walking movements. Indeed, her comment regarding her use of a walking cane is that it helps her to achieve exactly that and not to propel or to steady her gate. In this respect it is interesting to observe that subject AA's movement coordination when using a walking cane is remarkably similar to that of her unaided gait (Figs 7-9).

4 Conclusions

Correlation analysis, may prove to be a valuable tool for describing the spatiotemporal evolution of the motions of the human body. The analysis of simple aspects of single-directional movement permits the speculation that, when this type of analysis is extended to more complex movements of the human body and into higher orders of correlation, the critical links that connect simple motor programs together to form strategies of movement may be revealed. Further work will assess the potential of the method in this respect and it will clarify whether correlation analysis will join the rest of the gait analysis techniques.

References

Benecke, R., Meinck, H. M., and Conrad, B. (1985) Rapid goal-directed elbow flexion movements limitations of the speed control system due to neural constraints. Exp. Brain Res. 59 (3), 470-7.

Benecke, R., Rothwell, J. C., Day, B. L., Dick, J. P. R., and Marsden, C. D. (1986) Motor strategies involved in the performance of sequential movements Exp. Brain Res. 63 (3), 585-95.

Benecke, R., Rothwell, J. C., Dick, J. P. R., Day, B. L., and Marsden, C. D. (1987) Disturbance of sequential movements in patients with Parkinson's disease. Brain 110, 361-79.

Ferrigno, G. and Pedotti, A. (1985) ELITE: A digital dedicated hardware system for movement analysis via real-time TV signal processing. IEEE Trans. Biomed. Eng. 32 (11), 943-9.

Flowers, K. A. (1976) Visual "closed-loop" and "open-loop" characteristics of voluntary movement in patients with Parkinsonism and intention tremor. Brain 99, 269-310.

Rothwell, J. C., Traub, M. M., Day, B. L., Obeso, J. A., Thomas, P. K., and Marsden, C. D. (1982) Manual motor performance in a deafferented man. Brain 105, 515-42.

Stearns, S. D. (1983) Digital signal analysis, Hayden Book Co, N.J.

Plasticity of Primary Motor Areas of the Brain after Stroke - A Motor Cortex Stimulation Study

G. Rapisarda, E. Bastings, A. Lozza, A. Maertens de Noordhout, P.J. Delwaide.
University Department of Neurology, Hôpital de la Citadelle, Liège, Belgium

Abstract - We have used transcranial magnetic stimulation of the motor cortex with a focal, figure-of-eight stimulating coil to map bilaterally the topographic representation of the FDI muscle in the motor cortex of 17 right-handed and 5 left-handed normal subjects, and 3 patients having recovered hand function after stroke. In right-handed normals, the FDI muscle representation was broader in the dominant hemisphere, which was also more excitable. Such differences were not observed in left-handed subjects. In stroke patients after recovery, the affected hemisphere was more excitable, although it was the non-dominant one and in one of them, we observed a significant displacement of the FDI representation zone towards frontal regions, which we believe could represent an illustration of motor cortex plasticity.

1 Introduction

In recent years, the development of sophisticated neuro-imaging techniques (functional MRI, PET, etc...) has allowed in vivo studies of various functions of the cerebral cortex in normal man and their modifications in neurological or developmental diseases. Besides this, new electrophysiological tools have also been developed for functional studies of motor tracts. Transcranial magnetic stimulation (TMS) of the motor cortex allows non-invasive functional studies of cortico-motoneuronal pathways in conscious man (Barker et al. 1985). By means of surface EMG recordings, quantitative informations about latency, amplitude and morphology of muscle responses to TMS can be easily obtained. Moreover, the recent development of focal stimulating coils has opened the possibility to draw topographic maps of the cortical representation of a single muscle in primary motor areas (Wasserman et al. 1992; Wilson et al. 1993). Besides physiological studies, this method can be also used to investigate the possibilities of plasticity of primary motor centers in neurological diseases.

2 Methods

We have used the new tools described above to study the cortical representation of the first dorsal interosseous muscle of the hand in 17 right-handed and 5 left-handed normal subjects (14 men and 8 women, mean age: 41 years, range: 24-71).

We have also studied 3 patients (1 man, 2 women, ages: 37, 46 and 69 years) having fully recovered motor function of the hand after a massive ischaemic stroke of the middle cerebral artery territory, in order to determine whether some plasticity of primary motor centers can occur after such a cerebral insult. The major difficulties of motor cortex mapping procedures are linked to the following points.

First, a system has to be devised which gives reliable and reproducible coordinates of the coil position over the head. Therefore, we have used a slightly extensible rubber cap placed over the head with its surface divided in 1 cm^2 squares. This cap is positioned over each subject's head with reference to the Cz position of the international 10-20 EEG standard. With this system, the coil position over the head can be reported on a map with X and Y coordinates with very little intra- and interindividual variability. Indeed, this 2-D representation induces a distorsion of actual 3-D maps, but it was considered sufficiently accurate for the purposes of this study.

Secondly, mapping of the cortical representation of a given muscle requires the use of a figure of eight coil, which allows very focal stimulation of a given cortical region. Previous studies have indicated that the optimal orientation of the induced electrical field to activate hand motor areas was postero-anterior with a 30° upward tilt (Wasserman et al. 1992). However, we simply used a postero-anterior orientation without tilt which renders the mapping procedure much easier and does not require a much higher stimulus intensity. Due to the fact that the stimulation is delivered through the skull, the maps obtained remain less focal than with direct stimulation of the brain surface with electrical stimuli. However, preliminary studies conducted on 2 patients before and during tumor surgery have shown a good correlation between the optimal stimulation sites obtained with transcranial magnetic and direct electrical stimulations of the brain surface.

Thirdly, the activation threshold of a given muscle by the stimulations can differ considerably between individuals, as can the amplitudes of responses elicited. Moreover, it is well known that the level of background muscle activity has a strong influence on the morphology of responses elicited (Maertens de Noordhout et al. 1992). For these reasons, responses to TMS were recorded with fully relaxed target muscles and amplitude of the first negative peak was expressed as percentage of the negative peak of the muscle response evoked by supramaximal stimulation of the corresponding motor nerve (TMS/M max ratio). To take into account response fluctuations caused by individual threshold variations, two different stimulation intensities were chosen: 10% of the stimulator output above motor threshold and maximal output of the device. For each position of the coil over the head, five consecutive responses were collected and averaged.

With this technique, a cortical representation map of the fisrt dorsal interosseous muscle of the hand was drawn on the dominant and non-dominant sides of each normal subject and on the normal and affected side of stroke patients, taking handedness into account. Each individual map represents the brain area from which a muscle response can be elicited by the stimulation, as well as the peak-to-peak amplitude of the response evoked for each point expressed as a ratio to M max. From these data, the optimal stimulation site can also be defined with precision for each subject on both sides.

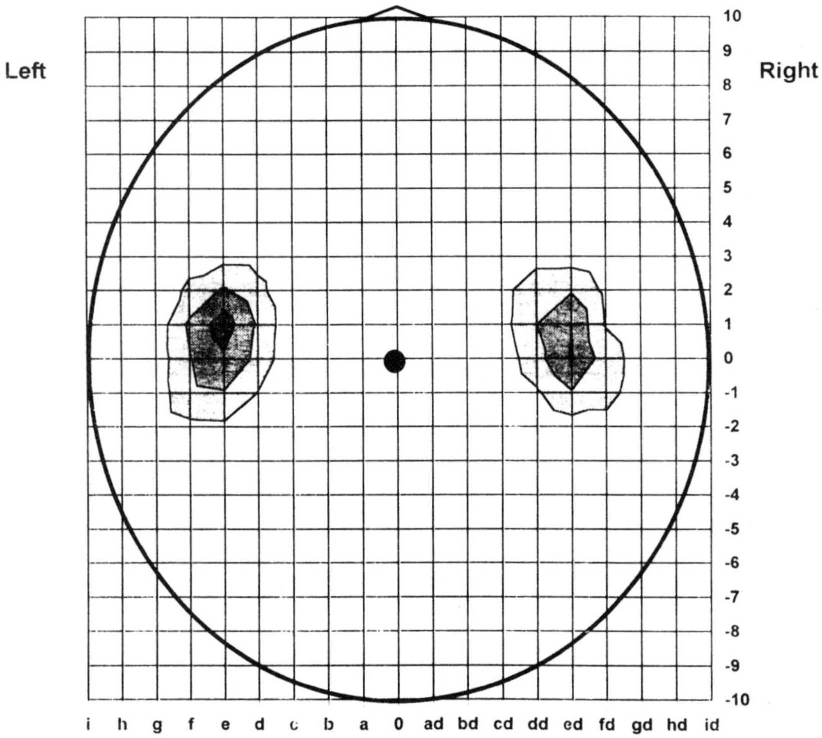

Fig. 1. Average representation maps of the left and right FDI muscles of 17 normal subjects, with a stimulus intensity of 10% above motor threshold, showing symmetrical location of maps on both sides. However, the maximal Mep/M max amplitude is larger and the map is slightly braoder on the dominant side. Each iso-curve represents 10% of M max.

3 Results

3.1 Normal subjects

Cortical mapping procedures were successfully completed in all 17 right-handed and 5 left-handed normal subjects. There was no significant difference of activation threshold of the FDI muscle by magnetic cortical stimulation (expressed as percentage of the maximal output of the stimulator) between the dominant and non-dominant sides in both groups (45 ± 4.8%. vs 47.3 ± 6.1% in right-handed subjects, 48 ± 11.1% vs 49 ± 8% in left-handed subjects). The amplitude of the maximal muscle response expressed as percentage of M max was also comparable on both sides (22 ± 9.5 ms vs 24.1 ± 9.8 % in right-handed, 23.4 ± 4.7 vs 28.4 ± 12.8% in left-handed). The optimal cortical stimulation sites to elicit maximal FDI responses ("hot spots") were strictly symmetrical over the head on the average maps of both groups (5 cm lateral and 0.7 cm frontal to Cz). Moreover, individual maps indicate that there is very little inter-individual variability of the optimal stimulation sites (< 1 cm in the X or Y axis). However, in right-handed subjects, several parameters indicate that the dominant hemisphere is more excitable than the non-dominant one. First, the maximal cortical area from which a muscle response could be elicited was significantly broader on the dominant than non-dominant side (24.6 ± 3.9 vs 20.6 ± 6.9 sq.cm, $p < 0.03$, Wilcoxon). Secondly, the amplitude ratio between responses elicited at 10% above motor threshold and at maximal stimulator output was significantly higher on the dominant versus non-dominant side (55.5 ± 24.1% vs 35.4 ± 22%). Results obtained in left-handed subjects fail to indicate similar differences between dominant and non-dominant side. The mean motor cortical representation area of both FDI muscles of 17 right-handed patients is shown in figure 1.

3.2 Stroke patients

Three right-handed stroke patients were studied after having fully recovered motor hand function following a massive ischaemic stroke in the non-dominant middle cerebral artery territory. The mapping procedure was undertaken between 6 and 23 months after the stroke. In all 3, FDI electro-myographic responses could be elicited from stimulation of the affected and normal motor cortices. In all patients, amplitudes of the maximal responses evoked by stimulation of the affected and normal sides were comparable. In case 1, the motor activation threshold was similar on both sides while in cases 2 and 3, threshold was higher on the affected side. However, in these 2 patients, the cortical area from which a response could be elicited was broader on the affected than on the normal side, in spite of the fact that the latter was the dominant one. One example of these findings in given in figure 2.

In patients 2 and 3, the optimal stimulation sites were symmetrical and located in the same region as in normals. The last patient (n°1) showed a different pattern with a considerable anterior shift (2.5 cm) of the representation map of the FDI on the affected side when compared to the normal side or to maps collected in normal subjects. This is illustrated in figure 3.

4 Discussion

With the method described above, it proved easy to delineate the motor cortical representation areas of a given muscle. Our results are comparable to those of previous studies (Wasserman et al. 1992; Wilson et al. 1993), at least for thresholds and optimal stimulation sites. There is also a good concordance with data obtained with direct electrical stimulation of the exposed motor cortex (Penfield and Boldrey, 1937). However, due to use of transcranial magnetic stimuli, the representation maps obtained in this study are broader than with direct stimulation. This is likely due to dispersion and attenuation of the stimulating current induced by the transient magnetic field, when it passes through the skull,

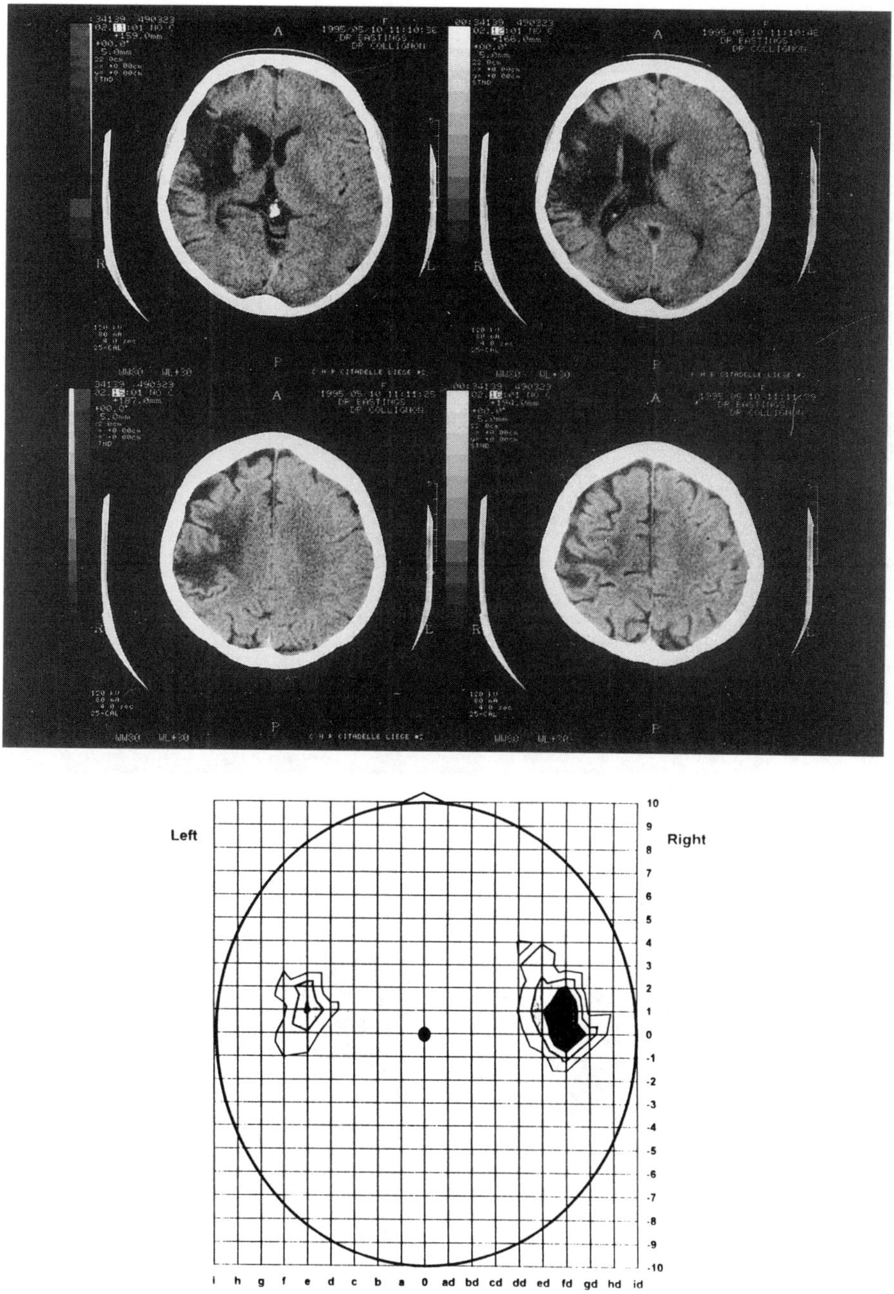

Fig. 2. CT-scans and representation maps of both FDI muscles of patient 2. Despite massive infarction of the MCA territory, the representation map of the right, affected FDI is broader than on the normal side and the amplitude of responses is greater. However, the hot spots remain symmetrical. On CT-scans, the left side is represented on the right.

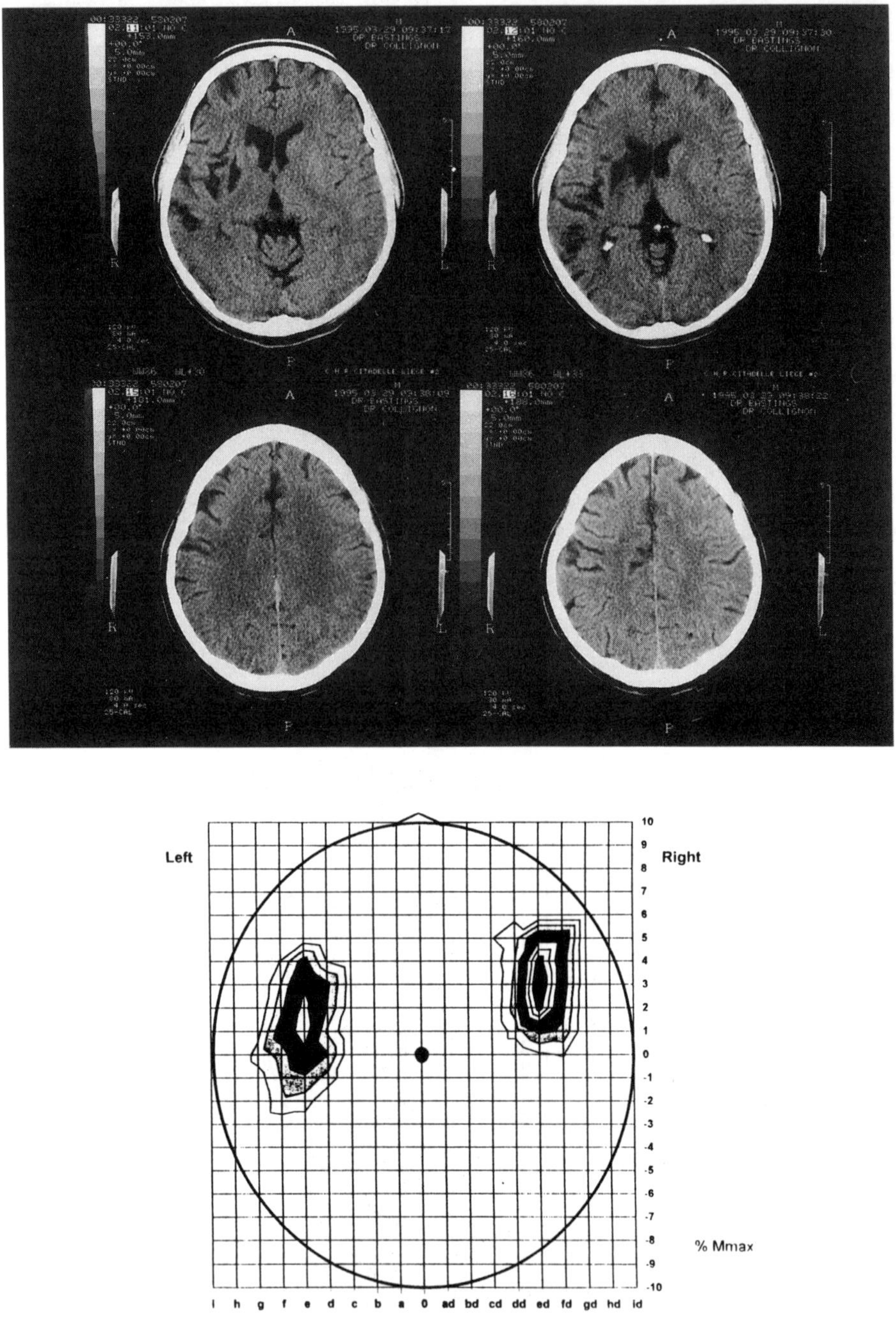

Fig.3. CT-scans and maps of patient 3, with considerable anterior shift of the FDI representation on the affected side. In this example, the iso-curves represent 5% of M max. On CT-scans, the left side is represented on the right

cerebrospinal fluid and meninges. The use of smaller stimulating coils might allow to draw more focal maps but due to physical properties, small coils are less efficient to activate deeply located structures than large ones. As the motor cortex lays some 15 mm under the skull surface, smaller coils could fail to activate excitable structures, particularly in some neurological diseases where a reduced cortical excitability is expected.

In normal right-handed subjects, there was no significant difference of motor thresholds, maximal muscle responses or optimal stimulation sites between the dominant and non-dominant hemisphere. However, the FDI representation maps were significantly broader on the dominant side, and contralateral muscle responses were also significantly larger when the dominant hemisphere was stimulated 10% above motor threshold. These findings suggest that the dominant hemisphere is more excitable in right-handed subjects, and confirm results obtained by Wilson et al. (1993). However, like these authors, we failed to find significant interside differences in left-handed subjects. Indeed, the latter group was more restricted, whi9ch causes statistics problems. Clearly, a confirmation in a larger group would be welcome.

In 2 patients with a full recovery of hand function after stroke, we observed that the FDI activation threshold was lower and the representation area was broader on the affected side, although it was the non-dominant side in both cases. These findings indicate that the affected hemisphere is more excitable in spite of the lesion caused to the brain (see CT-scan on figure 2). This can reflect adaptative mechanisms of the brain to overcome the initial cortical dysfunction or a phenomenon of denervation supersensitivity, presumably secondary to a damage caused to afferent pathways from the thalamus or primary sensory areas. However, the role of such pathways remains controversial in the literature (Lemon, 1979, Lemon and Van der Burgh, 1979). Whatever the final explanation, this phenomenon indicates that some functional plasticity of the motor cortex can occur even in adults.

In all normal subjects tested, the optimal stimulation sites ("hot spots") were symmetrical on the dominant and non-dominant sides. in none of them did the interside difference exceed 1 cm in the X or Y axis. Similarly, the individual hot spots were always located within 1 cm from the mean position for the group. This was also the case in 2 of the stroke patients tested but in the last one, there was a significant anterior shift (2.5 cm) of the FDI representation area on the affected side when compared to the normal side or to reference values of normal subjects. Besides this, muscle responses evoked on both sides of this patient showed comparable morphologies, but amplitude was larger on the affected side, in spite of the sutructural ischaemic lesion of the brain.

There could be several explanations to these topographic changes. First, anatomical destruction of some parts of the motor cortex could modify the optimal orientation of the coil to excite the remaining functional structures. Indeed, it is well known that exitation is more likely to occur if the orientation of the induced electric field is parallel to the axons to be excited. Secondly, this modification of FDI representation could be caused by activation of other motor structures located more frontally, normally silent but which might have become functional after destruction of the main efferent motor zone. Another explanation would be a progressive functional replacement of damaged motor cells by adjacent ones. As we have not performed prospective serial studies on this patient, these explanations remain speculative but we are currently investigating these possibilities in other stroke patients.

From this preliminary work and metabolic brain studies, we conclude that there are several arguments in favour of the existence of functional or even anatomical plasticity within the motor cortex of adults, but these hypotheses need confirmation by prospective studies.

References

Barker, A. T., Jalinous, R., and Freeston, I. L. (1985) Non-invasive magnetic stimulation of the human motor cortex. Lancet i: 1106-1107.

Lemon, R. N. (1979) Short-latency peripheral inputs to the motor cortex in conscious monkeys. Brain Res 161: 150-155.

Lemon, R. N. and Van der Burgh, J. (1979) Short-latency peripheral inputs to thalamic neurons projecting to the motor cortex in the monkey. Exp Brain Res 6: 445-462.

Maertens de Noordhout, A., Pepin, J. L., Gérard, P., and Delwaide, P. J. (1992): Facilitation of muscle responses to motor cortex stimulation: effects of isometric voluntary contraction. Ann Neurol 32: 365-370.

Penfield, W. G. and Boldrey, E. (1937) Somatic motor and sensory representation in the cerebral cortex of man as studied by electrical stimulation. Brain 60: 389-443.

Wasserman, E. M., McShane, L. M., Hallett, M., and Cohen, L. G. (1992) Noninvasive mapping of muscle representations in human motor cortex. Electroenceph clin Neurophysiol 85: 1-8.

Wilson, S. A., Thickbroom, G. W., Mastaglia, F. L. (1993) Transcranial magnetic stimulation mapping of the motor cortex in normal subjects. J Neurol Sci 118: 134-144.

Locomotor Capacity of Spinal Cord in Paraplegic Patients

L. Jensen, G. Colombo, V. Dietz
Paraplegic Centre, University Hospital Balgrist, Zurich, Switzerland

Abstract - The induction of complex bilateral leg muscle activation combined with coordinated stepping movements is demonstrated in patients with complete paraplegia. During the course of a daily locomotor training program, the amplitude of gastrocnemius electromyographic stance phase activity increased significantly. In about half of complete paraplegic patients with low muscle tone, no beneficial effect of the training was seen. This may be due to an inhibitory effect on spinal neuronal activity by drugs patients were taking. In this study intrathecal application of clonidine drastically reduced locomotor muscle EMG activity, while epinephrine enhanced it.

1 Introduction

The spinal generation of coordinated leg muscle EMG activity and movements on a moving treadmill in the low spinal cat is a well documented observation (Forssberg et al. 1980, for review see Grillner 1981). In humans step-like movements are present at birth and can be initiated spontaneously or by peripheral stimuli. The EMG activity underlying this newborn stepping has been shown to be centrally programmed and, as it has also been observed in anencephalic children, it is probable that spinal mechanisms generate the EMG activity (Forssberg 1986). Nevertheless, there are indications that in humans spinal interneuronal circuits exist which are involved in the generation of locomotor EMG activity in the leg muscles (for review see Dietz et al. 1987), similar to those described for the cat (Grillner 1981). The aim of this study was to show the degree to which locomotor EMG activity and movements can be both elicited and trained in leg muscles of both complete and incomplete paraplegic patients. In addition, it was of interest to know the degree to which the spinal locomotor pattern can be influenced by the application of noradrenergic substances.

2 Methods

All patients (10 with complete paraplegia and 3 patients with incomplete paraplegia) underwent daily locomotor training on the treadmill (approximately 300m of walking) after a period of 4-5 weeks post-trauma. In complete paraplegic patients and at the beginning of the training in all incomplete patients, stepping movements could only be induced with partial unloading of body weight and assistance in feet movement by physiotherapists.

Electromyographic (EMG) recordings were made using surface electrodes from the biceps femoris, rectus femoris, medial gastrocnemius and tibialis anterior muscles of both legs. Ankle and knee joint movements were monitored using mechanical goniometers. A force plate was used to provide a record of the force exerted on the treadmill. Individual step cycles were normalized to a relative time scale of one step cycle starting and ending with the right heel strike according to the force signal, and averaged over 20 step cycles. To investigate changes in EMG activity as a function of training, the signal energy (RMS=Root Mean Square) has been determined for a 20% interval of the step cycle ending 5% before end of stance phase when gastrocnemius activation was expected to occur. The knee joint signal was used to trigger the end of the stance phase. To allow intersubject comparison of changes in gastrocnemius activity as a function of training within a given interval, the individual RMS-amplitude and the time scale were normalized.

3 Results

Figure 1 shows typical examples of the EMG pattern of lower leg muscles of a patient with incomplete (level C7) (A) and a patient with complete paraplegia (level C5/6) (B). For comparison the group averages of five healthy subjects are displayed (C). Basically, the timing and coordination of the EMG pattern with an activation of gastrocnemius muscle during stance and tibialis anterior during swing were similar in patients and healthy subjects. The main difference consisted in a broader and less modulated gastrocnemius activity and, in the complete paraplegic patient a considerable lower level of EMG. After the training period in both patients gastrocnemius activity was bigger. For the tibialis anterior, an inappropriately timed EMG activity during the stance phase was reduced in both patients after the training period. In Figures 2 and 3 the normalized amplitudes of gastrocnemius EMG-stance-phase-activity over the training period from all incomplete and complete (group A) paraplegic patients are summarized. All these patients benefitted from the training with respect to the gastrocnemius EMG activity during the stance phase of locomotion. The relative increase per day amounted to 0.44% ($r=0.52$, $n=94$) in the incomplete, and to 1.38% [$r=0.74$, $n=116$) in the complete patient group (slope of increase was significant for both groups of patients ($p<0.001$)].

In 6 of 10 complete paraplegics studied over several months, no benefit from training was seen in the EMG traces (group B; fig. 4). In contrast to the complete paraplegic patients who did benefit from training (group A) it became clear that four of them received noradrenergic drugs (prazosin and/or clonidine) and the other two took cannabinoids during the training period. There was a negative slope in EMG amplitude during the course of training (-0.16% per day; r=0.18, n=138).

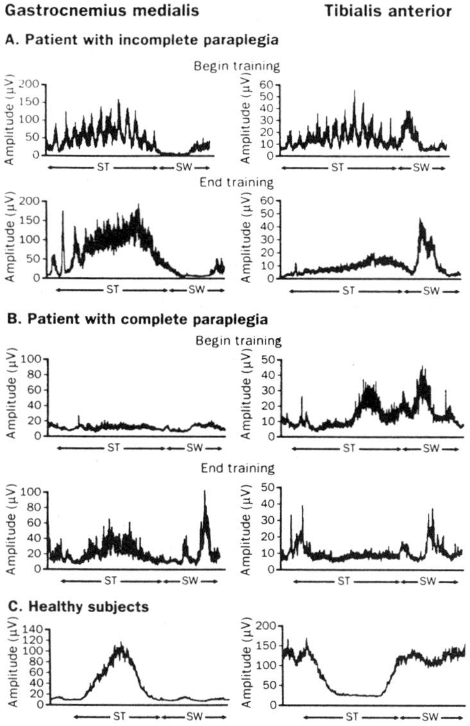

Fig. 1. Rectified and averaged EMG activity of lower leg muscles during slow locomotion (around 1.3km/h) of an incomplete (A) and a complete (B) paraplegic patient and group averages of five healthy subjects (C).

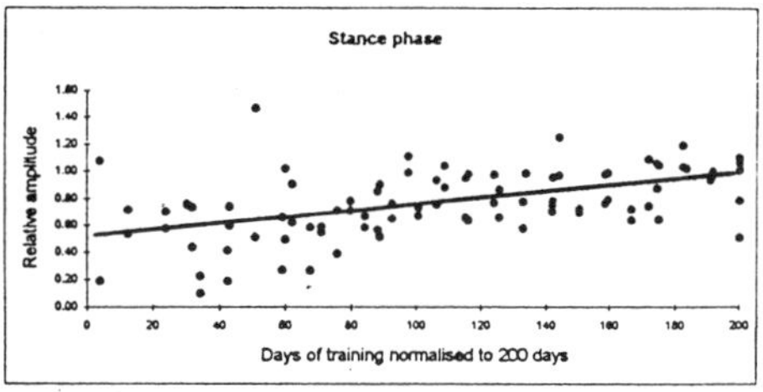

Fig. 2. Quantified gastrocnemius EMG during the stance phase as a function of the training period of the three incomplete paraplegic patients.

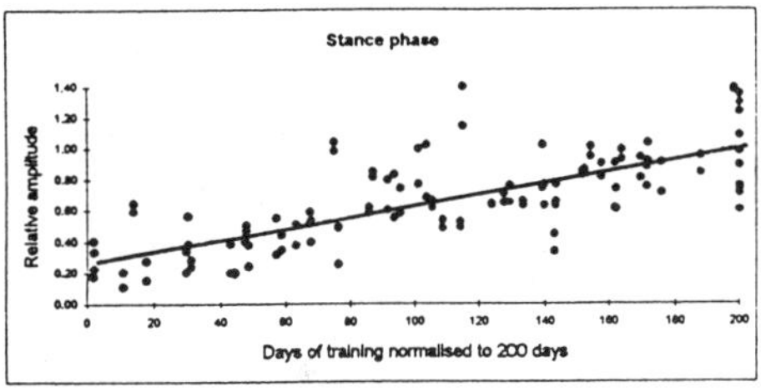

Fig. 3. 5 complete paraplegic patients (Group A).

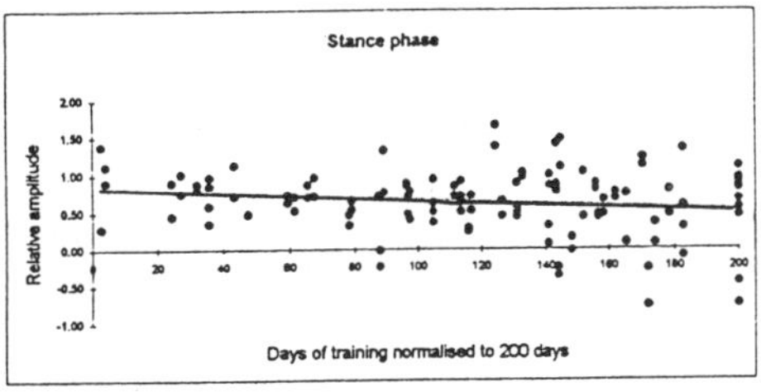

Fig. 4. 6 complete paraplegic patients (Group A).

In order to get further information about the effect of (nor)adrenergic substances on the locomotor activity, the effect of such substances was tested in a patient with complete paraplegia (A small dose of the sympathomimetic substance epinephrine (0.5mg) and, separated by 8 weeks, of the alpha-adrenoceptor agonist clonidine (75mg) was injected intrathecally and the locomotor pattern was recorded before and after the injection. After injection of epinephrine there was a clear increase (about one third) of gastrocnemius EMG-amplitude during the stance phase and a decrease during swing. After injection of clonidine there was a marked reduction of gastrocnemius and a loss of tibialis anterior EMG.

The main finding of this study is that coordinated leg movements and muscle activity could be induced by a moving treadmill in patients with either incomplete (demonstrated already earlier (Wernig et al. 1992)) or complete paraplegia. And an indication that human spinal locomotor activity can be influenced by pharmacological means. For a more detailed description of the results see Dietz et al. 1994 and Dietz et al. 1995.

References

Dietz V. (1992) Human neuronal control of automatic functional movements. Interaction between central programs and afferent input. Physiol Rev; 72: 33-69.

Dietz, V., Colombo, G., and Jensen, L. (1994) Locomotor activity in spinal man. The Lancet 1994;344;1260-1263.

Dietz, V., Colombo, G., Jensen, L., and Baumgartner, L. (1995) Locomotor Capacity of Spinal Cord in Paraplegic Patients. Annals of Neurology; 37; 574-582.

Forssberg, H., Grillner, S., Halbertsma, J., and Rossignol, S. (1980) The locomotion of the low spinal cat. II. Interlimb coordination. Acta Physiol Scand; 108: 283-95.

Forssberg, H. A. (1986) Developmental model of human locomotion. In: Grillner S, Stein PSG, Stuart DG, Forssberg H, Herman RM eds: Neurobiology of Vertebrate Locomotion, Wenner-Gren International Symposium Series, Vol. 45. London: Macmillan; 485 - 501.

Grillner, S. (1981) Control of locomotion in bipeds, tetrapods, and fish. In: Brookhart M and Mountcastle VB eds., Handbook of Physiology. The Nervous System. Vol. II, Motor Control part 2, Am Physiol Soc: Washington DC; 1179-1235.

Wernig, A. and Muller, S. (1992) Laufband locomotion with body weight support improved walking in persons with severe spinal cord injuries. Paraplegia; 30: 229-38.

Stretch Reflex Variations During Gait

J. B. Andersen, T. Sinkjær
Center for Sensory-Motor Interaction, Department of Medical Informatics and Image Analysis, Aalborg University, Aalborg, Denmark

Abstract - To be able to evaluate spasticity during a more functional situation and to determine the degree of which the nervous system regulates muscular mechanical properties, we have developed a method to investigate the electromyograhic and mechanical stretch reflex components during treadmill walking. A perturbation of the ankle joint was applied by a "stretcher" which consists of a mechanical joint attached to the subject's ankle joint. The mechanical joint was connected to a motor placed beside the treadmill by means of bowden wires.

1 Introduction

Electrophysiological investigations on the Hofmann (H) reflex in the Soleus muscle indicate a high modulation of spinal reflexes during walking (Frigo & Crenna 1987; Capaday & Stein 1986; Stein & Capaday 1988). The H-reflex study is a relatively easy way to achieve results of the spinal reflexes, however it is only possible to probe central factors, since the electrical stimulation bypasses the fusimotor system, and it is not possible to extract information about the biomechanical importance of the reflex modulation.

To study the electrophysiology and biomechanics during a naturally evoked stretch reflex of the human ankle extensors, a rapid stretch can be applied to the ankle joint during walking by a device attached to the ankle joint. It is of importance that the device does not influence the natural pattern of gait, i.e. the weight and the dimension of the system should be minimised. At any point of the gait cycle it should be possible to apply a well-defined stretch.

Several authors have attempted to investigate the stretch reflex during gait in humans. Yang et. al. (1988) developed a method to apply a muscle stretch during walking. It consisted of a pneumatic system that was able to apply a stretch to the triceps surae muscle. However, the system was limited to the early stance phase before push-off (Stein et. al. 1991). Llewellyn et. al. (1987) investigated the transmission of the human tendon jerk reflexes during stance and gait by incorporating a spring loaded hammer in the subject's shoe. The hammer was activated on the Achilles' tendon. So far, none of the traditional systems has been able to deliver a reproducible perturbation to explore the stretch reflex and the true kinetics of the human ankle joint during the entire gait cycle.

This paper reports on a new actuator system to investigate electrophysiological and biomechanical features around the human ankle joint during gait. The system is able of eliciting well defined stretches around the ankle joint during all phases of a step. The Soleus stretch reflex is compared with the Soleus H-reflex during normal walking in healthy subjects. It is our hope that such a system also can be used to evaluate spasticity during a more physiological situations such as walking.

2 Methods

Each subject was investigated on a treadmill. Stretch reflexes or H-reflexes were elicited during standing and walking.

2.1 Stretch reflex measurements

Stretch reflexes in the ankle extensors were elicited by a stretch machine which consisted of a functional joint attached to the subject's ankle joint and a motor system placed next to the treadmill. The functional joint revolves around the ankle joint and was connected to the motor by means of bowden wires (Fig. 1). The stretch velocity was limited to 600 °/s. An individual plaster cast of the leg was made for each subject. The weight of the total system attached to the leg of the subject was 0.9 kg. For details on the mechanical joint see Andersen & Sinkjær (1994).

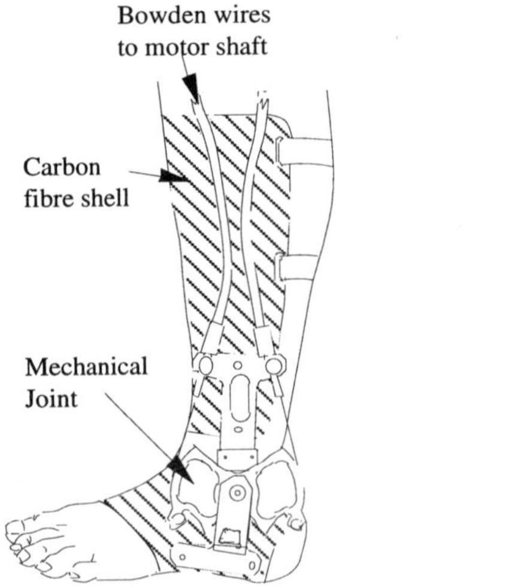

Fig. 1. Functional joint constructed with two joints aligned on a fixed axle. Three transducers are placed in this joint. A Whetstone strain gauge bridge is measuring the resulting perturbation force in the beam attached to the casing of the foot and two optical encoders is mounted in the functional joint. The first encoder measures the actual position of the ankle joint and the other encoder the position of the slip between the two joints (Figure adapted from Sinkjær, & Andersen 1993)

During a step, a stretch was imposed randomly between 8-10 time-segments. The EMGs, ankle position and torque during a stretch which arrived within the same segment, were averaged only if the size of the stretch and the velocity of the stretches were within a preset range and the stride length was within the average stride length ± 1 SD.

2.2 H-reflex measurements

The tibial nerve of the investigated leg was stimulated through a monopolar ball electrode with a diameter of 2 cm in the popliteal fossa, and an indifferent electrode above the patella on the anterior aspect of the thigh. The stimulations were square waves with a duration of 1 ms. A position of the ball electrode in which only the nerve to the Soleus muscle was stimulated, was chosen. Before the experiment and while the subject was standing on the treadmill, the stability of the registration electrode over the Soleus muscle was controlled by measurements of the M-wave during supramaximal stimulation while i) the subject varied the contraction level from a fully relaxed muscle to a strong, sustained contraction in the Soleus muscle, and ii) by asking the subject to rotate his/her ankle joint. If the size of the M-wave was not affected by the contraction and the ankle rotation, the position of the registration electrode was accepted.

During each experiment, the stability of the stimulation electrode was assessed from the constancy of the M-wave in the raw Soleus EMG of the investigated leg.

3 Results

3.1 The stretch reflex response during a step cycle

A step was divide into 8-10 intervals and a stretch of 8° with a velocity of 300°/s and with a hold time of 200 ms was applied infrequently at a rate of one perturbation every 5 to 10 strides in each interval. Figure 2A shows the change in ankle position to a stretch response in the stance phase in one subject walking at 4 km/h. Each trace shows superimposed averaged responses with control steps (heavy lines) and steps in which a stretch was elicited (thin lines). The EMG prior to the stretch matched the EMG in the control steps until approximately 45 ms after stretch onset (Figure 2B). At this time a distinct stretch reflex in the EMG was induced with a peak latency of approximately 60 ms (marked with an arrow). The onset and peak latencies are consistent with a short latency stretch reflex in the ankle extensors in man (Toft et al. 1991).

Figure 3A shows the modulation of the stretch reflex responses through the entire step when divided into 10 segments. The amplitude and velocity of the imposed stretch were kept constant throughout the step.

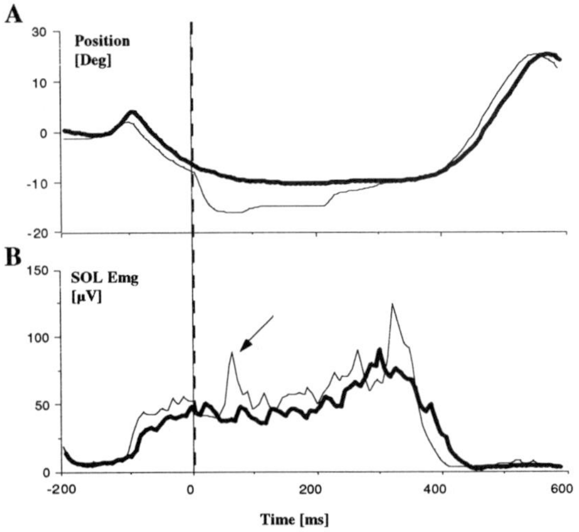

Fig. 2. Example of averaged, recorded data in control steps (heavy lines) and steps with a stretch of the ankle extensors (thin lines) in the stance phase (n=8). A) Ankle angle positions. B) Rectified and filtered Soleus muscle EMG. 4 km/h walking. Subject TS

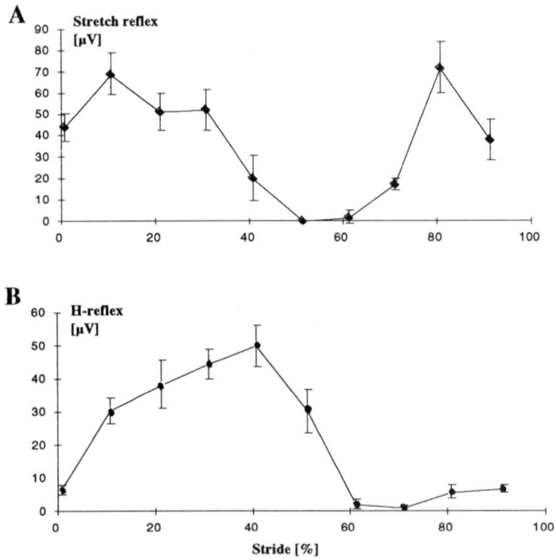

Fig. 3. Reflex modulation during an entire step at a walking speed 3.5 Km/h. A) The amplitude of the short latency stretch reflex B) The H-reflex amplitude. Subject JN. Each point is an average of eight trials ± 1SD.

In the stance phase (from heel-contact until toe-off), the stretch reflex nearly parallelled the background Soleus EMG. In the swing phase (from toe-off to heel contact), the reflex was suppressed to near zero. All subjects showed modulation of the short latency stretch reflex in the step cycle, but the modulation differed dependent on the stretch velocity and speed of walking.

To distinguish the central control of the reflex from the peripheral control, we also elicited the H-reflex during walking. Figure 3B shows the averaged H-reflex modulation during a 8% Mmax stimulation in one subject.

4 Discussion

Here we have demonstrated that it is possible to impose a rotation of the ankle joint during any point of the gait cycle. The joint is perturbed by a strong motor which is linked by a Bowden mechanism, to a mechanical joint strapped to the foot and the shine. When the system imposes a dorsiflexion during walking, the ankle extensor muscles on top of the normal stretches and unloadings are stretched. This stretch induces additional EMG with a latency which would be expected for a monosynaptic stretch reflex in the human ankle extensor muscles.

During maintained ankle extension in the sitting subject, the EMG response in the Soleus muscle to an imposed dorsiflexion of the ankle consisted typically of two peaks, labelled M1 and M2 (Toft et al. 1991) with mean peak latencies of 52 ms and 73 ms. The M1 response is consistent with the short latency reflex described here. Seldom we observed the M2 response during walking. This can either be due to a different stretch in this study (a 10-15% overshoot in the displaced position) or to another type of reflex modulation appearing in the walking subject compared to the sitting subject.

The variation in the stretch reflex amplitude during a step might be caused by i) a central modulation of the afferent input caused by the imposed stretch, ii) a variation in the afferent input due to the fusimotor system or iii) a variation in the stretch taken up by the proprioceptors, primarily the muscle spindles.

Studies on the H-reflex have demonstrated a distinct, centrally controlled modulation of the reflex during walking; with a suppression in the swing phase and an excitation in the stance phase of a step independent of the strength of the H-reflex (Frigo & Crenna 1987; Capaday & Stein 1986; Stein & Capaday 1988). The preliminary findings in this study suggest that the Soleus stretch reflex is modulated in a similar fashion as the H-reflex. The variation in late swing shows that the stretch reflex strength is most likely also influenced by other neural components.

5 Acknowledgement

The authors wish to express their gratitude to Associate Professor Svend Hvid Nielsen, Inst. of Production, PhD. Michael R. Hansen, Assistant Professor Orla Jensen, and Laboratory technician Leif Jacobsen, Inst. of Machine Construction,

Aalborg University, for ideas and construction of the functional joint. A special acknowledgement to Orthotics Jens Ditlev, Sava, Aalborg, for ideas and construction of carbon fibre supports. The authors would also like to thank M.Sc.EE Knud Larsen for development of the data collection software and his quick service whenever needed. This work was supported by CAMARC-II, The Society for Treatment of Multiple Sclerosis, and The Danish National Research Foundation.

References

Andersen, J. B. and Sinkjær, T. (1995) An actuator system to investigate electrophysiological and biomechanical features around the human ankle joint during dynamic conditions *IEEE - Transactions on Biomedical Eng., vol.3 No.4*

Capaday, C. and Stein, R. B. (1986) Amplitude Modulation of the Soleus H-Reflex in the Human During Walking and Standing *J. Neuroscience Vol.6(5):1308-1313*

Frigo, C. and Crenna, P. (1987). Neural control of locomotion: Some recent advancements in methodological approach. In Proceedings of the topical workshop: Restoration of walking aided by functional electrical stimulation. *Ed. Ja. A. VanAlster. Edizione Profucentuk - Milano.*

Llewellyn, M., Prochazka, A. and Vincent, S. (1987) Transmission of human tendon jerk during stance and gait *J. Physiol. 382:82P*

Sinkjær, T. and Andersen, J. B. (1993) A method to apply an external perturbation to the human ankle joint during any point of the gait cycle. *Abstracts Society for Neuroscience. 23rd Annual Meeting. Washington, D. C., November 7-12, 1993, p. 989, no. 404.1.*

Stein, R. B. and Capaday, C. (1988) The modulation of human reflexes during functional motor tasks. TINS, *vol 11 No. 7,328-332*

Stein, R. B., Yang, J., Edamura, M. and Capaday, C.(1991) Reflex Modulation during Normal and Pathological Human Locomotion *Nerobiological Basis of Human Locomotion : 335-346*

Toft, E., Sinkjær, T. and Rasmussen, A. (1991) Stretch reflex variation in the relaxed and the pre-activated quadriceps muscle of normal humans. *Acta Neurol Scand 84: 311-315*

Yang, J. F, Stein, R. B. and James K.(1988) A method to apply muscle Stretch during walking in Humans *Can. Soc. Biomech., Ottawa meeting, 5:42-43.*

Correspondence

Research Council Professor Thomas Sinkjær, Ph.D., Center for Sensory-Motor Interactions, Department of Medical Informatics and Image Analysis, Aalborg University, Fredrik Bajers Vej 7D, DK-9220 Aalborg, Denmark, Phone + 45 98 15 85 22, FAX + 45 98 15 40 08, e-mail: ts@miba.auc.dk.

Modulation of the Hoffmann Reflex of Soleus During the Walking Cycle in Stroke Patients and Associated Control of Ankle Joint Movement

M. Garrett, B. Caulfield
University College Dublin, School of Physiotherapy,
Movement Analysis Laboratory, Mater Hospital, Dublin, Ireland

Abstract - This study was carried out to investigate the pattern of modulation of the monosynaptic Hoffman (H) reflex of soleus during the walking cycle in a group of ten stroke patients and associated control of ankle joint movement in walking. Previous studies on normal walking using the Hoffmann reflex have shown that reflex excitability of soleus is increased by 188% in the stance phase of walking, and reduced by 40% in swing, compared to control conditions (Garrett et al., 1981). This pattern of modulation of the H-reflex in normal walking is associated with very repeatable ankle joint movement during walking. In the present study maximum H-reflex amplitude was measured at 50% of both the swing and stance phases of walking and under control conditions (soleus completely relaxed). H-reflexes were obtained from soleus and an electrogoniometer monitored angular displacement at the ankle at 50% of each phase of walking. The results demonstrated a significant increase in reflex excitability of soleus at mid stance (162%) but no decrease at mid swing (112%), compared to control. The pattern of modulation of H-reflex amplitude was different than that observed in normals. Differences in angular displacement at the ankle joint at 50% of swing and stance in successive gait cycles during the test represented the level of repeatability of ankle joint movement. Patients exhibited irregularity of ankle joint movement. However no clear relationship could be found between the level of repeatability of ankle joint movement and the level of modulation of H-reflex amplitude in the walking cycle within the group of stroke patients.

1 Introduction

A regular and well coordinated pattern of muscle activation is used to bring about the postural stability and movement of body parts which are necessary for normal walking in humans. This pattern of muscle activation is a learned behaviour and is thought to be under the control of neural networks known as Central Pattern Generators (CPGs) (Grillner and Wallen, 1985). These CPGs control movement patterns by means of a variety of neural mechanisms. One such mechanism is the stretch reflex, the purposive nature of which was first described by Liddell and

Sherrington (1924). Authors have used the monosynaptic Hoffmann (H) reflex to demonstrate that excitability of the reflex arc of soleus is increased greatly in the stance phase of walking and decreased in the swing phase (Garett *et al.*, 1981; Capaday and Stein, 1986). This pattern of modulation of reflex excitability of soleus is of functional importance in the walking cycle.

Following a cerebrovascular accident (CVA) many patients experience difficulty in walking which may contribute to problems in maintaining independence in the community. This arises from a disturbance to the normal pattern of walking which may come about as a result of disruption in the pattern of activation of the muscles involved in the walking cycle. The CPGs and the neural mechanisms through which they operate are not functioning properly. One such mechanism which may exhibit abnormal functioning following a CVA is the pattern of modulation of reflex excitability of soleus during the walking cycle as seen in normal walking. The present study used the H-reflex to examine reflex excitability of soleus at 50% of stance and swing during treadmill walking in a group of ten CVA patients. Then the relationship between the level of modulation of reflex excitability of soleus in walking and repeatability of ankle joint movement in successive gait cycles was examined to see the level of reflex control of walking was related to the level of control of ankle joint movement.

The H-reflex of the human soleus muscle utilises the same neural pathways as the stretch reflex (Fig. 1) and can be used to examine excitability of the stretch reflex arc under different functional conditions (Schiepatti, 1987). It is elicited by electrical stimulation of the posterior tibial nerve in the popliteal fossa. Two responses will result in the muscle following stimulation (Murray *et al.*, 1964). At low stimulus intensities there is a low threshold monosynaptic response called the H-reflex or H-wave. This is mediated by the Ia afferent fiber which synapses in the spinal cord with the alpha motoneuron, and its latency is approximately 40 msec. At higher stimulus intensities there is a direct motor response called the M-wave. This is mediated by the alpha motoneuron and its latency is 5-10 msec.

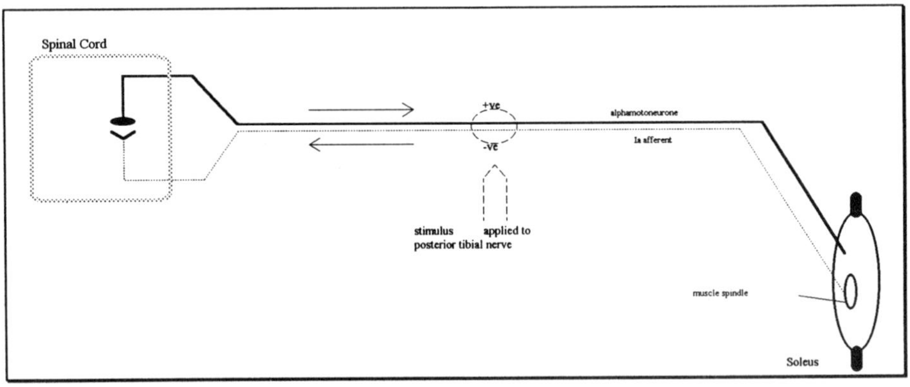

Fig. 1. Pathways involved in the Hoffmann Reflex

Figure 2 shows H and M responses at different stimulus intensities, increasing as one moves down the graph. The y-axis represents the amplitude response, in milivolts, of the M and H waves. The x-axis is the time scale, which is 50 msec; and each division corresponds to 5 msec. As can be seen from the graph, at low stimulus intensities there is no M-wave and a small H-wave, as the H response has a lower threshold of excitation. Then, as the stimulus intensity increases, the M-wave appears and begins to increase with higher intensities. As the M-wave increases the H-wave begins to decrease as there are fewer fibres available for recruitment in the long latency response. The H-wave is completely obliterated when the M-wave reaches its peak.

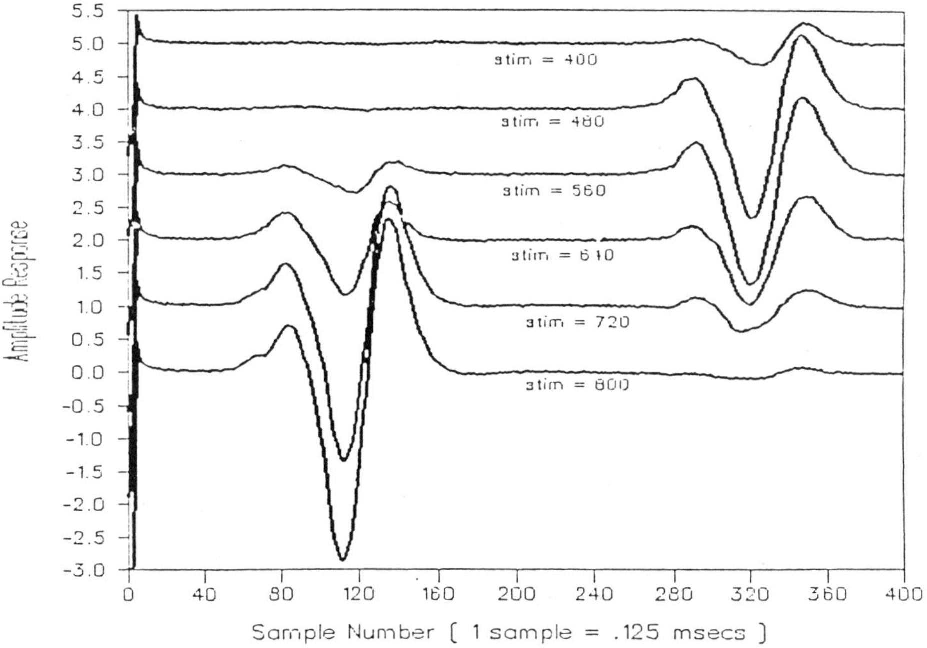

Fig. 2. Hoffman Reflex Study. M and H responses at different stimulation intensities.

The amplitude of the peak m wave for a given stimulus intensity will be the same under all conditions. However, the amplitude of the H-wave will vary under different functional conditions for a given stimulus intensity. So, transmission at the synaptic junction of the reflex arc must undergo some modulation from outside influences under different functional conditions. Transmission of impulses across the synaptic junction may be facilitated or inhibited. Therefore, the ratio between the peak H- and M- waves, the Hmax/Mmax ratio, can be used to indicate the level of excitability of the reflex arc in different activities, for example walking.

A previous study showed a modulation of reflex excitability in the walking cycle in a normal population (Garrett *et al.*, 1981). The Hmax/Mmax ratio midway through the stance phase of walking was nearly twice that obtained under control conditions. The Hmax/Mmax ratio midway through the swing phase was less than half that of control. Reflex excitability in the swing phase, therefore, was 25% that in the stance phase. These findings have been confirmed by other authors (Capaday and Stein, 1986).

This modulation of reflex excitability is of functional importance in the walking cycle. In the stance phase high reflex excitability in soleus is necessary in order to resist the soleus stretch which occurs as the body weight rotates about the ankle in the rollover phase and also to assist soleus to generate the large turning moment which is necessary for push-off. Low excitability of the reflex arc of soleus in the swing phase enables the dorsiflexion and resultant soleus stretch which is needed for toe clearance as the leg swings forwards towards the next heel strike. It is evident that loss of the pattern of modulation of reflex excitability as described above could contribute to the problems experienced by CVA patients during walking.

2 Materials and Methods

The pattern of modulation of reflex excitability of soleus in walking was investigated in ten CVA patients in an attempt to quantify the disturbance to reflex control of walking following a CVA. The test station is illustrated in Fig. 3. The affected side of each patient was tested. A direct current stimulus, of 0.5 msec duration, was delivered via the cathode at the popliteal fossa. The stimulating electrode was secured to the patient using elastic bands. An indifferent pad electrode was placed on the upper thigh, and the resultant activity in soleus was measured using two silver chloride E.M.G. electrodes (Diameter - 7mm). Footswitches timed the swing and stance phases of walking and an electrogoniometer measured the position of the ankle joint at the time of stimulus in successive walking cycles. Patients walked at a comfortable speed on the treadmill.

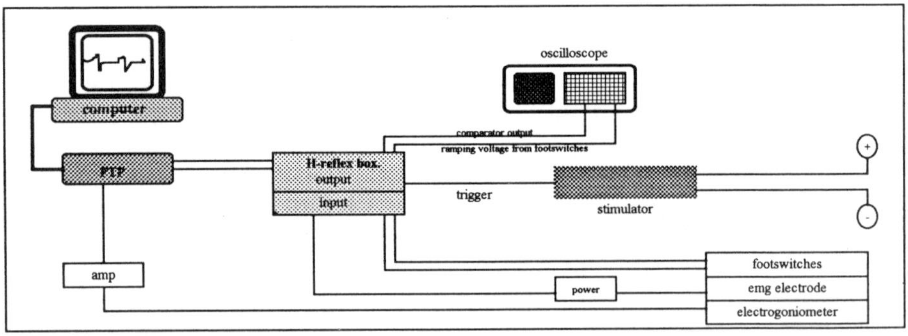

Fig. 3. Experimental Design

H-reflexes were elicited under control conditions, which entailed the soleus muscle being completely relaxed, and at 50% of the swing and stance phases of walking. Hmax/Mmax ratios for swing, stance, and control conditions were obtained. To eliminate intersubject differences the Hmax/Mmax ratios for swing and stance were expressed as a percentage of that of control for each patient.

3 Results and Discussion

The mean h/m ratio for stance was 162% that of control. This shows a statistically significant difference between reflex excitability under both conditions ($p<0.05$). The level of excitability in swing was 112% that of control, however the difference was not statistically significant. These results show differences from those obtained in a normal group. Figure 4 illustrates differences between the results obtained by the patients in the present study and the normals of a previous study (Garrett *et al.*, 1981). There is an increase in reflex excitability of soleus in the stance phase of walking in the stroke patients but not as much an increase as in the normals. There was no decrease in the swing phase as in normals, in fact there was a slight increase. This absence of a reduction in excitability of the reflex arc during swing in the stroke patients was the most marked difference between the two groups.

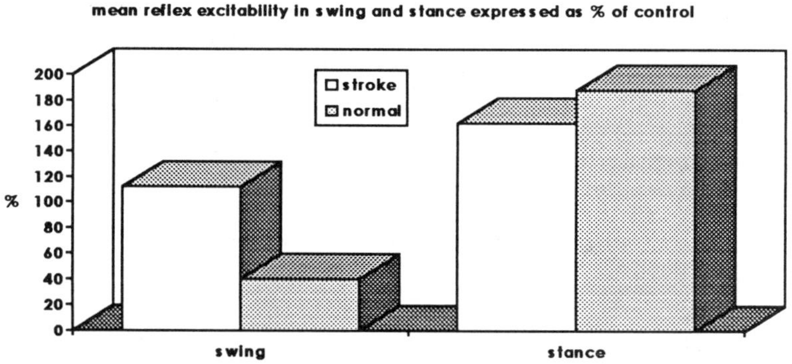

Fig. 4. Comparison of results obtained by CVA patients in the present study and a normal group in a previous study (Garrett *et al.*, 1981).

It was proposed that the ratio between the peak h/m ratio for the swing phase and that for the stance phase be used as an Index of Reflex Excitability (IRE). This index represents the degree of change of reflex excitability of soleus throughout the walking cycle. The lower the score on this index of reflex excitability the greater the level of reflex control of walking. The mean ratio for the stroke patients in this study as 72% compared with a mean ratio of 25% observed in a normal group of a previous study (Garrett *et al.*, 1981). Differences between the two groups are illustrated in Figure 5. It is evident that significant differences exist between the two groups. The level of modulation of reflex excitability of soleus from higher centres is diminished during walking in the stroke patients.

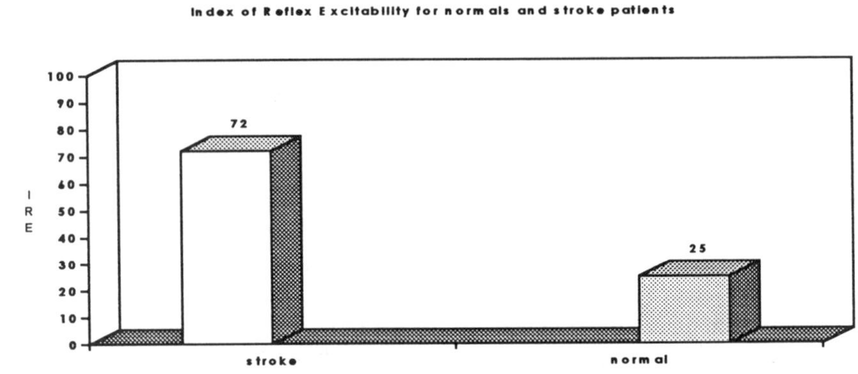

Fig. 5. Comparison of Index of Reflex Excitability exhibited by CVA patients in present study and a normal group in a previous study (Garrett *et al.*, 1981).

Ankle joint position at the time of stimulus was measured for each patient throughout the test and five readings midway through both swing and stance were selected at random for each patient. Figure 6 details ankle joint position at 50% of the swing phase for each patient. Gait studies on normal populations (Murray *et al.*, 1964) have demonstrated that the position of the ankle joint midway through the swing phase should be between 0 and 5 degrees of dorsiflexion. These stroke patients clearly show disordered ankle joint movement as nearly all lie outside this range.

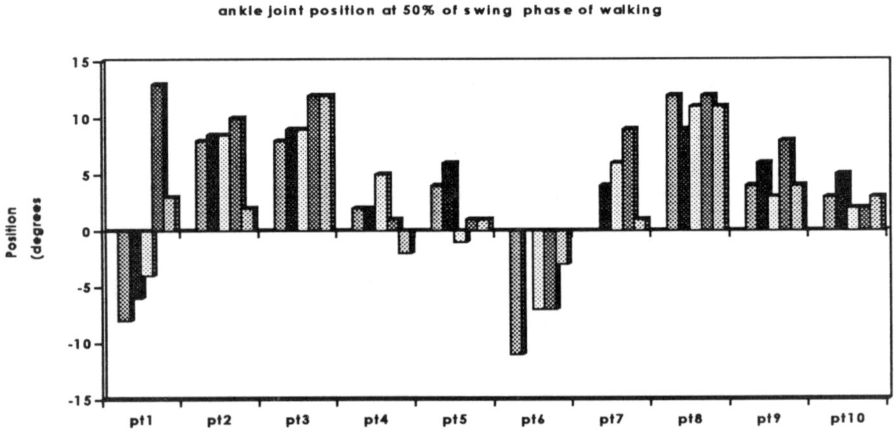

Fig. 6. Angular displacement at ankle joint at mid-swing during test. Positive values represent dorsiflexion; Negative values indicate plantarflexion.

Anova tests conducted on these results demonstrated highly significant differences in angular displacement at the ankle joint at mid swing and stance both between individual patients and within each patient. It is important that differences in angular displacement mid swing and stance were demonstrated within each patient as this shows that the patient could not rely on a constant pattern of ankle joint movement with each successive step. This is in contrast to the highly repeatable gait patterns which are found in normals. Repeatability of ankle joint movement is essential for a stable gait pattern. Similar results were found when the ankle joint position midway through stance was examined (Fig. 7).

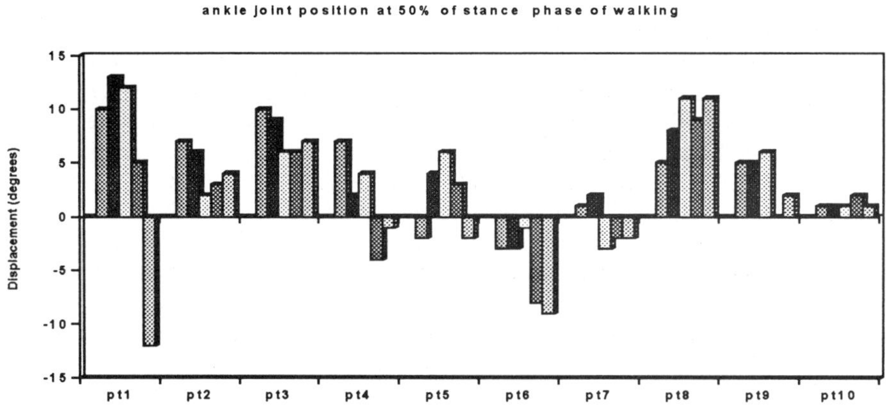

Fig. 7. Angular displacement at ankle joint at mid-stance during test. Positive values represent dorsiflexion; Negative values indicate plantarflexion.

Poor repeatability of ankle joint movement indicated a low level of control of ankle joint movement during the walking cycle. Regression analysis was carried out to investigate the relationship between the level of control of ankle joint movement and the index of movement control as measured using the H-reflex within the group of stroke patients. However, within the group, correlation between the two variables was very low ($r = 0.02$). This low correlation coefficient may be due to the limited number of patients tested in this study. It is evident, however, that diminished modulation of reflex excitability of soleus in the stroke patients as a group is associated with poor control of ankle joint movement. It is hoped that the results of an analysis, which is currently under way, of these two variables in a normal group, will show that high repeatability of ankle joint movement is associated with a low index of movement control.

4 Conclusion

In summary, it was found that an altered pattern of modulation of reflex excitability of soleus in the walking cycle existed in this group of stroke patients. They did exhibit an increased level of excitability of the reflex arc of soleus midway through the stance phase of walking as has been reported previously in normals (Garrett *et al.*, 1981; Capaday and Stein, 1986). Thus, the stroke patients had increased resistance to soleus stretch during the stance phase of walking, which aids in controlling the rotation of body weight about the ankle.

However, the stroke patients did not show a decrease in the level of reflex excitability of soleus midway through swing, as is exhibited by normals. No decrease in resistance to soleus stretch is apparent during the swing phase of walking. It could be postulated that absence of reduced resistance to soleus stretch would lead to the appearance of unwanted plantarflexion at the ankle joint during swing, yet, as Figure 6 illustrates, this was not the case in the group of stroke patients tested in the present study.

The stroke patients showed poor repeatability of ankle joint position at mid swing and mid stance in successive gait cycles throughout the test. This poor repeatability of ankle joint movement could result in an unstable gait pattern which could, in turn, lead to lack of confidence in walking. No clear relationship could be found between the level of repeatability of ankle joint movement during walking and the level of modulation of reflex excitability of soleus throughout the walking cycle within the group of patients. However, it is evident that the group of stroke patients as a whole exhibit diminished modulation of reflex excitability of soleus in walking and also exhibit a poor level of repeatability of ankle joint movement during walking. It is necessary to investigate these variables in greater detail on a larger population of stroke patients and on a group of normal subjects in order to come to a conclusion on the functional consequences of the pattern of modulation of reflex excitability of soleus in the walking cycle in stroke patients.

References

Akazawa, K., Aldridge, W. J., Steeves, D. J., and Stein, R. B. (1982) Modulation of stretch reflexes during locomotion in the mesencephalic cat. J Physiol, 329: 553-67.

Capaday, C. and Stein, R. B. (1986) Amplitude modulation of the soleus H-reflex in the human during walking and standing. J Neurosci, 6 (5): 1308-13.

Garrett, M., Luckwill, R.G., and McAleer J. J. A. (1981) The sensitivity of the monosynaptic reflex arc in the leg extensor muscles of the walking man. In: International series on Biomechanics, Eds Morecki A, et al, Vol. 3, University Park Press, Baltimore, 95-99.

Grillner, S. and Wallen, P. (1985) Central pattern generators for locomotion, with special reference to vertebrates. Ann. Reviews of Neuroscience, 8: 233-61.

Liddell, E. G. and Sherrington, C. S. (1924) Reflexes in response to stretch (myotatic reflex). Proceedings of the Royal Society, London, 96, 212-42.

Murray, M. P, Drought, A. B., and Kory, R. C. (1964) Walking patterns of normal men. J Bone Joint Surg, 46A (2): 335-60.

Schieppati, M. (1987) The Hoffmann Reflex: A means of assessing spinal reflex excitability and its descending control in man. Prog. in Neurobiology, 28: 345-76.

Chapter 2

Contraction and Fatigue of Stimulated Muscles

Muscle Recruitment with Surface and Implanted Electrodes

E. Rabischong
Centre Propara, Parc Euromedecine, Montpellier, France

Abstract - We have measured the relationship between pulse amplitude and force output in the electrically stimulated muscle by means of surface and implantable electrodes (epimysial and neural cuff). In each configuration, the slope of recruitment appeared rather steep. However, the slope value increased from surface to neural electrodes (from 0.07 to 11.9). Considering the epimysial electrodes the closer the electrode to the entry point of the nerve the higher the slope value and the force output. It remained possible, in a moderate extent, to modulate the gain of recruitment by placing the electrodes more or less close to the nerve which also modified the force output. The amount of current at threshold was the lowest for neural cuff (0.25 mA). It was ten times higher for epimysial electrodes and 100 times higher for surface electrodes. Nevertheless, the range on which a control could be applied, i.e. the slope of recruitment, is the lowest with cuff electrodes.

1 Introduction

Since many years now the electrical stimulation can be used to help the paraplegic patients to remain upright and in some cases to walk with a walking frame. But then the problem of the control of these actions arises, and the need for precise control and regulation grows. In general, no control system is used. One of the main reasons is that the muscle is a difficult actuator to control when electrically activated. In this case, its output is highly non linear, time-variable and position-dependent.

We have been interested in studying the recruitment of the muscle stimulated by means of three different types of electrodes; surface and implantable electrodes (epimysial and neural cuff, MXM company, Antibes, France)

Some studies (Crago *et al.*, 1980; Mc Neal *et al.*, 1989; Mc Neal and Bowman, 1985) reported the modulation of frequency or pulse width or amplitude of the pulses. The relation between force and either stimulus parameter was non-linear, with region of high slope separated by region of low slope. Muscle tension can be controlled by fixing pulse duration and varying pulse amplitude or by fixing pulse amplitude and varying pulse duration. There was little difference between pulsewidth and pulse amplitude modulation in terms of overall shape of the curves being essentially congruent over the whole modulation range. In the frame of the CALIES project we decided to explore the amplitude modulation.

2 Method

Three different types of electrodes were used;

- self-adhering electrodes (8cm x 10cm, PALS, Axelgaard Manufacturing Co., Ltd., Fallbrook, CA, USA) were placed on the quadriceps muscle of spinal cord injured patients.
- pimysial electrodes designed in the frame of the CALIES project (MXM company, Antibes, France) which consisted in a Pt-Ir disk (10 mm of diameter) placed in silicone and reinforced with dacron. The multistrand stainless steel wires were in a silicone tubing. The epimysial electrodes were sutured on the muscle belly close to the entry point of the nerve (motor point). Some tests have been done to determine the best position. The electrodes were used during tendon transfer surgery in tetraplegics and four of this electrodes were implanted in paraplegic patients during 8 months.
- neural cuff electrodes (also designed by MXM company). It consisted of four platinum pieces facing each other by pair in a silicone cuff. We recorded data in one baboon during acute tests. The neural cuffs were placed around the peroneal nerve after a careful dissection of the sciatic nerve. The tendon of the tibialis anterior was cut and attached to the force transducer.

In all cases we have used a stimulator delivering biphasic charge-balanced pulses we developed in the unit 103 of INSERM. The maximal output was 150 mA under 2.2 kW. Pulse trains lasting 1 s at 20 Hz with a pulse width of 300 ms have been applied to the muscle or the nerve through the electrodes. These parameters are generally used for functional electrical stimulation. A 30 to 45 seconds rest period have been respected between two stimulations. The mechanical output has been recorded by means of a force transducer placed on the anterior aspect of the lower leg in case of surface electrodes, and in series on the tendon for implantable electrodes (epimysial and neural). In fact, in this last case the tendon was cut and deinserted from the bone. We have modulated the pulse amplitude all the other parameters remaining constant (Frequency, PW). The increment of current was 5 mA for surface electrodes, 1 mA for epimysial electrodes and 0.05 mA for neural electrodes.

Acquisition was made through an analog/digital, and timing I/O board for PC (12 bits resolution). Data were sampled at 50 Hz. The steady-state force was calculated by averaging the samples taken during the last 0.3 s of the 1 s stimulus train.

The variables computed were the slope value, the threshold and the saturation in the output (table 1).

3 Results

Concerning the epimysial electrodes in acute condition (table 1, fig. 1) we recorded a variable slope value depending on the muscle stimulated. The highest value (0.44 s-1) was recorded during posterior deltoid to triceps transfer in quadriplegics. In brachio radialis transfer the gain of recruitment was lower. Electrodes of the same dimensions, but at different locations in the muscle gave different recruitment characteristics. If the slope was different from case to case, the threshold was always close to 2 mA. For the saturation, the values recorded ranged from 16 to 20 mA. In this test condition the electrical resistance of the system was measured and the mean resistive value was around 1.2 kW.

Type of electrode	Slope (max) s-1	Threshold mA	Saturation mA
Epimysial (acute condition)	0.44	2	15
	0.16	2	20
Epimysial (implanted)	0.2	2	10
	0.16	2	8
	0.2	4	15
Neural cuff	11.9	0.25	0.35
Surface	0.07	25	60
	0.03	25	100

Table 1. Summary of the different parameters recorded.

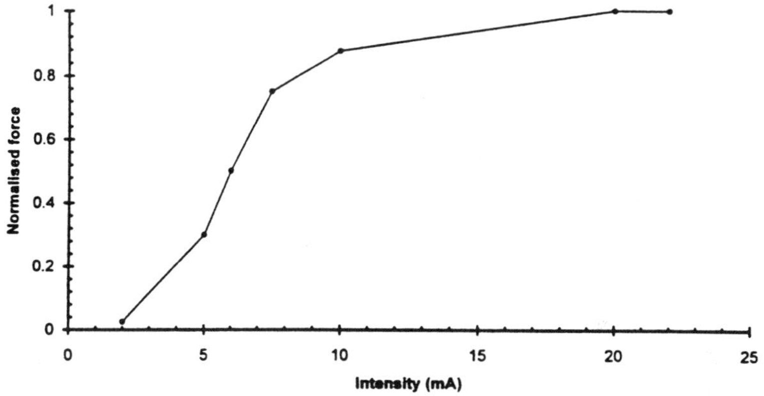

Fig. 1. Recruitment curve with epimysial electrode.

Concerning the implanted epimysial electrodes (n=4) we recorded a maximum slope value about 0.2 s-1. The recorded threshold were of comparable value (2 mA). The mean resistive value ranged from 1.2 to 1.8 kW depending on the time post implantation. The resistivity after surgery increased during 2 to 3 weeks to reach a plateau about 1.5 to 1.8 kW. During this time course the threshold of recruitment was very stable.

Concerning the neural cuff tested in the baboon the slope values were the highest we recorded (11.9 s-1). However, the recruitment curves (fig. 2) were very reproducible. The current intensity was ten times lower (0.25 mA) compared to epimysial electrodes. The mean resistive value was about 3 kW.

Concerning the surface electrodes (fig. 3) we recorded the lowest slope value (0.07 s-1). The amount of current was the highest (25 mA at threshold) which was 100 times higher than cuff electrodes and 10 times higher than epimysial. In some patients we noticed several plateau in the recruitment curve. This phenomenon also occurred one time during acute surgery with epimysial electrodes. It seemed related to the movement of the electrode during the contraction relative to the nerve position. This carried an instability in the output.

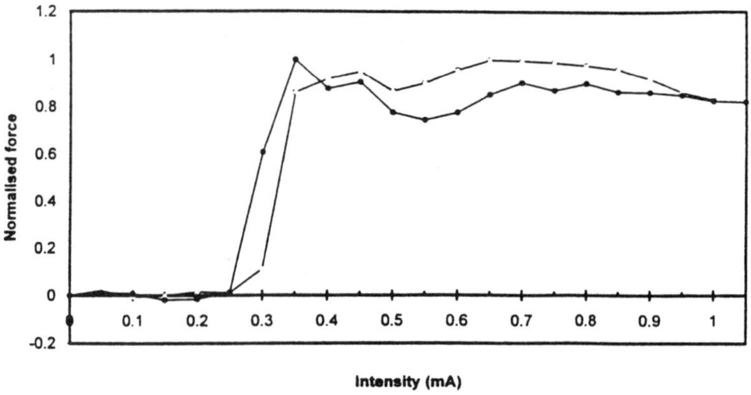

Fig. 2. Recruitment curve with neural cuff.

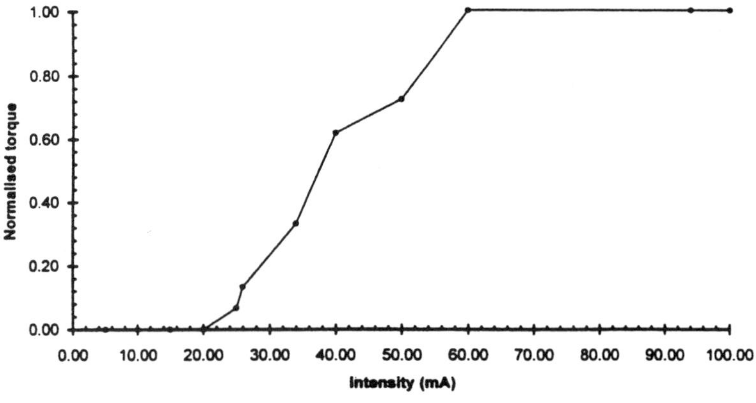

Fig. 3. Recuitment curve with surface electrode.

4 Discussion

Linearity simplifies the analysis and design of the controller and low gain allows better controllability. Unfortunately, the steep relationship between stimulus pulse amplitude and muscle force results in limiting force grading possibilities. The non linearity of muscle recruitment results mainly from reverse recruitment order, i.e. larger motor units are excited before smaller. Large axons have the lowest input resistance and are recruited at low stimulus strength. Therefore, the fast-fatigable fibre (IIb or FF) are recruited at the lowest stimulus threshold. Attempts have been made to reverse the recruitment order in electrically activated muscle by using either dc or high frequency blocking techniques (Baratta *et al.,* 1989) or by using special pulses (Fang and Mortimer, 1991 a and b). These current pulses consisted of a square leading edge and a plateau phase of approximately 350 ms followed by an exponential trailing phase with a fall time (90-10%) of approximately 600 ms. The recruitment order of small-to-large a fibre was observed in most of the cases studied.

The non-linear input-output relationship between stimulus amplitude and the muscle force depends on muscle length (Crago *et al.,* 1980). Our results are in accordance with most reports of the literature which show simple sigmoidal curves which usually have a region which can be approximated by a first order equation. However, some authors (Gruner and Mason, 1989) reported relationship containing "plateaus" resulting from the recruitment of fascicles at different thresholds during nerve stimulation. Recruitment order is influenced by electrode position, in addition to stimulus parameters as predicted by some models (Veltink *et al.*, 1991).

References

Baratta, A., Ichie, M., Hwang, S., and Solomonow, M. (1989) Method for studying muscle properties under orderly stimulated motor units with tripolar nerve cuff electrode, J. Biomed. Eng., 11, 141-147.

Crago, P. E., Peckham, P. H., and Thrope, G. B. (1980) Modulation of muscle force by recruitment during intramuscular stimulation, IEEE Transactions on BME, 12.

Fang, Z. P. and Mortimer, J. T. (1991 a) A method to effect physiolofgical recruitment order in electrically activated muscle, IEEE Transactions on BME, 38, 175-179.

Fang, Z. P. and Mortimer J.T. (1991 b) Selective activation of small motor axons by quazitrapezoidal current pulses, IEEE Transactions on BME, 38, 168-174.

Gruner, J. A. and Mason C. P. (1989) Nonlinear muscle recruitment during intramuscular and nerve stimulation, J. Rehabilitation Research and Development, 26, 1-16.

Mc Neal, D. R., Baker, L. L., and Symons, J. (1989) Recruitment data for nerve cuff electrodes: implications for design of implantable stimulators, IEEE Transactions on BME, 36, 301-308.

Mc Neal, D. R. and Bowman, B. R. (1985) Selective activation of muscles using peripheral nerve electrodes, Med. & Biol. Eng. & Comput., 23, 249-253.

Veltink, P. H., Van Alsté, J. A., and Boom, H. B. K. (1991) Multielectrode intrafascicular and extraneural stimulation, Med. & Biol. Eng. & Comput., 27, 19-24.

The Effect of Contractile Activity on the Damaged Skeletal Muscle and the Application on Paraplegic Locomotion

T. Seene, M. Umnova, P. Kaasik, J. Järva, K. Alev, R. Puhke, A. Pehme, M. Pääsuke
Institute of Exercise Biology, University of Tartu, Tartu, Estonia

Abstract - Striated muscle tissue cannot adequately resist to chronic disuse and overexertion. The main reason for this is the disturbance of functions caused by the changes in the structure of myofibrillar apparatus. Myopathies of different genesis are to smaller or greater extent caused by the injury of myofibrillar apparatus. The common feature of muscular disturbance despite its genesis is the fact that pathogenesis of myofibrillar apparatus depends to great extent upon oxidative potential of a muscle fibre. Furthermore, the effect of muscular activity has the same effect on restoration of function of muscular contractile apparatus also depends on oxidative potential of muscle. In this respect the character of muscular activity is essential, either in the form of exercise or while using functional electrostimulation. The turnover rate of skeletal muscle contractile proteins in the type 1 and 2A fibres reflect the physiological and morphological state of contractile apparatus, have good correlations with the activation of satellite cells, reorganisation of neuromuscular junctions and may be regarded as a manifestation of the functionally determined adaptive process caused by an increase in the muscular activity.

1 Introduction

The concept of functional electrical stimulation (FES) is based on a simple fact that the muscles with intact reflex are electrically excitable and it was thought that this property could be used to provide all the three basic requirements, i.e. stability, mobility and control, necessary for locomotion. Long and Laerton (1955) defined physical activity goals for patients with spinal cord injury (SCI) and related these goals to the level of injury. It appears that there are many physical factors which determine whether a paraplegic can achieve functional ambulation or not, the most important being the anatomical level of the lesion. The relationship between motor status at admission and functional ability at discharge is statistically significant and motor status predicts functional outcome (Laurikainen, Piirainen, 1993). Muscle atrophy as well as deformities of the spine on the extremities and the need of appliances were specifically noted in the physical examination of polio-patients. The loss of motor units was evaluated during maximal voluntary contraction and changes in the motor unit potentials were noted during weak contraction of these patients. The dysfunction of the neuro-muscular junction, some distal branches of neural axons cannot deliver the neural impulse to the muscle fibres with certainty (Seppäläinen, Luisto, 1993). Long-term training with electrically induced bicycling in SCI individuals results in increased whole body aerobic capacity and in an increased leg bone mass and bone mineral density in the proximal tibia. This indicates that exercise training of paralysed leg muscle can reverse local bone mineral loss as well as the cardiovascular deconditioning often seen in SCI (M.Kjaer, et al., 1993).

Artificial increase of the muscle mass by functional neuromuscular stimulation (FNS) reduce this risk, and may be of some help even if the muscle remains paralysed (Lannen, Berstad, Lilleas, 1993). It is furthermore known that SCI in both man and other species results in fibre type transformation from type I to type II fibres. After electrically induced bicycling for 30 min 3 times per week for one year increase in fibres co-expressing myosin HC isoform IIA/IIB, and only expressing myosin HC isoform IIA was observed. After 6 months a small percentage of fibres co-expressing myosin HC isoform I/IIA was found , indicating a shift in myosin HC expression from myosin HC IIB towards myosin HCI (Mohr, et al., 1993). There is evidence to assume that exercise in combination with electrostimulation gives still greater effect on restoration of muscular function.

2 Methods

In the research we use people who are suffering from disturbance of function of skeletal muscle, like myopathies of different genesis, disturbance of contraction in result of muscular disfunction, etc. In addition to exercise we also use electro-stimulation of different character. Before and after muscular activity the properties of muscle contraction are registered. Laboratory animals are used to experiment the changes in the properties of muscle contraction throughout myopathies of different genesis and to study hypo- and hyperfunction. The experiments are approved of by the ethical commission of the Medical Faculty of Tartu University, licence No. 193.

2.1 Electrical Stimulation of Rat Muscles

Rats are anaesthetised and then needle-type electrodes are inserted into both gastrocnemius muscles of rats. The tibia and foot of one leg are fixed at right angles to each other with a knee clamp and foot strap, and electrically stimulated. The contralateral leg of each rat is neither fixed nor stimulated for the purpose of control. Rectangular pulses are of 2-ms duration, 10 V at 20-100 Hz. The use of different frequency in the experiment enables to learn comparatively the effect of electrostimulation with low and high frequency. These stimulation pulses are given for 2s, followed by 5s rest. One set consists of ten such stimuli. Three sets at 5-min intervals to each rat each day.

2.2 Electrical Stimulation on Human Muscles

We use direct electrostimulation m.quadriceps femoris. Two broad plate-like electrodes are laid on muscle belly with the interval of 10 cm. Stimulation regimen - 1 ms rectangular stimulus with frequency of 25 Hz is lasting for 2 s. These stimulation pulses are given for 2 s, followed by 5-s the rest. One set consists of ten such stimuli. 10 sets are given at 3-min intervals to each person each day. Electrostimulation for humans as well as laboratory animals is carried out within the period of 6 weeks.

2.3 Measurement of Contractile Properties of the Rat Skeletal Muscles

Contractile properties of the stimulated muscles are measured according to the Morteni et al. (1987). Isometric twitch: contraction time (CT), relaxation time (RT) and peak twitch (P_t). Tetanic contraction, 100 Hz, 1 s: maximal isometric tetanic force (P_o), maximal rate of force development (+dF/dt), maximal rate of relaxation (-dF/dt) and electromechanical delay (EMD). The contractile properties of quadriceps femoris of the humans are measured by percutaneous electrical stimulation using submaximal stimulation of 25 Hz lasting for 1 s. The intensity of contraction is approximately 25% of maximal voluntary contraction (MVC) of muscle. The following properties are measured: isometric tetanic force (PF), +dF/dt and -dF/dt. Isokinetic dynamometry is used for testing.

2.4 Exercise Training

In case of running at the speed of 35 m/min the intensity of this run corresponds to about 70% VO_2 max or, in other words, this is endurance training in an aerobic zone. In the first week of training the total work is 4.294± 117J and in the 6th week 27.950±1050 J. The total energy expenditure during 6 weeks of exercise training is 25.000 Cal. The intensity of exercise during this period rises from 1.30±0.04 to 1.58±0.07 W. In case of running at the speed of 65 m/min the intensity of this speed corresponds to about 130% VO_2 max. This is anaerobic exercise, meant for endurance development. In the first week of training the total work is 3.990±140 J and in the 6th week 10.370±487 J. The total energy expenditure during six weeks of exercise training is 11.390 Cal. The intensity of exercise during this period rises from 1.71±0.06 to 2.90±0.13 W. In case of running at the speed of 95 m/min the intensity of this speed corresponds to about 190% VO_2 max. This is training of anaerobic nature, meant for speed development. In the first week of training the total work is 1.870±60 J and in the 6th week 1.620±81 J. The total energy expenditure during 6 weeks of exercise training is 2.570 Cal. The intensity of exercise training during this period rises from 2.60±0.08 to 4.1±0.2 W.

Male rats of the Wistar strain, 16-17 weeks old, are maintained on a constant diet SDS-RM 1 (C) 3/8 (SDS, Witham, Essex, England). Food and water are given ad libitum. The rats are housed four per cage in plastic cages at 12/12h light/dark period. Different types of muscle fibres are separated as described by us previously (Seene, Alev 1991). At the ultrastructural level the types of muscle fibres are determined on the basis of their morphological differences (Seene, Umnova, 1992). Dynamics of the turnover rate of contractile proteins is estimated by single and double isotope method (Seene, Alev, 1991).

3 Results and Discussion

3.1 The Effect of Exercise on the Skeletal Muscle

Exercise influences the whole organism, including the muscular system. Repeated exercise makes the organism adapt itself to it. Adaptive changes in the organism and in the skeletal muscles depend on the nature of exercise. The muscular system is characterised by a dynamic state, reflected in the continuous processes of protein synthesis and degradation in the muscular tissue. These processes guarantee the renewal or turnover of muscle proteins. The turnover rate of contractile proteins in muscle fibres is different. In type 1 and 2A fibres it is faster than in the 2B fibres (Seene, Alev, 1991). The fact that in the type 1 muscle fibres which participate in comparatively low-intensive sluggish movements and during static loads, the myofibrillar proteins have a faster turnover rate than in other types of fibers, has set us thinking that the character of exercise might influence the turnover rate of contractile proteins (Seene,Alev, 1991). In mixed muscles in case of low-intensive exercise the type 1 muscle fibres are the first to be recruited. As the exercise intensity increases, also type 2A muscle fibres and, in case of especially vigorous contractions, type 2B muscle fibres become involved. This increase in work intensity is also characterised by the intensity of glycogenolysis in different muscle fibers. Thus, in aerobic regime running rats (70% VO_2 max) the intensity of glycogenolysis in type 1 and type 2A muscle fibres was about four times higher than in the type 2B muscle fibres. With the increase in running speed (130% VO_2 max) the intensity of glycogenolysis in the I type of muscle fibres rose about four times, in the type 2A muscle fibres about 40 times, and in the type 2B muscle fibres about 140 times. Further rise in the work intensity increased the intensity of glycogenolysis only in the type 2B muscle fibres. In endurance exercised rats 24 hours after the last exercise session in all types of skeletal muscle fibers, the myosin heavy chains (MHC) turned over faster than in control animals. In sprint exercised animals the MHC turned over faster only in type 2A and type 2B fibres. Differences in the turnover rate of MHC between endurance and sprint trained animals, the turnover rate of myosin light chains (MLC) remained at the control animals' level 24 hours after the last exercise. It is surprising that the different training protocols did not have different effect on the turnover rate of actin in muscle fibers. A comparison of the actin turnover rate in sprint and endurance-trained animals showed that there were more rapid turnover rates in both groups in comparison with the control group. After sprint and endurance exercise we did not observe any significant changes in the turnover rate of MLC. During long-lasting exhaustive exercise the turnover rate of MHC in mixed muscles fell significantly.

There were no significant changes in the turnover rate of MLC and actin this time. However, 12 hours after exercise MLC 2 and 3 and actin had a faster turnover rate than it was in the control rates. During endurance exercise, synthesis of skeletal muscle contractile proteins is suppressed and the breakdown of these proteins is increased. During recovery after exercise the synthesis rate of contractile proteins increases but this process depends on the character of exercise and the type of skeletal muscle fibers.

3.2 Changes in Ultrastructure of Skeletal Muscle in Exercise

24 hours after the last endurance exercise training session some destructive changes in the myofibrils could be observed at the ultrastructural level in type 1 and 2A muscle fibres. The lesions in actin and myosin filaments, mostly located in peripheral myofibrils, are typical examples of these changes. Some myosin filaments can be absent in the A-disk on the border of H-zone where myosin and actin filaments overlap. As the whole A-disk of myofibrils has often been lysed we get the impression that lesions of actin filaments are fewer in number than those of myosin. Although the focal destruction of myofibrils is characteristic of both types of muscle fibres, it is more frequently manifested in 2A muscle fibres. A complete degeneration and lysis of myofibrils are registered only in a few of both types of muscle fibres. In type 1 muscle fibres of m.soleus the trained rats streaming Z-line can be seen more often if compared with the controls (Fig.1). Mitochondria show changes in the density of their matrix: most organelles have a sparse matrix; in some of them cristae are lysed, part of mitochondria change into vacuoles. In muscle fibres with damaged myofibrils, mitochondria located under plasmalemma are degenerated as well: their size has diminished, dense structure cristae are packed close to each other, matrix cannot be seen. Secondary lysosomes, autophagic vacuoles with degenerating mitochondria and membranous remnants occur in the sarcoplasm of both type of muscle fibres. This shows that in both types of skeletal muscle fibres the lysosomal system has been active, a process that ensures the complete disintegration of damaged structural elements. Penetration of macrophages under the plasmalemma of myofibres is not frequently observed. Likewise can be dilatation of the terminal cisternae of sarcoplasmic reticulum and the tubules of the T-system included in the destructive changes in the skeletal muscle cell; this may be a process of recurrent nature. Traces of regular exercises can also be found in the muscle blood vessels: the cytoplasm of endotheliocytes contains lysosome-like and residual bodies, lots of pinocyte vesicles. Sometimes the endotheliocyte cytoplasm is swollen closing lumen of capillary.

Concomitantly with the above-described destructive processes taking place in the muscle fibres of the endurance trained rats, simultaneous signs of intracellular regeneration can be registered in the muscle fibres. An example of that can be accumulation of mitochondria under plasmalemma in both types of muscle fibres (Fig. 2). In clusters of mitochondria among large forms there are also small ones with occasional cristae, presumably newly formed mitochondria. The intensive

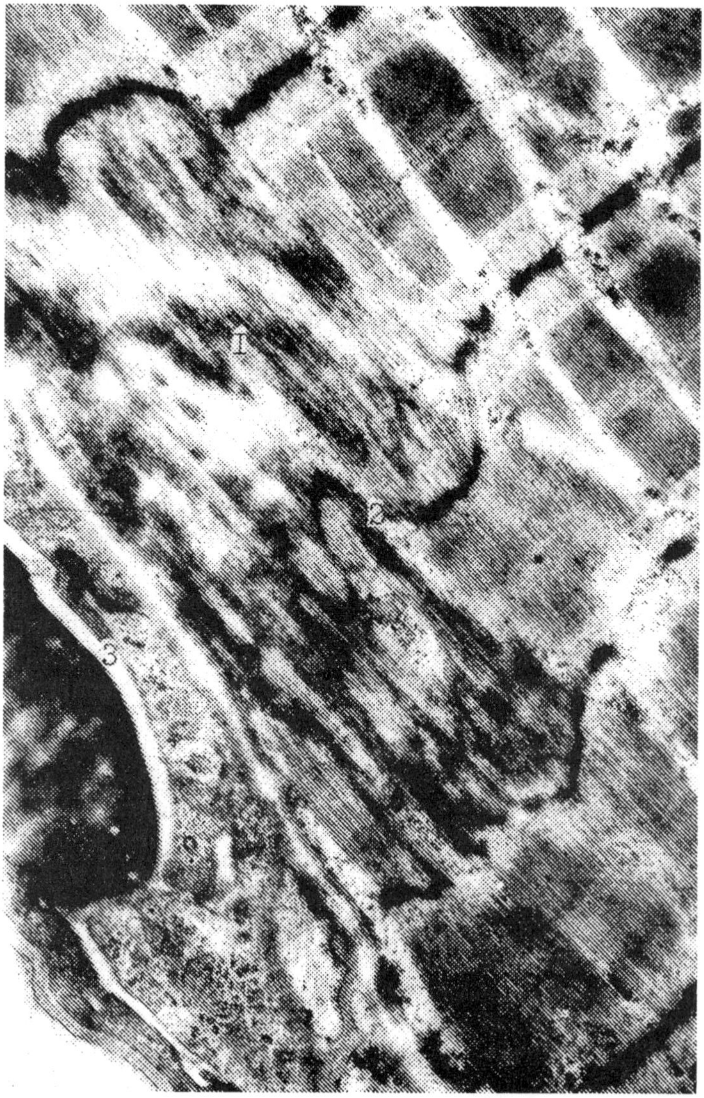

Fig. 1. Electron micrograph of a fragment of slow-twitch oxidative muscle fibre of endurance trained rat. 1 - destruction of the structure of some myofibrils; 2 - Z-line has become wavy ; 3 - capillary. Magnification x 21 600.

development of the mitochondrial apparatus in the post-training period vividly reflects the adaptive processes to endurance exercises which develop as a result of evaluated energy requirements of skeletal muscle cells. In peripheral sarcoplasm of trained rats there occur many different organelles which allow to evaluate the increased protein synthesis: free ribosomes, polysomes, rough endoplasmic reticulum and well developed Golgi complexes, difficult to identify in control rats. The smallest Golgi apparatus usually consists of 3-4 cisternae and its function is connected with processing of proteins. Protein secretion gets into the Golgi complex from the granular sarcoplasmic reticulum, moves from one cisternae to another where it is packed into vesicles and transported further. The complete maturing of the plasmic membrane proteins as well as that of secretory and lysosomal proteins takes place in the Golgi apparatus. Thus, for instance, the phosphate group and several aminoacids are added to lysosomal proteins in Golgi complexes.

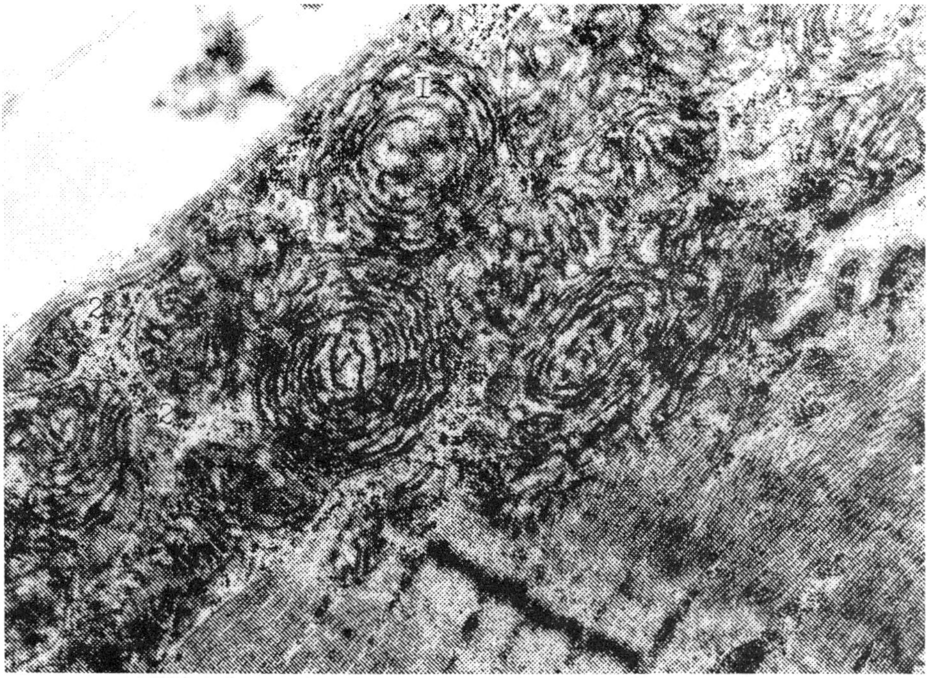

Fig. 2. Electron micrograph of fast-twitch oxidative-glycolytic muscle fibre of endurance trained rat. 1 - mitochondria with conventrically located cristae; 2 - polyribosomes. Magnification x 20 750.

The satellite cell frequency in the 2A muscle fibres in endurance trained rats is 9.59±1.09% which is over 2.5-fold higher in comparison with the controls. Satellite cells located between basal lamina and plasmalemma of muscle fibre are at the distinct stages of differentiation (Appell, Forsberg, Hollmann, 1988). Many of them have augmented nucleus-cytoplasmic ratios and numerous organelles : lots of ribosomes, extensive branching granular endoplasmic reticulum with substance of middle electron density, some small and large mitochondria, well developed Golgi complex, multivesicular bodies; centrioles are present in the sections of many satellite cells. Some satellite cells contain short bundles of filaments in perinuclear sarcoplasm: their origin is unknown. Small groups of satellite cells are concentrated under the basal lamina of trained rats. Several fragments of satellite cells can be observed in the same sites of muscle fibres. Sometimes the basal lamina penetrates between the muscle fibre and satellite cell separating these different structural formations which earlier existed in close topographic and trophic connections. Ultrastructural features and the behaviour reaction of satellite cells connected probably with their increased proliferative activity and other factors may reflect functional state of skeletal muscle fibres.

Individually trained rats show the appearance of single juvenile muscle fibres in red deep portion of m.quadriceps femoris. Newly formed small muscle fibre and the adjacent mature presumably parent muscle fibre are surrounded by a common basal lamina in some sites. A small compact body with short filaments similar to the developing Z-line system can be seen in the new muscle fibre sarcoplasm filled with numerous filaments located around nucleus occupying the central position.

Partial detachment of satellite cells from the surface of muscle fibre by manner of the invagination of a basal lamina and also the formation of new muscle fibres reveal the possibility of hyperplasia of type IIA muscle fibres in some trained animals. As the process of appearance of new muscle fibres is rarely observed in trained rats there is evidence to believe that activated satellite cells merge with differentiated muscle fibres probably causing the hypertrophy of muscle fibre under used training regimen. The tendency towards the increase of rat skeletal muscle mass is registered after endurance exercise.

As endurance training results in over 2.5-fold increase in the number of satellite cells as well as intensification of protein synthesis in 2A muscle fibres largely on account of biosynthesis of sarcoplasmic proteins, there are grounds to believe that satellite cells in trained rats replenish the fraction of sarcoplasmic and myofibrillar fractions. Therefore, the elevated incorporation of labelled leucine into sarcoplasmic fraction of 2A muscle fibres may be caused by satellite cells in which the involvement of aminoacid probably more intensive than in muscle fibres (Seene, Umnova, 1992).

3.3 Changes in the Ultrastructure of Neuromuscular Junctions of Skeletal Muscle in Exercise

The ultrastructure of neuromuscular junctions seems to be of special interest because they are essential in respect to the transfer of both motor phasic impulses and neurotrophic signals. The changes in the axonal terminals of the synapses are of great interest. The type 1 muscle fibres have small-sized round-shaped axonal terminals, surrounded by a number of rather short junctional folds are separated from each other with sarcoplasm. The type 2A muscle fibres have a more elongated shape of axonal terminals. After a week's training already one can see abundance of terminals, possibly resulting from their intensive branching off after beginning of the training programme (Fig.3).

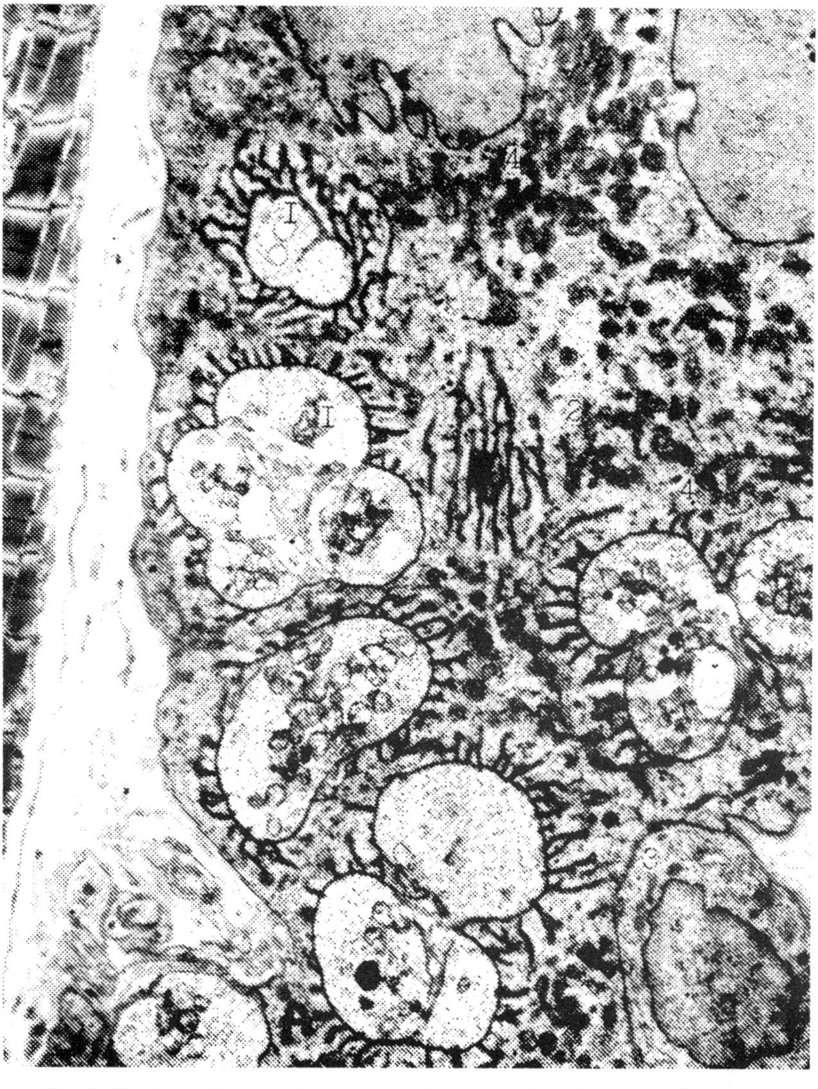

Fig. 3. Electron micrograph of neuromuscular junctions (1) on the fast-twitch oxidative-glycolytic muscle fibre (2) in a rat with one week endurance training. Hyperinnervation of muscle fibre, satellite cell (3) in the synaptic region, mitochondria (4) in the postsynaptic sarcoplasm. Magnification, x 5 600.

One axonal terminal may be divided into 2-4 branches at the sectional level: some of them contain secondary lysosomes and myelin-like bodies. The number of axonal terminals in trained animals at the ultrathin section may exceed the limit of 10-13. Six weeks after the endurance training in the same animal axonal terminals have heterogeneous structure: a part of axonal terminals is rich in smooth light synaptic vesicles while the others contain, besides light vesicles with smooth surface, several coated vesicles which are not frequently met in the control rats. The appearance of coated vesicles is suggested to be connected with the resynthesis of acetylcholine after active synapse function (Bruner, Bursztajan, 1986). Lysosome-like bodies, autophagosomes, containing involvements of tubular form and large extensive membrane structures are seen in axonal terminals of both type of muscle fibres after endurance exercises. In those terminals synaptic vesicles are almost completely absent. In addition to them, some axonal terminals are completely destroyed and old synaptic grooves with exposed junctional folds may be seen. We consider such cases as manifestation of partial denervation of some sites of muscle fibres in endurance trained rats. it is possible that the focal denervation of some muscle fibres is caused at the level of axonal terminals; that is why the regeneration of new terminals is completed by the end of the training process in most cases. The heterogeneous structure of axonal terminals in the same trained rat is an indicative of the injury of terminals in different periods of the training cycle. With the damage of axonal terminals at a long distance from muscle fibre even in the early period of the work the process of reinnervation of the neuromuscular junctions is not entirely completed by the end of training. In this case reduced junctional folds surround old synaptic groove. When some rats refused to complete the training programme one week earlier than the others their axonal terminals were separated from muscle fibres by collagen fibrils, penetrating into delated primary synaptic cleft. In the future, part of those terminals may be destroyed and phagocytosed with Schwann cell processes sometimes penetrating into primary synaptic cleft. The signs of focal degeneration of axonal terminals of the type 1 and type 2A muscle fibres are one of the notable destructive features caused by the prolonged running on treadmill. It is assumed that partial degeneration of some axonal terminals probably caused decrease in the whole area of synaptic contact in the neuromuscular junction (Cardasis, 1983).

The focal degeneration of some muscle fibres under endurance exercises is in most cases reversible and is accompanied by the regeneration of axonal terminals. The newly-formed axonal terminals ingrowing into pre-existing synaptic grooves are smaller in size than the destroyed ones at the sites where they appear. That is why in one old synaptic groove there may be some new regenerative terminals. Pre-existing synaptic groove may contain small newly formed terminal established contact with muscle fibre by the means of short junctional folds and some axonal sprouts ingrowing into it. Quite often two small newly formed axonal terminals are located in the same primary synaptic cleft separated from each other by Schwann cell cytoplasm. Therefore, the new neuromuscular contacts are characterised by small size and the presence of some terminals at one primary synaptic cleft. The process of renewal of the axonal terminals under endurance training programme is similar to the regeneration of terminal after the instrumental injury of nerve (Miledi, Slater, 1968; Manolov, 1975) and to the age reorganisation of rat m.soleus neuromuscular junctions (Cardasis, Padycula, 1981; Cardasis, 1983).

It is shown that in normal rats there is an age-dependent rearrangement of m.soleus neuromuscular junctions with the formation of exposed junctional folds (Cardasis, 1983). This process is probably connected with the increasing load to the muscle apparatus due to the growth in the body mass of the animals (Barker, Ip, 1966; Taffery, 1971). In rats it occurs at the age of 37-43 weeks (Cardasis,

Padycula, 1981). However, since we have not revealed substantial changes of pre- and postsynaptic structural formations, we believe that the process of reorganisation of neuromuscular junctions in endurance trained rats about six months old can be explained by the effect of increased muscle activity. Endurance exercises cause both destruction and restoration of organelles in the region of neuro-muscular junctions with the renewal process prevailing here. Perisynaptic satellite cells connected with motor end plates and locating in the vicinity of axonal terminals can be seen in trained rats more often than in the controls, locating in the vicinity of axonal terminals. The fact that satellite cells are observed in the postsynaptic zones, especially after work-load, is a probable evidence of the great plastic and metabolic significance of this region in muscle fibre. When necessary such a cell can possibly join the muscle fibre and increase the synapse area and the number of nuclei there. In some sites the basal lamina may penetrate into the space between satellite cell and muscle fibre (Fig. 4). We consider this fact as one of some possibilities for satellite cells to leave muscle fibre and form a new population of myogenic cells, later developing in new muscle fibres. Besides, it may also be suggested that the postsynaptic area is the site of muscle regenerative activity because new muscle fibre can be formed in the interstitial space in the vicinity of motor end plates.

One of the factors for activation of satellite cells may be focal partial degeneration of muscle fibres as we observed in trained rats. Some authors have proved that in case compensatory hypertrophy of rat m.soleus is combined with its denervation, the number of satellite cells increased 5-fold in comparison with the normal muscle (Hanzlikova et al., 1975). In case of endurance trained rats there occur transition of junctional folds into the tubules of T-system connected with transferring nerve impulse along muscle fibre. Usually these pictures are seldom met at the level of axonal terminal sections in rats.

In the postsynaptic sarcoplasm of m. soleus in trained and control rats, there are organelle-complexes consisting of many bundles of regularly or irregularly packed thin filaments and located among dark bodies of intensive electron density; these organelles seem to be typical of slow-twitch skeletal muscle. Sometimes these structures are involved into junctional nuclei sarcoplasm invaginations after work-load as in normal rats.

Thus, ultrastructural adaptive peculiarities in skeletal muscle fibres of both types in endurance trained rats are correlated with biochemical data. Increased RNA/DNA ratio is confirmed by existence of numerous organelles usually involved into the protein synthesis located in peripheral sarcoplasm of muscle fibres, postsynaptic areas, satellite cells, newly formed muscle fibres (Seene, Umnova, 1992). Hence, changes in the turnover rate of muscle contractile proteins in the type 1 and the type 2A muscle fibres in endurance trained rats reflect the physiological and morphological state of contractile apparatus, have good correlations with the activation of satellite cells, reorganisation of neuromuscular junctions and may be possibly regarded as a manifestation of the functionally-determined adaptive process caused by an increase in the rat muscular activity (Seene, Umnova, 1991).

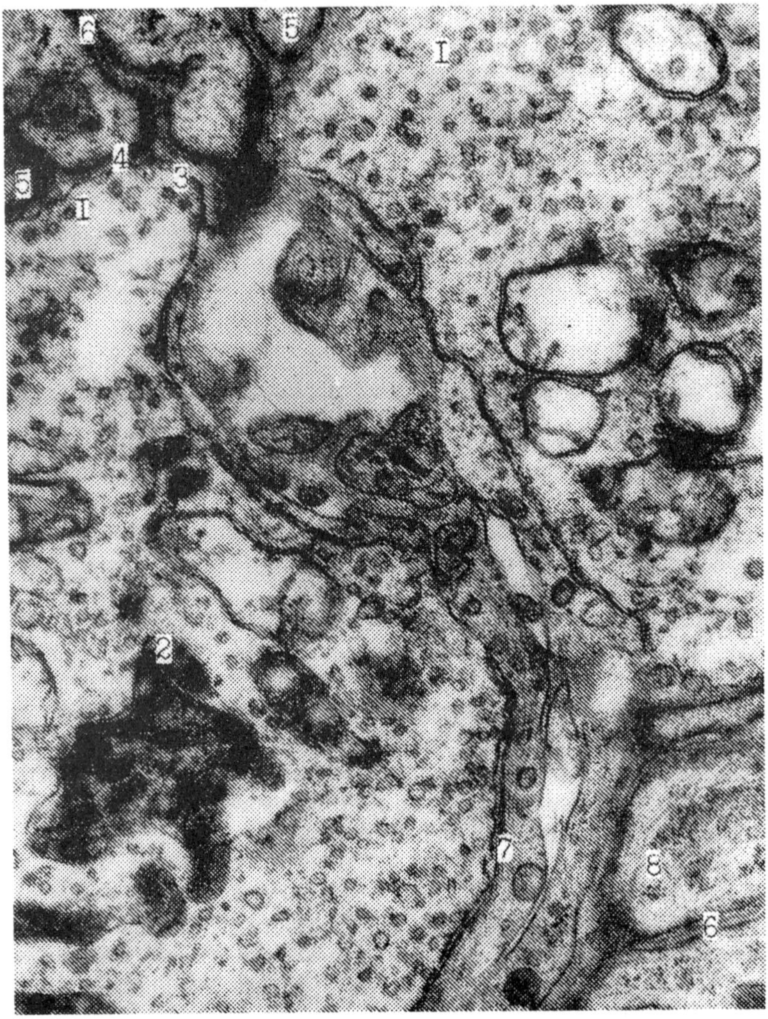

Fig. 4. Fragment of satellite cell (1) in the synaptic region (2), satellite cell nucleus (3), mitochondria (4), granular endoplasmic reticulum (5), autophagic vacuole (6) and complex Golgy (7). Magnification, x 16 000.

References

Apell, H. J. (1984) Proliferation of motor end-plates induced by increased muscular activity. *Int.J.Sports Med.* 5: 125-129.

Barker, D. and Ip, M. (1966) Sprouting and degeneration of mammalian motor axons in normal and de-afferentated skeletal muscles. *Proc.Roy.Soc. (London),ser.B.* 163: 538-554.

Bruner, J. and Bursztajan, Sh. (1986) Acetylcholine receptor clusters are associated with nuclei in rat myotubes. *Dev.Biol.* 115: 35-43.

Cardasis, C. (1983) Ultrastructural evidence of continued reorganization at the aging (11-26 months) rat soleus neuromuscular junction. *Anat.Rec.* 207: 399-415.

Cardasis, C. and Padykula, H. (1981) Ultrastructural evidence indicating reorganization at the neuromuscular junction in the normal rat soleus muscle. *Anat.Rec.* 200: 41-59.

Hanzlikova, V., Mackova, E. and Hnik, P. (1975) Satellite cells of the rat soleus muscle in the process of compensatory hypertrophy combined with denervation. *Cell Tiss.Res.* 160: 411-421.

Kjaer, M., Mohr, T., Christensen, P., Beyer, N., Podenphant, J., Galbo, H., and Biering-Sorensen, F. (1993) Adaptation to long-term FES-induced bicycle training in tetra and paraplegic individuals - effect on aerobic capacity and bone mineral density. *Abstracts 3rd Scientific Meeting Scandinavian Medical Society of Paraplegia.* Lahti, Finland, Septembe p.30.

Lannen, A., Berstad, J., and Lilleas, E. (1993) Change in paralysed gluteal muscle after use of functional neuromuscular stimulation (FNS). *Abstract 3rd Scientific Meeting Scandinavian Medical Society of Paraplegia.* Lahti, Finland, September 9-11 p. 29.

Laurikainen, S. and Piirainen, E. (1993) Patients with incomplete spinal cord injury - their muscle strength and functional ability during rehabilitation. *Abstracts 3rd Scientific Meeting Scandinavian Medical Society of Paraplegia.* Lahti, Finland, September 9-11

Long, C. and Laerton, E. B. (1955) Functional significance of spinal cord lesion level. *Arch.Phys.Med,* 36: 249-255.

Manolov, S. (1975) Ultrastructural studies of regeneration of neuromuscular synapses of rat plantaris muscle. *Compts.Rendus d l'Academie Bulgare des Sci.,* 28: 853-855.

Miledi, R. and Slater, C. (1968)Electrophysiology and electronmicroscopy of rat neuromuscular junctions after nerve degeneration. *Proc.Roy.Soc.,* 169: 289-306.

Mohr, T., Andersen, J., Pedersen, H., and Biering-Sorensen, F. (1993) Effect of electrically induced bicycle training on muscle volume and myosin heavy chain expression in spinal cord injured individuals. *Abstract 3rd Scientific Meeting Scandinavian Medical Society of Paraplegia.* Lahti, Finland, September 9-11 p.31.

Seene, T. and Alev, K. (1991) Effect of muscular activity on the turnover rate of actin and myosin heavy and light chains in different types of skeletal muscle. *Int. J. Sports. Med.,* 12: 204-207.

Seene, T. and Umnova, M. (1992) Relations between the changes in the turnover rate of contractile proteins, activation of satellite cells and ultra-structural response of neuromuscular junctions in the fast-oxidative-glycolytic muscle fibres in endurance trained rats. *Basic and Applied Myology,* 2: 34-46.

Seppäläinen, A. and Luisto, M. (1993) Electromyography in the diagnosis of post olio syndrome. *Abstracts 3rd Scientific Meeting Scandinavian Medical Society of Paraplegia.* Lahti, Finland, September 9-11, p. 28.

Umnova, M., Seene, T. (1991) The effect of increased functional load on the activation of satellite cells in the skeletal muscle of adult rats. *Int.J.Sports Med.,* 12:501-504.

A Dynamic Model of Electrically Stimulated Knee Muscles in Healthy and Paraplegics

M. Ferrarin[1,2], P. Iacuone[1], A. Mingrino[1,2], C. Frigo[1,2], A. Pedotti[1,2]
[1]Dipartimento di Bioingegneria, Politecnico di Milano, Italy
[2]Centro di Bioingegneria, Fnd. Pro Juventute, Politecnico di Milano, Italy

Abstract - Goal of this study is to find the dynamic model representing the relationship between the electrical stimulation applied on rectus femoris muscle and the produced muscle torque on the knee joint, in order to characterize artificial muscle contraction under dynamic conditions. The dynamics of the system is represented with a non linear second order model, whose passive parameters are identified from kinematic data collected during free pendular movement of the leg. A one pole transfer function is proposed to identify the relationship between stimulation intensity and induced muscle torque. Results about five healthy and three paraplegic patients are here reported.

1 Introduction

The Functional Electrical Stimulation (FES) allows patients with motor disorders derived from a spinal cord lesion to restore some motion activities through the application of electrical stimulation at a peripherical level that artificially supply to the physiological stimulus not present because of the lesion. The knowledge of the relationship between the stimulation parameters and the induced movement is an important point towards the definition of an optimal stimulation strategy adapted to the single patient characteristics. Several studies have been done in this frame considering in vitro experiments (Baratta et al. 1990) and/or isometric condition (Levy et al.1990), but a general procedure able to provide these informations in dynamic condition for a specific subject is still to be defined. This is due to the complexity of the system: non linearity, multiple input and output variables, time dependence. In our approach the input variable is the stimulation signal acting on a muscle or on a group of muscles, and the output is the induced joint torque. Purpose of this study is the identification of the relation existing between the main stimulation parameters (pulse width and frequency) and the intensity of the joint moment produced by the artificially activated muscles.

In order to reach this goal an experimental procedure and a mathematical model have been developed and applied to the knee joint. The choice of this joint is due to its importance in the main motor activities (standing up, sitting down, walking, standing, climbing stairs, etc.). The experimental procedure is divided into two main phases: in a first phase, a passive pendulum test was performed in order to estimate the unknown parameters of the viscous-elastic joint model; in the second phase, the rectus femoris muscle was stimulated and resulting torque about the knee joint was computed using kinematic data acquired during the artificially induced movement. These data were used to estimate the transfer function between the electrical stimulus and the generated torque on the basis of an ARX model whose order was found with optimization technique.

2 Method

The mechanical model of the lower limb is supposed to be composed by two rigid segments: the thigh and the shank-foot complex. Movements of the ankle joint were not considered in order to limit the total number of degree of freedom and to avoid modification of the passive characteristic of the knee due to change in length of biarticular muscles (gastrocnemius). For this reason during the experiments the ankle of each subject was maintained in a fixed position with a plastic AFO (Ankle Foot Orthosis).

The passive properties of the knee joint were represented respectively with a non linear (exponential) elastic component and a linear viscous component, as proposed by several authors (Yoon et al. 1982, Audu et al. 1985, Franken et al. 1993).

From a mathematical point of view the dynamic equilibrium of the above system is expressed by the following equation of motion:

$$J\ddot{\Theta} = -mgl \cdot sin(\Theta_{rv}) + \lambda \cdot e^{-E\Theta}(\omega - \Theta) - B\dot{\Theta} + Me \tag{1}$$

where:

J = inertial moment of shank-foot complex;
Θ = flexion/extension knee angle (angle between shank and thigh);
$\dot{\Theta}, \ddot{\Theta}$ = angular velocity and acceleration;
m = mass of shank-foot complex;
g = gravitational acceleration;
l = distance between knee and centre of gravity of shank-foot complex;
Θ_{rv} = angle between shank and vertical direction;
λ, E = elastic parameters;
ω = resting elastic knee angle;
B = viscous coefficient;
Me = knee torque due to electrical stimulation.

In equation (1) the kinematic variables (angular displacement Θ, Θ_{rv} and derivatives $\dot{\Theta}, \ddot{\Theta}$) were computed from the data collected using the ELITE motion analysis system (Pedotti et al. 1985). For this purpose three retroreflective markers were glued respectively on hip, knee and ankle joint centers and their 3-D coordinates were collected during movement with a 100 Hz sample rate. The anthropometric parameters J, m and l were estimated starting from subject height and weight and using regression equations (Zatsiorsky et al. 1983), while the viscous-elastic parameters (B, λ, E and ω) were derived using the data acquired during passive pendulum tests of the lower limb (Lin et al. 1991, Campisi et al. 1993). During these tests the subject was lying supine on a bench with the legs hanging over the edge: after the operator extended completely the subject's knee, the lower leg was left free to oscillate passively (Ferrarin et al. 1996). By substituting these kinematic data in equation (1), in which the Me term due to stimulation is absent, and using non linear optimization techniques (SQP methods, Andrew Grace 1992) to minimize the mean square deviation between first and second member, the viscous-elastic parameters were computed. Trials with voluntary or spastic muscular activity (detected with surface Electromyography) were rejected, in order to assess only the real passive joint component.

Kinematic acquisition during experiments performed with electrical stimulation on rectus femoris muscle were then performed with the same experimental set-up used in the passive pendulum test. In order to generalize the procedure, we used two different stimulation patterns (step and ramp) each of them applied at four pulse frequencies (20, 25, 33 and 50 Hz). Pulse amplitude was always maintained at the same precalibrated value while pulse width was modulated according to the selected pattern. Pulse width in the step pattern had a constant value of 220 μs for 3 s, while in the ramp pattern it was rising linearly from 80 to 220 μs in 2 s and then it was maintained constant at 220 μs for the following 2 s.

The electrical stimulation was provided by a programmable stimulator developed at the Bioengineering Unit of Strathclyde University, Glasgow, a constant current pulses generator with the following characteristics (Phillips 1988):

pulse amplitude:	<150 mA;
pulse width:	20-500 μs;
pulse rate:	20-50 Hz;
shape:	monophasic rectangular current pulses.

Pulse rate and width were controlled by software while pulse amplitude was controlled by potentiometers.

Torque due to electrical stimulation was computed entering in the following equation the viscous-elastic parameters derived from the passive pendulum test and the kinematic values derived from the data acquired during the muscle stimulation:

$$Me = J\ddot{\Theta} + mgl \cdot sin(\Theta_{rv}) - \lambda \cdot e^{-E\Theta}(\omega - \Theta) + B\dot{\Theta} \qquad (2)$$

Finally, through a parametric identification procedure based on an ARX model, we estimated the transfer function between stimulus and induced torque. To choose the best order of the ARX model we used the MDL (Minimum Description Length) Rissanen criterium, that supplies a compromise between model complexity and accuracy (Ljung 1987).

The above procedure was applied to five healthy and three paraplegic male subjects with age ranging from 26 to 32 years.

3 Results and Discussion

For each subject the viscous-elastic parameters (λ, E, B and ω) were computed as the average of ten different pendulum tests. Results for healthy (H) and paraplegic patients (P) are shown in table 1:

Tab. 1. Viscous-elastic parameters (averaged on ten trials)

subject	age	λ [N·m/rad]	E [1/rad]	B [N·m·s/rad]	ω [rad]
H1	27	1.2	-0.486	0.377	2.548
H2	27	4.679	0.041	0.311	2.427
H3	27	3.658	-0.031	0.4	2.711
H4	26	4.49	0.257	0.305	2.701
H5	27	3.889	-0.079	0.332	2.413
P1	30	41.208	2.024	0.27	2.918
P2	32	3.761	1.317	0.302	2.52
P3	25	15.352	1.645	0.289	3.896

From the above data the following comments can be expressed:

- the intersubject variability of the viscous coefficient B as well as of the resting elastic angle ω are lesser than the variability of the elastic coefficient λ;
- the elastic coefficient λ can assume very high values in paraplegic patients (P1, P3), probably due to changes in rehologic characteristics of paralized muscles;
- the exponential coefficient (E) is near to zero in healthy subjects and it is larger than one in paraplegic patients: it means that the elastic component is almost linear in healthy muscles and approximately exponential in paralyzed muscles.

As a validation of the obtained viscous-elastic model, the comparison between data acquired from pendulum test on subject H2 (dashed line) and numerical integration of differential equation (1) with his estimated passive parameters (solid line) is shown in fig.1.

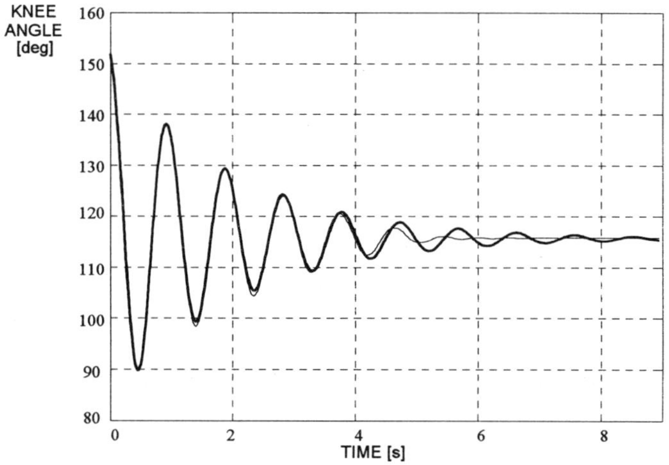

Fig.1. Comparison between real data of subject H2 (solid line) and data simulated with his viscous-elastic estimated model (bold line).

By using the estimated viscous-elastic parameters of each subjects and the kinematic data acquired in experiments with electrical stimulation, the torque Me due to stimulation was computed from equation (2). The torque Me for step and ramp stimulation pattern respectively is shown in fig.2 and 3 for all stimulation frequencies (subject H4).

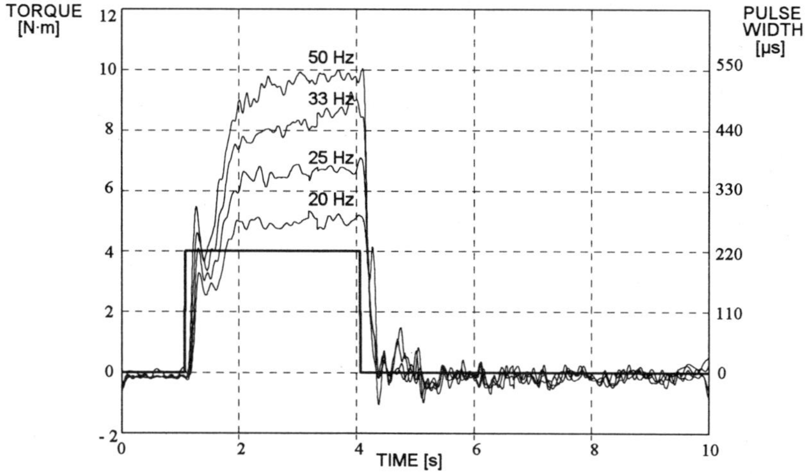

Fig. 2. Joint torque Me (solid line, left scale) generated by a step stimulation pattern (bold line, right scale) at different stimulation frequencies for subject H4.

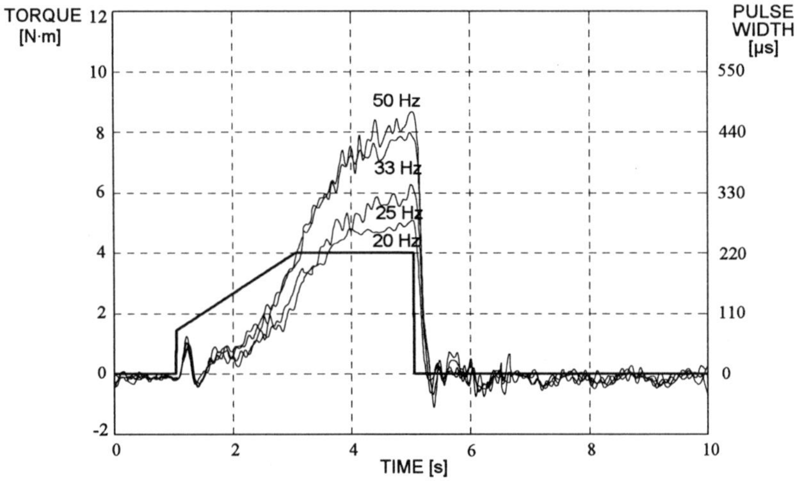

Fig. 3. Joint torque Me (solid line, left scale) generated by a ramp stimulation pattern (bold line, right scale) at different stimulation frequencies for subject H4.

Contraction and decontraction phases were separately considered; only the results concerning the contraction phases are presented in this paper.

The parametrical identification with ARX models was performed at each stimulation frequency considering the stimulus pattern (step or ramp) as input and the obtained Me torques as output. We can assume that the optimal model according to MDL Rissanen criterium was always a first order model (one pole). Only in a very few instances infact the best agreement was obtained for models with two poles and one zero characterized by high probability of cancellation between poles and zeros and so reducible to one pole model too. It is therefore possible to represent in the following single pole form the transfer function for each subject, where the parameter values depend on stimulation pattern and frequency:

$$H(s) = \frac{G}{1 + s\tau} \tag{3}$$

where:
τ = time constant of the pole;
G = static gain.

Pole time constants result not to be correlated to the stimulation frequency, then it was possible to use the values averaged over the different frequencies. On the contrary statistically significant differences of pole time constants corresponding to step and ramp stimulations were found.

The resulting time constant τ for both stimulation patterns are presented for each subject in table 2.

Tab. 2. Time constant of poles [s]

subject	step	ramp
H1	0.454	0.916
H2	0.426	0.72
H3	0.491	0.735
H4	0.406	1.749
H5	0.438	2.057
P1	0.769	7.38
P2	0.203	0.574
P3	0.215	1.094

It is evident from table 2 that step and ramp pattern dynamic responses are different in a significant way. We found infact faster response (smaller time constant) for step than for ramp stimulation.

As to concerns the static gain G, it was found that it depends on the stimulation frequency. The relations between G and frequency for the step pattern are shown in figure 4 and 5 for healthy and paraplegic subjects respectively. Similar trends were found for ramp pattern.

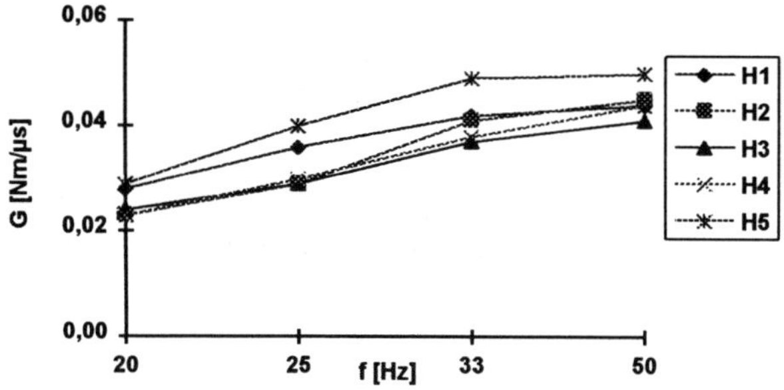

Fig. 4. Static gain at the various frequencies for healthy subjects, with a step pattern.

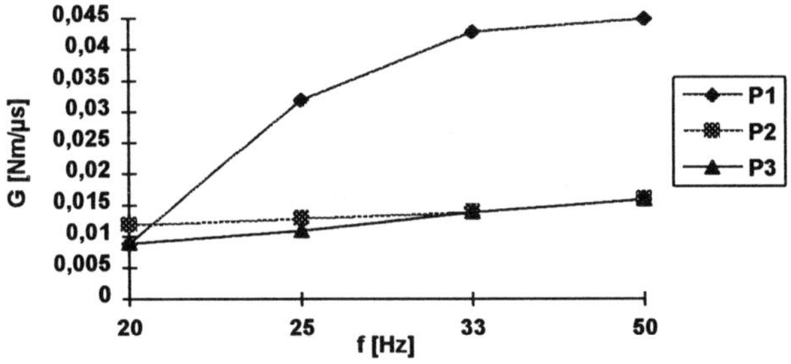

Fig. 5. Static gain at the various frequencies for paraplegic patients, with a step pattern.

As it was to be expected the gain is directly dependent on stimulation frequency. In fact frequency increase corresponds to increase of electric charge delivered to the muscle, this increases muscle contraction and as a consequence the produced joint torque Me.

Finally the comparison between muscle torque Me estimated by the first order model and that obtained from real data for an healthy subject (H2) are shown in figure 6 and 7 for a step and a ramp pattern respectively at all stimulation frequencies.

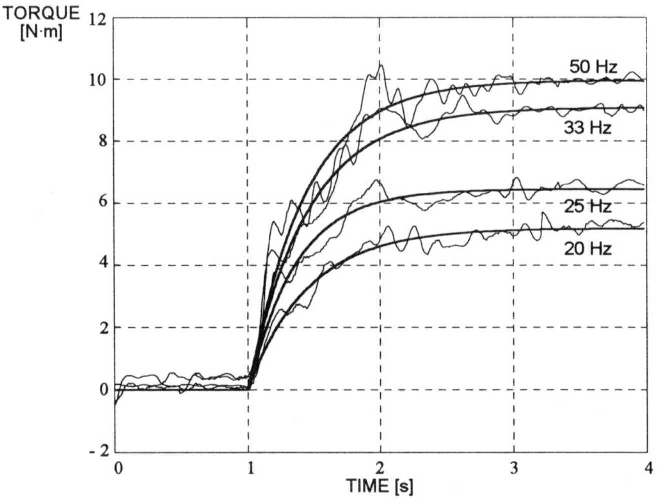

Fig.6. Knee torque (Me) estimated by the model (bold line) for a step stimulus at different pulse frequencies compared to real data (solid line) in subject H2; x axis represents time in seconds, y axis is the knee torque in Nm.

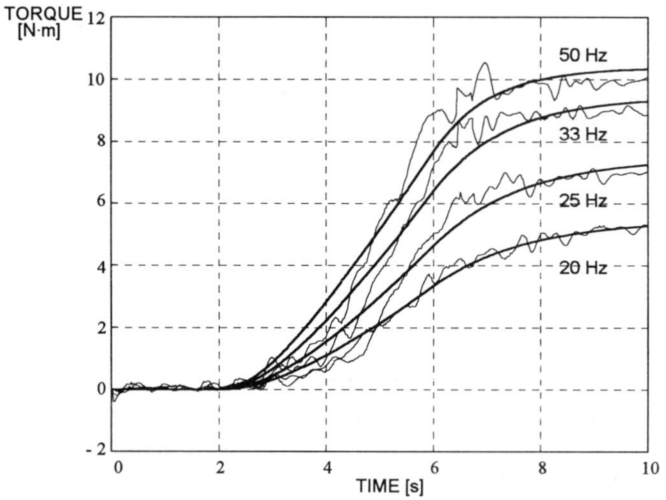

Fig.7. Knee torque (Me) estimated by the model (bold line) for a ramp stimulus at different pulse frequencies compared to real data (solid line) in subject H2. Axes and scales are the same as in fig.6.

4 Conclusions

Movement restoration in paraplegic patients by means of Functional Electrical Stimulation is an important but difficult task if functional results must be achieved. One main problem in clinical applications of FES system is finding out the optimal stimulation pattern related to the single patient characteristics. In the present study we developed an experimental and analytical procedure suitable to identify the transfer function between stimulation pattern and induced joint torque in dynamic conditions. Knowledge of this relationship allows to predict the effect of a given stimulation pattern on joint movement and therefore to optimize it by means of simulation models defined on the basis of patient specific characteristics. Moreover such a model can be used in the setting-up of control scheme for closed loop stimulators where signals detected with sensors are used to regulate stimulation pattern.

It was shown that a passive model of the knee joint including exponential elastic and linear viscous components is suitable to fit both healthy and paraplegic subjects data with a more evident exponential elastic behaviour in paraplegics than in healthy. Further investigations to understand the reason of this differentiation in muscolar characteristics must be carried on.

A simple single pole model with static gain dependent from stimulation frequency was found to identify rather accurately the relationship between stimulation and produced joint torque. Both gain and pole time constant are dependent on stimulation patterns (step or ramp) and on the sign of stimulation variation (increase or decrease), showing the presence of non linearity in the system. Intra and intersubject variability of model parameters is quite high particularly in paraplegic subjects. We expect it should decrease with implanted stimulators, where electrode movements and any external disturbance are very limited and therefore the model should apply in a more consistent way.

References

Andrew, G. (1992) Constrained optimization: Sequential Quadratic Programing (SQP). In: *Optimization Toolbox for use with Matlab*. The Math-Works inc, pp.22-32.

Audu, M. L. and Davy, D. T. (1985) The influence of muscle model complexity in musculoskeletal motion modeling. *Journal of Biomechanical Engineering,* **107**: 147-157.

Baratta, R. and Solomonow, M. (1990) The dynamic response model of nine different skeletal muscles. *IEEE Transaction on Biomedical Engineering*, **37**: 243-251.

Campisi, A., Baglioni, P., Ferrarin, M., Rabuffetti, M., and Pedotti, A. (1993) Evaluation of the torque at the knee joint due to electrical stimulation using kinematic analysis. In: R. Jaeger, T. Bajd (eds.) *Proceedings of The Ljubljana FES Conference*, Slovenia, August 25-26, 1993, pp.115-118.

Ferrarin, M., Osio, M., and Abello, G. (1996) A new biomechanical approach to Pendulum Test for spasticity evaluation. This book.

Franken, H.M. and Veltink, P.H. (1993) Identification of passive knee joint and shank dynamics in paraplegics using quadriceps stimulation. *IEEE Transaction on Rehabilitation Engineering,* **1**(3): 154-164.

Levi, M., Mizrahi, J., and Susak, Z. (1990) Recruitment, force and fatigue characteristics of quadriceps muscles of paraplegics isometrically activated by surface functional electrical stimulation. *Journal of Biomedical engineering,* **12**:150-156.

Ljung, L. (1987) System identification. Theory for the users. Prentice-Hall, pp.192-195.

Lin, D. C. and Rymer, W. Z. (1991) A quantitative analysis of pendular motion of the lower leg in spastic human subjects. *IEEE Transaction on Biomedical Engineering,* **38**: 906-918.

Pedotti, A. and Ferrigno, G. (1985) ELITE: a digital dedicated hardware system for movement analysis via real-time TV signal processing. *IEEE Transaction on Biomedical Engineering,* **32**: 943-949.

Phillips, G. (1988) Strathclyde Research Stimulator User Manual.

Yoon, Y. S. and Mansour, J. M., (1982) The passive elastic moment at the hip. *Journal of Biomechanics,* **15**: 905-910.

Zatsiorsky, V. and Seluyanov, V. (1983) The mass and inertia characteristic of the main segments of human body. *Biomechanics VIII-B*, University Park Press: 1152-1159.

A Model for an Artificially Activated Musculoskeletal System

S. J. Dorgan, M. J. O'Malley
Department of Electronic and Electrical Engineering,
University College Dublin, Belfield, Dublin 4, Ireland.

Abstract - A new physiologically based mathematical model for a human musculoskeletal system is presented. The presented model incorporates a novel musculotendon model developed specifically for skeletal muscle activated by Functional Electrical Stimulation, (FES). A new heterogeneous model structure is utilised that overcomes many of the problems which arise when attempting to describe all possible contraction modes. Also presented is a simple knee joint model that permits determination of the quadriceps force as a function of active knee moment. These physiologically based models are intended as alternatives to those currently available in the literature. They will be of use to those conducting research into the modelling, control and optimisation of FES generated motion.

1 Introduction

The usefulness of non-linear coupled systems in modelling non-isometric contractions has recently been demonstrated (Shue et al. 1995). With this in mind physiologically based non-linear models for FES activated human skeletal muscle, the human knee joint, and shank dynamics have been combined to produce a novel musculoskeletal system model. The model has stimulation frequency and intensity (pulse width or pulse amplitude) as inputs, with both force developed and thus the resulting limb motion as outputs. This model will be valuable in the design and testing of control and fatigue minimisation strategies for FES activated skeletal systems. The complete structure of the musculoskeletal system and the interactions between the constituent models are illustrated in Fig. 1.

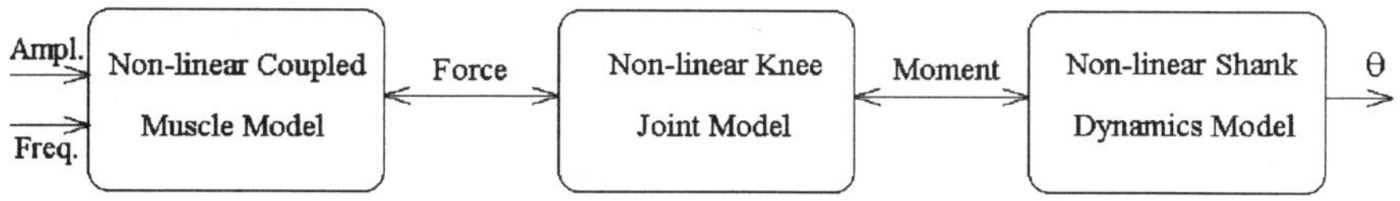

Fig. 1. Structure of the Musculoskeletal Model.

2 Musculoskeletal Model

The model used to capture the shank dynamics exhibited by the freely swinging shank is (Franken et al. 1993)

$$M_n = \ddot{\theta} + \lambda_1 \dot{\theta} + \lambda_2 \sin(\theta) + \lambda_3 \left[e^{\lambda_4 \theta} - 1 \right] \tag{1}$$

The usual pendular assumption that sin(θ) ≈ θ is not made, while the final term captures the non-linear joint dynamics. The entire system is normalised w.r.t. the shank inertia, giving M_n, the normalised active knee joint moment.

Making the assumption that the patella is a rigid body, and the patellar ligament is inextensible one finds, performing a mechanical analysis of an idealised knee joint (van Eijden et al. 1985) that

$$\frac{F_q}{F_r} = \frac{\cos(\theta + \alpha + \varepsilon)}{\sin(\theta + \alpha + \delta)} \tag{2}$$

$$\frac{F_q}{F_{pl}} = \frac{\cos(\theta + \alpha - \varepsilon)}{\sin(\delta + \varepsilon)} \tag{3}$$

where F_q, F_{pl} and F_r are the quadricep tendon, patellar tendon and patellar compression forces respectively, while the angles α, δ, ε and θ are defined as previously by van Eijden et al. (1985). Each of the above ratios may be calculated for any angle of flexion, θ, if the functions defining α, δ and ε in terms of θ are known. Such fuctions have indeed been found from experimental data (van Eijden et al. 1985). Combining this with a function defining the non-linear moment arm variation as a function of knee angle one has a simple physiologically based knee model capable of giving the quadriceps force developed as a function of active knee moment.

The new FES muscle model presented is inspired by previous physiological modelling efforts (Hatze 1978). The model structure utilised here is also new to muscle modelling attempts, it is heterogeneous (Kuipers and Åstrom 1994) with weighting functions for the recruiting, de-recruiting, and static states as in Fig. 2.

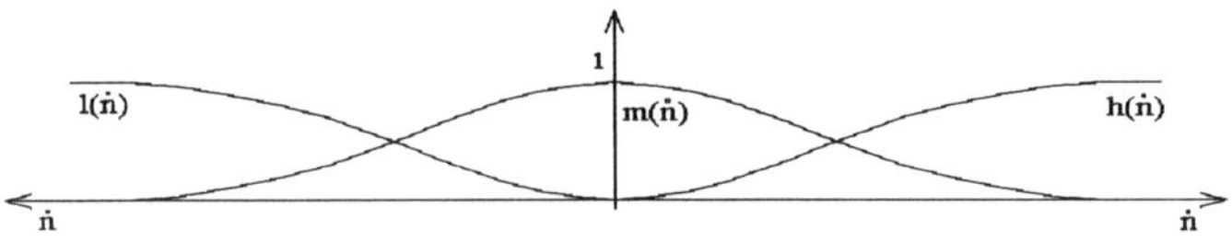

Fig. 2. Heterogeneous weighting functions $l(\dot{n})$, $m(\dot{n})$ and $h(\dot{n})$ for use within the FES muscle model. As n is the number of active motor units these functions represent the muscle's membership of recruiting, de-recruiting or static states.

Considering the inverse recruitment dynamics and the other muscular physiological mechanisms the model state equations (4-12) are obtained. A full derivation of this FES musculotendon model may be found elsewhere (Dorgan and O'Malley 1995).

$$\dot{n} = \overline{m}\left[z(a) - n\right] \tag{4}$$

$$\dot{r} = -\dot{n}.\,f(r,\dot{n}) - r - \frac{r}{log\left(1 + q_0 + c.\,\phi/_{q_0}\right)} \tag{5}$$

$$\dot{\psi} = l(\dot{n})\dot{\psi}_l + m(\dot{n})\dot{\psi}_m + h(\dot{n})\dot{\psi}_h \tag{6}$$

$$\dot{\phi} = l(\dot{n})\dot{\phi}_l + m(\dot{n})\dot{\phi}_m + h(\dot{n})\dot{\phi}_h \tag{7}$$

$$\dot{\psi}_l = m_n(cv - \psi) \tag{8}$$

$$\dot{\psi}_m = \dot{\psi}_h = m_n(cv - \psi) - \bar{c}\dot{n}\frac{\left[1 - e^{\rho_0(\varepsilon)(\psi - \phi)}\right]}{\rho_0(\varepsilon)\left[1 - e^{\bar{c}n}\right]} + \dot{\phi} \tag{9}$$

$$\dot{\phi}_l = \dot{\phi}_m = -\phi m_r e^{\bar{c}n} + \frac{\dot{\psi}}{\psi}\phi + \bar{c}\left[\dot{r} + \dot{n}\left(1 - e^{\bar{c}r}\right)\right]\frac{\left[1 - e^{\rho_0(\varepsilon)(\phi - \psi)}\right]}{\rho_0(\varepsilon)\left[e^{\bar{c}r} - 1\right]} \tag{10}$$

$$\dot{\phi}_h = -\phi m_r e^{\bar{c}n} \tag{11}$$

$$\dot{\varepsilon} = -\frac{\bar{\dot{\lambda}}_0}{\bar{\lambda}}\left\{a_2 + \frac{1}{a_1}tanh^{-1}\left[\frac{\left(F^{se}/_{\bar{F}\,sin\theta(\varepsilon)} + b_1.\,e^{-a_6(\varepsilon - 1)}\right)b_2}{\upsilon(t)k(\varepsilon)} - 1\right]\right\} \tag{12}$$

3 Results

Fig. 3(a) and Fig. 3(b) illustrate the ability of the presented non-linear knee model to predict the ratios of F_q/F_{pl} and F_r/F_{pl} experimentally determined for the human knee joint (Nisell 1985).

Parameters were identified using the Levenberg-Marquardt optimisation method for the pendular dynamics of the shank. In Fig. 3(c) a comparison is presented between the predicted and experimentally determined non-linear shank dynamics.

The ability of the muscle model to predict force generation by the quadriceps group during skeletal motion is illustrated in Fig. 3(d). The stimulus waveform used is a linearly increasing pulse amplitude, with constant pulse width and frequency, while the shank is free to swing.

The normalised errors between the model predictions and experimental results indicate the model's ability to capture the dynamics of this very non-linear system with high accuracy. This illustrates the return achieved from the development of physiologically based as opposed to black box musculoskeletal models.

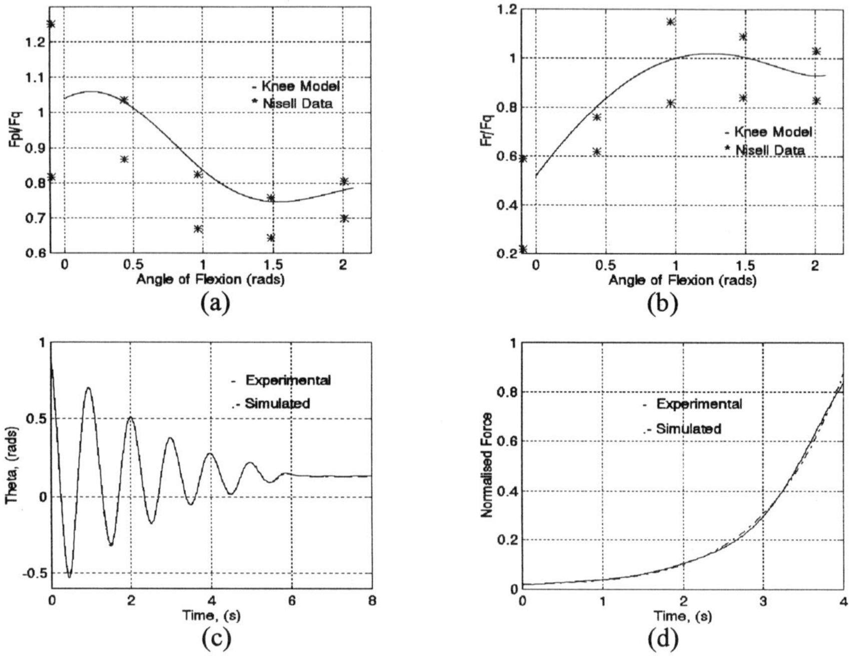

Fig. 3. Performance of (a), (b) Knee Model; (c) Shank dynamics model, normalised error=0.025; and (d) Complete musculoskeletal model, normalised error=0.029.

References

Dorgan, S. J. and O'Malley M. J. (1995) A Physiologically Based Mathematical Model of Electrically Stimulated Muscle, *In Review - IEEE Trans Rehab. Eng.*

Franken, H. M., Veltink, P. H., Tijsmans, R., Nijmeijer, H. and Boom, H. B. K. (1993) Identification of Passive Knee Joint and Shank Dynamics in Paraplegics Using Quadriceps Stimulation, *IEEE Trans. Rehab. Eng.*, **1**: 154-164.

Hatze, H. (1978) A General Myocybernetic Control Model of Skeletal Muscle, *Biological Cybernetics*, **28**: 143-157.

Kuipers, B. and Åström, K. (1994) The Composition and Validation of Heterogenous Control Laws, *Automatica*, **30**, pp. 233-249.

Nisell, R. (1985) Biomechanics of the Knee. A study of Joint and Muscle Load with Clinical Application, *Acta Orthop. Scand.*, **56**, Suppl. 216: 1-42.

Shue, G., Crago, P. E., and Chizeck, H. J. (1995) Muscle-Joint Models Incorporating Activation Dynamics, Moment-Angle and Moment-Velocity Properties, *IEEE Trans. Biomed. Eng.*, **42**: 212-223.

van Eijden, T. M. G. J., de Boer, W., and Weijs, W. A. (1985) The Orientation of the Distal Part of the Quadriceps Femoris Muscle as a Function of the Knee Flexion-Extension Angle, *J. Biomechanics*, **18**, pp. 803-809.

Physiologically Based Multi-Input Model of Muscle Activation

R. Riener[1], J. Quintern[2], E. Psaier[1], G. Schmidt[1]
[1]Dept. of Automatic Control Engineering, Technical University Munich, Germany
[2]Neurological Clinic, Klinikum Grosshadern, University of Munich, Germany

Abstract - A physiologically based model of muscle activation is presented which accounts for major effects that occur during artificial stimulation of human muscle under isometric conditions. Inputs of the model include interpulse interval, pulse width, and pulse amplitude. The model is divided into two submodels. One submodel characterizes the dynamic relationship between pulse interval and force generated in a single motor unit. Among other aspects this part also accounts for muscle fatigue and recovery. The second submodel uses a nonlinear recruitment characteristic to compute the number of recruited motor units as a function of pulse width and pulse amplitude. Total muscle force depends on the force developed in the single motor units (temporal summation) and the number of units recruited (spatial summation). Different motor units (slow and fast twitch units) with different contraction, recruitment, and fatigue properties are distinguished. The model was evaluated qualitatively by comparing the isometric force output with experimental data from the literature and our own measurements. This model is proposed for designing effective FES control strategies, e.g., in which pulse rate and recruitment are modulated simultaneously.

1 Introduction

Muscle force induced by functional electrical stimulation (FES) can be controlled by adjusting pulse width or amplitude (recruitment modulation) and pulse frequency (rate modulation). Although Chizeck *et al.* (1991) have shown that simultaneous modulation of both recruitment and rate can improve controller performance, most investigators control muscle force by applying only recruitment modulation. Another advantage of using simultaneous recruitment and rate modulation is that the stimulation pattern can be adjusted so that minimum fatigue occurs, and rapid force generation and fused tetanus are performed when necessary.

The principal objective of this study is to develop a multi-input model that describes major characteristics of artificially stimulated muscle. Such characteristics are, for example, the force-frequency (Mortimer, 1981; Binder-Macleod and McDermond, 1992) and the recruitment characteristic (Crago *et al.*, 1980 a), the doublet effect (Karu *et al.*, 1995; Kwende *et al.*, 1995; Jarvis, 1996), also known as nonlinear summation (Stein and Parmiggiani, 1981), and the fatigue characteristic as a function of different continuous stimulation inputs (Mortimer, 1981; Binder-Macleod and Barker, 1991; Rabischong and Ohanna, 1992; Karu *et al.*, 1995).

A model that accounts for these effects can assist in optimizing open- and closed-loop control strategies, where effective muscle contraction is achieved by simultaneously modulating more than one input quantity (e.g., pulse width and pulse frequency). We believe that such a controller is a promising potential component of neural prostheses for restoring functional movement in paralyzed individuals.

2 Methods

2.1 Model

Muscle force is controlled by the number of motor units activated and the amount of force generated in these units. Thus, the model is divided into two submodels (Fig. 1). A *static recruitment model* determines the motor units recruited (spatial summation). Input to this submodel includes the pulse width $d(t)$ and pulse amplitude pattern $A(t)$, which are generated by the stimulator. A discrete-space *dynamic motor unit model* computes the normalized, isometric muscle force $F(t)$ produced by n motor units. The force developed in a single motor unit depends on the input train of nerve potentials and can be adjusted only by the pulse frequency $f(t)$ (temporal summation), which is equal to the inverse of the interpulse interval T. Further input to the motor unit model is the "on/off" information $j_i(t)$ of a single unit i determined in the static recruitment model.

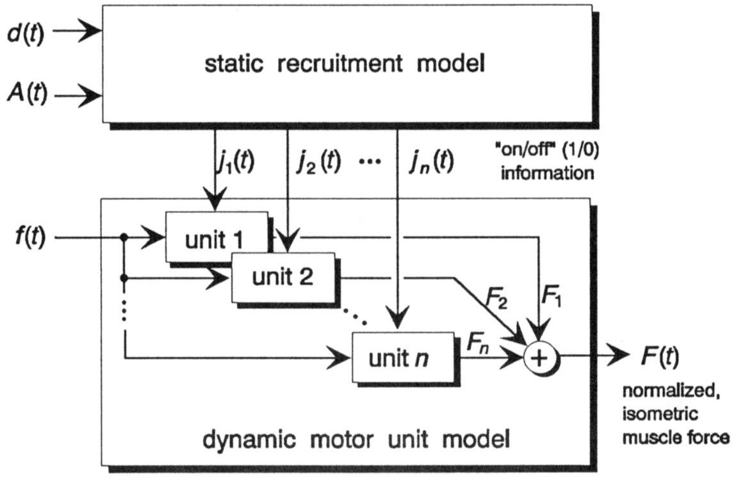

Fig. 1. Total activation dynamics model. Normalized, isometric muscle force F is calculated from the stimulation signal, which is characterized by pulse width d, pulse amplitude A, and pulse frequency f.

2.1.1 Dynamic Motor Unit Model

To describe the force-output in a single motor unit as a function of the stimulation frequency f, we derived a model on the basis of Hatze's (1977) myocybernetic control model (Fig. 2). If a motor unit i is recruited (j_i=1), the impulse generator produces a train of nerve impulses (action potentials) occurring at variable intervals $T=1/f$. If the pulse interval of two pulses is lower than the refractory period, no action potential is generated. Mihelin et al. (1991) found the mean refractory period of human muscle to be 4.1 msec. Each nerve impulse has the same shape and is approximated by a half-sine wave with a half-period of 1 ms.

As described by Hatze (1977), motor endplate and sarcoplasmic reticulum are modeled as lumped second order systems. In these parts of the model different contraction and relaxation times of fast and slow motor units are taken into consideration.

In order to describe the effect of muscle fatigue and recovery, we introduced the following fitness function $fit(t)$:

$$\dot{fit}(t) = 1/T_{fat}\,(fit_{\min} - fit(t))\,\bar{\gamma}^*(t) + 1/T_{rec}\,(1 - fit(t))\,(1 - \bar{\gamma}^*(t))$$
$$fit(t),\ \bar{\gamma}^*(t) = 0 \ldots 1 \qquad (1)$$

The value $\bar{\gamma}^*(t)$ represents the normalized ($\bar{\gamma}^*(t)$=0...1) concentration of free calcium ions in non-fatiguing muscle. T_{fat} and T_{rec} are the time constants for fatigue and recovery, respectively. They differ in fast and slow motor units. The minimum fitness is given by fit_{min}. The optimal agreement with fatigue experiments was obtained by placing the fatigue model right after the model of the sarcoplasmic reticulum, where it reduces the concentration of free calcium ions (see Riener *et al.*, 1996 a,b for comparison). This is justified also from a physiological point of view, for it has been demonstrated in the literature that the amplitude of the calcium ion transient decreases as fatigue develops (Westerblad and Allen, 1991; Fitts, 1994). This decrease might be explained by a blockage of the T tubular action potential, a reduced intramembranous T tubular charge movement, an inhibition of the calcium release channel in the sarcoplasmic reticulum, or depletion of releasable calcium ions from the sarcoplasmic reticulum.

The concentration of free calcium ions in fatiguing muscle $\gamma(t)$ is obtained by

$$\gamma(t) = fit(t) \cdot \gamma^*(t)\,. \qquad (2)$$

For the binding process of calcium ions to the troponin-tropomyosin complex in the presence of a varying calcium concentration, we applied a nonlinear function as described by Hatze (1978). This function determines the active state $a(t)$ of muscle from the concentration of free calcium ions $\gamma(t)$. Hatze defines the active state a "to be the relative amount of calcium bound to troponin" (Hatze, 1977).

To obtain the normalized force $F_i(t)$ in a single motor unit i, we introduced the following first-order relation, which smooths $a(t)$ due to friction and gliding effects in the muscle fibres:

$$\dot{F}_i(t) = 1/T_g\,(a(t) - F_i(t)),\tag{3}$$

where T_g denotes the gliding time constant.

Note that in general there are time delays between the onsets of the nerve potential $\alpha(t)$, the depolarizing potential on the muscle $\beta(t)$, the calcium concentration $\gamma(t)$, and the active state $a(t)$, due to finite conduction velocities in the membrane system and limitations in the rates of the chemical reactions involved. Using the model presented for designing control strategies, we propose that a total delay (time between stimulus pulse to the onset of force production) be considered within the impulse generator.

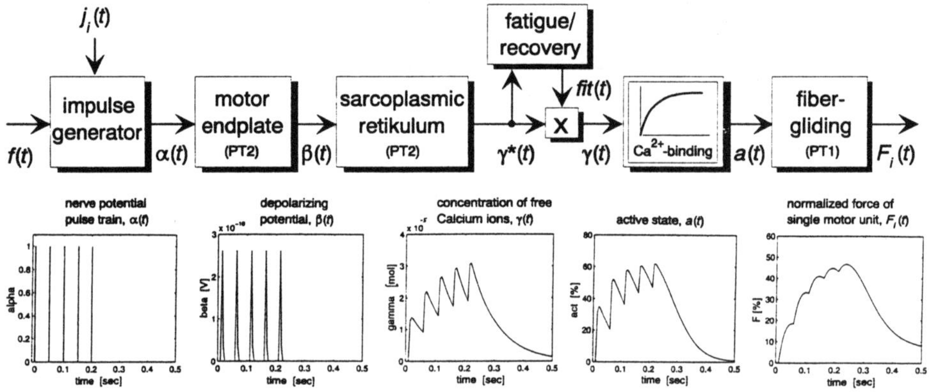

Fig. 2. Dynamic model of the activation dynamics in a single motor unit. Input to the model is the pulse frequency $f(t)$; output is the normalized force $F_i(t)$ developed in a single motor unit.

2.1.2 Static Recruitment Model

Instead of adjusting muscle force by rate modulation, muscle force can also be controlled by modulating pulse width or amplitude. Pulse amplitude modulation is, in effect, equivalent to pulse width modulation, since an increase in either recruits more motor units (Crago *et al.*, 1980 a). We developed a static recruitment model that determines the motor units recruited (Fig. 3). For a given pulse width d and pulse amplitude A, the percentages of the recruited slow (corresponding to muscle fibre type I) and fast (corresponding to type II) motor units can in a first step be computed on the basis of the muscle's recruitment curve (Fig. 4). This curve can be approximated using the following equation, which relates the stimulation pulse width d to the percentage of recruited motor units p_{rec} (Note that in this case the pulse amplitude was held constant, A=1):

$$p_{rec}(d) = c_1\{\,(d-d_{thr})\arctan[\kappa_{thr}(d-d_{thr})] - (d-d_{sat})\arctan[\kappa_{sat}(d-d_{sat})]\,\} + c_2 \tag{4}$$

The parameters d_{thr} and d_{sat} denote pulse width values corresponding to threshold and saturation, respectively (see Fig. 4). The curvatures of the recruitment curve in the area of threshold and saturation can be adjusted by changing κ_{thr} and κ_{sat}, respectively. The recruitment curve is scaled by the constants c_1 and c_2 in order to satisfy the conditions $p_{rec}(0) = 0$ and $p_{rec}(d \to \infty) = 100\%$.

After computing the absolute number of recruited slow and fast motor units, $n_{rec,s}$ and $n_{rec,f}$, respectively, threshold functions determine which units are recruited or not (Fig. 3, on the right). As soon as the number of recruited units $n_{rec,s}$ (for slow units) exceeds the threshold value related to a unit i, this unit starts to be recruited and obtains the value j_i=1. If $n_{rec,s}$ decreases below the threshold value, then this unit is not recruited anymore, and becomes j_i=0. However, it still develops force, since free calcium ions can be bound to troponin as long as they are not fully reuptaken by the sarcoplasmic reticulum - the unit is semi-active (see decreasing part of graphs in Fig. 2). This period is also called the relaxation period.

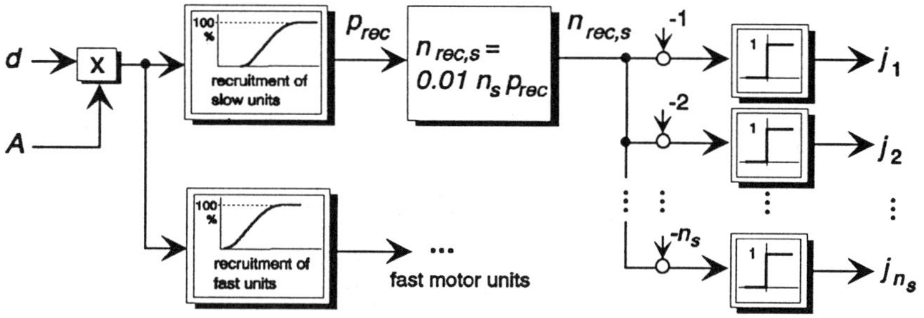

Fig. 3. Static recruitment model. We distinguished between slow and fast motor units. Each type has its own recruitment curve. p_{rec} represents the percentage of recruited fibres and n_s is the total number of slow units that are assumed in the model. $n_{rec,s}$ is a 'real' type variable that expresses how many of the slow motor units are recruited. Note that in this study the pulse amplitude A was held constant (A=1).

Note that high threshold values correspond to motor units that are remote from the electrodes (and thus from the electrical field developed by the electrodes). They are recruited less often during recruitment modulation (during frequency modulation the number of recruited units is constant), which enables them to recover better than units closer to the electrodes. This way of modeling is important in order to describe the effect of fatigue in a realistic way.

We distinguished between fast and slow motor units in both submodels (the existence of other types, e.g. IIa and IIb, was neglected for this version of the model), because many characteristics of artificially stimulated muscle, such as the inverse size-order recruitment (Gorman and Mortimer, 1983; Heyters et al., 1994) (Fig. 4) and the shape of the fatigue characteristic (Edström and Kugelberg, 1968; Mortimer, 1981; Rabischong and Ohanna, 1992), can be attributed to the existence of different motor units with different properties. In our model fast motor units differ from slow ones in lower contraction and relaxation times, lower pulse widths for threshold and saturation (Eq. 4, Fig. 3), and higher fatigue rate (lower T_{fat}, Eqs. 1). The percentages of fast and slow motor units in the stimulated muscle were estimated from the literature (Johnson *et al.*, 1973). In view of the high variability of fibre distributions among individuals, we suggest that muscle biopsies be used in order to adjust the model to an individual subject.

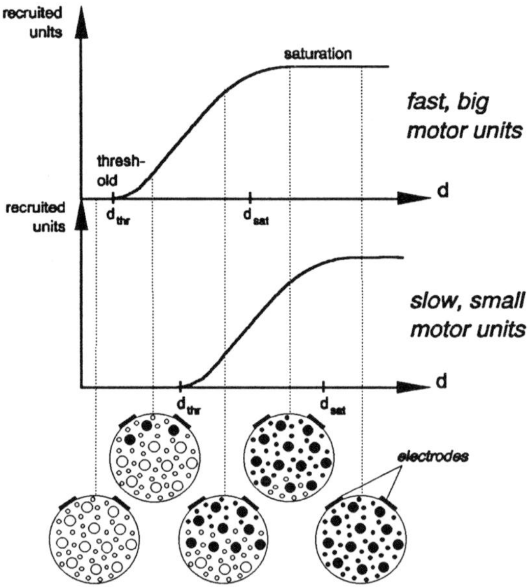

Fig. 4 Inverse size-order recruitment characteristic of artificially stimulated muscle (surface electrodes). Big, fast motor units close to the electrodes are the first, whereas small, slow motor units far from the electrodes are the last recruited. Recruited units are represented by filled circles. All motor units of one group (type I or II) are modeled as if they had identical properties.

2.2 Measurements

Stimulation experiments were performed in one patient with complete thoracic spinal cord injury. The patient gave his informed consent to participate in the study. The subject laid supine with the thigh supported. Measurements were performed under isometric conditions. The shank was fixed to a strain-gauge-based torque transducer (shank position perpendicular to the thigh). The quadriceps muscle was stimulated with surface electrodes. Balanced bipolar stimulation pulses were delivered by a computer-controlled stimulator. Data were digitized and stored in a computer (sampling rate: 200 Hz).

The experiments were driven by a "pattern definition file", which enabled the user to define any train of pulses. Each pulse is characterized by its position in time, pulse width, and pulse amplitude. The same file is also used as input for the computer simulation.

3 Results

The activation dynamics model presented was evaluated by comparing simulation results with experimental data from the literature and from our own measurements. Parameters were adjusted in the model so that the computed muscle force during the stimulation produced by the model would qualitatively agree with isometric measurements (see Table 1 in the Discussion).

The model describes the force characteristic of single twitches sufficiently well (see also Hatze, 1977). It is possible to show how twitch force depends on the interpulse interval (Fig. 5), when the muscle is activated by doublet stimulation (a pair of closely spaced stimulus pulses). For relatively short pulse intervals even nonlinear summation (doublet effect) was observed in the simulation. That is, in fast motor units the twitch force amplitude resulting from doublet excitation is more than twice the amplitude of twitches produced by singlet stimulation. This phenomenon has been demonstrated in stimulation experiments with mammalian muscles (Stein and Parmiggiani, 1981; Karu *et al.*, 1995; Kwende *et al.*, 1995; Jarvis *et al.*, 1996). We compared our simulation results with experimental data from Karu et al. (1995) who used surface stimulation of the quadriceps muscle to produce isometric knee joint torque (Fig. 5). Model parameters of the differential equations describing mainly the properties of the sarcoplasmic reticulum, were adjusted in such way that the doublet effect showed the same intensity as in the experiments. However, the maximum amplitude per pulse of the resulting twitch occurred at higher interpulse intervals in the simulation ($PI \approx 9$ msec) than in the experiment ($PI \approx 5$ msec, see Karu *et al.*, 1995).

Comparing the force response in experiments and in the simulation, we identified a total delay of $T_{tot} \approx 25$ msec for the time between stimulus pulse to the onset of force production. This result agrees with delay times mentioned by others (Phillips *et al.*, 1994; Karu, 1992).

The model also allows accurate prediction of the force-frequency characteristic during stimulation at different frequency levels (Fig. 6). Muscle relaxation in the simulation was a little bit slower than in the experiments (performed by Binder-Macleod and McDermond, 1992). We also generated force responses for linearly increasing pulse frequency (Fig. 7), obtaining good agreement with data from the literature (Reid *et al.*, 1993).

Good agreement between measurement and simulation was also obtained for the force response to a stimulation pattern with arbitrary pulse parameters. For example, we stimulated the quadriceps continuously with constant pulse parameters (f=20 Hz, d=320 μsec) and increased the pulse width of single pulses or added intermediate pulses every second (Fig. 8). Skipping only one or two pulses resulted in a significant collapse of the force plateau in the simulation as well as in the experiment.

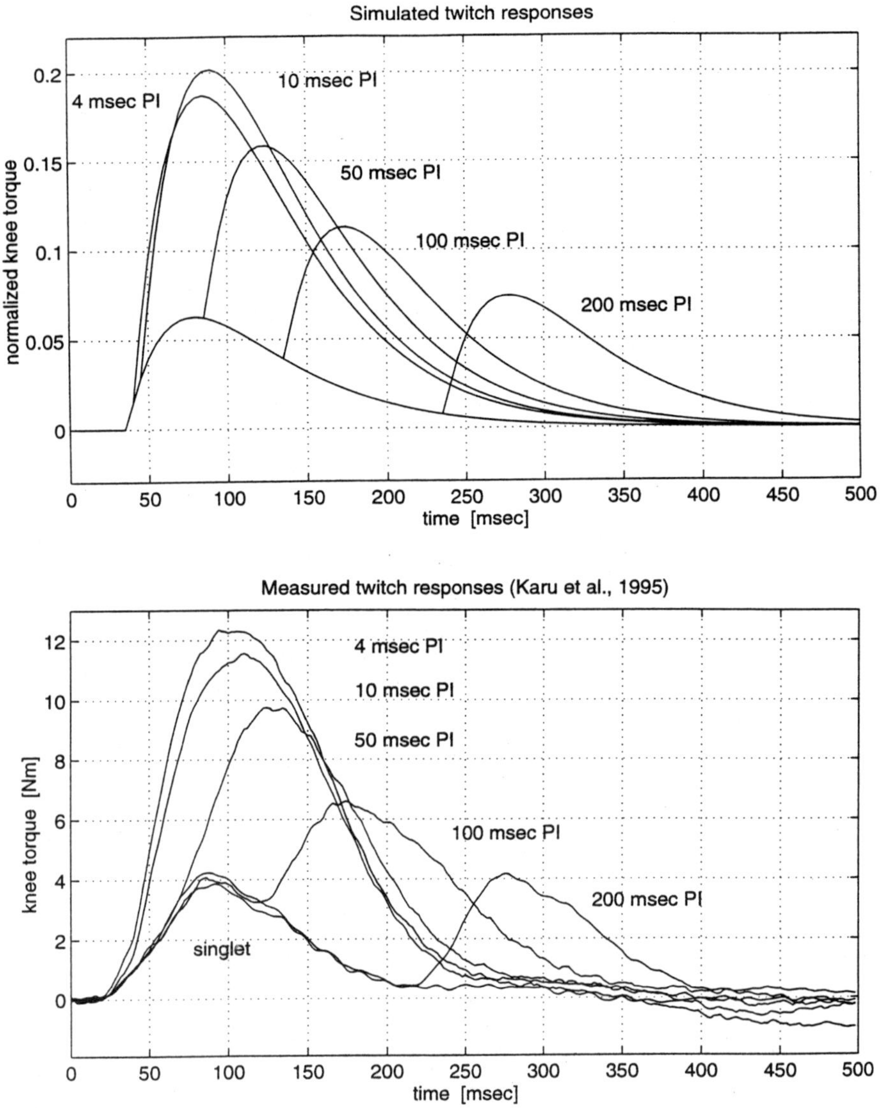

Fig. 5. Twitch response to singlets and doublets with different pulse intervals. In the experiments human quadriceps muscle of a healthy subject was stimulated using surface electrodes. The abbreviation *PI* means pulse interval. Experimental data is shown with permission of Karu *et al.* (1995) (zzkaru@mit.edu).

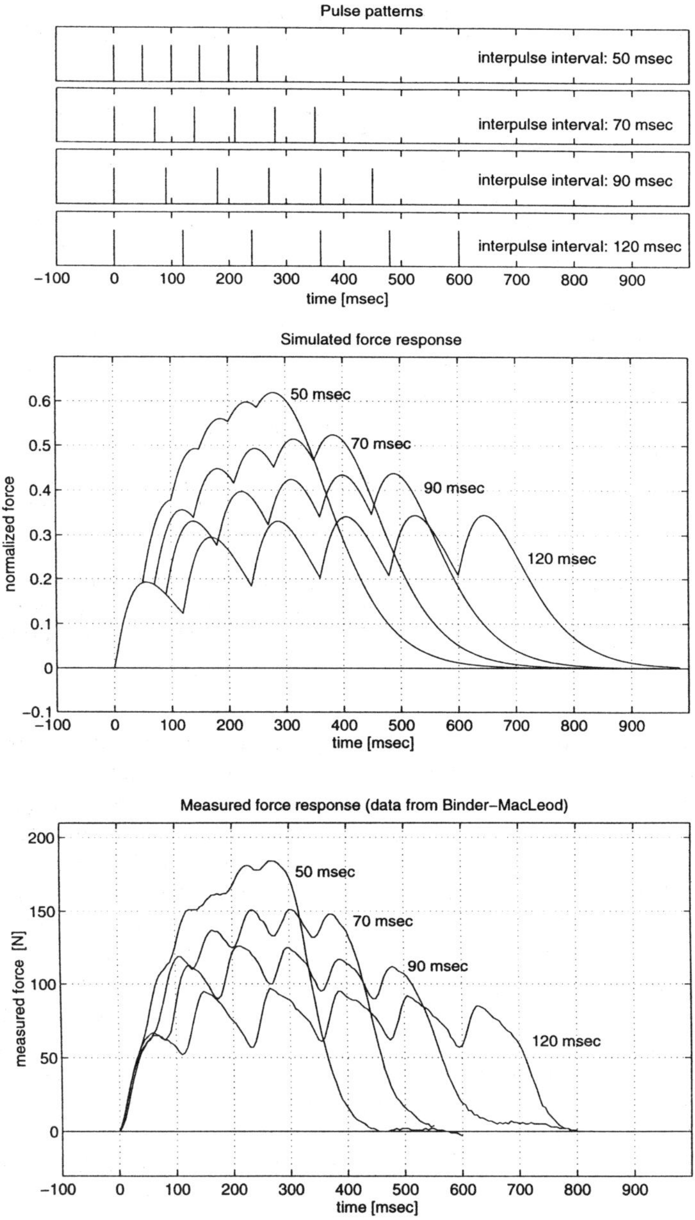

Fig. 6. Simulated and measured force responses at pulse trains with various interpulse intervals. All trains contain six pulses. Fatigue was "switched off" in the simulation. In the experiments human quadriceps femoris muscle was stimulated. Experimental results were kindly provided by Binder-Macleod (see also Binder-Macleod and McDermond, 1992).

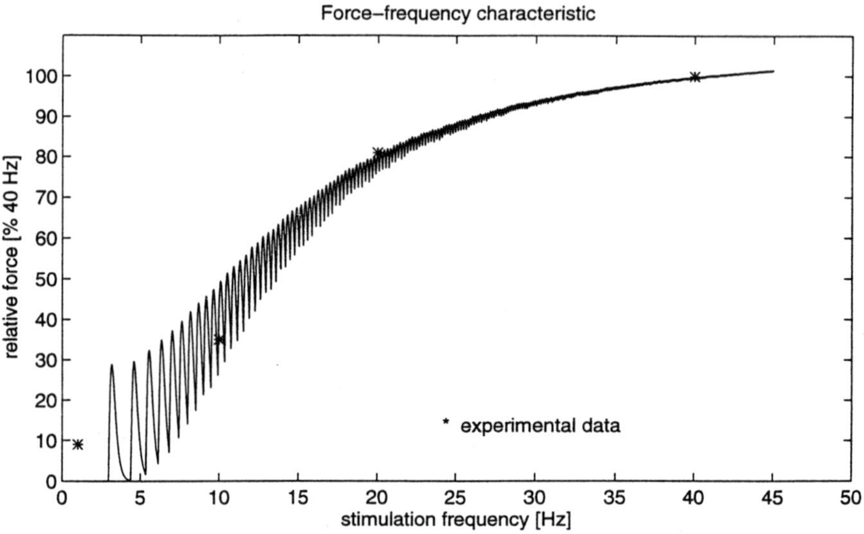

Fig. 7. Simulated force-frequency characteristic when stimulating with linearly increasing pulse width (f = 1...45 Hz, increased within 5 sec). The stars depict relative forces from experiments evoked by stimulating human anterior tibialis muscle (Reid *et al.*, 1993).

Furthermore, the model shows considerably good correspondence with measured recruitment characteristics of fatigued and non-fatigued muscles (Fig. 9). This is not only due to the application of a nonlinear recruitment characteristic (Eq. 4), but also due to the differentiation of fast and slow motor units. In most of our experiments we observed a sudden drop in the slope of the torque at about d=350μsec, but only for non-fatigued muscle (see arrows in Fig. 9). In our simulations we reconstructed this effect by assuming that the recruitment characteristic of fast motor units shows a lower saturation pulse width than that of slow units. Another typical phenomenon observed in simulations and experiments of fatigued muscle is that threshold is increased compared to that of non-fatigued muscle (Fig. 9, two graphs on the bottom). This can be explained by the fact that the activity of fatigue-resistant slow motor units, which have higher threshold values than fast ones (inverse size-order recruitment), dominate in a fatigued muscle with mixed fibre distribution.

Our model predicts muscle fatigue characteristics sufficiently well. Both simulation and experiments (Karu *et al.*, 1995) showed that muscle fatigue depends on the pulse frequency. During continuous stimulation, high frequency stimulation in both simulation and experiment leads to a faster decrease of force and to a lower force plateau than low frequency stimulation (Fig. 10).

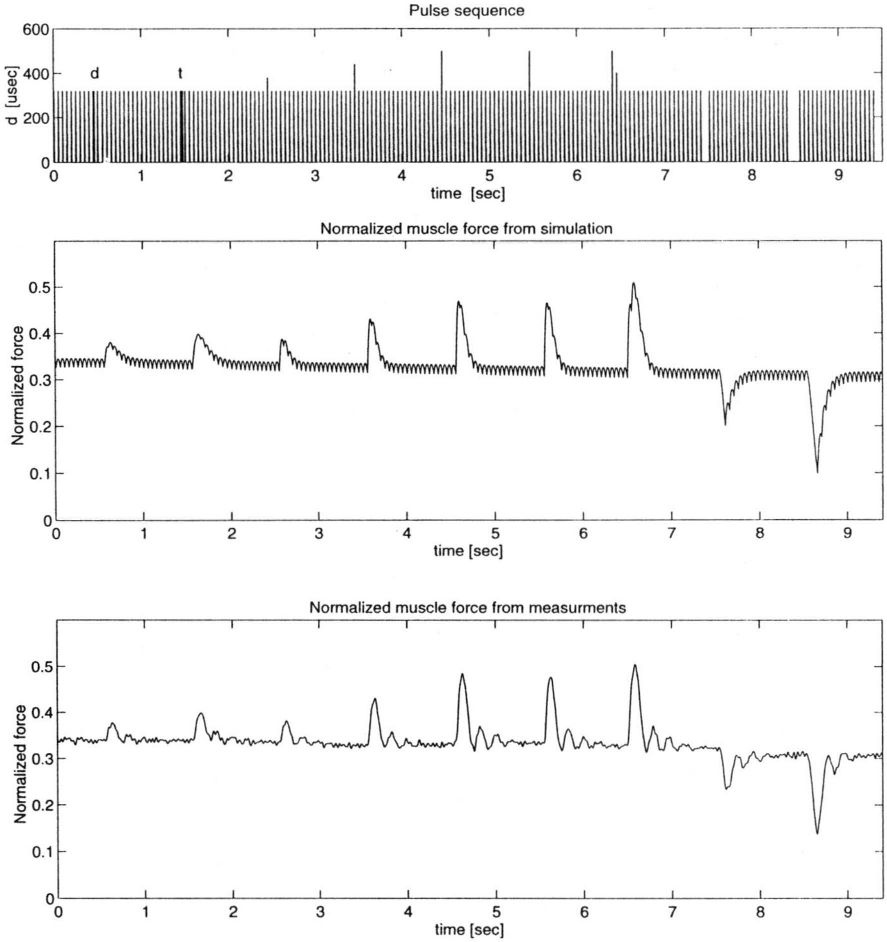

Fig. 8. Comparison of simulated and measured isometric muscle force with predefined stimulation pattern. Quadriceps was stimulated at 320 μsec with 20 Hz (own measurements). At periodic times (1 sec) pulses were added, were deleted, or changed in pulse width. At 'd' and 't' the singlet is changed by a double and triple pulse, respectively. Note that the small oscillations in the measurements after each pulse are due to bending effects in the torque transducer.

Furthermore, the model permitted us to show which strategy - pulse width modulation or frequency modulation - is more effective with respect to fatigue resistance. We performed simulations with two different pulse patterns. In one pattern pulse width and in the other pattern pulse frequency was modulated while the other stimulation parameters remained constant. Both patterns were

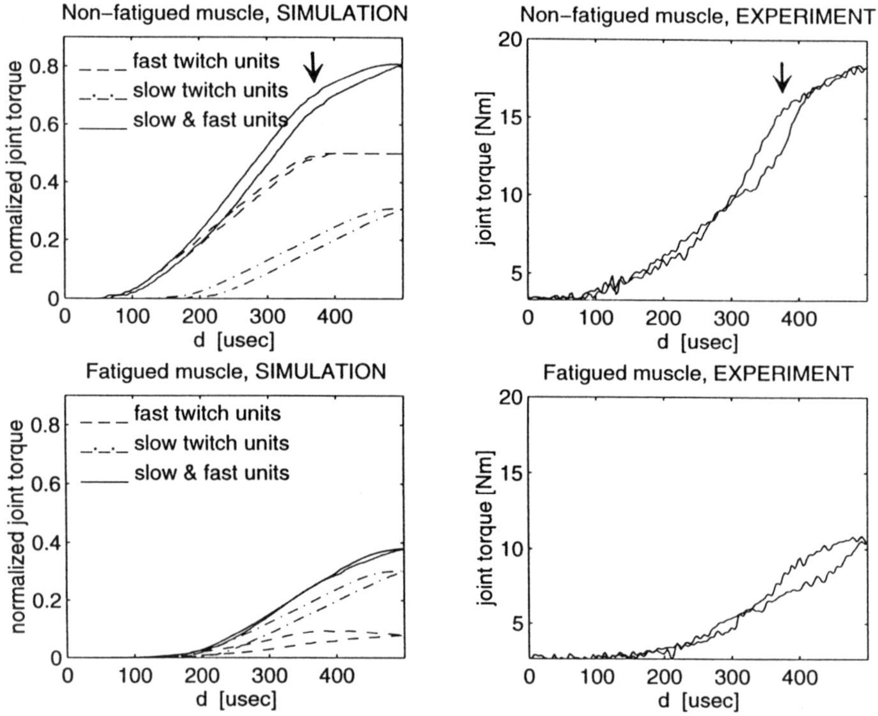

Fig. 9. Recruitment characteristics of fatigued and non-fatigued muscles. Thresholds and saturations and their dependence on muscle fatigue in simulation show good correspondence to measured recruitment characteristics (own measurements). The arrow marks the often observed sudden drop in the slope of the torque.

constructed so that the number of pulses and the average force developed by the non-fatigued muscle were the same, (i.e., both force outputs looked very similar). However, when fatigue was taken into consideration by "switching on" our fitness model, the simulation showed that frequency modulation led to a faster decrease of muscle fitness than pulse width modulation. This phenomenon has already been observed in our experiments and can be explained by the fact that during frequency modulation the same motor units are always recruited. However, during pulse width modulation, the number of recruited units changes incessantly, so that units - especially the ones remote from the electrodes - have time to recover while they are not being recruited.

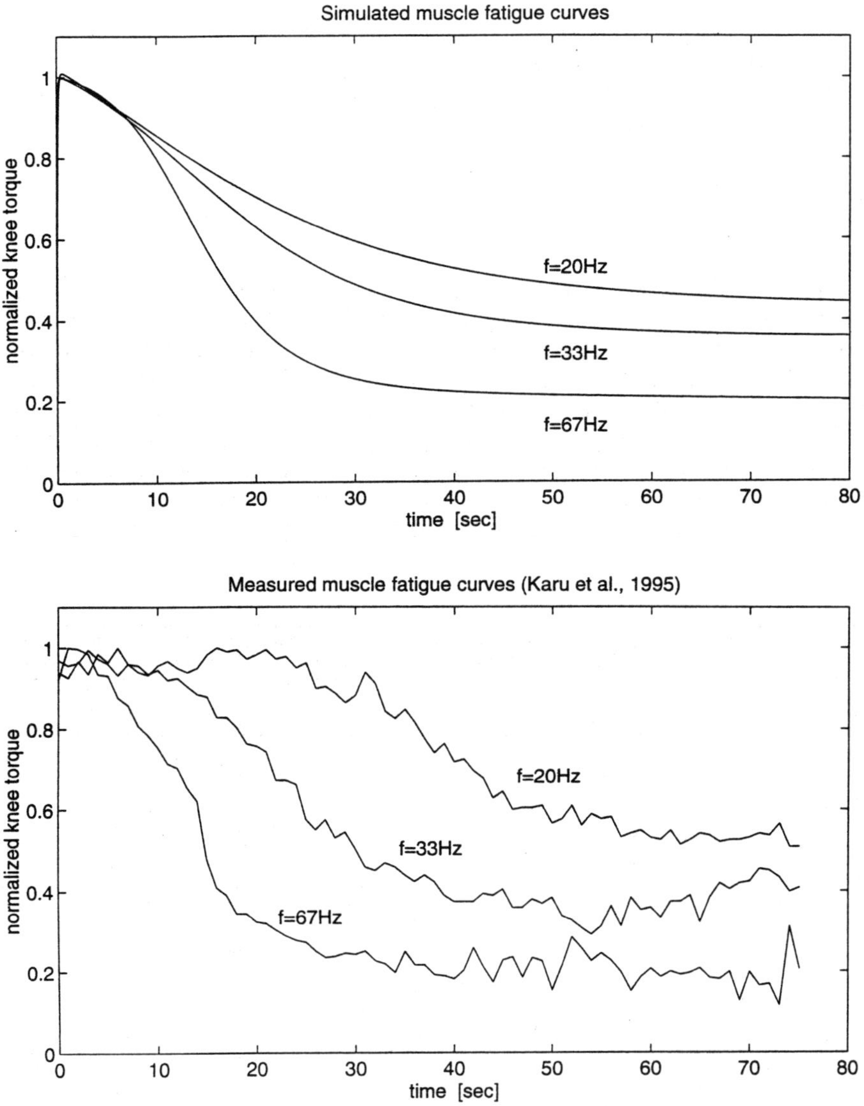

Fig. 10. Simulated and measured muscle fatigue characteristics for different pulse frequencies. In the experiments human quadriceps muscle was stimulated using surface electrodes (d=300μsec). Experimental data are shown with permission of Karu *et al.* (1995) (zzkaru@mit.edu). As soon as fast motor units, which have lower fatigue resistance than slow ones, are fatigued, a constant force plateau is reached (see also Edström and Kugelberg, 1968; Mortimer, 1981).

4 Discussion

The presented model accounts for major effects occurring during electrical neuromuscular stimulation under isometric conditions. The model was evaluated by comparing it with experimental data from the literature and our own measurements. There was good agreement between measured and simulated muscle force outputs.

4.1 Parameter Identification

Isometric force production was taken into consideration, where muscle length was assumed to be constant (tendon elasticity was neglected). Therefore, neither body-segmental dynamics nor velocity-dependent characteristics such as the force-velocity relation of muscle or viscous properties in muscle, tendon, and connective tissue were treated in this study. Also static relations that depend on muscle length (e.g., force-length relation of muscle) or joint angle (e.g., nonlinear moment arm) were not taken into consideration. Instead, a constant factor, which accounts for major static relations, has to be adjusted in the model so that the absolute joint torque produced by the model during stimulation of the muscle agrees with the measurements.

Physiological part of the model =>	motor endplate	sarcoplasmic reticulum	fatigue/ recovery	calcium binding	fibre gliding	relation of fast to slow	motor unit recruitment
Parameters =>	c_4 c_5 Hatze '77	c_1 c_2 Hatze '77	T_{fat} T_{rec} fit_{min}	ρ Hatze '78	T_g	n_f / n_s Johnson *et al.*'73	d_{thr} d_{sat} K_{thr} K_{sat}
single twitch shape (Fig. 5)	X X	X X	-	X	X	X	-
doublet effect (Fig. 5)	- X	X -	-	X	-	X	-
force-freq. char. (Figs. 6 and 7)	X X	X X	-	X	X	X	-
recruitment char. (Figs. 8 and 9)	- -	- -	-	-	-	X	X
fatigue curve shape (Fig. 10)	- -	- -	X	-	-	X	X
fatigue-frequency relation (Fig. 10)	X X	X X	X	-	-	X	-

Table 1. Important parameters and their main influences on different effects occurring during FES under isometric condition (existing dependence is marked by "X"). Parameters c_1, c_2, c_4, c_5, and ρ are explained in Hatze (1977, 1978). Fiber type percentages are taken from Johnson *et al.* (1973)

Note that in this study the model parameters were determined separately for each comparison shown in Figs. 5-10. One set of subject-specific parameters, valid for all comparisons shown in this section, could not be generated, because the measurements were performed on different subjects and insufficient experimental data were available for one subject. However, current investigation has shown that a single set of subject-specific parameters can be identified by a series of experiments where the muscle is stimulated by certain pulse patterns (singlets, doublets, linear increase of pulse width and frequency, fatigue test, etc.).

Table 1 gives an overview of important subject-specific model parameters and their influences on different effects occurring during FES. This table shows the force characteristics for identifying major subject-specific parameters used in the model.

4.2 Comparison with other Models

Unlike *black box approaches* (Donaldson *et al.*, 1995) our model is more complex. It has the disadvantage of requiring more parameters, which have to be estimated by experiments or taken from the literature. However, the greatest advantage of our *physiologically based model* is the insight it gives into the muscle's biomechanical and physiological connections, thus elucidating certain phenomena such as recruitment and fatigue. For example, with this approach we were able to show that the fatigue dependence of threshold and saturation in the recruitment characteristic of muscle can be described by the existence of motor units with different properties (Fig. 9).

Several other models describe muscle activation dynamics in more or less detail. Many investigators derived first- or second-order models to estimate muscle force induced by electrical stimulation (Khang and Zajac, 1989; Schutte *et al.*, 1993; Bobet *et al.*, 1993; Phillips et al., 1994). Hannaford (1990) developed a more complex phasic excitation-activation model of the process of motoneuron excitation and the resultant activation and force development of a motor unit. Model input is the amount of depolarizing current (e.g., when injected with an intracellular electrode), and the model output is muscle force. The model was evaluated by measured data.

However, none of the mentioned models can be used to design controllers where recruitment and pulse frequency are modulated simultaneously. Another model presented by Bernotas *et al.* (1986) also used two model elements simlilar to our model: a static nonlinear element, which describes the relationship between pulse width and steady state force, and a linear dynamic second-order element, which accounts for temporal summation of force. The model parameters were identified in cat soleus and plantaris muscles. The authors propose their model for the design of closed-loop strategies.

A more detailed model of muscle activation in humans with two control inputs (stimulation rate and motor unit recruitment) was presented by Hatze (1977 and 1978). His model is capable of accurately predicting many phenomena of natural muscular force-output. Parts of this model are used in ours.

No general model was found in the literature that accurately predicts major phenomena, which occur during artificial multi-input stimulation (e.g., simultaneous pulse width and frequency modulation), such as the doublet effect, force-frequency relation, recruitment and fatigue characteristic. Since muscle fatigue is an especially significant problem occurring during FES, it should not be neglected when designing control strategies.

4.3 Modeling Fatigue

Fatigue models in the literature describe how muscle force decreases during continuous stimulation without any change in the stimulation input (Giat *et al.*, 1993; Rabischong and Guiraud, 1993; Boom *et al.*, 1993). Our fatigue model involves a more general approach, which has the additional advantage that it can be applied to any shape of stimulation input.

As stated in the literature (Karu *et al.* 1995; Crago *et al.*, 1980 b) and also shown in the model, fatigue depends on the pulse frequency. High frequency stimulation leads to a faster decrease of force and to a lower force plateau than low frequency stimulation (Fig. 10). However, when pulse width d or pulse amplitude A increases, the shape of the normalized fatigue characteristic does not change significantly, in either measurements or simulation. This can be easily explained: the individual pulse pattern in a recruited motor unit does not change when increasing d or A; only the number of recruited units increases. The force plateau in the normalized fatigue curve will be even higher when stimulating with increased d or A values, because more fatigue-resistant slow motor units are recruited at higher pulse width or amplitudes (inverse size-order recruitment, see Gorman and Mortimer, 1983; Heyters et al., 1994). Of course, at higher recruitment levels the fitness of the entire muscle decreases, since more units are affected by fatigue.

As mentioned in the Methods section, the concentration of free calcium ions is reduced in our fatigue model, which is justified from a physiological point of view (Westerblad and Allen, 1991; for review see Fitts, 1994). This fatigue-induced decrease of calcium ions has many different causes (blockage of the T tubular action potential, reduced intramembranous T tubular charge movement, inhibition of the calcium release channel in the sarcoplasmic reticulum, depletion of releasable calcium ions from the sarcoplasmic reticulum, etc.). However, there are some further effects that lead to fatigue and thus to a decrease of muscle force, but are not reflected in the concentration of free calcium ions. Such effects are, for example, changes in the ATP supply for force generation by the myosin cross-bridges or anaerobic production of lactic acid from glycose and glycogen (Fitts, 1994). These effects were not taken directly into consideration, since the determined fatigue parameters (T_{fat}, T_{rec}, fit_{min}) approximate the overall, temporary behavior of muscle fatigue which occurs during the fatigue experiment.

Note that the current version of our activation dynamics model fails to predict the effects of high-frequency and low-frequency fatigue (also observed in experiments performed by others). Low-frequency fatigue is characterized by a loss of force at low stimulation frequencies despite recovery of the force generated at a high stimulation frequency (Edwards, 1981). High-frequency fatigue was demonstrated by Jones *et al.* (1979). They performed experiments on human adductor pollicis muscle under ischemic conditions, during which an 80 Hz stimulation was periodically interrupted by a 20 Hz burst. Initially, the 20 Hz interruption produced less force than the corresponding 80 Hz train, but after several seconds of stimulation, switching to the 20 Hz train produced an increase in force, thus indicating high-frequency fatigue.

4.4 Doublet Effect

Stein and Parmiggiani (1981) have suggested that an increase in muscle stiffness resulting from the first pulse can considerably facilitate transmission of force generated internally. This is in addition to any facilitation arising from calcium release mechanisms or nonlinearities in the calcium-troponin binding process, which cause the observed doublet effect (they call it nonlinear summation).

The fact that in our model the doublet response can be adjusted mainly by the parameters c_5 (calcium release in the sarcoplasmic reticulum) and ρ (calcium-troponin binding) supports our assumption that the doublet effect can be attributed to the calcium-release or calcium-troponin binding mechanisms, respectively (Table 1). However, other muscle properties that might also be responsible for this effect, have not been taken into consideration in this study (e.g., length-tension effects, increased muscle stiffness, or interaction between contractile elements and series elastic elements such as tendons).

In our own measurements we observed that the doublet effect occurred even at pulse widths where muscle force was saturated (i.e. when all motor units are recruited). We therefore excluded the possibility that the doublet effect is due to additional recruitment of (partially excited) motor units during the second pulse.

4.5 Use of the Model for the Design of Control Strategies

Our model can describe many relevant characteristics of artificially stimulated muscle under isometric conditions, such as the shape of single twitch responses and the doublet effect (Karu *et al.*, 1995; Kwende *et al.*, 1995; Jarvis *et al.*, 1996; Stein and Parmiggiani, 1981), the force-frequency relationship (Mortimer, 1981; Binder-Macleod and McDermond, 1992), the recruitment characteristic for fatigued and non-fatigued muscles (Crago *et al.*, 1980 a), and the behavior of muscle fatigue (Mortimer, 1981; Binder-Macleod and Barker, 1991; Rabischong and Ohanna, 1992; Karu *et al.*, 1995). The model also has the potential of predicting the qualitative muscle force response for an arbitrary train of pulses with varying input parameters (pulse width and pulse frequency).

Since the model satisfactorily accounts for relevant characteristics of artificially stimulated muscle, we conclude that it can be used to design optimal FES control strategies. For example, simultaneous recruitment and frequency modulation could contribute to better fatigue resistance and more effective force production. The strategy we propose would perform priority recruitment modulation and adjust the pulse frequency to the actual situation. In general, pulse frequency should be as low as possible - just above a certain value to ensure a fused tetanus - in order to reduce the effects of fatigue due to high-frequency stimulation (Fig. 10) (Karu *et al.*, 1995; Crago *et al.*, 1980 b). However, for fast movements (high accelerations), or as soon as external or internal disturbances occur (e.g., heel strike or spasticity) and increase the tracking error, the frequency could be increased for a short period of time (e.g., by adding single pulses into the stimulation pattern) in order to achieve faster force production and, hence, better control of motion. Another reason for following such a strategy is that both high-frequency and low-frequency fatigue (Jones *et al.*, 1979; Edwards, 1981) are reduced by keeping pulse frequency variable.

The muscle activation dynamics model presented here is relatively complex. The complexity will increase when the model is combined with nonlinear contraction and multibody dynamics in order to describe movements induced by stimulating several muscles of the lower extremities. The computational effort, especially of such an extended version, will be considerably high. However, such a complex model, which describes relevant effects in a realistic way, is initially required for a better understanding of neurophysiologic processes during FES and for the study of the effects of different FES control strategies. In the future, simpler models can be easily derived from this comprehensive model, e.g., for use in *model-based* FES control algorithms. A simplified model will also allow on-line adapting of certain model parameters during the control of FES-induced movements.

Currently we are developing specific off-line parameter identification procedures for automatic adjustment of the model to an individual. This will allow the user to adapt an effective feedback control strategy to each individual, so that the model can predict subject-specific control parameters. Thus, trail-and-error adjustments can be avoided or at least shortened and the number of experiments in humans reduced, both of which should accelerate the development of neural prostheses.

5 Acknowledgements

We are indebted to Z. Karu and S. Binder-Macleod for providing experimental data. Further, we thank S. Volz for his support during the measurements and J. Benson for copyediting the manuscript. The experimental part of this work was supported by the German Federal Department of Education and Research (BMBF, project number 01K094026).

References

Bernotas, L. A., Crago, P. E., and Chizeck, H. J. (1986) A discrete-time model of electrically stimulated muscle, *IEEE Trans. Biomed. Eng.*, **33**, 829-838.

Bobet, J. Stein, R. B., and Oguztöreli, M. N. (1993) A linear time-varying model of force generation in skeletal muscle, *IEEE Trans. Biomed. Eng.*, **40**, 1000-1006.

Binder-Macleod, S. A. and Barker, C. B. (1991) Use of a catchlike property of human skeletal muscle to reduce fatigue, *Muscle and Nerve* **14**, 850-857.

Binder-Macleod, S. A. and McDermond, L. R. (1992) Changes in the force-frequency relationship of the human quadriceps femoris muscle following electrically and voluntarily induced fatigue, *Physical Therapy* **72**, 14-23.

Boom, H. B. K., Mulder, A. J., and Veltink, P. H. (1993) Fatigue during functional neuromuscular stimulation, *Progress in Brain Research*, **97**, 409-418.

Chizeck, H. J., Lan, N., Palmieri, S. P., and Crago, P. E. (1991) Feedback control of electrically stimulated muscle using simultaneous pulse width and stimulus period modulation, *IEEE Trans. Biomed. Eng.* **38**, 1224-1234.

Crago, P. E., Peckham, P. H., and Thrope, G. B. (1980 a) Modulation of muscle force by recruitment during intramuscular stimulation, *IEEE Trans. Biomed. Eng.*, **27**(12), 679-684.

Crago, P. E., Mortimer, J. T., and Peckham, P. H. (1980 b) Closed-loop control of force during electrical stimulation of muscle, *IEEE Trans. Biomed. Eng.*, **27**, 306-312.

Donaldson, N. N., Gollee, H., Hunt, K. J., Jarvis, J. C., and Kwende, M. K. N. (1995) A radial basis function model of muscle stimulated with irregular interpulse intervals. *Med. Eng. Phys.* **17**, 431-441.

Edström, L. and Kugelberg, E. (1968) Histochemical composition, distribution of fibers and fatiguability of single motor units. *J. Neurol. Neurosurg. Psychiatry* **31**, 424-433.

Edwards, R. H. T. (1981) Human muscle function and fatigue. In: R. Porter and J. Whelan (eds), Human Muscle Fatigue: Physiological Mechanisms, 1-18. Pitman Medical, London.

Fitts, R. H. (1994) Cellular Mechanisms of muscle fatigue. *Physiological Reviews* **74**, 49-94.

Giat, Y., Mizrahi, J., and Levy, M. (1993) A musculotendon model of the fatigue profiles of paralyzed quadriceps muscle under FES, *IEEE Trans. Biomed. Eng.*, **40**, 664-673.

Gorman, P. H. and Mortimer, T. (1983) The effect of stimulus parameters on the recruitment characteristic of direct nerve stimulation. *IEEE Trans. Biomed. Eng.* **30**, 407-414.

Hannaford, B., (1990) A nonlinear model of the phasic dynamics of muscle activation, *IEEE Trans. Biomed. Eng.*, **37**, 1067-1075.

Hatze, H. (1977) A myocybernetic control model of skeletal muscle, *Biol. Cybern.* **25**, 103-119.

Hatze, H. (1978) A general myocybernetic control model of skeletal muscle, *Biol. Cybern.* **28**, 143-157.

Heyters, M., Carpentier, A., Duchateau, J., and Hainaut, K. (1994) Twitch analysis as an approach to motor unit activation during electrical stimulation. *Can. J. Appl. Physiol.*, **19**, 451-461.

Jarvis, J. C., Gollee, H., Kwende, M. M. N., Salmons, S, and Murray-Smith, D. J. (1996) Towards an optimized muscle controller (*this volume*).

Johnson, M. A., Polgar, J., Weightman, D., and Appleton, D. (1973) Data on the distribution of fibre types in thirty-six human muscles: an autopsy study, *J. Neurological Sciences*, **18**, 111-129.

Jones, D. A., Bigland-Ritchie, B., and Edwards, R. H. T. (1979) Excitation frequency and muscle fatigue: Mechanical responses during human voluntary and stimulated contractions. *Experimental Neurology*, **64**, 401-413.

Karu, Z. Z. (1992) Optimization of force and fatigue properties of electrically stimulated human skeletal muscle. *Master thesis*, MIT, May 1992.

Karu, Z. Z., Durfee, W. K., and Barzilai, A. M. (1995) Reducing muscle fatigue in FES applications by stimulating with N-let pulse trains. *IEEE Trans. Biomed. Eng.* **42**, 809-817.

Khang, G. and Zajac, F. E. (1989) Paraplegic standing controlled by functional neuromuscular stimulation: part I. - computer model and control-system design, *IEEE Trans. Biomed. Eng.*, **36**, 873-884.

Kwende, M. M. N., Jarvis, J. C., and Salmons, S. (1995) The input-output relations of skeletal muscle. *Proc. R. Soc.Lond.*, **261**, 193-201.

Mihelin, M., Trontel, J. V., and Stalberg, E. (1991) Muscle fiber recovery functions studied with double pulse stimulation. *Muscle Nerve* **14**, 739-747.

Mortimer, J. T. (1981) Motor prostheses. In: V.B. Brooks (ed), *Handbook of Physiology, Nervous System II*. Bethesda, MD: American Physiological Society, **2**, 155-187.

Phillips, G. F., Donaldson, N., deN., and Barr, F. M. D. (1994) Artificial control of balance by electrical stimulation of the plantarflexors for unsupported standing in paraplegia. In: Control of Ambulation using FNS, P. H. Veltink and H. B. K. Boom (eds.), RAFT Workshop, Enschede, December, 1994.

Rabischong, E. and Ohanna F. (1992) Effects of Functional Electrical Stimulation (FES) on evoked muscular output in paraplegic quadriceps muscle, *Paraplegia* **30**, 467-473.

Rabischong, E. and Guiraud, D. (1993) Determination of the fatigue in the electrically stimulated quadriceps muscle and relative effect of ischaemia, *J. Biomed. Eng.*, **15**, 443- 450.

Reid, M. B., Grubwieser, G. J., Stokic, D. S., Koch, S. M., and Leis, A. A. (1993) Development and reversal of fatigue in human of tibialis anterior, *Muscle and Nerve* **16**, 1239-1245.

Riener, R., Villars, S., Quintern, J., and Schmidt, G. (1996 a) Biomechanical simulation and animation of the lower extremity for the design of neural prostheses (*this volume*).

Riener, R., Quintern, J., Schmidt, G. (1996 b) Biomechanical model of the human knee evaluated by neuromuscular stimulation, *Journal of Biomechanics*, in press.

Schutte, L. M., Rodgers, M. M., Zajac, F. E., and Glaser, R. M. (1993) Improving the efficacy of electrical stimulation-induced leg cycle ergometry: an analysis based on a dynamic musculoskeletal model. *IEEE Trans. Rehab. Eng.*, **1**, 109-125.

Stein, R. B. and Parmiggiani, F. (1981) Nonlinear summation of contractions in cat muscles. I and II. *J. Gen. Physiol.* **78**, 277-311.

Westerblad, H. and Allen D. G. (1991) Changes of myoplasmic calcium concentration during fatigue in single mouse muscle fibers. *J. Gen. Physiol.* **98**, 615-635.

Novel Stimulation Strategies for the Recruitment of Paralysed Muscle

D. J. Maxwell[1], M. H. Granat[1], R. H. Baxendale[2]
[1]Bioengineering Unit, University of Strathclyde, Glasgow, Scotland
[2]Institute of Physiology, University of Glasgow, Scotland

Abstract - Three alternative strategies are described which employ non-uniform stimulation patterns to maximise the output of isometrically contracting muscle. As muscle fatigue seems to be a function of the number of pulses delivered any strategy which will allow a greater muscular output for the same number of stimulus pulses should be useful in Functional Electrical Stimulation (FES) systems. When a single extra pulse was inserted at the beginning of the stimulus train the enhancement produced was most pronounced at sub-tetanic stimulation frequencies. By the repeated insertion of short inter pulse intervals it was possible to greatly increase the muscle output for the same average number of pulses. A third strategy attempted to define an optimum series of IPIs to maximise the force time integral produced per stimulus pulse. This strategy confirmed that muscle output could be increased by using a non-uniform stimulation pattern containing some short intervals. While this approach has obvious potential for FES systems it is still not clear how the optimum IPIs for a particular muscle can be elucidated.

1 Introduction

Functional Electrical Stimulation (FES) systems employ a subject's paralysed muscles to produce useful forces or movements. The force generated by the stimulated muscle will vary with the intensity of stimulation. The stimulation takes the form of discrete pulses applied to the motor-nerve of the muscle. The intensity of stimulation may be modulated in two ways. By increasing the magnitude of each individual pulse a spatial summation of force will be produced as an increasing number of axons, and consequently motor units, are recruited. Secondly, by increasing the frequency of application of the stimulus pulses a temporal summation of force will occur within each recruited motor-unit. The mechanism underlying the spatial summation of force is easily understood. However the mechanism underlying the temporal summation of force within the motor unit and its relationship to stimulation frequency is more complex.

Practical demonstrations of FES systems have typically used constant frequencies of stimulation. The choice of stimulation frequency is constrained by the need to achieve a smooth tetanic contraction of the muscle with minimum fatigue. As muscle fatigue increases with stimulation frequency the lowest frequency which gives a smooth force output is normally chosen. Although higher frequencies of stimulation would result in greater force output the muscle would also fatigue much more rapidly. Ideally, FES applications require a sustained (low fatigue) and high force output for functional purposes. It has been demonstrated that, in some situations, by inserting a few closely spaced stimulus pulses at the beginning of the stimulus train the benefits of higher frequencies of stimulation (rapid, high force development) can be achieved without the fatigue associated with high frequencies of stimulation (Burke *et al.*, 1970; Andrews *et al.*, 1990). This rationale is further supported by the observation that each stimulus pulse is associated with energy expenditure at both the neuro-muscular junction and in calcium cycling within the muscle. Hence any strategy which reduces the number of stimuli delivered for a given functional output is attractive. However it has been the view that the benefits to be gained from employing non-constant stimulation frequencies have not been shown to be sufficient to outweigh the practical difficulties of implementation, not least of which is the choice of what actual pattern of stimulation to use.

In order to evaluate these strategies we must have a method of quantifying the functional output of the muscle. In a static (isometric) contraction no work is done although the force generated by the muscle may be high. In FES systems isometric contractions can be functionally useful for example in the maintenance of standing. However the maximum force produced is a poor indicator of functional output as sustained force production is often a more important requirement. The work done by a muscle is the product of force and distance. However as there is no work done during an isometric contraction, the product of force and time can be used to quantify the muscle output. This measure is obtained by evaluating the area under the force time graph (Force Time Integral, FTI).

This study presents some strategies we have evaluated for improving the FTI produced by a fixed number of stimulus pulses.

2 Method

Three successive strategies were experimentally evaluated in terms of the FTI produced per stimulus pulse (Figure 1). Three different kinds of muscle (normal human, paralysed human, and rabbit) were used to evaluate the strategies. The long term aim is to identify stimulation strategies which will be useful for paralysed muscle. The other kinds of muscle were used to establish the existence of the phenomena.

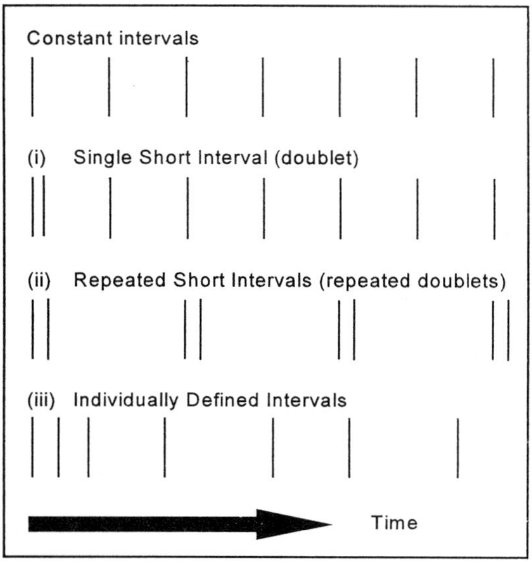

Fig. 1. Illustration of the three different stimulation strategies evaluated in the study

The stimulation strategies were controlled by computer (IBM PC) and this was also used for data acquisition and processing. For each of the different kinds of muscle the computer was used to control an appropriate stimulation device and sample the force record. In the case of the human subjects the knee moment produced by stimulating the quadriceps muscle group was recorded. The Strathclyde Research Stimulator (Bioengineering Unit, University of Strathclyde) was used to deliver the stimulation while the subject was restrained in a dynamometer chair. Animal experiments were performed on deeply anaesthetized rabbits. The force produced by isometrically contracting rabbit tibialis anterior was recorded and a proprietary stimulator (Neurolog,Digitimer Ltd, England) delivered the stimulation directly onto the common peroneal nerve. In each case muscle length was set in the central portion of the muscle's length-tension curve.

(i) Insertion of Single Short Interval.

The first strategy employed a single short inter pulse interval (doublet) at the beginning of a constant frequency stimulus train. One extra pulse was inserted 10ms after the first pulse of the stimulus train. Each doublet test was paired with a control test with no initial doublet. The frequency of the stimulus train was varied between tests.

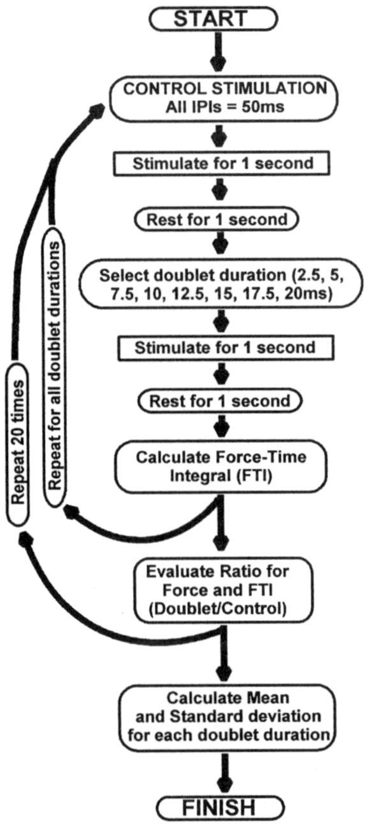

Fig. 2. A flow chart describing the stimulation protocol for strategy (ii).

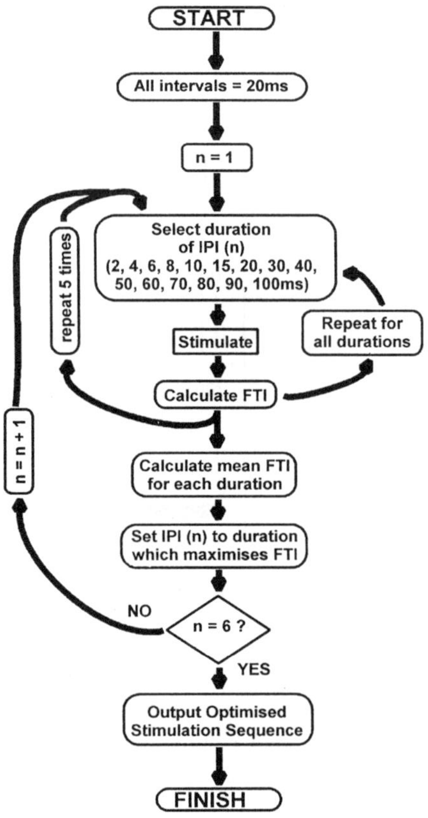

Fig. 3. A flow chart describing the stimulation protocol for strategy (iii).

(ii) Repetitive Insertion of Short Intervals.

The second strategy employed repetitive short inter pulse intervals (IPIs) separated by a longer IPI (Figures 1 and 2). In each test the same number of pulses (20) were delivered in the same time (1 second). Hence there were 10 doublets delivered in each test and for each doublet test there was a control test consisting of 20 equally spaced stimulus pulses (20Hz).

(iii) Serial Optimisation of Stimulation Intervals.

The third strategy used an iterative technique to define an optimum stimulus pattern (Figures 1 and 3). Initially a train of seven pulses were applied with all 6 IPIs of the same duration. In a sequential manner, starting with the first IPI, each IPI was varied to determine the IPI at which it would give the maximum enhancement of the FTI. When this duration had been determined the IPI became fixed at this optimum value and the next IPI would be varied with the remaining

IPIs retaining their initial duration. In this manner all six IPIs were optimised for maximum FTI.

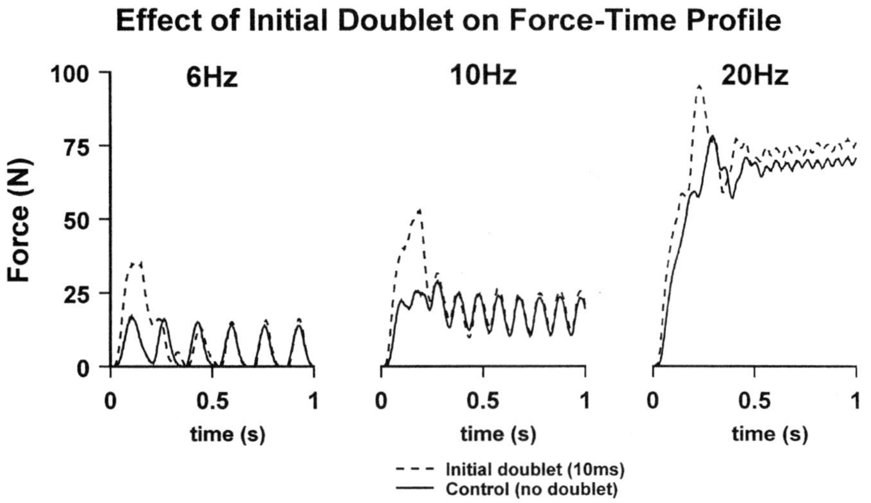

Fig. 4. Isometric contraction in quadriceps of a complete lesion (C7) SCI subject. Effect of insertion of a single extra pulse (10ms after first stimulus pulse) on force record.

3 Results and Discussion

(i) Insertion of Single Short Interval.

The effect of an initial doublet is illustrated in Figure 4. It can be seen that the insertion of a pulse doublet results in enhanced force development. The force enhancement is prolonged despite the return to longer IPIs. The magnitude of the force enhancement achieved depends on the length of the following IPIs. The observation that, even with 20Hz stimulation, the potentiating effect of the extra pulse carried over a number of subsequent longer intervals prompted the question of what would happen if extra pulses were added repeatedly. This was the rationale for the second stimulation strategy.

(ii) Repetitive Insertion of Short Intervals

The Maximum Force and the FTI generated by the test stimulation in 1 second was compared on each occasion with the output from the control stimulation (the same number of pulses equally spaced) and the ratio calculated. The results of this series of tests are given in Figure 5. The results illustrated are for normal human quadriceps. A ratio of one represents no improvement over the control stimulation. We have previously demonstrated that the inclusion of a single doublet will greatly enhance maximum force. For this pattern of stimulation a large increase in FTI was also found. This indicated that the higher force level was being maintained for the period of the contraction. The results shown seem to indicate an optimum duration of 5ms for the doublet. This result is similar to that recently reported by Karu and Durfee (1993) where they too found an optimum of 5ms for normal quadriceps. To investigate this further the third stimulation strategy was devised. This strategy aims to define each interval in a short stimulus train.

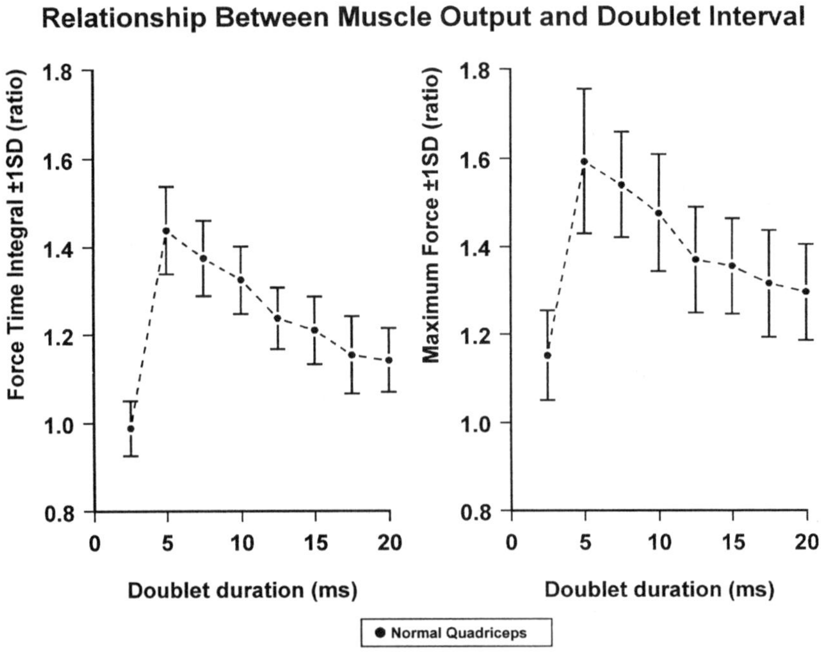

Fig. 5. Means and Standard deviations (n=20) are shown for all IPI durations. The results are for a non-motor impaired male subject.

(iii) Serial Optimisation of Stimulation Pattern

Results are presented in Figure 6 for all three muscle types (paralysed quadriceps, normal quadriceps and rabbit tibialis anterior) demonstrating the effect on the FTI produced by optimising the stimulus train for maximum FTI. The results are expressed as ratios of the constant-frequency control stimulation. The points are joined to show the trend for each muscle. The value on the abscissa indicates the number of IPIs which have been optimised. For example, the FTI for interval three is the resulting output after the first three IPIs have been optimised. The remaining three IPIs in the stimulus train retain their initial value.

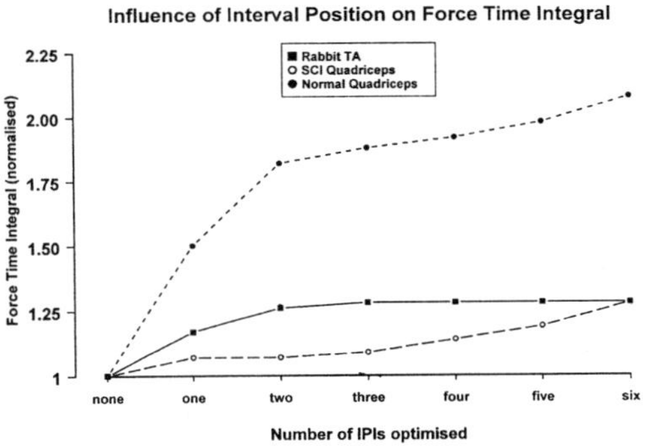

Fig. 6. The influence of each successive IPI on muscle output (FTI). Each data point represents the maximum achieved by successively optimising each interval. The output has been normalised to that produced by a constant frequency train.

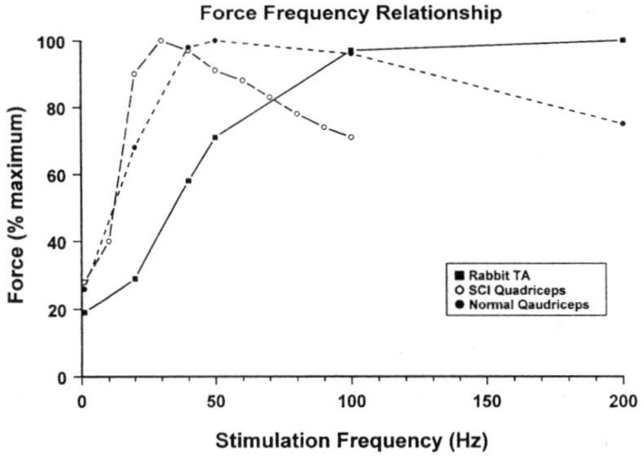

Fig. 7. Force Frequency Relationship for the three different muscles.

Force-frequency curves are given for the three muscles in Figure 7. The stimulation strategy requires the six IPIs to be of equal duration initially and this initial value was taken to be representative of the constant stimulation frequency employed in FES systems. In the human muscle this is normally of the order of 20Hz (equivalent to 50ms between pulses). The rabbit TA is much the fastest of the three muscles. The force frequency curve indicates that it has a fast twitch time and summation of twitches into a useful tetanic contraction does not occur at the frequencies used for human quadriceps. The IPIs had to be reduced to 20ms (equivalent to 50Hz) for the rabbit TA to achieve a similar type of fused contraction. This may be a factor in why the rabbit muscle only achieves a 25% increase in FTI compared to the 100% increase realised by the normal quadriceps. The force frequency curve for the quadriceps muscle of the spinal cord injured subject shows a marked decline in force at short IPIs (high stimulation frequencies). This is surprising as it is commonly assumed that the fibre-type of paralysed muscle will have reverted to a fast type-II due to the absence of any chronic neural discharge to the muscle. This lower response to higher frequencies of stimulation may explain the difference in behaviour of the SCI quadriceps to the optimisation procedure. The force-frequency graph (Figure 7) shows the SCI quadriceps already producing 90% of its maximum force at 20Hz stimulation the normal quadriceps and rabbit TA only produce about 70% of their maximum at the constant frequency from which the optimisation was started (20Hz and 50Hz respectively).

The optimised pulse train gives an enhanced FTI over that achieved with a constant frequency of stimulation. The optimised pulse train tends to have short IPIs at the beginning of the train although the actual duration determined for individual IPIs is variable.

It appears from the results that the paralysed muscle is the least susceptible of the three muscles to this approach.

4 Conclusions

It is clear that there is a potential benefit from employing a non-uniform stimulation pattern. It is not however clear what form this pattern should take, other than that it should contain some short IPIs. Some investigators have attempted to use stimulation patterns employed successfully on one subject on other subjects with mixed results (Binder-Maclead and Barker, 1991). It may be that each muscle has its own optimum pattern and, given that the force frequency response of a muscle is related to its fibre-type composition, the fibre-type may have a major influence. This would also suggest that as the muscle fatigues the optimum stimulation pattern will change.

References

Burke, R. E., Rudomin, P., and Zajac, F. E. (1970) Catch property in single mammalian motor units. Science 168: 122-125

Andrews, B. J., Granat, M. H., and Kirkwood, C. A. (1990) Observation of the catch property in human quadriceps muscle. Journal of Physiology 429 P

Karu, Z. Z. and Durfee, W. K. (1993) Using pulse doublets to enhance muscle force for FES. Proceedings of 14th Annual International Conference of IEEE Engineering, Medicine and Biology Society. Paris Oct 19 - Nov 1, pp 1356-1357.

Binder-Macleod, S. A. and Barker, C. B. (1991) Use of a catchlike property of human muscle to reduce fatigue. Muscle and Nerve 14: 850-857.

Towards an Optimized Muscle Controller

J. C. Jarvis[1], H. Gollee[2], M. M. N. Kwende[1], S. Salmons[1], D.J. Murray-Smith[2]
[1]Dept. of Human Anatomy and Cell Biology, The University of Liverpool, UK
[2]Dept. of Electronics and Electrical Engineering, The University of Glasgow, UK

Abstract - The use of skeletal muscle ventricles to assist the failing heart is a potential solution to the problems associated with cardiac transplantation - donor shortage, tissue rejection and its suppression, and high cost. In this new approach, circulatory assistance would be provided by an auxiliary pump (skeletal muscle ventricle or SMV) formed from the patient's own back muscle and activated by an implanted controller. We do not yet have sufficient understanding of the function of SMVs to use them safely and effectively in humans, but the feasibility of the technique has been established - SMVs have worked for up to two years in dogs.

Skeletal muscle itself is a highly complex linear motor. Its passive mechanical properties, the relationship between its neural input and its mechanical output, and the dependence of its mechanical output on its loading conditions, are all non-linear. Together with the geometrical complexities of thick-walled pumping chambers, these factors preclude analytical modelling of SMVs from first principles. A new approach is needed to link these many interacting factors together. Developments in systems engineering and computer science in terms of local linear network models (LLNMs), and new methods of controller design based on LLMNs, have considerable potential for this application. LLMN methods have evolved recently from the more general field of artificial neural networks.The ultimate goal of this project is to generate controllers for SMVs based on LLMNs. Such controllers would elicit pumping work from the assist device, with due regard to the history of activation of the muscle, and with the fewest possible neural impulses. The latter condition must be met in order to maintain the balance between the desirable increase in endurance and the undesirable reduction in speed and power that are both consequences of activation of skeletal muscle in the long-term.

1 Introduction

Many force controllers designed for use in FES operate as graded recruitment controllers in which the amount of muscle tissue recruited (and therefore the force) is adjusted by amplitude or pulse-width modulation of constant-frequency trains of pulses. Such muscle controllers treat the muscle fibres as either on or off.

In fact, muscle fibres have a highly non-linear activation characteristic, that has been gradually characterized over the past 20 years. Although the intracellular mechanisms underlying these non-linearities are not yet fully understood, we wished to embark on the development of a controller that would take these non-linearities into account. Observation of natural motor unit firing patterns shows that in eliciting a tetanic contraction, motoneurones often produce a few initial action potentials at a high frequency, with subsequent spikes at a lower frequency. We have now shown (Kwende, Jarvis and Salmons, 1995) that such patterns are in fact optimized in the sense that they elicit more mechanical output per action potential than any constant frequency, and may therefore be associated with a lower rate of fatigue, although the latter point still awaits direct experimental verification.

2 Methods

We have recently reported the results of experiments to characterize the activation characteristics of whole fast and slow rabbit muscles (Kwende, Jarvis and Salmons, 1995) The slow muscles were fast muscles whose properties had been transformed by long-term continuous electrical stimulation. We confirmed the presence of the doublet effect in fast muscle; this term refers to a more than linear summation of force-time integral (FTI) from two closely-spaced pulses and is best presented in a diagram in which FTI per pulse (FTIpP) is plotted against inter-pulse interval (Figure 1).

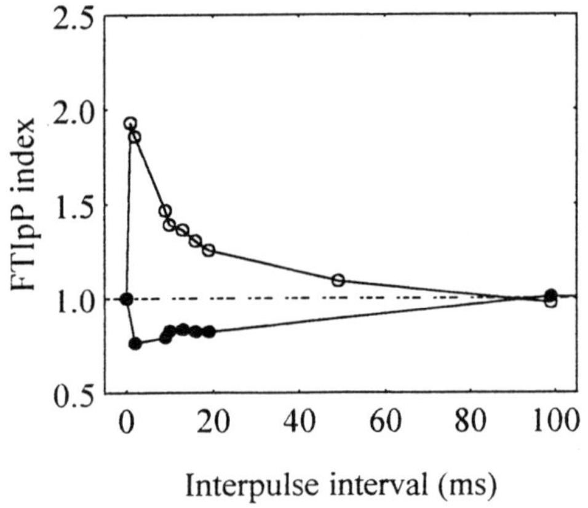

Fig. 1. Force-time integral per pulse versus inter-pulse interval

The value of the FTI resulting from a single pulse is taken as unity. Then any value of FTI produced by two pulses that is greater than 2 (equivalent to an FTIpP greater than 1) is evidence for the presence of the doublet effect, as seen in the curve for fast muscle (open circles). Figure 1 also shows, however, that muscle that had received chronic electrical stimulation at 10Hz for a number of weeks (filled circles) did not show the doublet effect. Indeed, there was a less than linear summation of FTI when two pulses were delivered at a short inter-pulse interval (see footnote[1]) We have developed a series of models to try to describe this behavior. The models were developed and refined using part of the data set that was collected for the description of the input/output characteristics of skeletal muscle described in Kwende, Jarvis and Salmons (1995). The rest of the data was used as test data for the model. The data set consisted of isometric force records elicited by random trains of supramaximal pulses with the following constraints: interpulse intervals were integer values between 1 and 100 ms, and the total length of the train was limited to 600 ms. The set of random patterns was delivered to rabbit tibialis anterior muscles either in the natural, fast, state, or after several weeks of continuous stimulation that rendered the muscle slow.

3 Results

It was found not to be possible to obtain a satisfactory characterization of the muscles with a single linear model (Donaldson *et al.* 1995). But a better fit with the experimental data was obtained by generating a radial basis function model (described in the same paper). This model was the first, to our knowledge, that incorporated the non-linearity of muscle activation, but it was not sufficiently robust. Although it gave close predictions of the force output produced by random patterns similar to those used in the training set, it did not predict well the force response to a sustained constant frequency. We have had more success with a type of model known as a local linear model network (Gollee et al. 1994). With this type of model, the behavior of the muscle is described by a series of functions (in this specific case, linear ARX models) whose validity, or contribution to the model output, depends on the operating region defined by a scheduling variable. A useful illustration would be the description of the relationship between the movements of the control surfaces of an aircraft and the effect on the orientation of the aircraft itself. The relationship would certainly depend on the speed of the aircraft, which would be used as the scheduling variable, but within a certain speed range, the relationship might be described by a relatively simple model. The models were created progressively from an initial stock series of validity

[1]As an aside, this result appears to argue against the use of optimized stimulation patterns for applications such as cardiac assistance in which chronic repetitive stimulation is unavoidable. If the doublet effect is lost after chronic stimulation, there would surely be no benefit in using optimized stimulation patterns? In fact, our preliminary results suggest strongly that the doublet effect can, in fact, be preserved with chronic optimized stimulation.

functions that could be refined by unifying adjacent models if they were similar. The great appeal of such a model structure is that the local models can be very simple (in this case linear), and so the computational overhead is much smaller than for a typical neural network. Furthermore, the characteristics of the real system are reflected in the set of local models. Local linear model networks therefore have great potential as the basis for controllers that could be implemented in implantable devices. We are presently working on methods of developing such models so that we could use them in the "reverse" direction to calculate the optimal stimulus pattern that would generate a particular force trajectory.

Models have now been made for both fast and slow muscle. The models were tested by performing on the models the same experiments as were performed on actual muscle in Kwende, Jarvis and Salmons (1995). The fidelity of the models is striking; the models give a close fit to actual data not only for the random patterns of stimulation but also for fixed frequency bursts. When a series of random patterns was delivered to the fast and slow models and ranked in terms of FTI per pulse, the models selected the best and worst patterns for fast and slow muscles just as reported for the real muscles (Kwende, Jarvis and Salmons 1995) The output generated by the models for a series of fixed frequencies appears entirely authentic (Figures 2 and 3). The lower fusion frequency and the "negative doublet effect" of the slow muscle were reproduced in the behavior of the model. We have also begun to investigate the possibility of adding further dimensions to the model structure. Muscles do not, of course, develop only force. We wish to extend the models to the description of dynamic contractions. If the model structures can be validated for this case, then an extension to the description of skeletal muscle ventricle function in terms of activation pattern, pressure and flow would seem feasible.

4 Conclusion

We have shown that local linear model networks can describe the force response of rested muscle, accommodating the non-linearity of muscle activation. This opens the way for further development of the models, with the aim of predicting the work output of shortening contractions and taking account of slow changes in muscle properties such as potentiation and fatigue.

Since models of non-linear systems can be made by concatenating locally-valid linear models the computational overhead is much lower than that for other types of neural network. Inverse LLMNs therefore have the potential for implementation as implantable skeletal muscle controllers.

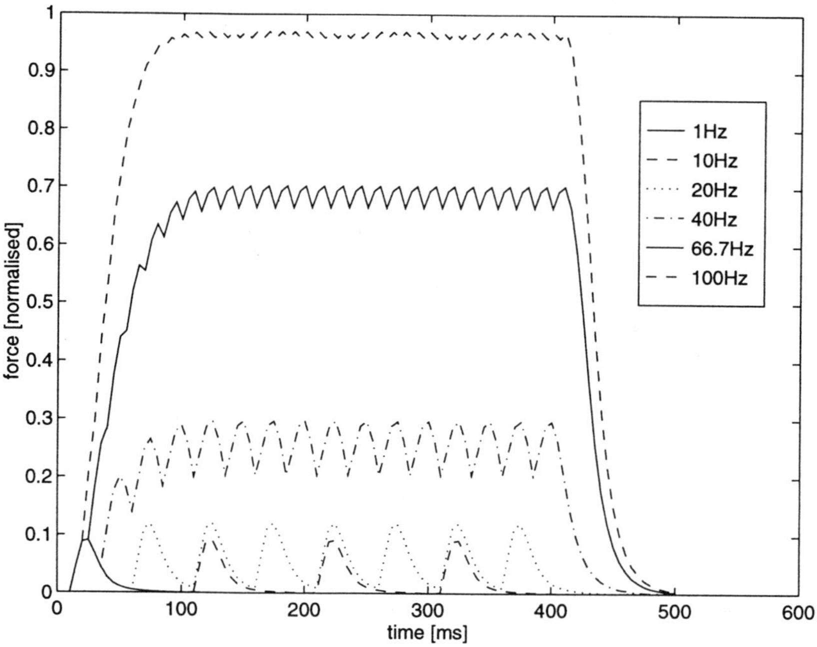

Fig. 2. Constant frequency inputs, fast muscle

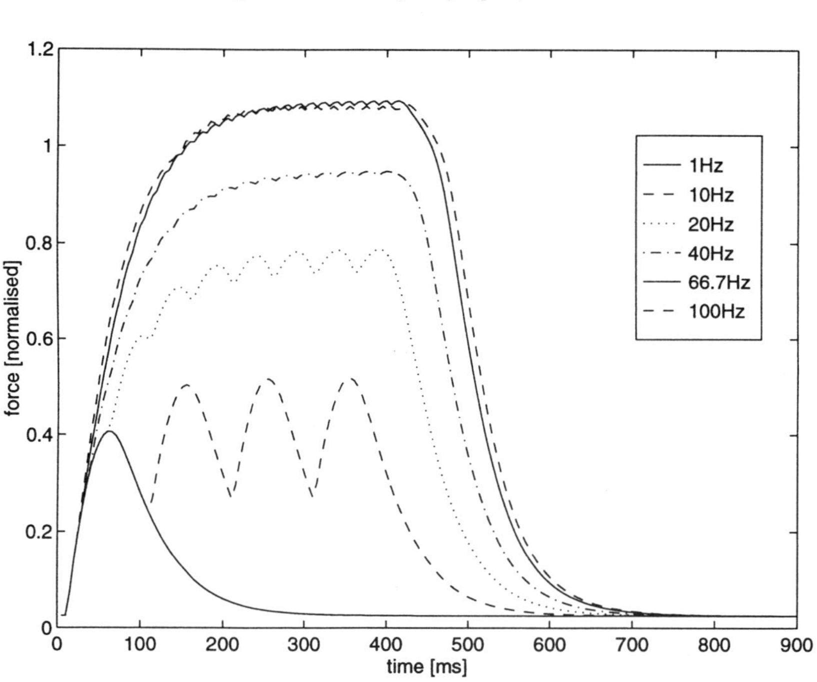

Fig. 3. Constant frequency inputs, slow muscle

References

Donaldson, N. de N., Gollee, H., Hunt, K. J., Jarvis, J. C., and Kwende, M. M. N. (1995) A radial basis function model of muscle stimulated with irregular inter-pulse intervals. *Journal Medical Engineering and Physics* 17: 431-441

Gollee, H., Hunt, K. J., Donaldson, N. de N., Jarvis, J. C., and Kwende, M. M. N. (1994) A mathematical analogue of electrically stimulated muscle using local model networks. *Proceedings of IEEE Conference on Decision and Control*, December 1994, Orlando, Florida, 1879-1880.

Kwende, M. M. N., Jarvis, J. C., and Salmons, S. (1995) The input-output relations of skeletal muscle. *Proceedings of the Royal Society London,* Series B 261: 193-201

The Function of Neuromuscular Junction in Upper Motor Neuron Weakness

J. V. Trontelj, J. M. Fernandez, M. Mihelin, D. Rugelj
University Institute of Clinical Neurophysiology,
University Medical Centre, Ljubljana, Slovenia

Abstract - Hemiplegic muscles often show abnormally fast fatigue when stimulated through their nerves. Single fibre EMG with axonal microstimulation was used to examine the possible contribution of neuromuscular transmission impairment. The study was performed in normal and paralysed limbs of 24 hemiparetic patients with a recent ischemic stroke. The mean jitter values were mildly but definitely abnormal on the affected side in 18 patients, suggesting some degree of transsynaptic lower motor neuron dysfunction during early stages of upper motor neuron paralysis. This degree of impairment, however, does not seem to play any significant role in the abnormal fatigue of muscles affected with upper motor neurone weakness.

1 Introduction

Muscles paralysed due to corticospinal tract lesions are often abnormally fatigable when stimulated with repetitive supramaximal electrical stimuli. This may be due to a number of different mechanisms, including unreliable nerve depolarization and conduction, impaired neuromuscular transmission, abnormal depolarization-contraction coupling, as well as altered biomechanics of muscle contraction. The weakness is commonly associated with some degree of muscle atrophy, as well as signs suggestive of partial denervation, such as low amplitude compound muscle action potentials (CMAPs) (McComas et al. 1973), reduced number of functioning motor units, fibrillation potentials and positive sharp waves (Cruz Martinez 1983, Brown et al. 1990). Some studies reported decremental response to repetitive nerve stimulation (McComas et al. 1973, Cruz Martinez 1983), possibly suggesting impaired neuromuscular transmission (NMT). This possibility was examined more in detail in the present study, using axonal microstimulation with SFEMG (Trontelj, Stålberg 1992, Stålberg et al 1992), a highly sensitive technique, capable of detecting even subtle changes in the motor units. Part of the study has been published before (Trontelj et al. 1995).

2 Methods and Patients

2.1 Methods

Axonal microstimulation was performed in the extensor digitorum communis muscle and the responses were recorded by a single fibre EMG electrode. The method has been described in detail elsewhere (Trontelj and Stålberg 1992) and will only briefly be summarised here. It is based on rather selective stimulation with a pair of thin needle electrodes (Medelec MF37) insulated to a few mm from the tip. They were inserted into the muscle near the motor point and a position was found from which it was possible to elicit fine twitches in a small portion of the muscle while using relatively weak stimuli of 0.05 ms duration and 1-30 Volts amplitude. A single fiber EMG electrode was then inserted into the twitching part of the muscle and manipulated so as to record from a single or a few responding muscle fibers with well defined and properly separated action potentials. Stimulus intensity was carefully adjusted to be well above the threshold for the responding motor axon. Jitter was measured at 10 Hz using the technique and the precautions to avoid errors, particularly directly stimulated muscle fibers, were observed, as described in detail previously (Trontelj et al. 1992). At least 20-40 neuromuscular junctions were assessed on each of the two sides, each during one or several series of 50-100 stimuli. The recording and analysis were performed on a Medelec MS6 and Mystro electromyographs, (in case of MS6, connected to a home-made jittermeter - Mihelin et al., 1975).

2.2 Patients

Altogether 24 patients with hemiplegia were included in the study , 17 males and 7 females, aged 25 to 83 years (median 64 years). They were examined 7 to 150 days (median 26 days) after an ischemic stroke in the irrigation area of the middle cerebral artery, resulting in a typical clinical picture including predominantly upper limb weakness. The nature and localisation of the lesion were confirmed by a CT scan. None of the patients had suffered any major manifestation of a cerebrovascular disease before. At the time of the study, all were alert and able to understand and cooperate. None had any evidence of a peripheral nerve or muscle disorder. Patients with diabetes, history of alcohol abuse or any other possible cause of focal or systemic neuropathy were carefully excluded. Motor and sensory conduction velocities were normal; however needle EMG of the affected limb muscles showed fibrillation potentials, consistent with previous studies.

Nineteen patients had no voluntary movement in the EDC muscle on the affected side, 3 had a rating of 1, and the remaining 2 patients had -3 and 3, respectively, on the MRC scale. The study was approved by the National Medical Ethics Committee, and all of the patients gave an informed consent.

3 Results

A summary of the results is shown in Figs. 1 and 2. In 18 patients, the median jitter (MCD) value on the diseased side was greater than that on the normal; in the remaining 6 it was either equal or slightly lower (by up to 4 μs, Fig.1). Of the 18 patients, 4 had their median MCD on the paretic side within the limits of normal (< 25μs), however still significantly higher than on the normal side. Some of the neuromuscular junctions (NMJs) with MCD values above 60-70 μs (only recorded on the paretic side) also showed intermittent blocking.

When the mean jitter values of the two sides *in individual patients* are compared, the difference is quite significant ($p = 0.001$). When comparison is made between the normal and the paretic side *for the pooled data* from all patients, there is a difference significant at $p < 0.0001$ (Fig. 2). However after exclusion of all abnormal individual values (MCD > 40 μs), so called outliers (Stålberg et al. 1994), the difference between the pooled data for each side was only slight (although still statistically significant, $p = 0.013$), suggesting that a large majority of the NMJs in the paretic muscles remained practically unaffected.

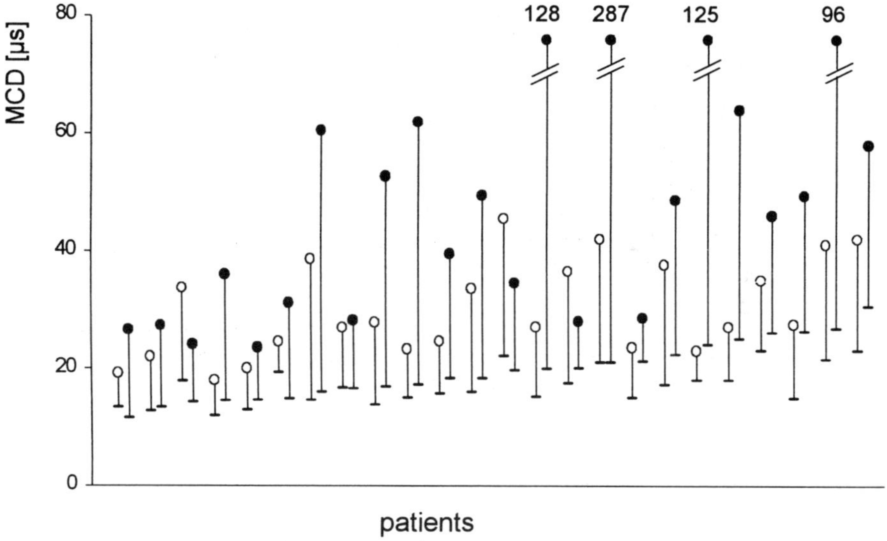

Fig. 1. Jitter values in EDC of the individual patients, plotted in order of increasing median value on the affected side. Median values are shown as dashes, upper 95th centiles (after eliminating most extreme 5% of the data) as circles: empty normal side, closed paretic side.

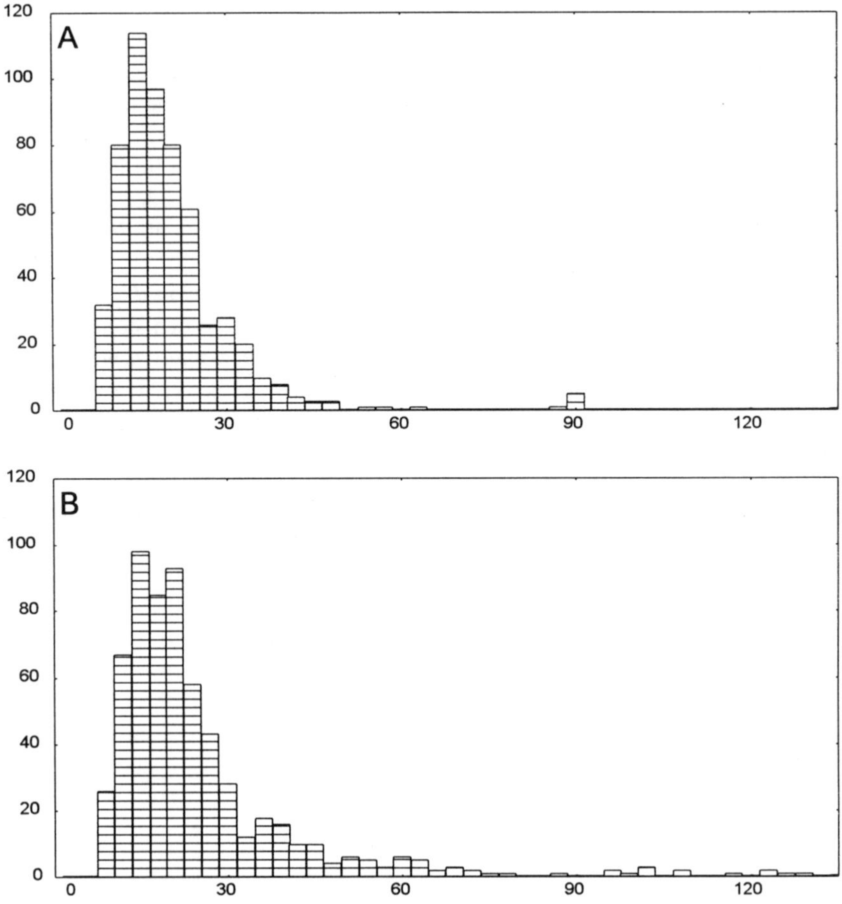

Fig. 2. Pooled jitter values of individual EDC NMJs of the normal (A) and paretic side (B). The data for the normal side do not differ from those collected in control subjects.

4 Discussion

Some authors suggested that the neurogenic changes seen in muscles of the weak limbs after a stroke may be due to *pressure or traction neuropathies* sustained during coma (e.g. Chokroverty et al. 1978). We do not believe that peripheral nerve lesion could have been responsible for the abnormal findings in our series of patients as none of them was in coma after their stroke, and they received proper care during the acute stage; thus we estimate that the possibility of inadvertent stretch or pressure damage to their nerves was small. Furthermore, in all of the patients who had motor and sensory conduction velocity and F-wave studies the findings were normal and symmetrical. Similarly, the sensory nerve action potential amplitudes were normal on both sides, and short latency components of the SEPs were reported to be normal, as they were in the study by Brown et al. (1990).

Inactivity of the paralysed muscles might be another possibility to account for some of the abnormalities. Ultrastructural changes such as the appearance of extrajunctional ACh receptors and even features of denervation, have been observed in muscles immobilised for prolonged periods of time (Eldridge et al. 1981). However, part of these findings may have been due to inadvertent nerve lesions produced by the immobilisation techniques. Inactivity *per se* is unlikely to be the cause of impaired NMT in human patients, as disuse alone does not seem to give rise to increased jitter (Stålberg and Sellman, unpublished observation).

A third possibility to explain the neurogenic changes in the paretic muscles on the side of hemiplegia is so-called *transsynaptic degeneration* (McComas et al 1973, Brown et al. 1990), a phenomenon known to occur in the CNS (Eidelberg et al. 1989). This could take a form of partial loss of lower motor neurons compensated later by collateral sprouting of the surviving ones. The findings supporting such loss include the reduced M-wave amplitude, fibrillation potentials and subsequent reorganisation of motor units, presumably resulting from collateral reinnervation. Alternatively, it could be manifested as a transient dysfunction of the lower motor neurons due to loss of some supraspinal trophic influence, leading, among other things, to impaired neuromuscular transmission and fibrillation activity. Which of the two mechanisms is in fact responsible for these observations is conjectural.

Single fiber jitter has been shown to be related to the safety factor of the individual NMJs (Stålberg et al. 1975). The neuromuscular jitter is increased in a variety of pre- and postsynaptic disorders, including denervation and reinnervation (Stålberg and Trontelj 1994). During the latter two processes, the jitter may be abnormal at two different stages: first, at a phase of Wallerian degeneration, which is probably short, lasting hours or days at the most (Trontelj and Stålberg, unpublished observation); and second, during reinnervation, after new NMJs had been established by the axonal sprouts; this phase has been shown to last several weeks to months after a known partial peripheral nerve lesion, when the newly reinnervated muscle fibres showed increased jitter and intermittent blocking (Massey et al. 1992), until their NMJs have functionally matured.

The results of this study demonstrate that a large majority of NMJs in the paretic muscles of our stroke patients had normal jitter, indicating a normal safety factor, nearly symmetrical to that on the unaffected side. Indeed, in 6 out of the 24 patients we have found no abnormality at all. However, a small but significant proportion of the NMJs on the paretic side showed increased jitter: about 13 %, compared to only 2 % on the unaffected side in the pooled material (about 2% is acceptable in the normal muscle). The increased jitter was sometimes (in 4% of all NMJs) associated with intermittent blocking. It should be added that large jitter alone does not result in weakness or fatigue; motor output is only reduced when blocking is manifested. Thus, neuromuscular transmission impairment does not appear to a major factor in fatigue of muscles paralysed by an upper motor neuron lesion.

As disturbed transmission may have occurred either at reinnervated NMJs or at the original NMJs of degenerating motor neurons, abnormal jitter in itself cannot help in distinguishing between the two situations. However, in case of a recently reinnervated NMJ, the response latency is prolonged due to slower impulse conduction in the new terminal axonal sprout and along the still atrophic muscle fiber, as well as due to a longer NMT time. In this study, correlation between the abnormal jitter values and response latency was not found. Furthermore, the abnormal jitter was recorded as early as 7 days after stroke in one patient. Such short time is probably insufficient for collateral reinnervation. Therefore, the abnormal jitter values may have been obtained from degenerating rather that reinnervating NMJs.

On the other hand, the probability of abnormal jitter seemed to increase with the duration of the condition in the 6 cases who had repeat studies. This suggests that at least some of the abnormal jitter values in the later stages of hemiplegia may have been derived from reinnervated NMJs.

In conclusion, the present study shows normal NMT at a large majority of NMJs even in completely paralysed muscles after recent stroke. Increased jitter and blocking seen at a small percentage of the NMJs in most of our patients may have occurred both in degenerating and reinnervating motor units. We cannot reliably distinguish between the different possible causes, i.e. withdrawal of a hypothetical trophic function of the upper motor neurone, followed by either postsynaptic dysfunction or the actual death of the lower motor neurons. At any rate, fatiguing response to electrical nerve stimulation in paretic muscles after an upper motor neuron lesion appears to be largely due to mechanisms peripheral to neuromuscular junction.

4 Acknowledgement

This study was performed in collaboration with the Institute for Rehabilitation of Disabled, Ljubljana, and the Department of Neurology who kindly referred their patients, and was supported by the Ministry of Science and Technology of the Republic of Slovenia, grant P3-5258-0312, by the Commission of the European Communities, grant PL93-1033, and Fondo de Investigaciones Sanitarias of Spain, Grant 92/0978 (JMF).

References

McComas, A. J., Sica, R. E. P., Upton, A. R. M., and Aguilera, N. (1973) Functional changes in motoneurones of hemiplegic patients. *J Neurol Neurosurg Psychiatry* **36**: 183-193.

Cruz Martinez, A. (1983) Electrophysiological study in hemiparetic patients. Electromyography, motor conduction velocity, and response to repetitive nerve stimulation. *Electromyogr clin Neurophysiol* **23**: 139-148.

Brown, W. F. and Snow, R. (1990) Denervation in hemiplegic muscles. *Stroke* **21**: 1700-1704.

Trontelj, J. V. and Stålberg, E. (1992) Jitter measurement by axonal stimulation: guidelines and technical notes. *Electroencephal clin Neurophysiol* **85**: 30-37.

Stålberg, E., Trontelj, J. V. and Mihelin, M. (1992) Electrical microstimulation with single-fiber electromyography: a useful method to study the physiology of the motor unit. *J. Clin. Neurophysiol.* **9**: 105-119.

Trontelj, J. V., Fernandez, J. M., Mihelin, M., Rugelj, D., and Stålberg, E. (1995) Neuromuscular transmission is mildly disturbed in hemiplegic muscles. *Zdrav. Vestn.* (in press).

Mihelin, M., Trontelj, J. K., and Trontelj J. V. (1975) Automatic measurement of random interpotential intervals in single fiber electromyography. *Int. J. Biomed. Comput.* **6**: 181-191.

Stålberg, E., Bischoff, C., and Fokk B. (1994) Outliers: a way to detect abnormality in quantitative EMG. *Muscle Nerve* **17**: 392-399.

Chokroverty, S. and Medina, J. (1978) Electrophysiological study of hemiplegia. *Arch Neurol* **35**: 360-363.

Eldridge, L., Liebhold, M., and Steinbach, J. H. (1981) Alterations in cat skeletal neuromuscular junctions following prolonged inactivity. *J Physiol* **313**: 529-545.

Eidelberg, E., Nguyen, L. H., and Polich, R., et al. (1989) Trans-synaptic degeneration of motoneurons caudal to spinal cord lesions. *Brain Research Bulletin* **22**: 39-45.

Stålberg, E, Shiller, H.H., and Schwartz, M.S. (1975) Safety factor in single human motor end-plates studied *in vivo* with single fibre electromyography. *J. Neurol. Neurosurg. Psychiatry* **38**: 799-804.

Stålberg, E. and Trontelj, J. V. (1994) *Single Fiber EMG. Studies in healthy and diseased muscle.* Second edition, Raven Press, New York.

Massey, J. M. and Sanders. D. B. (1992) Single-fiber EMG demonstrates reinnervation dynamics after nerve injury. *Neurology* **41**: 1150-1151.

Fatigue Indices in the Electrically Stimulated Quadriceps Muscle with Surface Electrodes

E. Rabischong[1,2], D. Guiraud[1]
[1]Centre Propara, Parc Euromédecine, Montpellier, France
[2]INSERM U 103, Appareil Moteur et Handicap, Montpellier, France

Abstract - Muscle fatigue using surface electrical stimulation represents a reproducible phenomenon in spinal cord injured patients. We recorded the torque output coming from the quadriceps muscle electrically activated. The fatigue curves exhibited three parts; first, a plateau of short duration, followed by a more or less steep slope and then a second plateau which was maintained for a long time. We fitted this phenomenon using a non linear regression analysis and introduced four parameters that outlined the muscle behavior. A set of fatigue indices was defined to characterize the asymptotic value, the slope, the coordinates of the inflexion point, the time constant and the vertical amplitude of the curve recorded. Two populations were studied; a group of 11 thoracic level of injury paraplegic patients and a group of ten able-bodied control subjects. The mean torque output did not differ between the two populations until 25 seconds has elapsed, but from 30 seconds onwards it was markedly lower in paraplegics. The mean residual torque output was 19.1±1.5% in the paraplegic group while it was 59.5±3.1% in the control group. We also studied the effect of blood supply in the production of fatigue, by repeating the same tests using a tourniquet at the groin level. The residual torque became 13.3±1.7% in the paraplegic group and 42.2±6.4% in the control group.

1 Introduction

Muscle fatigue represents a limiting factor for the different investigational groups working on surface electrical stimulation for the lower extremity. The muscular actuator is unable to maintain a steady torque of high value for very long; after a few seconds, it rapidly decreases to reach a value so low that it is functionless (Levy *et al.*, 1990; Rabischong and Ohanna, 1992). It appeared possible to extract a set of regression-based indices of fatigue which should provide information about the amount and rate of change in the muscular output. Non invasive fiber typing, at a gross level, could result from the analysis of these parameters. In this way, the effects of a directed training on fatigue resistance could be assessed.

2 Method

2.1 Population

We studied two groups. One consisted of 11 paraplegic patients (8 males, 3 females). All patients had complete thoracic level lesions (range: T4 to T11). The mean age was 27 (range: 23 to 40). No patient had severe spasticity or intermittent spasms which would impede the tests. The time post injury was extended from 8 to 18 months. The second group was composed of ten able-bodied subjects (9 males, 1 female, mean age 30, range: 24 to 41) who served as a control sample.

2.2 Measurement

The subjects sat in a special chair with the hips flexed to 90° and the knee to 60°: this corresponds to the position where the maximum isometric torque has been recorded in paraplegics using electrical stimulation (Levy *et al.*, 1990; Rabischong and Ohanna, 1992). We designed a force transducer (bridge of strain gauges) which we placed on the anterior aspect of the leg. It was padded to avoid polysynaptic withdrawal reflexes due to pain. The signal was low-pass filtered (30 Hz).

2.3 Current generator

We designed a two channel current regulated electrical stimulator which delivered biphasic charge-balanced pulses of 150 mA for maximum output. Pulse amplitude was adjusted to obtain saturation of the output in the recruitment in paraplegic patients and was dependent on pain threshold in control. Two self-adhering electrodes (8cm x 10cm, PALS, Axelgaard Manufacturing Co., Ltd.) were placed on the quadriceps muscle. Pulse width was set at 300 ms and frequency at 20 Hz. Both quadriceps muscles were stimulated for 110 seconds in both populations (n=22 in the patient group, n=20 in the control group).

The effect of blood supply was assessed by means of a tourniquet placed at the groin level. The groups were reduced to 6 persons for the paraplegic group (4 males, 2 females) and 5 for the control group (5 males). All subjects gave their informed consent for the use of tourniquet. The tourniquet was inflated at 300 mm of Hg. The test began two minutes after the tourniquet was inflated.

2.4 Off-line data analysis

Since the fatigue curves were highly reproducible and had a very comparable shape (two plateaus separated by a slope), we fitted the phenomenon using non linear regression analysis (Rabischong and Guiraud, 1993):

$$T_{(t)} = a\tanh(bt - c) + d \quad \Rightarrow \quad T_{(t)} = \frac{a\,(e^{bt-c} - e^{-bt+c})}{e^{bt-c} + e^{-bt+c}} + d\,, \tag{1}$$

where T was the torque developed as a function of time t (expressed in seconds), tanh the hyperbolic tangent and e the exponential of t.

The four parameters were determined by successive iterations on a compatible computer. Estimated coefficients were obtained by minimizing the residual sum of squares.

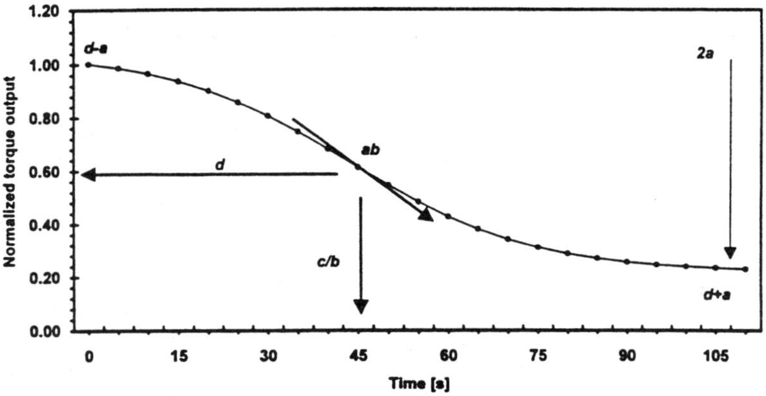

Fig. 1. The different fatigue indices computed.

Concerning the amount of decrease (fig. 1) three indices were computed: the asymptotic value ($d+a$), i.e. the residual isometric torque output, the total decrease ($2a$), the output at the inflexion point (d).

Concerning the rate of decrease (fig. 1) three indices were calculated: the slope value at the inflexion point (ab), the time constant t ($1/b$), the time coordinate of the inflexion point.

For all the results the torque was normalized to 1 with respect to initial value, and the time (t) was expressed in seconds. Values are expressed plus or minus one standard-error.

3 Results

3.1 Fatigue test without tourniquet

The recorded fatigue curves show the non linearity of muscle output with time (fig. 2). They exhibit three parts; the first part consists of a short plateau, the second one represents the main slope, and the last one forms a long plateau which is maintained for long time.

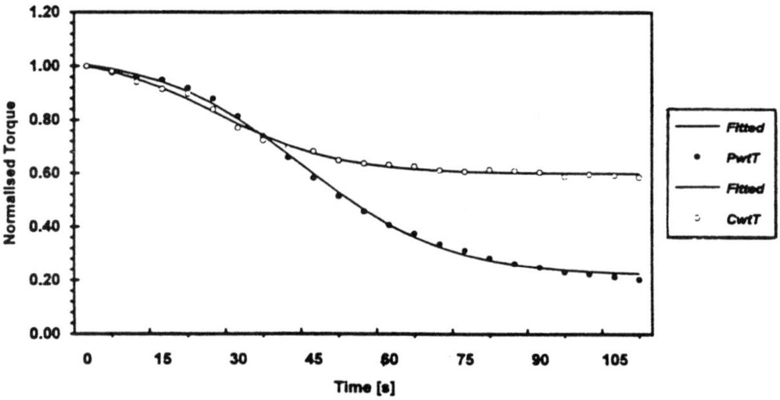

Fig. 2. Values measured in both groups without the tourniquet. CwtT is noted for control subjects without the tourniquet use, and PwtT for paraplegics without the tourniquet use.

In the patients group, the mean residual torque output that we measured at the end of the 110-seconds test was of low value with 20.3±2.21 % of the maximum output. The mean value of the computed asymptotic values (n=21) was 19.1±1.5 (Table 1, 2). In the control population we recorded curves with comparable shape. However, the second plateau exhibited a higher residual torque output measuring in average of the recorded value 58.5±3.2 % of the maximum output. The average of the computed asymptotic values (n=20) was 59.5±3.1.

The quadriceps muscle produced comparable relative output during the first 25 seconds (inflexion point for the able-bodied group) in both groups when electrically activated. During this time interval, the output was maximum.

Fatigue indices

	Without tourniquet		With tourniquet	
	Group 1	Group 2	Group1	Group 2
Asymptotic value (x100)	19.1±1.5	59.5±3.1	13.3±1.7	42.2±6.4
Output at the inflx pt. (x100)	63.3±1.5	81.8±2.6	57.6±1.6	69.9±3.6
Total decrease (x100)	-88.5±3.4	-0.45±1.5	-88.5±0.5	-55.4±5.7
Inflexion point	42.6±2.1	26.1±2.1	56±7.8	43±5.5
Slope (x100)	-1.6±0.13	-1±0.2	-1.5±0.14	-1.7±0.3
Time constant	33.2±5.2	24.7±5	29.3±2.4	17.1±2.1

Table 1. Mean value of the fatigue indices computed with equation [1] in both groups. Values are expressed plus and minus one standard error.

Regression parameters				
	Without tourniquet		With tourniquet	
	Group 1	Group 2	Group 1	Group 2
a	-0.41	-0.22	-0.44	-0.28
b	0.035	0.042	0.034	0.053
c	1.5	1.09	1.94	2.33
d	0.63	0.82	0.58	0.7
r^2	0.998	0.995	0.999	0.996

Table 2. Regression parameters computed for the mean curves of both groups.

3.2 Fatigue test adding a tourniquet

In the spinal cord injured group, the curve which was measured during the use of the tourniquet differed from that obtained without tourniquet, especially in the residual values of torque output (mean value recorded 14.7±1.3, mean asymptotic value computed 13.4±1.7).

The residual value of torque in the able-bodied group (mean value measured 42.9%±6.3, mean asymptotic value computed 42.3%) decreased notably when the tourniquet was applied but remained higher than that seen in the paraplegic subjects (fig. 3).

Results obtained with tourniquet use were not extremely different between the two groups concerning the first part and the main slope (the first 60 seconds) if relative values of torque were considered. The difference appeared after this time. The effects of the tourniquet were more evident in control than they were in paraplegic subjects. Nevertheless, the tourniquet always affected the residual torque.

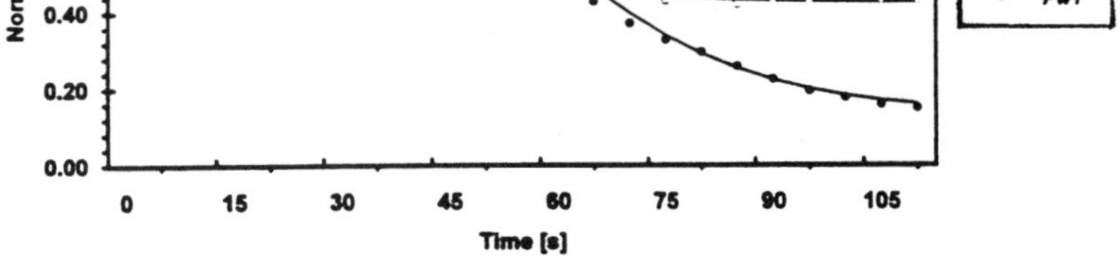

Fig. 3. Values measured in both groups with the tourniquet use. PwT is noted for paraplegics with the tourniquet use, and CwT for control subjects with the tourniquet use.

4 Discussion

Fatigue indexes, calculated as the decrease in output over a fixed period (Robinson *et al.,* 1990) (60 seconds) did not provide enough sensitivity to characterize muscle fatigue, even mechanically. The values of torque after 60 s were, in the present study, far from the asymptotic value in both groups of subjects studied. Therefore, only a rough approximation could be obtained using such indexes.

It appears that, the different parts of the curves represent a temporal change in the different metabolic phases involved in muscle output. From 0 to 10-20 s the output was not truly affected by the addition of the tourniquet in either population. Therefore, the metabolism of such fibers is anaerobic and dominant at this level. The duration of their output, nearly 20 s, is accorded to the physiology of FF fibers (Burke *et al.,* 1973) whose metabolism is, in fact, almost exclusively oriented to anaerobic glycolysis with a very moderate fitness for aerobic metabolism. After about 20 s, they stopped their activity. Moreover, they have the lowest entry impedance and, thus, are first recruited with electrical stimulation (Henneman and Mendell, 1981; Mortimer, 1981; Burke, 1981). They develop the highest mechanical tension compared to the other types of fibers. Those facts are consistent with an anaerobic alactic oriented metabolism. Other authors agree with this point (Hainaut and Duchateau, 1989). However, the output was not maintained in a steady state during these 10 to 20 seconds.

Thereafter, the metabolism became anaerobic lactic. The decrease of the output could be due to the production of lactate and the accumulation of H+ ions with a resulting pH decrease. The accumulation of products of anaerobic glycolysis inhibits rate-controlling enzymes with a resulting reduction of ATP supply for the contractile process. The relationship of pH decrease and fatigue are well documented (Sahlin, 1991).

The tourniquet had, as mentioned, a true effect on the residual values of torque; in other words, this plateau represents an output generated by fibers requiring blood supply. The S fibers, contrarily to the FF fibers, have almost exclusively an aerobic oriented metabolism and a very low aptitude for anaerobic glycolysis. It appears consistent that, to a large extent, the tourniquet keeps them from providing their maximal tension output. Jammes et al. (1990) recorded comparable behavior in the adductor pollicis longus muscle in humans with a cuff inflated to higher than systolic blood pressure. We consider the main slope as a reflection of the FR fibers' output; they have an intermediate metabolism between the FF and the S types; they have the same aptitude as the FF fiber for anaerobic glycolysis but they also have a significant aptitude for aerobic metabolism. It is important to notice that the values obtained with tourniquet use are higher for the first plateau and the main slope.

If the duration determines which fiber type is active, the output amplitude gives an idea of the number of active fibers. As the main slope becomes steeper and the asymptotic value lower, the output of FR and S fibers is less pronounced in paraplegic subjects. The data using the tourniquet confirms this point; the first part remains unchanged.

Salmons and Henriksson (1981) reported a significant increase in the number of FF fibers in spinal cord injured patients. It is likely that, due to non use, the fibers return to a state closer to the initial distribution where fast fibers are dominant.

Therefore, our fatigue indices give information concerning the fatigue-resistant fiber population. Non invasive fiber typing, at a gross level, resulted from the fatigue indices analysis. Asymptotic value and vertical amplitude most closely represent the actions of the S fibers. The slope value, time constant and coordinates of the inflexion point represent the action of FR fibers. The lower *d+a*, *t*, and/or the higher *ab*, *c/b*, *2a* the lower the resistance to fatigue.

The deprivation of blood supply does not explain the decrease in torque output in paraplegic subjects. This decrease in torque is better explained by the change in muscle fiber population and by the recruitment mode using electrical stimulation.

References

Burke, R. E., Levine, D. N., Tsairis, P., and Zajac, F. E. (1973) Physiological types and histochemical profiles in motor units of the cat gastrocnemius, J Physiol, 234: 723-748.

Burke R. E. (1981) Motors units: anatomy, physiology, and functional organization. In 'Handbook of Physiology, The nervous system II', V.B. Brooks (Ed), American Physiological Society, Bethesda, Maryland, 2: pp 345-422.

Hainaut, K. and Duchateau, J. (1989) Muscle fatigue, effects of training and disuse. increased use, Muscle & Nerve 4: 94-105.

Henneman, E. and Mendell, L. M. (1981) Functional organization of motoneuron pool and its inputs. In 'Hanbook of Physiology, The nervous system II,' V.B. Brooks (Ed), American Physiological Society, Bethesda, Maryland, 2: pp 423-507.

Jammes, Y., Badier, M., and Guillot, Ch. (1990) Oxygen transport and muscle fatigue. In: Muscle fatigue. Biochemical and physiological aspects. G. Atlan, L. Beliveau, P. Bouissou (Eds), Masson, Paris, pp 73-89, 1991.Vollestad N.K., Wesche J., Sejersted O.M.: Gradual increase in leg oxygen uptake during repeated submaximal contractions in human, J. Appl. Physiol. 68(3): 1150-1156.

Levy, M., Mizrahi, J., and Susak, Z. (1990) Recruitment, force and fatigue Muscle & Nerve 12: 660-669.

Mortimer, T. (1981) Motor prostheses. In 'Hanbook of Physiology, The nervous system II', V.B. Brooks (Ed), American Physiological Society, Bethesda, Maryland 1981, 2: pp 155-187.

Rabischong, E. and Ohanna, F. (1992) Effects of FES on evoked muscular output in paraplegics, Paraplegia, 30: 467-473.

Rabischong, E. and Guiraud, D. (1993) Determination of fatigue using surface electrical stimulation, J. Biomed. Eng., 15: 443-450.

Robinson, L. R., Mustovic, E. H., Lieber, P. S., Haidet, P. M., Irgang, J. J., McLane, T., and Nicholas, J. J. (1990) A technique for quantifying and determining the site of isometric muscle fatigue in the clinical setting, Arch. Phys. Med. Rehabil, 71: 902-904.

Sahlin, K. (1991) Role of intracellular pH in fatigue. In G. Atlan, L. Beliveau, P. Bouissou (eds), Muscle fatigue. Biochemical and physiological aspects, Masson, Paris, pp 27-39.

Salmons, S. and Henriksson J. (1981) The adaptative response of skeletal muscle to characteristics of quadriceps muscles of paraplegics isometrically activated by surface functional electrical stimulation, J Biomed Eng, 12: 150-156.

Muscle Fatigue Facing Continuous and Intermittent Stimulation and Recovery from Fatigue

E. Rabischong, M. Gaviria
Laboratory of Clinical Neurophysiology, Centre Propara , Montpellier, France

Abstract - In the present study, we compared muscle fatigue of the electrically stimulated quadriceps induced with continuous (120 s) and intermittent (300 s, 1 s on, 2 s off) stimulation and the recovery from fatigue tests (15 minutes). Torque output and surface action potentials were recorded and compared in both conditions. Force production and surface action potentials appeared to be more affected by continuous stimulation. The residual output was lower, the decrease in amplitude and increase in duration of the recorded surface action potentials were higher. By the end of the 15 minutes recovery period, the torque output never exceeded 50% of the values recorded prior to the fatigue test while the temporal parameters returned to values close to initial one.

1 Introduction

Muscle fatigue is considered to be an inability to maintain force output during sustained or repetitive contractions (Enoka et al. 1988). This failure to maintain force is usually gradual and time-dependent changes are noted (Merletti et al. 1991, Rabischong et al. 1993). These changes, i.e. amount and rate, lead to myoelectric manifestations of muscle fatigue. The mechanisms which cause skeletal muscle fatigue are not fully understood, although considerable evidence indicates that it is most probably due to excitation-contraction coupling failure (Edwards et al. 1991). Intermittent tests are generally conducted to measure fatigue (Duchateau et al. 1987, Enoka et al. 1992, Hainaut et al. 1989, Robinson et al. 1991), even though continuous tests could appear, in some cases, more appropriate to characterise muscle fatigue with functional purposes. For some authors, the electrical changes encountered during fatigue are not well related to the mechanical changes (Enoka et al. 1992, Hainaut et al. 1989, Merletti et al. 1991). In different investigations a number of muscles have been studied: soleus (Burke 1991), gastrocnemius (Merletti et al. 1991), adductor pollicis (Duchateau et al. 1987, Hainaut et al. 1989, Moussavi et al. 1989), tibialis anterior (Moussavi et al. 1989), quadriceps (Franken et al. 1993, Rabischong et al. 1992, 1993). The quadriceps muscle deprived of voluntary control represents an interesting isolated functional contractile tissue independent of motivational factors and of central nervous system drive modifying force output. It represents the main actuator to stand up and keep standing in paraplegics with electrical stimulation. Therefore, it appeared important to characterise its behaviour facing sustained and intermittent contraction and its recovery from fatigue.

2 Material and Methods

2.1 Population

Tests were performed on 4 paraplegic patients never trained with electrical stimulation. All of the spinal cord injured patients had complete thoracic level lesions (range from T8 to T10) verified by clinical examination. No patient had severe spasticity or intermittent spasms which would have impeded the tests, and the quadriceps reflex was present in each patient. The time after injury was extended from 15 to 36 months. The mean age was 27 (±3). All subjects gave informed consent to participate in this investigation.

2.2 Measurements

We measured both the torque output and the surface action potentials (SAPs) of the electrically stimulated quadriceps muscle in two different conditions: continuous (CS) and intermittent stimulation (IS) in all the patients. To assess recovery from fatigue, we recorded prior to the fatigue test a single twitch considered as the reference for the output and for the SAPs. Then the fatigue test was conducted. After this test twitches were recorded every minute for 15 minutes.

The subjects sat in a special chair with the hip flexed at 90° and the knee to 60°. We used a force transducer (bridge of strain gauges) to measure the torque output in isometric condition. The signal was amplified (Tektronics, AM 502) and filtered (DC-30 KHz).

The muscle was supramaximally stimulated through a pair of Nicolet electrodes (0.9 cm diameter, 3 cm between electrodes) placed on the femoral nerve at the groin level. The cathode was proximaly located. The electrodes were connected to a current-regulated electrical stimulator that delivered biphasic charge-balanced pulses of 150 mA for maximum output. The recorded duration of the twitches (prior and after the fatigue test) was 300 ms. For this recording a single pulse of 300 μs was applied to the femoral nerve. The duration of the fatigue test was 120 s with CS and 300 s with IS (duty cycle 1 s on and 2 s off). The frequency was set at 20 Hz and pulse width at 300 μs, which corresponds to the usual parameters for functional electrical stimulation.

For the SAP recording we used skin surface electrodes (Beckman, 0.8 cm of internal diameter) placed on the vastus medialis and separated by 3 cm. The ground electrode was placed around the mid part of the thigh between the stimulating and the recording electrodes. The SAPs were amplified with a differential amplifier (Tektronix AM 502) and filtered (bandpass 10 Hz to 1 kHz).

Software written in Labview (National Instrument Co., Austin, TX, USA) in conjunction with a library we developed was used for the acquisition. Signals coming from the force transducer and from the surface electrode were acquired through an I/O board for PC (12 bits resolution). Data were stored to a personal computer. For the twitches recording, the time acquisition window was 300 ms. For the fatigue test, the signal was segmented in subsequent epochs lasting 100 ms each, 0.8 s apart with CS and 3 s apart with IS. Within each epoch the signal was sampled at 5 kHz.

2.3 Off-line data analysis

Concerning the torque output, a mean value of the signal obtained through the force transducer during the 100 ms acquisition window was computed. We used a non linear function (1) we described (Rabischong et al. 1993) to fit the torque production relative to time:

$$\xi_{(t)} = \frac{a\left(e^{bt-c)} - e^{-bt+c}\right)}{e^{bt-c} + e^{-bt+c}} + d\,,\ with\ b = \frac{1}{\tau} \qquad (1)$$

where $\xi_{(t)}$ represents the torque output as a function of time *t*. $\xi_{(t)}$ is normalised with respect to initial value. *e* is the exponential, *t* the time, and τ the time constant.

Concerning the amount of decrease, the asymptotic value $(d+a)$ was computed. The parameter $(d\text{-}a)$ represents the initial value and provides information concerning the potentiation. Concerning the rate of decrease two indices were calculated: the maximum slope value (ab) and the time constant τ $(1/b)$. All those parameters are representing the set of fatigue indices.

The beginning and end of the twitches were determined at 5 % of the maximum value. We computed the onset of the twitch (O in ms), the end of the twitch (E in ms), the duration (D in ms), the maximum value (Max in V), the rising time to peak (RTP_t in ms), the decreasing time (DT in ms), and the half relaxation time (1/2R in ms).

The beginning of the SAP was determined at 5% of the first peak. We computed the peak to peak amplitude (PTP_a in mV). To discriminate the conduction velocity along the nerve fibers and along the muscle fibers we studied three different parameters:

- the latency (L) from the onset of stimulation to the onset of the SAP (5 % of maximum) were the nerve conduction velocity (NCV) and the neuromuscular junction transmission (NMJT) were studied,

• the rising time to peak (RTP) from the onset of the SAP to the maximum amplitude of the first peak and

• the peak to peak duration (PTP_d) from the maximum to the minimum of the SAP were the muscle fiber conduction velocity (MFCV) was studied.

The same model was used to fit the data. Therefore $\xi_{(t)}$ represented either L, RTP or PTP_d as a function of time t. We also computed the surface of the two peaks (S1 and S2 in mV*ms). All the data were normalised with respect to the initial value.

3 Results

3.1 Fatigue test

3.1.1 Torque output

The recorded fatigue curves revealed the non-linearity of muscle output as a function of time. As a general behaviour, the initial output rapidly increased (potentiation) during the first seconds of the test reaching a maximum after which the output decreased with a slope which varied among patients. However, this increase was limited. Neither the level of injury nor the length of time after injury correlated with residual output or maximum torque. Considering the model, the value of the coefficient of determination (r^2) was very high in all the patients (from 0.971 to 0.999).

Fig. 1. Torque output in the same patient with CS (left graph) and with IS (right graph). The solid line represents the values computed by the model. AS is noted for asymptotic value and TC for time constant.

As a general result, all the variables computed showed a better resistance to fatigue with IS. The asymptotic value and the time constant were higher and the slope of decrease lower.

3.1.2 Surface action potentials (SAPs)

3.1.2.1 Peak-to-peak amplitude (PTP)

It is clear from fig. 2, that SAPs underwent important changes along the fatigue test. However, the modifications of the shape was limited with IS compared to CS. This was noted in all the patients studied.

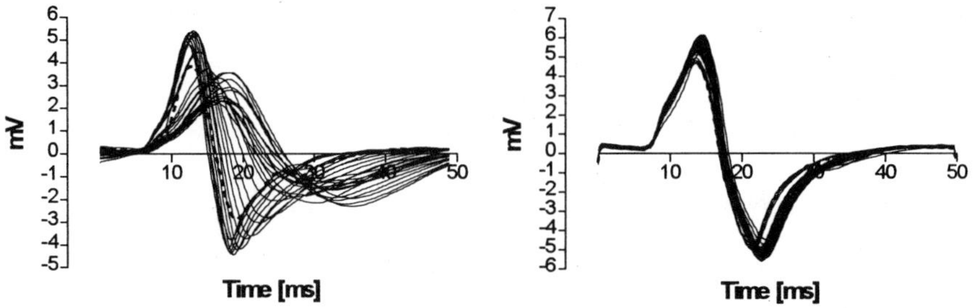

Fig. 2. Typical modifications of SAPs shape in the same patient along the fatigue test with CS (left graph) and IS (right graph). The discontinuous line indicates the first SAP.

The PTP amplitude was not related to the torque output. As a general behaviour with CS, it first increased to reach a maximum (from 1.14 to 1.5), then decreased to reach very low values (from 0.1 to 0.4) and increased again to reach values comprised between 0.3 and 1. During this late increase the torque output still decreased.

With IS, PTP increased to reach a maximum (from 1.05 to 1.25), and then decreased to reach final level by the end of the test (from 0.89 to 0.98). Therefore, no late increased was noticed and the reduction in amplitude was limited compared with CS.

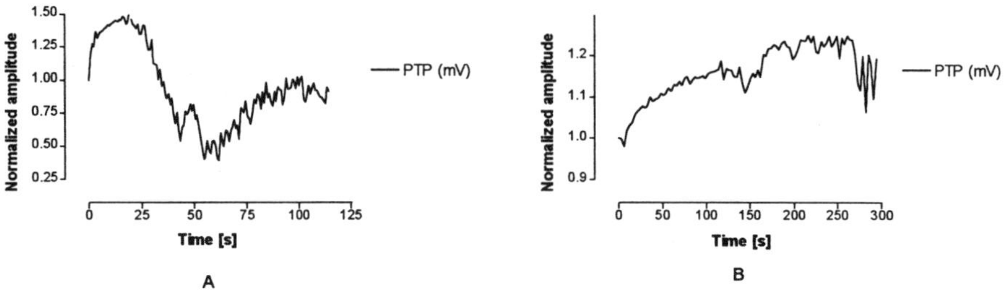

Fig. 3. PTP amplitude along the test with CS (A) and IS (B) in the same patient.

3.1.2.2 Peak-to-peak duration (PPD) and latency (L)

The PPD and L were extremely affected by the CS. To fit the data obtained in this condition the model provided excellent curve fitting (r^2 from 0.85 to 0.93). With CS, the increase of PPD, indicating a slowing in the muscle fiber conduction velocity, was comprised between 2.5 and 4. The increase of the latency, indicating a slowing in the nerve conduction velocity and/or neuromuscular junction transmission, was comprised between 1.15 and 1.3.

With IS, the increase of DPP was limited (from 1.07 to 1.64) and the latency did not increase. In all the patients the latency decreased during the first seconds (from 0.8 to 0.93).

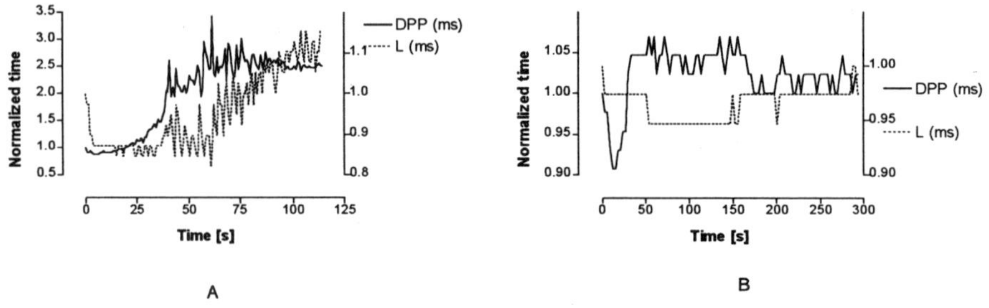

Fig. 4. DPP and L in the same patient with CS (A) and IS (B). DPP is scaled on the left axis and L on the right one.

3.1.2.3 Rising time to peak (RTP)

RTP continuously increased from initial value to reach values comprised between 2.4 and 2.6 with CS and between 1.2 and 1.5 with IS. Therefore, here again the SAPs were less affected by the stimulation in intermittent condition.

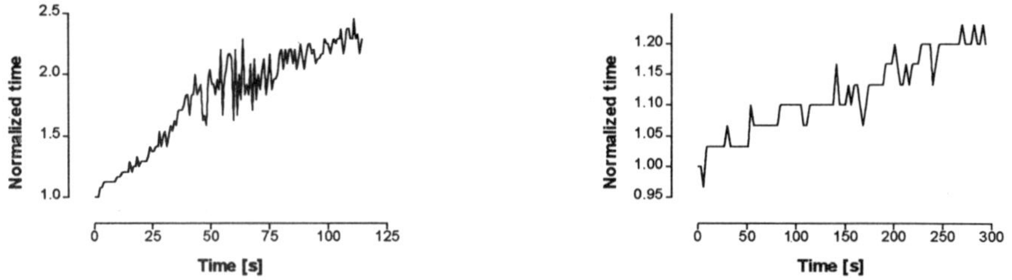

Fig. 5. RTP along the fatigue test with CS (left graph) and with IS (right graph) in the same patient.

3.1.2.3 Surface

In general, S1 and S2 presented a comparable shape and were not related to the torque production. With CS, surface first increased to reach value ranging from 1.67 to 1.83, then decreased to reach low value (from 0.27 to 0.89) and, then, increased again to reach values ranging from 0.97 to 2.3. With IS, the increase was limited (from 1.3 to 1.35).

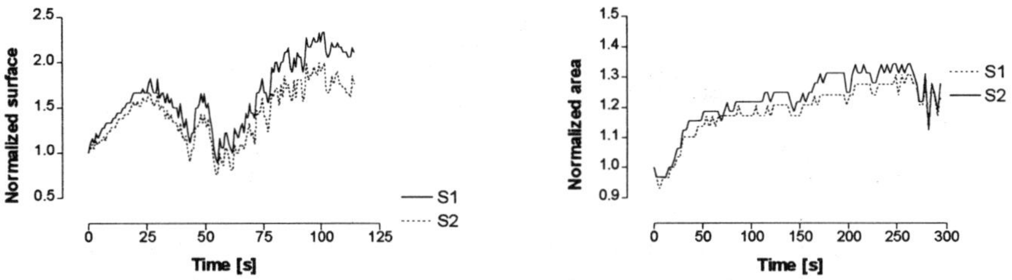

Fig. 6. Evolution of surface S1 and S2 with CS (left) and IS (right) along the fatigue test in the same patient.

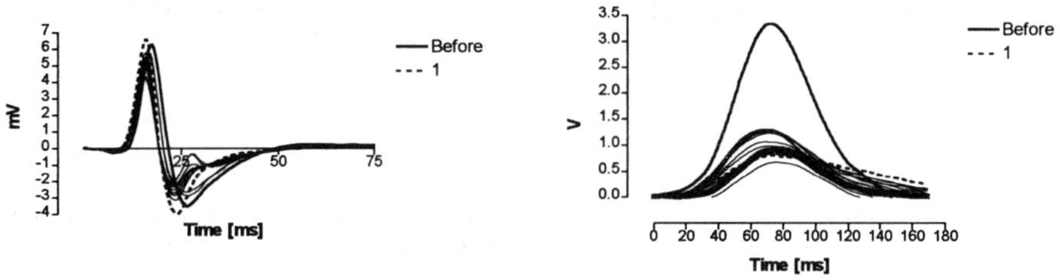

Fig. 7. Evolution of SAPs (left) and twitches (right) in the same patient after CS. Before is noted for the values recorded prior to the fatigue test and 1 for the values recorded one minute after the fatigue test.

3.2 Recovery from fatigue

3.2.1 Twitch

After CS the different temporal variables returned close to initial values by the end of the 15 mn recovery. Some of those variables indicating fatigue, e.g., 1/2R were extremely increased after the test. The torque output, in all the patients, never exceeded 50 % of initial values and obviously, the surface remained reduced during this phase of recovery. After IS, the temporal variables returned to initial faster than after CS. However, the torque output and the surface never reached 50 % of initial value by the end of the 15 min recovery phase.

Considering the SAPs, after both type of tests the latencies appeared to be shorter than initial values. But after CS, PTP continued to decrease while it was fairly stable after IS and close to initial values.

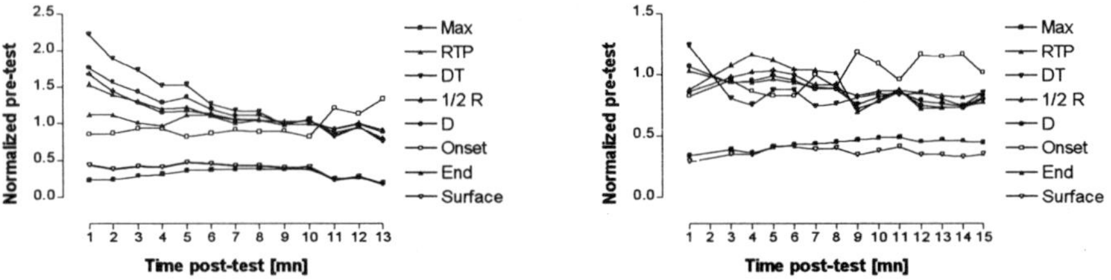

Fig. 8. Twitch values with CS (left) and IS (right) along the 15 minutes of recovery in the same patient. Data were normalised with respect to the twitch recorded prior to the fatigue test.

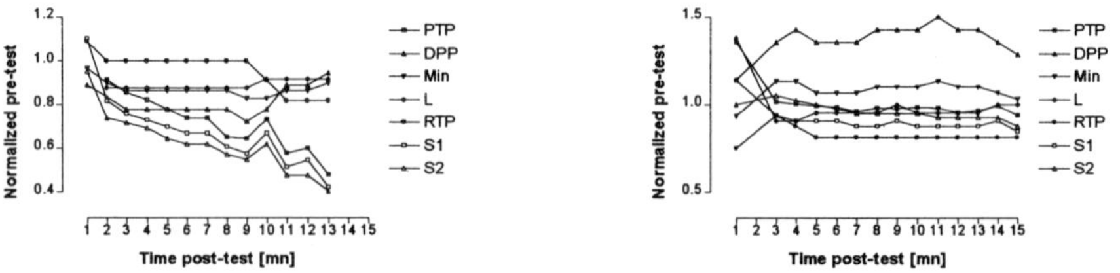

Fig. 9. SAPs values with CS (left) and IS (right) along the 15 minutes of recovery in the same patient. Data were normalised with respect to the twitch recorded prior to the fatigue test.

4 Discussion

Although significant differences were encountered among patients with respect to mechanical and electrophysiological measures, the general pattern of responses to electrical stimulation was similar. The resistance to fatigue appeared, in the present study, extremely variable among the patients. The muscle behaviour facing CS and IS was different. The force production and the related SAPs were more affected by CS. Nevertheless, if force production remained at higher level by the end of the test with IS, the recovery from this effort did not appeared to be extremely different with the recovery obtained after CS. The output remained affected and never exceeded half the value of the initial twitch. With both test conditions, the fatigue curve remained with a sigmoid shape. Only the parameters characterising this shape were different.

The amplitude of the SAP first increased and then decreased which is in accordance with several studies (Enoka et al. 1992, Hainaut et al. 1989). The surface EMG is a weighted sum of all motor unit potentials within the pick-up area of the electrodes. Therefore the reduction of the amplitude could result either from the reduction in single-fiber events, i.e. a reduction in the number of contributing MUAPs, or a reduction in the amplitude of the MUAPs.

The muscle deprived from voluntary control is subject to changes in its fiber typing characterised by an increase in type IIb and a decrease in type I fibers (Salmons et al. 1981). It appeared obvious that the muscles studied were very fatigable. Moreover, fatigable units usually displayed marked reduction in amplitude and area, whereas, fatigue-resistant motor units exhibited little or no change in the SAP (Enoka et al. 1992).

During fatigue test with CS, the increase in the computed latencies could result from the decrease in the conduction velocity or could be the reflect of the remaining slow fibers still activated. Units with low conduction velocities and low twitch tensions are more resistant to fatigue and might therefore be predominant in the EMG signal when progresses. This predominance will tend to decrease the average muscle fiber conduction velocity (Arendt-Nielsen et al. 1989). The nerve conduction velocity and the NMJ transmission appeared to be less affected than the muscle conduction velocity (RTP and PTPd). The slowing of the conduction was identified by the broadening of the action potential. The decrease in muscle fiber conduction velocity represents a normal behaviour during sustained contractions (Arendt-Nielsen et al. 1989, Merletti et al. 1991). The slowing of velocity in currently stimulated units would tend to decrease the average muscle fiber conduction velocity.

By opposite, the parameters reflecting the conduction velocity were not extremely modified during IS. Nevertheless, the torque output decreased.
Differences in the time course of mechanical and electrical changes suggest that the change in SAPs was not the major determinant of the force change. In fact, the decline in the torque production of the muscle studied began well before any substantial depression of the SAP. For Hainaut et al. electrical changes do not closely control mechanical failure.

References

Arendt-Nielsen, L., Mills, KR., Forster, (1989) A. Changes in muscle fiber conduction velocity, mean power frequency, and mean EMG voltage during prolonged submaximal contractions. *Muscle & Nerve*, 12: 493-497.

Burke, R.E. (1981) Motors units: anatomy, physiology, and functional organization. In: V.B. Brooks (eds.) *Handbook of Physiology, The nervous system II*, American Physiological Society, Bethesda, Maryland, 2, pp. 345-422.

Duchateau, J., Hainaut, K. (1987) Electrical and mechanical changes in immobilized human muscle. *J Appl Physiol*, 62: 2168-2173.

Edwards, R.H.T., Gibson, H. (1991) Perspectives in the study of normal and pathological skeletal muscle. In: G. Atlan, L. Beliveau, P. Bouissou (eds.) *Muscle fatigue. Biochemical and physiological aspects*, Masson, Paris, pp. 3-15.

Enoka, R.M., Rankin, L.L., Joyner, M.J., Stuart, D.G. (1988) Fatigue-related changes in neuromuscular excitability of rat hindlimb muscles. *Muscle & Nerve,* 11: 1123-1132.

Enoka, R.M., Trayanova, N., Laouris, Y., Bevan, L., Reinking, R.M., Stuart, D.G. (1992) Fatigue-related changes in motor unit action potentials of adult cats. *Muscle & Nerve,* 14: 138-150.

Franken, H.M., Veltink, P.H., Fidder, M., Boom, B.K. (1993) Fatigue of intermittently stimulated paralyzed human quadriceps during imposed cyclical lower leg movements. *J Electromyogr Kinesiol*, 3: 3-12

Hainaut, K., Duchateau, J. (1989) Muscle fatigue, effects of training and disuse. *Muscle & Nerve,* 12: 660-669.

Merletti, R., Lo Conte, L.R., Orizio, C. (1991) Indices of muscle fatigue. *Journal of Electromyography and Kinesiology,* 1: 20-33.

Moussavi, R.S., Carson, P.J., Boska, M.D., Weiner, M.W., Miller, R.G. (1989) Nonmetabolic fatigue in exercising human muscle. *Neurology,* 39: 1222-1226.

Rabischong, E., Guiraud, D. (1993) Determination of fatigue in the electrically stimulated quadriceps muscle and relative effect of ischemia. *Journal of Biomedical Engineering,* 15: 443-450.

Rabischong, E., Ohanna, F. (1992) Effects of FES on evoked muscular output in paraplegics, *Paraplegia,* 30: 467-473.

Robinson, G.A., Enoka, R.M., Stuart, D.G. (1991) Immobilization-induced changes in motor unit force and fatigability in the cat. *Muscle & Nerve,* 14: 563-573.

Salmons, S., Henriksson, J. (1981) The adaptative response of skeletal muscle to increased use. *Muscle & Nerve,* 4: 94-105.

Fatigue of Intermittently Stimulated Human Quadriceps: Influence of Knee Angular Velocity

H. M. Franken, P. H. Veltink, H. B.K. Boom
Biomedical Technological Institute,
University of Twente, Enschede, The Netherlands

Abstract - During prolonged experiments the influence of knee angular velocity, and stimulation parameters (interpulse interval (IPI), duty cycle (DC), number of pulses per cycle (NP)) on fatigue-induced torque decline of paralyzed human quadriceps was studied. Identification of torque-angle and -angular velocity relations was also performed. The overall loss of maximum torque (MT) and torque-time integral (TTI) per cycle during sustained intermittent stimulation during isokinetic movement had a typical exponential decay reaching asymptotic values. Larger knee velocities resulted in a significantly faster and relatively larger decay of MT and TTI. The rate and relative magnitude of fatigue during concentric contractions are in direct relation to NP. The results may be valuable in the design of optimal control systems for FES which pursue minimisation of muscle fatigue.

1 Introduction

A major issue in the control of functional electrical stimulation (FES) of paralysed muscles is the decay of muscle force as a result of fatigue under sustained (continuous and intermittent) stimulation (Andrews et al. 1989, Boom et al. 1993, Levy et al. 1990). Stimulated paralyzed human quadriceps fatigue under isometric condition can be described by an exponential decay (Boom et al. 1993, Levy et al. 1990). In this study the torque of intermittently stimulated paralysed human knee extensors during (isokinetic) cyclical lower leg movements was investigated.

2 Methods

2.1 Subjects

The subjects who participated in this study were complete T5-T6 level spinal cord injured patients. All had normal excitable quadriceps muscle and had been enrolled in the FES training program of the rehabilitation center *'t Roessingh* (Enschede, The Netherlands).

2.2 Protocol

A protocol of 7 fatigue trials (FT) was designed to compare overall loss of tetanic torque at the knee joint during sustained intermittent stimulation at different isokinetic velocities.

The angle and velocity ranges were limited by the anatomical restrictions of the shank, the restrictions imposed by the dynamometer bench and the desire to maintain a constant cycle time (2 s.), comparable to a walking cycle. The experimental set-up is shown in fig. 1.

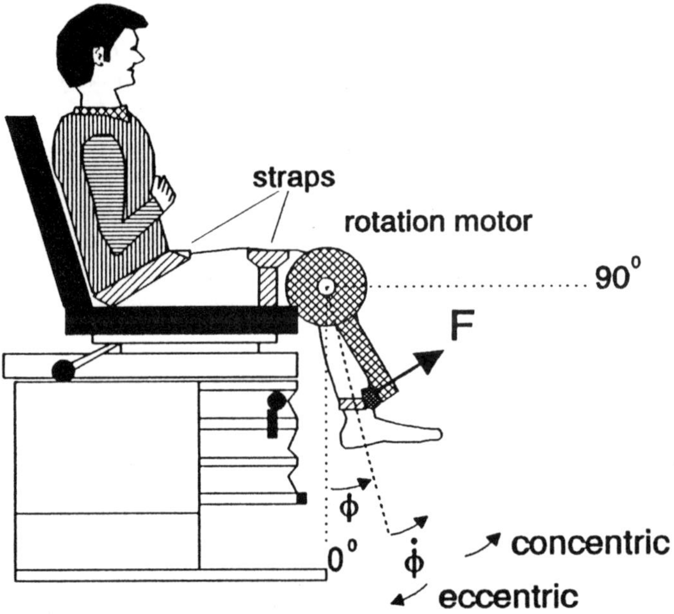

Fig. 1. Schematic of experimental set-up. The angular position and velocity, measured at the motor axis, are defined positive in extension motion with zero as indicated. The patient is strapped at the hip and knee to measure knee torque (at the tibia) only and to ensure static position of the body.

The influence of IPI (20 and 40 ms), DC ([ontime/cycle time]: 16 and 32 %) and NP ([ontime/IPI]: 16 and 32), at isokinetic joint movement, was investigated. Pulsewidth (PW = 300 μs) and stimulation amplitude (SA = 100 mA) were set to obtain maximal recruitment. Three muscle identification trials, determining the torque-angle (isometric measurement) and torque-angular velocity (isokinetically measured at 50 deg) relations, were performed. Force, knee angular position, and velocity were sampled at 100 Hz. These signals and stimulus data were stored on disk for off-line analysis.

2.3 Off-line data analysis

From the active torque, the maximum torque (MT) and torque-time integral per swing (TTI) are calculated. "Fatigue parameters", describing the decay of the MT and TTI as a function of time (one sample per cycle), were derived by curve-fitting the following equation to the data:

$$\xi(\tau) = \xi_{max} \left[(1-\xi_o) \exp(-t/\tau_\xi) + \xi_o\right] \tag{1}$$

where ξ is either MT or TTI, t is time, ξ_{max} is the maximum achieved in the considered trial, τ_ξ is the time constant of decay in ξ due to fatigue, and ξ_o is the relative asymptotic value to which $\xi(t)$ descends. The first part of the data (approximately 10 samples) which increases to ξ_{max} has been ignored. Equation (1) is fitted iteratively by minimizing the resulting RMS deviation from the experimental data (see also Boom et al. 1993).

3 Results

3.1 Measured and estimated signals

Fig. 2 displays a typical registration of measured and estimated signals for one cycle.

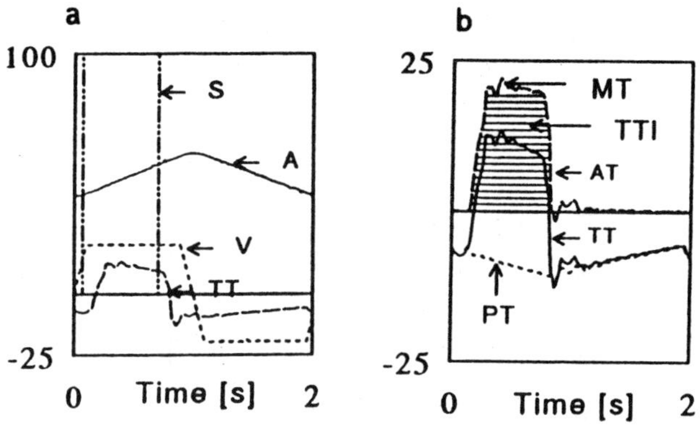

Fig. 2. a: Total knee torque (TT [Nm]), angular position (A [deg]) and velocity (V [deg/s]), and the applied stimulation burst (S [mA]), for one cycle with concentric contraction. **b**: Total (TT [Nm]), passive (PT [Nm]) and active knee torque (AT [Nm]). Estimated parameters TTI [Nms] and MT [Nm].

3.2 Fatigue parameters

Fig. 3 depicts the fatigue parameters estimated from the decay in TTI. TTI_{max} displays a Hill type dependence on velocity, indicating comparable muscle condition for each trial. The graphs for τ_{TTI} and TTI_o show that higher velocities result in a significantly larger and faster decay of TTI ($\alpha<0.05$). Varations in stimulation parameters indicated that the rate and magnitude of fatigue for concentric contractions are in direct relation to NP. The fatigue parameters for MT are similar.

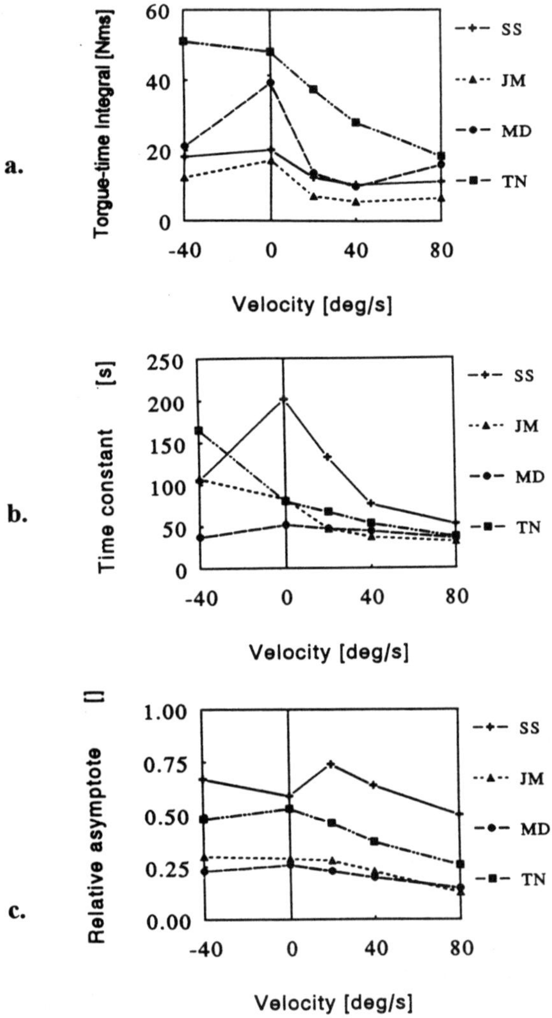

Fig. 3. Different velocities refer to seperate fatigue trials with identical stimulation parameters. (Subjects: SS, JM, MD, TN) **a**: Torque time integral ($TTI_{max)}$, **b**: Time constant (τ_{TTI}), **c**: Relative asymptote of TTI_o

3.3 Muscle dynamics

A typical Gaussian-type dependence of the isometrically generated torque on the knee angle was found (fig. 4a). The measured torgue-angular velocity relations supports the Hill equation. The relations alter due to fatigue. The decline in torque output due to fatigue is larger at higher velocities (see also fig. 3c).

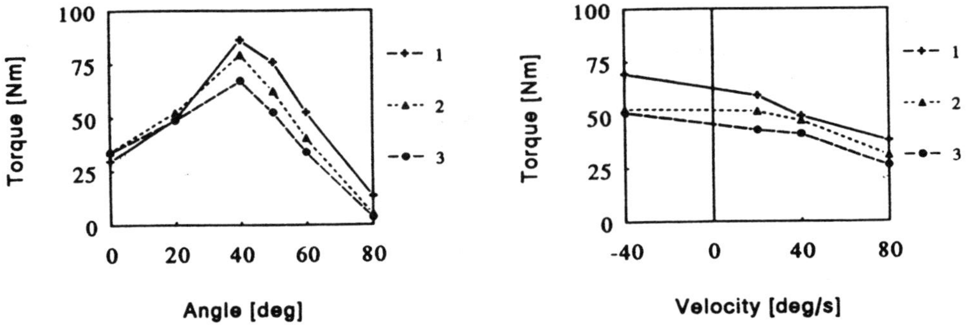

Fig. 4. Identification results of TN. (1): prior to fatigue trial 1, (2): after fatigue trial 3, (3): after fatigue trial 7. (IPI = 20 ms) **a**: Torque-angle relation. **b**: Torque-angular velocity relation.

4 Discussion

The apparent dependence of the quadriceps fatique curve on the isokinetic knee joint velocity has not been reported before. The dependence might be explained by lower metabolic efficiency (shortage in ATP or hihg IMP concentrations) of the total muscle or by complete exhaustion of fast twitch fibers, which are more susceptible to fatigue than slow twitch fibers.

Concering stimulation parameters, the results indicate that, within the boundary conditions for a given task, NP should be minimized to postpone fatigue. This can be accomplished by minimisation of DC and/or 1/IPI. The results may contribute to the derivation of an optimization criterion, describing muscle fatigue as a function of both joint movement and stimulation parameters.

References

Andrews, B. J., Barnett, R. W., Philips, G. F., and Kirkwood, C. A. (1989) Rule-based control of a hybrid FES orthosis for assisting paraplegic locomotion. *Automedica* **11**:175-199

Boom, H. B. K., Mulder, A. J., and Veltink, P.H. (1993) Fatigue during functional neuromuscular stimulation. *Progress in Brain Research* **97**: 409-418.

Levy, M., Mizrahi, J., and Susak, Z. (1990) Recruitment, force and fatigue characteristics of quadriceps muscles of paraplegics isometrically activated by surface functional electrical stimulation.. *J. Biomed. Eng.* **12**:150-156.

Chapter 3

Control Strategies in FES

A Comprehensive FES Control System for Mobility Restoration in Paraplegics

P. H. Veltink[1], W. de Vries[1,2], H. J. Hermens[2], G. Baardman[2], M. IJzerman[1,2], S. Heinze[1,2], A.V. Nene[2], G. Zilvold[2], H.B.K. Boom[1]
[1]Faculty of Electrical Engineering, University of Twente, Enschede, NL
[2]Roessingh Research and Development, Enschede, NL

Abstract - A comprehensive FES control system has been designed and partly tested, which controls Functional Electrical Stimulation (FES) to support the mobility tasks standing up, making a right or left step and sitting down. The control system features the detection of the intentions of the user by artificial sensory inputs and an intention detection finite state model of the tasks. No voluntary command input is required from the user during the use of the system. The control system is realised and tested as part of a hybrid system, consisting of a STEEPER Advanced Reciprocating Gait Orthosis (ARGO) and external stimulation of quadriceps, hip flexors and hamstrings using electrodes on the surface of the skin. The sensor system consists of spring preloaded switches in the crutches, which switch at a preset force, hip goniometers, hip and knee lock switches and accelerometers on trunc and upper leg. The sensors are integrated in the crutches or attached to the orthosis. The sensor and control system are to be further developed, such that it will be suitable for control of the CALIES implantable stimulation system.

1 Introduction

Stimulation systems have been developed for the restoration of mobility of paraplegic patients (Kralj et al., 1983; Marsolais and Kobetic, 1987; Solomonow et al., 1989). All of these systems need explicit control by the user during the performance of the mobility tasks. In most cases the control input is generated by the patient using manually operated switches. Andrews et al. (1989) introduced implicit intention detection using artificial sensors on the body used for the control of standing and gait. In this study we extend this principle of implicit intention detection also for the tasks standing-up and sitting-down and the automatic identification of the task to be performed.

2 Control System Design

The control system architecture has a multi-level architecture (see also Chizeck et al., 1988) (figure 1): the *high level intention detection*, the *intermediate task control level* and the *low level stimulation control*.

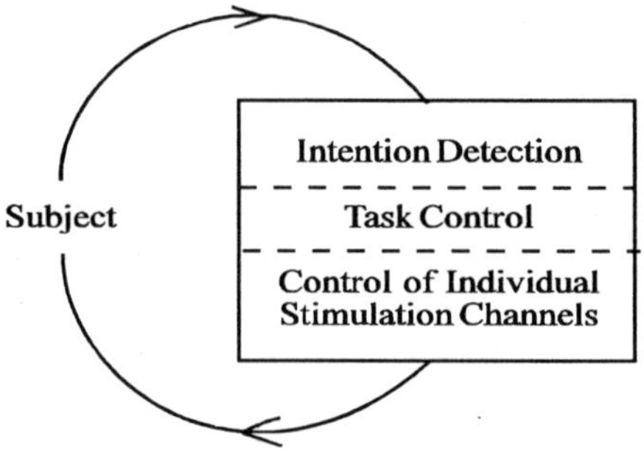

Fig. 1. Hierarchical structure of the FES mobility control system.

The structure of the *high level intention detection system* is shown in figure 2. The mobility tasks standing up, sitting down, making a right or left step are modeled as tranfers between stable states. The initiation of these state transfers is controlled by the intention of the user, which is implicitely detected by sensors on the orthosis and in the crutches:

transfer	detection conditions
stand up	- sitting posture - loading of crutches - anterior trunk movement
sit down	- standing posture - unlock of hip and knee locks of orthosis
step left	- right leg in front - loading of crutches
step right	- left leg in front - loading of crutches

In the current control system the patient has to transfer one of his/her legs in front by only upper body effort, before stimulation supported stepping is initiated. Stimulation support of the first step requires an extension of the current intention detection system.

Identification of the postures sitting and standing can be performed using tangentially directed accelerometers at the trunk and the upper leg (Veltink et al., 1993), statically measuring the inclinations of these body segments. The detection of the relative position of the legs during stance was performed by a goniometers at the hip, but can alternatively be performed by accelerometers on the upper leg.

At the *task control level* the coordination of a task is performed. Stimulation is only required during the dynamic transfer tasks standing up, sitting down, stepping left or right. The postures sitting and standing (both feet together, or one in front of the other) do not require stimulation, because the required stabilisation is realised by the orthosis.

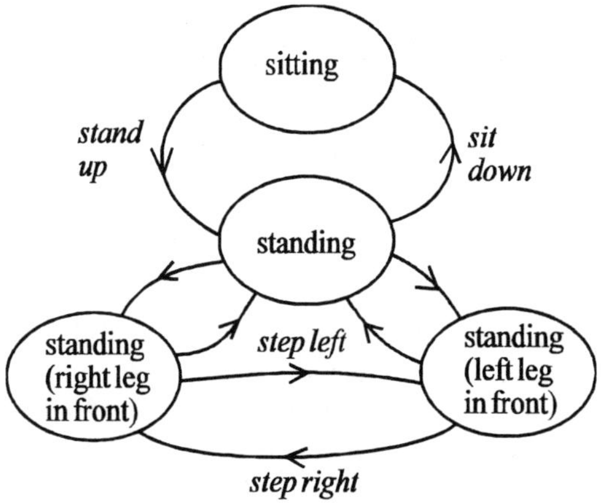

Fig. 2. Finite state model of mobility tasks. The mobility tasks standing up, sitting down, left step and right step are modeled as transfers between postures. The conditions for these transers are detected using artificial sensors on the orthosis and in the crutches.

The following muscle groups are stimulated during the performance of a transfer task:

transfer	stimulation
stand up	- quadriceps - hamstrings
sit down	- decay of quadriceps and hamstrings stimulation
step left	- left hip flexors - right hamstrings
step right	- right hip flexors - left hamstrings

In the current control system preset stimulation patterns are applied open loop, after the detection of the intention of a transfer task.

The *low level stimulation control* is in the current control system limited to stimulation of the muscles with fixed frequency, pulse width and pulse amplitude. Only the timing of the stimulation bursts are applied according to the commands from the intermediate layer.

3 Control System Realisation

The hybrid system consisted of a combination of surface stimulation and a STEEPER Advanced Reciprocating Gait Orthosis (ARGO). The control system required the following sensor set:

- Hip goniometer
- Spring preloaded switches in the crutches. The switches detect crutch loading above a preset force threshold.
- Hip and knee lock switches
- Upper leg and trunc accelerometers (tangentially mounted)

The hip goniometer, hip and knee lock switches and the accelerometers were attached to or integrated in the Steeper orthosis. Stimulation electrodes were mounted directly on the skin using self adhesive electrodes (Pals Axelgaard, 5x9 cm). The control system is first implemented on a portable controller/datalogger system (Infotronic Ultraflex) for initial testing, and subsequently in dedicated hardware. Two versions of the stimulator, designed at the Roessingh Research and Development, were used: an 8 channel programmable and a 4 channel non-programmable version.

4 Evaluation of the Control of Gait

Part of the control strategy has been tested up to now: control of gait (stepping right or left). The feasibility of intention detection for left and right steps on the basis of hip angles and crutch loading is illustrated in figure 3 to 5. Figure 3 illustrates the states which were defined for the coordination of making a step (on the intermediate task control level). The actual intention detection corresponds to the transfers from states 1 to 2 (left step) and from states 5 to 6 (right step). Figure 4 displays recordings from analog crutch force sensors and hip goniometers, on the basis of which the subsequent states could be detected (figure 5) (Franken et al., 1994).

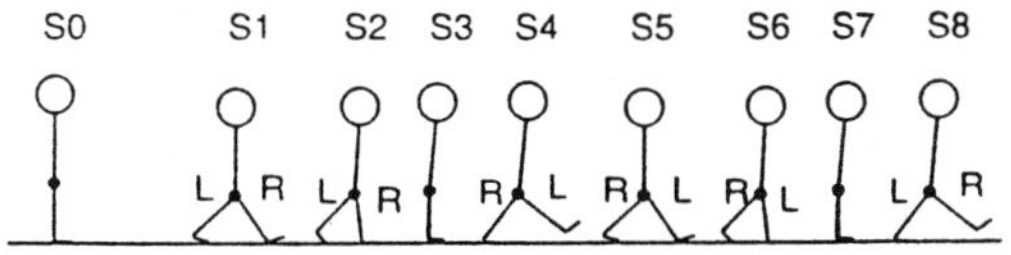

Fig. 3. Definition of 9 states for the finite state description of gait (Franken et al., 1994).

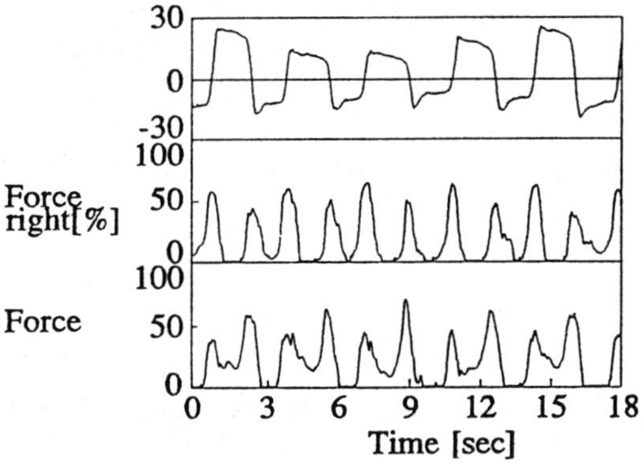

Fig. 4: Registration of the difference signal of the hip angles φ_d at both sides of the body measured by hip goniometers, and the crutch force signals measured by force transducers in the crutches during paraplegic locomotion (Franken et al., 1994).

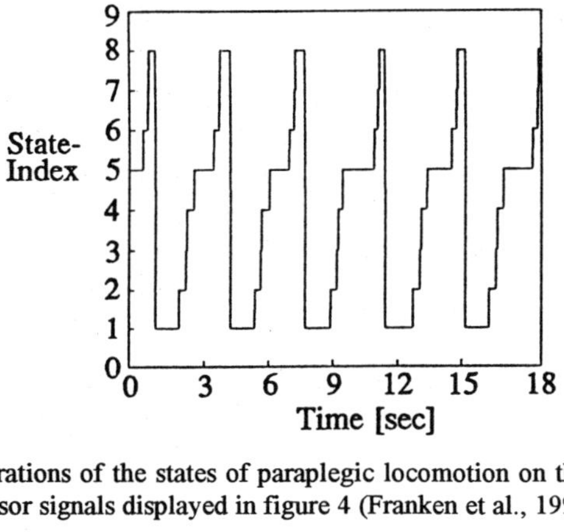

Fig. 5. Registrations of the states of paraplegic locomotion on the basis of the sensor signals displayed in figure 4 (Franken et al., 1994).

5 Discussion

In this paper, we presented a hierarchical control strategy, which requires minimal explicit attention from the user, because the intentions of the user with respect to the identification of the task to be perform and the moment of execution are automatically detected using a finite state model of the tasks and artificial sensors on the orthosis and on the crutches.

The total control strategy has to be further tested for evaluation of its performance and possible suggestions for improvements.

The control system has been designed in combination with an existing orthosis system and surface stimulation. Applicability of these principles in the control of implantable systems (e.g. the CALIES system) has to be investigated.

In the current control system preset stimulation patterns are applied open loop, after the detection of the intention of a transfer task. In future the stimulation patterns can be adjusted from step to step for gait, e.g. to control step length (Franken et al., 1994) or during transfers (e.g. Mulder et al., 1992; Veltink et al. 1994).

6 Acknowledgements

This research is supported by the European program INTERREG for regional development.

References

Andrews, B. J., Barnett, R. W., Phillips, G. F., and Kirkwood, C. A. (1989) Rule-based Control of a Hybrid FES Orthosis for Assisting Paraplegic Locomotion. *Automedica*, 11: 175-199.

Chizeck, H. J, Kobetic, R., Marsolais, E. B., Abbas, J. J., Donner, I. H., and Simon, E. (1988) Control of Neuromuscular Stimulation Systems for Standing and Locomotion in Paraplegics. *Proc. IEEE*, 76: 1155-1165.

Franken, H. M., Veltink, P. H., and Boom, H. B. K. (1984) Restoring Gait in Paraplegics by Functional Electrical Stimulation. *IEEE Engineering in Medicine and Biology Magazine*, 13: 564-570.

Kralj, A., Bajd, T., Turk, R., Krajnik, J., and Benko, H. (1983) Gait Restoration in Paraplegic Patients: a Feasibility Demonstration using Multichannel Surface Electrode FES. *J. Rehab. Res. and Dev.*, 20:3-20.

Marsolais, E. B. and Kobetic, R. (1987) Functional Electrical Stimulation for Walking in Paraplegia. *J. Bone and Joint Surgery*, 69-A: 728-733.

Mulder, A. J., Veltink, P. H., and Boom, H. B. K. (1992) On/off Control in FES-induced Standing Up: a Model Study and Experiments. *Med. & Biol. Eng. & Comput.*, 30: 205-212.

Solomonow, M., Baratta, R., Hirokawa, S., Rightor, N., Walker, W., Beaudette, P., Shoji, H., and D'Ambrosia, R. (1989) The RGO Generation II: Muscle Stimulation Powered Orthosis as a Practical Walking System for Thoracic Paraplegics. *Orthopedics*, 12: 1309-1315.

Veltink, P. H., Franken, H. M., de Vries, W., Baardman, G., and Boom H. B. K. (1993) Artificial Sensors in Feedback Control of FES supported Paraplegic Ambulation. *Proceedings of the Ljubljana FES conference*, Ljubljana, Slovenia, 85-88.

Veltink, P. H., Bussmann, H. B. J., Koelma, F., Martens, W. L. J., Van Lummel, R. C. (1993) The feasibility of Posture and Movement Detection by Accelerometry. *Proc. 15th Annual International Conference of the IEEE-EMBS*, San Diego, 1230-1231.

Veltink, P. H., Geerdink, B. M., Koopman, B. F. J. M., Huijing, P. A., and Boom, H. B. K. (1994) Control of FES-Assisted Standing-Up in Paraplegics - The Role of Mono- and Biarticular Muscles. *Proc. IEEE Eng. in Med & Biol. Soc. 16th Annual Int. Conf.*, Baltimore, November 3-6, 444-445.

Control of the First Generation CALIES Implants

J. H. Hermens, G. Baardman
Roessingh Research and Development Centre, Enschede - The Netherlands

Abstract - In May 1993 a special CALIES Technical Workgroup meeting took place in Enschede in The Netherlands, with representatives of INSERM Montpellier, Centre Propara Montpellier, Twente University Enschede and Roessingh Research & Development Enschede. The goal of this meeting was to make a proposal for the definition of the control system of the first generation of CALIES implants. This paper reflects the results of this meeting.

1 Introduction

1.1 General

The planned simultaneous implantation in five different countries in Europe necessitates a so called 'cook book' approach in order to standardize the peri-surgical procedures of all participating groups and, as a consequence, to insure comparability of the results. The cook book is meant for the national teams of rehabilitation physicians and technicians. It should provide the exact procedures according to which the patient has to be prepared, tested and evaluated and according to which the patient is provided with increasing functional possibilities of the CALIES system. This means that the cook book includes chapters like:

- procedures for testing, training and adjustment of stimulation parameters
- procedures for evaluation, including the evaluation forms.

In fact this is the same approach as used by the Rehabilitation group of the CALIES network. The clinicians work on an extensive description of the rehabilitation program. They have an additional reason for it: they need it for the Ethical Committee in order to get clearance for implantation.

It is to be expected that the control cook book will result in certain prerequisites for the rehabilitation program; a number of muscles have to be trained to reach a certain force and endurance.

The cook book must be constantly updated. This can be done best when a small project group works constantly on it. A structure is considered in which this project group is part of the technical group of the CALIES network coordinated by prof. Pedotti. The project group could function as clinical knowledge centre and provide guidelines to scientists working on design of control strategies.

1.2 Control

With respect to the first generation CALIES implants, the following starting points were agreed:

- The first implants will be applied in low lesion patients.
  The reason for this is that control becomes easier as the patient has some stability around the hip/trunk region.
- The patient will use at least ankle foot orthoses.
  At this moment we cannot foresee to what extent the patient needs an orthosis to stabilize the hip. The philosophy of the rehabilitation program is that after surgery the patient starts with a complete orthosis for safety reasons, but the goal is to minimize it to the use of only ankle foot orthoses.
- Only 'proven' technology will be used, meaning:
  - control strategies that were applied successfully in patients in experimental conditions
  - externally mounted sensors
- The system must be an extension of the neuromuscular system of the patient. This means that:
  - the system should behave in a predictable manner
  - training is essential

2 Control System Layout

The proposed control system is based on the -nowadays commonly applied- hierarchical control concept. Control is divided into two levels: patient controlled supervision of the programs (high level) and low level task control.

2.1 High level control

The high level concerns the coordination and selection of the programs incorporated in the first generation control system. It consists of a small number of programs, each subject to a rule base that defines the entry and exit criteria (transition rules). With this rule base, the possible routes through programs are established.

The rule base definition depends on the sensors and patient command interface (PCI) incorporated in the control system, and vice versa. The sensor and PCI inputs define a set of system states, each of which having a corresponding rule.

Also dependent on the sensors in the system, part of the high level control may be automated; starting point, however, is that the patient is always in supervision of the programs.

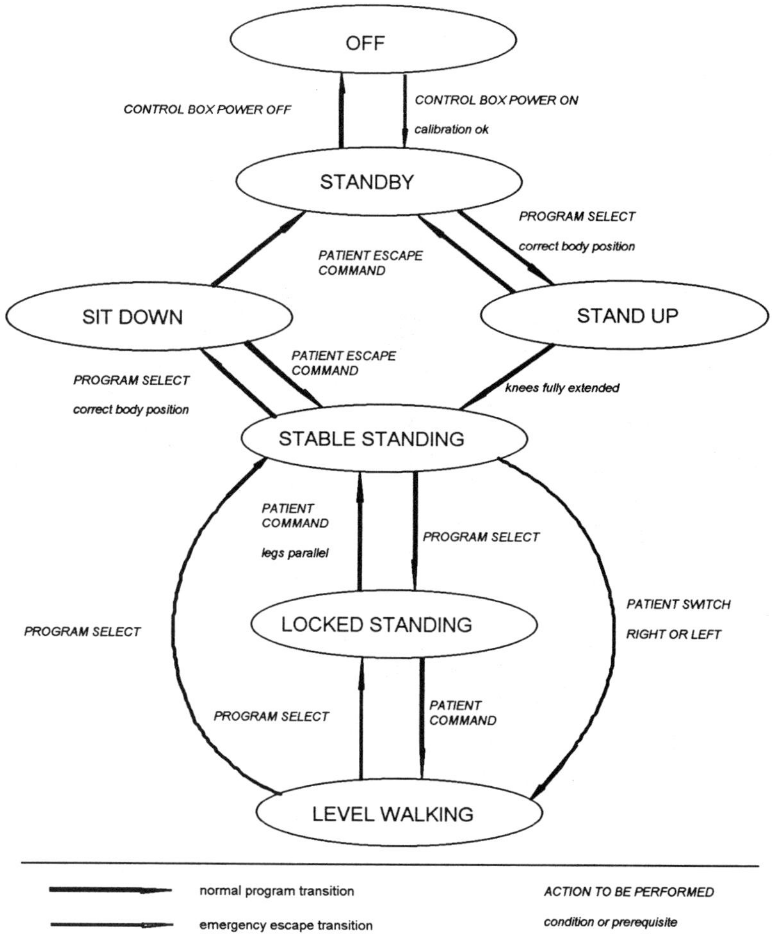

Fig. 1. Schematic representation of the control system's high level

The programs and transition rules of the high level control are shown in figure 1.

Beside the necessary programs for standing up, sitting down, standing and level walking, a seperate program is incorporated for so called *locked standing*. The difference between stable standing and locked standing is in the control: open loop during locked standing and closed loop for stable standing. The main reason for this additional program is the lack of knowledge of the performance of closed loop controlled stable standing. We cannot foresee whether this control is accurate enough to ensure the patient safe standing with one hand free or a quick turn on the spot.

Level walking is the more complex of the programs, i.e. it consists of a number of patient controlled states. Since the high level of control reaches into this program, it is elaborated seperately below.

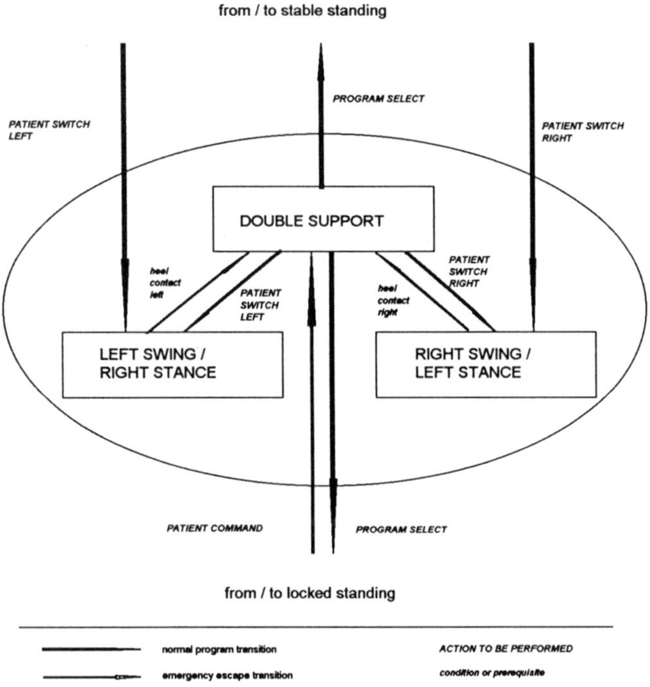

Fig. 2. Schematic representation of the LEVEL WALKING program

Three different states are discerned: double support, left swing and right swing. The swing states are entered by the patient pressing a switch. Both swing states will end in the double support state when heel contact of the swinging leg has been reached. It was chosen not to discriminate between left and right double support states, thus allowing the patient to step again with the same leg, e.g. when the step length is insufficient.

2.2 Low level control

The low level concerns the control of joint stability and movements within programs. This level of control operates without the patient's consciousness being necessary.

For each of the programs shown in figure 1, a low level control algorithm was defined in terms of control tasks. The main tasks in the different algorithms are described below.

2.2.1 Stand up

Before standing up, the patient has to get into a good position, which means: feet on the ground, crutches in front of him and than initiates a command. The system checks the correct body position and gives a sign back. At the moment that the patient loads his crutches the system will be activated and the quadriceps will be stimulated. This will be done in an open loop fashion.

When the knees are fully extended, the program transition to stable standing will be performed automatically.

2.2.2 Stable standing

Because of the well known dramatic effect of muscular fatigue, it is considered absolutely necessary to incorporate closed loop control in the stable standing program. Otherwise the patient will only be able to perform standing during 2 or 3 minutes. As we will use only technology that has proven to be feasible, there are 2 options:

- The finite state closed loop controlled hybrid system that was developed by Andrews (Andrews et al., 1989). In this control scheme either the extension force above the knee or the dorsal flexion force around the ankle (described in a previous system) has to be measured in order to detect stability of the knee.
- The modified on/off artificial reflex control system for the knee that was developed by Mulder at Twente University (Mulder et al., 1990). In this system two states are discerned: knee locked and knee unlocked. When the knee is locked the stimulation amplitude is decreased. The transition to the knee-unlock state is detected by the knee angle exceeding a treshold value. When this happens the stimulation amplitude is immediately increased upto a pregiven value. Knee-lock is detected by a zero knee angle velocity. The advantage of using the velocity is that it can be used to recalibrate the knee angle.

With respect to the hip we consider to use a similar artificial reflex control system. This means that if the hip flexion ankle exceeds a treshold, the hip extensors will be stimulated. In both knee and hip control systems the patient will be warned about insufficient performance by using for instance the locking velocity and the time or range of the instability situation.

With respect to performance of the closed loop system it is very important that the patient trains with it, as the efficiency of the system depends largely on the posture of the patient. In fact the patient has to learn to stand in the so called C-posture. Standing in the C-posture will cause the closed loop system to stop stimulating the muscles and therefore to avoid fatigue.

2.2.3 Locked standing

The locked standing program comprises open loop stimulation of hip and knee extensors. Since during this activity the muscles will fatigue very rapidly, acoustic warning to the patient will be started after 30 seconds.

2.2.4 Level walking

The low level control algorithm is depicted below.

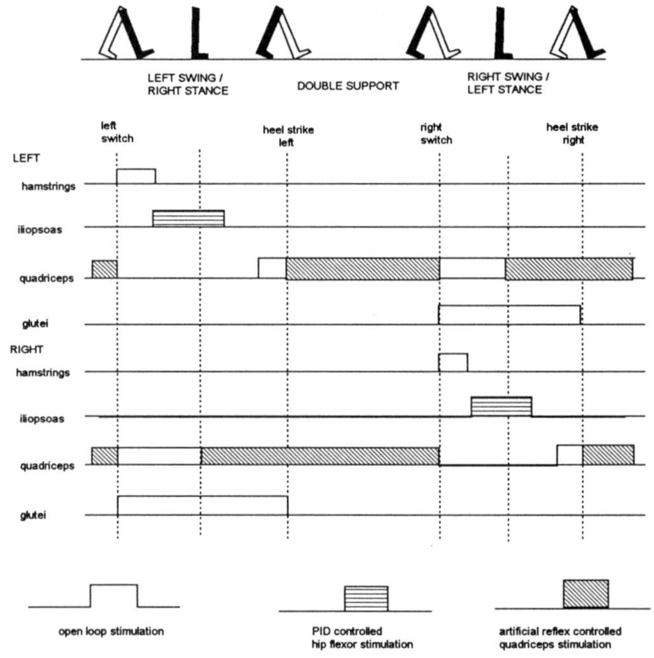

Fig. 3. Timing diagram of the LEVEL WALKING low level controller

The level walking control makes use of stimulation of quadriceps for knee stabilisation, gluteus for hip stabilisation and propulsion, hamstrings for effecting foot clearance at initial swing and iliopsoas for inducing a hip flexion moment during the swing phase of gait.

During the double support phase the same artificial reflex closed loop stimulation of the quadriceps muscles will be used as was described for stable standing.

Stimulation during the swing phase consists of preset stimulation of hamstrings, followed by PID controlled stimulation of iliopsoas and open loop quadriceps stimulation to obtain knee extension at terminal swing.

Iliopsoas stimulation is controlled by cycle-to-cycle PID control of the stimulation burst duration (Franken et al., 1993). Within one swing phase the stimulation parameters are fixed. At terminal swing, the established hip flexion angle (as measure for the obtained step length) is evaluated and new stimulation parameters are calculated according to preset criteria for the next swing phase. This swing phase controller was developed and tested during the past year at Twente University and Roessingh Research and Development.

Gluteus stimulation is on during the complete stance phase in order to increase propulsive forces and stabilize the stance leg's hip.

At initial stance, the quadriceps stimulation is switched to open loop for safety reasons; after the centre of gravity has passed the knee joint of the stance leg, control is reset to closed loop artificial reflex stimulation.

3 Sensors and Patient Command Interface

As was mentioned before, the layout and performance of both high and low control levels are strongly dependent on the configuration of the sensors and patient command interface.

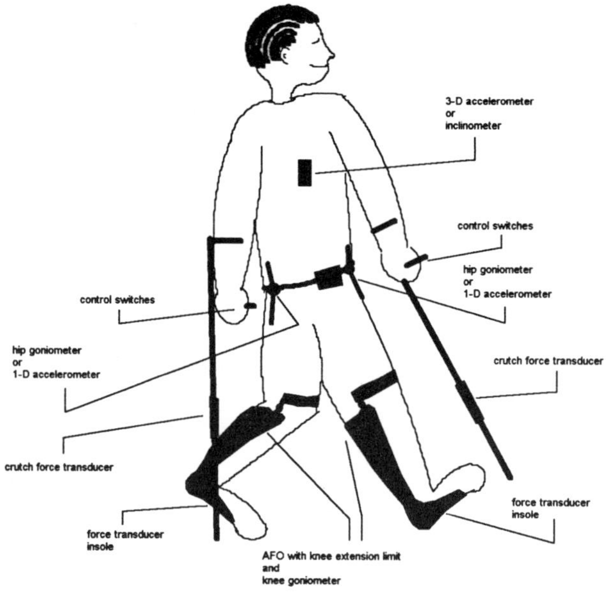

Fig. 4. Configuration of sensors

In general, a higher number of sensors results in a higher observability of the controlled system. However, from a user friendliness point of view, a low number of sensors is preferable. With the set of sensors depicted in figure 4, a compromise can be found that is sufficient for the control system layout described in the last section.

The patient command interface must be designed in such a manner that the necessary patient intervention can be established in a safe, simple and unambiguous way. There are no clear ideas yet about the actual make up of the interface. Nevertheless it is quite clear that the traditional interface, one push button at each crutch, is not enough. An ergonomic study will be performed on how the functions could be performed by the patient in an easy and very reliable way.

4 Conclusion

We can conclude that the first meeting was a very succesful one. The concepts and a global plan for the whole control were defined and seem feasible. We must be aware that this definition of the control system is meant to be a realistic plan for the first generation CALIES implants; later generations will necessitate and enable further sophistication of the control.

References

Andrews, B. J., Barnett, R. W., Phillips, G. F., and Kirkwood, C. A. (1989) Rule-based control of a hybrid FES orthosis for assisting paraplegic locomotion. *Automedica*, **11**, p. 175-199.

Franken, H. M., Veltink, P. H., Baardman, G., Redmeijer, R. A., and Boom, H. B. K. (1993) Optimized experimental control of FES-induced swing phase of paraplegic gait. *Proceedings of the Ljubljana FES Conference*, p. 69-71.

Mulder, A. J., Boom, H. B. K., Hermens, H. J., and Zilvold, G. (1990) Artificial-reflex stimulation for FES-induced standing with minimum quadriceps force. *Medical and Biological Engineering and Computing*, **28**, p. 483-488.

Description of the CALIES External Controller

D. Guiraud[1,2], M. Beliaeff[1], B. Gilbert[2], J. C. Repetto[1], E. Rabischong[3]
[1] MXM, Antibes, France
[2] INSERM U103, Montpellier, France
[3] PROPARA, Montpellier, France

Abstract - the first version of the CALIES external controller has been designed to give practicians a flexible and efficient tool. Then, it can be used with external (surface) or internal (implanted) stimulation during all the phases of CALIES implantation programme. It can also emulate the final portable version of the programmer, with the same hardware and software configurations.

1 Introduction

In the CALIES project, one of the most difficult problem is the design of the external controller. Following the discussions in the CALIES meeting in Dusseldorf (1992), we try to realise a dedicated but flexible system. We achieve a prototype now partially operational. This paper tries to explain the "philosophy" of the design and justifies the choices we have done.

2 General Description

The CALIES implantation procedure includes three important phases as far as stimulation type is concerned. The pre-surgical phase will concern only surface stimulation, the post-surgical phase only implanted stimulation, and during the surgery direct stimulation of the electrodes (with an external ASIC) must be available. These first considerations induce the following constraints:

1. Possibility of doing internal or external stimulations with the same protocol and same material, to avoid errors on result's interpretation, and to simplify practician's work.
2. Portability of the system. No card in the PC, only optocoupled RS transmissions. This feature allows us to use portable computer or any other one without problems. This ensures the total safety of the patient.
3. Autonomous functioning without PC to use in the post-surgical phase and to simulate the final CALIES portable programmer.
4. Flexibility of reprogramming to implement new control strategies.

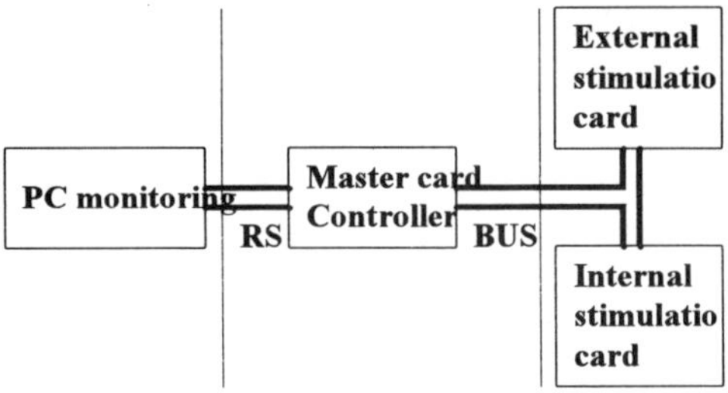

Fig. 1. CALIES controller 3-levels architecture.

To achieve these goals, we decide to make a three levels hardware and software architecture as it is shown on figure 1.

The low level concerns what we call slave cards dedicated to each type of stimulation. They receive common type of orders like "stimulation on the channel n with this kind of pulse pattern", so that the upper level sees only little differences between both stimulation types (only number of channels and range of stimulation intensity change). These cards are programmed one time for ever, and a new implantation of algorithms does not concern them.

The second level includes the real intelligence of the system. It contains all the control strategies and stimulation protocols as fatigue or recruitment measurements. This card can run in an autonomous mode without any connection to PC, and provides the five CALIES movements selected by the patient himself. In this mode, the patient characteristics must be totally determined. When the card is connected to a PC via optocoupled RS232C, a dialogue can be established. This mode includes an important variety of protocols controlled by the PC (choice of parameters, interpretation of the results) but effectively done by the master card (time control, intensity ramp, data acquisition...) so that the RS232C is used only to exchange parameters and results, not to control the stimulator. This mode can be used to evaluate patient characteristics (fatigue, recruitment, pendulum test,...), to check the system integrity (electrode impedances both implanted and surface, tests of ASIC, ...); to store patient characteristics in the master card (computed by the PC), to monitor the final implanted system functioning in real conditions, ...

The third level is the PC itself. This level is used to do off-line computation, data archiving, adjustments of control parameters, experimental mode,...

The system is very flexible and easy to use because there is no hardware or software modifications to do on both slave cards. A new function or control strategy consists in modifying master card software and if necessary, PC software menu extensions. The only constraint is to respect dialogue protocol between the master card and the slave cards, and between the master card and the PC. Finally, the hardware architecture of the cards is shown on the figure 2.

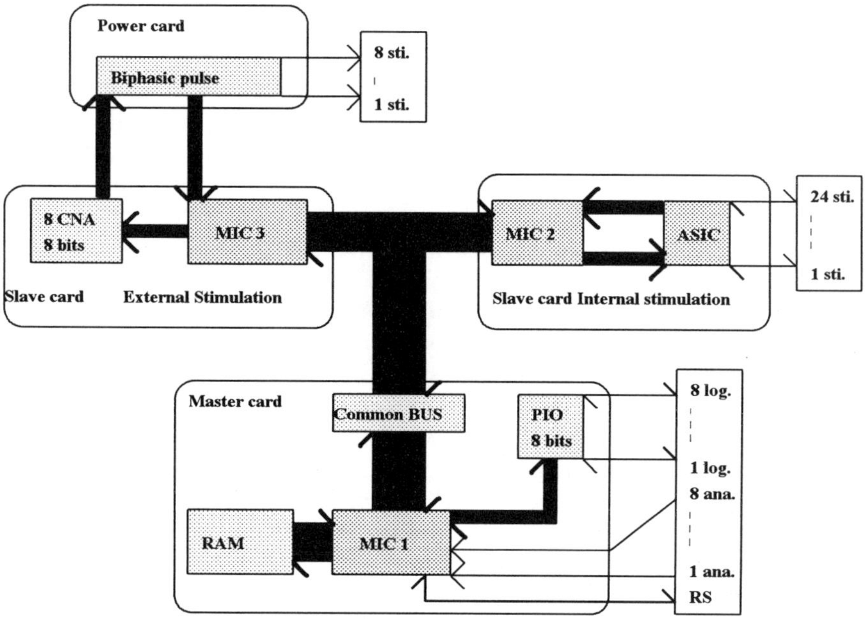

Fig. 2. CALIES controller architecture.

The characteristics of the external stimulation delivered by the stimulator are:

1. Eight channels biphasic 300µs pulses with a maximum intensity of 180mA (1.5 kΩ load).
2. The current is measured and controlled.
3. Stimulation pattern (4 groups of 2 channels) can be simplet, cyclic doublet, cyclic triplet, with programmable frequency of stimulation and programmable interpulse time within a doublet or a triplet.

The characteristics of the internal stimulation are:

1. 24 channels stimulation (14 bipolar, 10 monopolar), pulse width modulation (0-500µs).
2. ranges of intensity (0-2mA 0-20mA).
3. Same stimulation pattern as above (4 groups of 6 channels).
4. Programmable interpulse delay between cathodal phase and anodal recovery phase.

The master card includes 8 analogue inputs (10 bits) and 8 logic IO.

3 Function

Different functions are already available : measurement of electrode impedances, hardware testing, edition and visualisation of patient characteristics, simple stimulation on one channel with the selection of all stimulation parameters, fatigue and recruitment curves with calculation of models, pendulum test with second order model evaluation (for the hips and the knees), PID control of the swinging leg (for the hips and the knees). All these parameters are stored in a file for each patient.

We are now developing the part of the software devoted to autonomous functioning including the five CALIES basic movements : stand up, seat down, keep standing, walking, go up or downstairs. For the moment, only the control strategies for the first three movements are known. The practician has to choose which channel controls which of the five necessary muscles, and must do all the tests for these ten muscles (fatigue, recruitment, pendulum test on the four joints), then the computer evaluates the optimal control parameters that can be adjusted by the practician. This part of the software is not yet available and still in development.

4 Conclusions

A first version of the CALIES external controller was developed. Some work has to be finished, in particular on the master card we have to implement all the software for autonomous functioning. Moreover we have to develop some extra softwares for the slave card dedicated to the ASIC (implanted part). The product has been tested on patients and has done very good results, in particular due to the accurate current control. The portability of the system and the flexibility of the software allow a very simple use and reproducible experiments. We are studying new technologies to reduce the dimensions of the master card and the slave cards, and we hope to obtain the size of a walkman.

References

Veltink, P. H. (1991) Control of FES induced cyclical movements of the lower leg. *Med. & Biol. Eng. & Comput.*, **29:** NS8-NS12.

Guiraud, D. (1993) Thesis Système de contrôle du mouvement du membre inférieur à base de réseaux de neurones artificiels : restauration de la marche chez le paraplégique, Ecole Centrale de Paris.

Guiraud, D., Gilbert, B., and Rabischong, E., (1995), The use of new technologies in the restoration of gaitin paraplegic patients. *Proc. of IEEE Conference on Systems, Man and Cybernetics*, Vancouver, 22-25 October.

Design of a Multi-Sensor Closed-Loop Neurostimulator Part A: Communication Unit with Wireless Data Link and Digital Signal Processor

M. Keller[1], P. Krauß[1], G. Hoch[2], J. Quintern[3]
[1]Department for Data Processing, Technical University, Munich, Germany
[2]Neurological Clinic Bad Aibling, Bad Aibling, Germany
[3]Neurological Clinic, Klinikum Grosshadern, University of Munich, Germany

Abstract - A versatile neurostimulator was developed to permit complex closed-loop applications of functional electrical stimulation (FES) via surface electrodes. The mobile unit carried by the patient consists of a data acquisition unit, a stimulation unit, a digital signal processor (DSP) unit, a communication unit, and a user interface. The DSP unit with fast static random access memory provides enough calculation power for sensor signal processing and complex closed-loop stimulation algorithms. Additionally, non-volatile flash-memory allows fail-safe data-logging in the mobile unit. These features allow the mobile unit to operate in stand-alone operation mode. For remote control of the mobile unit and data transmission to the laboratory PC, two different kinds of data exchange with the laboratory PC were employed. A wireless radio-frequency data link provides high flexibility inside and outside the laboratory. For operation in noisy environments an additional fiberoptic data connection was implemented. The whole system will be submitted for approval for clinical use according to the standards of the European Union (EU).

1 Introduction

Today clinically applied motor neural prostheses are still open-loop systems with preprogrammed stimulation patterns. The feasiblity and superiority of closed-loop control have been proven in a variety of experiments (Quintern et al. 1989). Other methods to improve current FES systems such as automatic intention detection (Veltink et al. 1996) and model-based control (Quintern et al. 1996) cannot be accomplished with the hardware presently approved for clinical application.

The design of this new stimulation system was motivated by the desire for a versatile neurostimulator which enables complex open-loop and closed-loop FES applications not restricted to the laboratory environment. Since stimulation programs should be easy to change for experimental purposes, bidirectional data transmission lines were used to allow a remote-control operation mode with the controller implemented in the laboratory PC. A wireless data link provides complete galvanic isolation from the PC and a high data transfer rate combined with optimal spatial flexibility. As a backup for use in a noisy environment, a fiberoptic connection is also available. When the mobile unit is used as a stand-alone device, real-time execution of closed-loop algorithms requires a high processing speed, which is provided by a 32 bit digital signal processor (DSP) unit. With 32 analog inputs, 8 digital I/O channels, and 16 completely independent stimulation channels (Weiss et al. 1996) even complex closed-loop FES applications are possible. The system will be submitted for approval for clinical use according to the European standards EN 60601-1 and EN60601-2-10.

2 Methods and Results

2.1 Structural Overview

The complete stimulator system consists of two parts: the basic unit and the mobile unit carried by the patient.

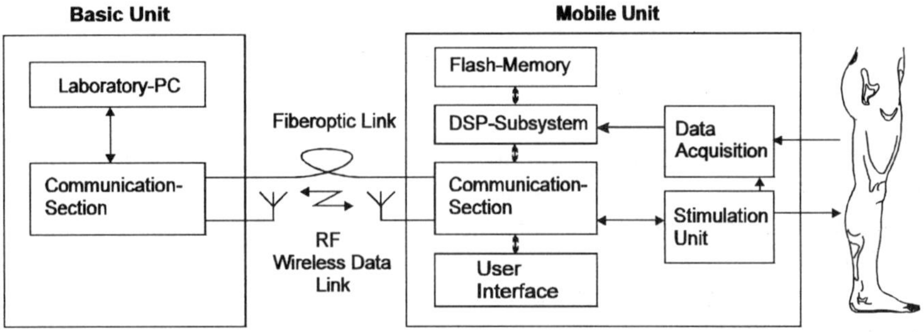

Fig. 1. Block diagram of the stimulation system

2.2 Operation Modes

The stimulator can operate in stand-alone mode as well as in data-coupling to the laboratory PC. The following three operation modes are possible.

2.2.1 Remote control

In the remote-control mode the laboratory PC uses the mobile unit for data acquisition and for output of stimulation pulses according to the transmitted commands. In this case the stimulation controller is implemented in the PC. If measured data from all analog input channels have to be transferred at a high rate from the mobile unit to the PC and the stimulation commands in the opposite direction, the required data rate may be higher than the wireless RF-link can handle (625 kbit/s). A fiberoptic connection solves the restricted data rate problem.

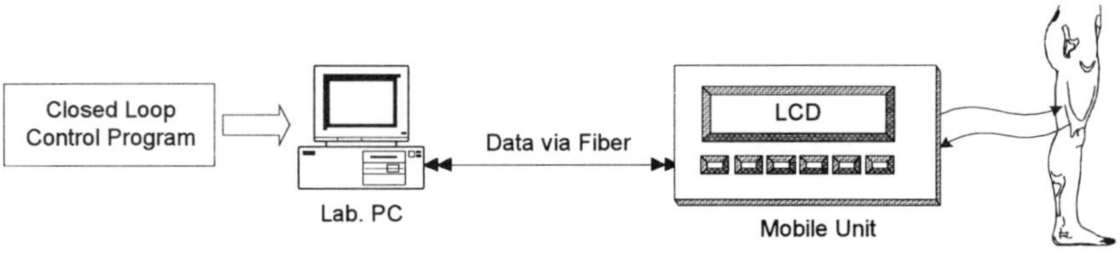

Fig. 2. Remote control operation mode

2.2.2 Stand-alone operation mode with data transmission

During stand-alone operation the integrated digital signal processor provides enough computational power for complex closed-loop stimulation programs to operate in real-time. Datalogging is performed in the PC, which receives the data via the data link. The control program is developed on the PC using cross-compiler software and then loaded into the digital signal processor memory.

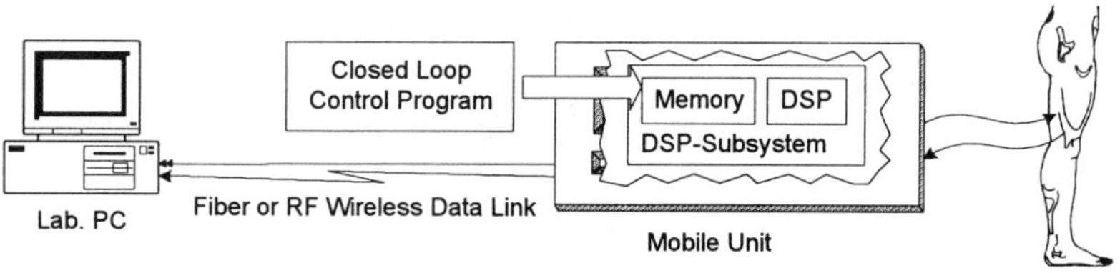

Fig. 3. Stand-alone operation mode with data transmission

2.2.3 Stand-alone operation mode (without data transmission)

In this operation mode the mobile unit works independently. This mode is useful for carring out a training program or for testing stimulation strategies outside the laboratory environment. User dialogue takes place via keyboard and alphanumeric display. For datalogging there is a non-volatile flash memory in the mobile unit.

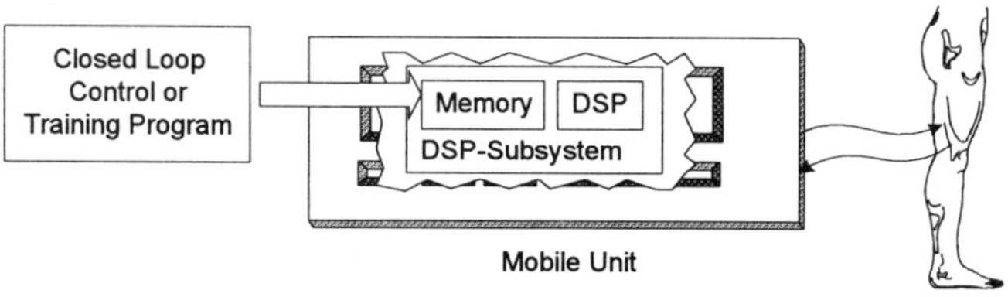

Fig. 4. Stand-alone operation mode

2.3 Safety considerations

The most important safety issue is to prevent harm to the patient in case of technical failure. When the neurostimulator is used for locomotion, there are two main risks: (1) the risk of damage to the patient by inadequate electrical currents and (2) the risk of falling due to a malfunction of the device.

To prevent the first risk, the device was designed according to the concept of passive safety (see part B, Weiss et al. 1996). The complete, galvanic isolation of the communication unit from the PC and mains current supply was achieved by using radio-frequency or optic data-transmission instead of conventional cable.

The second risk, a fall of the patient, could be caused by a failure of data transmission. The following modes of failure have to be considered with respect to data transmission:

I. *Break-down of transmission.* If no further stimulation commands are transmitted, the microcontroller in the output stage switches to an emergency routine. This usually consists of stimulation of the anti-gravity muscles, thus preventing the patient from falling.

II. *Error during transmission.* In case of an error in transmission, the communication protocol detects the false data block with help of the included error checking (CRC-CCITT). The respective block will be ignored and retransmitted. As a result, risk II is not critical as long as the transmission of the stimulation commands succeeds at the right time. Otherwise, the emergency routine operates (I.).

2.4 Hardware and software realization

2.4.1 Communication section

The communication section is responsible for data and command transfers between the basic unit and the mobile unit. A radio-frequency part and a fiberoptic interface are located in this section.

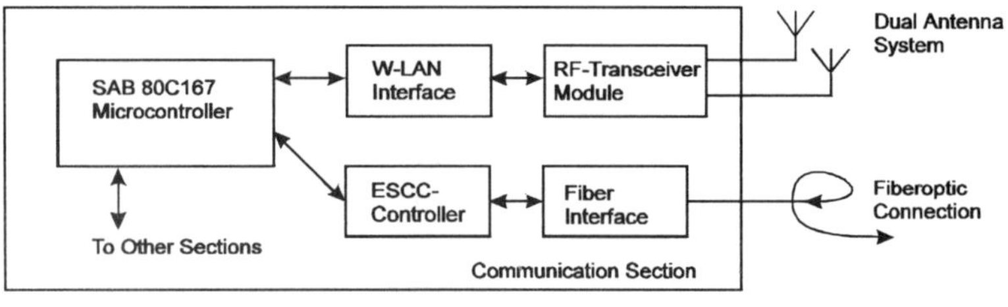

Fig. 5. Communication section

Wireless data link at 2.4 GHz in the license-free ISM band

The requirements of a high data transmission rate combined with small size and low power consumption can be fulfilled only at a very high carrier frequency. The wireless frequency band used lies in the range of 2.4 to 2.5 GHz and is called the *ISM* band for *I*ndustrial, *S*cientific and *M*edical purposes. It can span more than 50 meters, transmitting a maximum uncoded data rate of 625 kbit/s. The RF-transceiver module (GEC Plessey DE6003) looks like a credit card and is about 4 mm thick; the miniature antennas are about 35 mm long.

The problems of interference and fading are always present in mobile wireless applications. The spread spectrum frequency hopping technique (Dixon 1994) with dual diversity provides high resistance to fading by using two antennas at different places in the electromagnetic field, e.g., for $\lambda = 124$ mm at a distance of 93 mm. High resistance to interference is achieved by the receiver's ability to select the best transmission channel by frequency hopping.

A special wireless LAN-circuit converts data according to a protocol. Its functionality covers several requirements, for example, the Cyclic Redundancy Check for error detection. The software of the microcontroller features media access and packet protocol. Special hardware codec-devices (e.g., Viterbi FEC) can be easily integrated to improve error correction.

Fiberoptic data transmission

The bidirectional fiberoptic connection achieves a maximum data rate of 2 Mbit/s full-duplex. It works according to the HDLC-standard with packet-orientated serial synchronous data transmission (Spragins 1992). The plastic duplex light wave leader used as fiber results in a thin, light, and robust cable which is inexpensive.

2.4.2 Basic Unit

The basic unit consists of a laboratory PC and an AT-bus card with the communication section. The PC interface is supported by a microcontroller on the AT-bus card to reduce PC load.

2.4.3 Mobile Unit

The mobile unit contains the communication section, DSP-system, input and output stage, and a user interface. User dialogue to the patient is established with an alphanumeric LC-display and a keyboard for inputs. A buzzer signals alarm situations.

Digital Signal Processor Subsystem with Flash Memory

A floating point digital signal processor TMS 320C32 is used as calculator for the stimulation programs or for sensor data pre-processing. Processing speed is 50 MFLOPS working up to 40 bit precise floating point operands. The processor is designed for highly parallel operations and contains 2 Kbytes internal single-cycle dual access RAM and a separate instruction cache. One Mbyte of fast static external memory in a SIMM module is included together with 8 Mbytes non-volatile flash memory. The latter provides sector erase and write, e.g., for data logging or program storage. This configuration is the result of a compromise between power consumption and performance in a battery-driven mobile unit.

The DSP software is developed with a cross-compiler on the PC and is then loaded via a boot loader from the PC into the flash memory of the mobile unit. This ensures comfortable software development.

Input and output stage

The input and output stages are described in Part B (Weiss et al. 1996).

3 Conclusions

The flexible design of this neurostimulator and its data links permit a broad spectrum of applications. The fiberoptic link makes the system an ideal tool for FES experiments and the testing of new control strategies in the laboratory. The 32 sensor inputs and 16 stimulation channels are a prerequisite for the development of complex closed-loop FES systems. Due to the powerful built-in DSP, the stimulator can be used as a stand-alone device, which can perform complex control algorithms such as model-based control. The DSP and the user interface allow use of the neurostimulator outside research laboratories, e.g., in a hospital or a patient's home. The wireless link permits observation of the patient indoor and outdoor during training sessions; alternatively data can be logged in the flash memory. After the system will have been approved by an authorized institution, a small number will be built for laboratory experiments and clinical studies.

References

Dixon, Robert C. (1994) Spread Spectrum Systems with Commercial Applications, John Wiley & Sons, Inc., New York

Quintern, J., Minwegen, P., Mauritz, K.-H. (1989) Control mechanisms for restoring posture and movements in paraplegics. In: J.H.J Allum, M. Hulliger (eds.) *Progress in Brain Research*, **80**, Elsevier, Amsterdam, pp. 489-502.

Quintern, J., Riener, R., Volz, S., Rupprecht, S., Straube, A. (1996) Inverse models for control of movements. This volume, pp. 255-262.

Spragins, D. (1992) Telecommunications, Protocols and Design, Addison-Wesley, New York.

Veltink, P.H., de Vries, W., Hermens, H.J., Baardman, G., Ijzerman, M., Heinze, S., Nene, A.V., Zilvold, G., Boom, H.B.K. (1996) A comprehensive FES control system for mobility restoration in paraplegics. This volume, pp. 163-170.

Weiss, A., Krauß, P., Hoch, G., Quintern, J. (1996) Design of a Multi-Sensor Closed-Loop Neurostimulator. Part B: Input and Output Stage. This volume, pp. 189-193.

Design of a Multi-Sensor Closed-Loop Neurostimulator Part B: Input and Output Stage

A. Weiß[1,3], P. Krauß[1], G. Hoch[2], J. Quintern[3]
[1]Dept. of Data Processing, Technical University, Munich, Germany
[2]Neurological Clinic Bad Aibling, Germany
[3]Neurological Clinic, Klinikum Grosshadern, University of Munich, Germany

Abstract - A multichannel neurostimulator was designed for closed-loop applications of functional electrical stimulation (FES) using surface electrodes. The device has 32 analog inputs, 16 output amplifiers, high calculation power and a communication unit with wireless data link to the laboratory computer. The device is intended to be approved for clinical application according to the European standards for medical devices EN60601-1 and EN60601-2-10.

1 Introduction

In countries of the European Union (EU) not only commercially available electrical nerve stimulators, but also neurostimulators which are used in clinical studies and laboratory experiments have to be approved according to the European standards for medical devices (EN 60601-1 1991; EN60601-2-10 1989). These standards considerably influence the design of the stimulator, especially the design of the output stages. Two design strategies guarantee that the electrical parameters stay within the required limits: active control and passive safety. Active control requires at least two independent electronic circuits that control the output parameters of the stimulator, and switch it off if critical values are exceeded. The control circuits themselves have to be controlled during power-up. If microcontrollers or other programmable devices are part of the control structure, the whole software has to undergo a costly approval process by an authorized agency. In contrast to active control, passive safety is based on a self-limiting design. One problem of this concept is that the safety margins, which are needed to guarantee the observance of the limits in the case of malfunctioning parts, may restrict performance of the device.
The aim of our project was to design a versatile closed-loop functional electrical stimulation system suitable for clinical application (Keller et al. 1996). To enable multijoint feedback control, a system with 32 analog input channels, 16 independent output stages, and high calculation power was planned. The system had to provide high performance reserves despite strict safety regulations, which have to be observed for approval for use in Europe.

2 Methods

2.1 Safety requirements for patient protection

The risk analysis (tab. 1) shows that most restrictions affect the output stage.

A	output current limit for an equivalent 500Ω-load: DC: **I < 80 mA** f < 400 Hz: **I < 50 mA** f < 1500 Hz: **I < 80 mA** f > 1500 Hz: **I < 100 mA** To fulfill these requirements without considering each frequency range, we chose a maximum power output of 1.25 W ($P = I^2 * R$, I = 50 mA) over the complete frequency range.
B	output energy limit for pulses with a maximal length of 0.1s for an equivalent 500Ω-load: $\mathbf{E_{puls} < 300mJ}$
C	output voltage limit: $\mathbf{U_{max} < 500V}$
D	current between two electrode pairs (input or output) is limited to 500μA
E	fail-safe design to prevent the patient from falling

Tab.1. Rules for a safe stimulator design according to EN60601-2-10

For the development process we used the fault tree analysis method in accordance with the German Industry Norm DIN 25424 (DIN 25424). With this method the undesired results have to be defined first; then all possible combinations of reasons for this undesired result have to be analyzed. For example, one of the undesired results is a pulse output energy above 300 mJ. This error can arise due to the following reasons: 1) output voltage too high, 2) capacity of output capacitor too high, 3) short-circuit of output capacitor and pulse duration too high. In this example only the second reason can be excluded, since the capacity of a (electrolytic) capacitor does not increase by itself. For all remaining reasons (e.g., output voltage too high) three-fold logically AND connected safety systems (e.g., three Zener-diodes in parallel to exclude an overvoltage) or two-fold AND connected safety systems with continuous surveillance of their functioning are required to exclude a possible error.

2.2 Realization

2.2.1 Data acquisition unit / input stage

The input stage was designed to ensure a very flexible data acquisition unit, which can be individually adapted to different applications. The data acquisition unit consists of 32 multiplexed analog inputs, which are digitized with a fast analog-to-digital (A/D) converter (MAXIM MAX120). The precision is 12 bit and the conversion rate is up to 500k samples per second (sum of all channels). The amplifier has a programmable gain for each input; the analog inputs are protected against overvoltage. In addition, the input stage has 8 latched digital inputs with programmable sample time for external keybuttons and foot-switches.

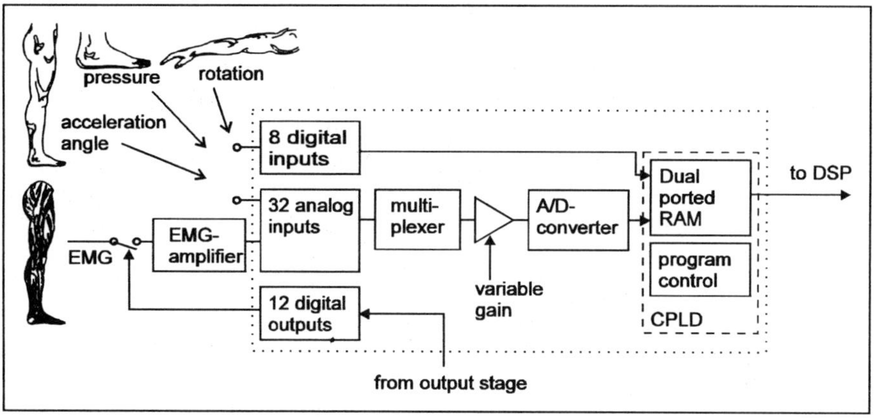

Fig. 1. Input Stage

A complex in-circuit programmable logic device (CPLD) controls the multiplexer and the A/D-converter. The conversion program can be changed by the lab PC. One part of the CPLD is configured as static random access memory (SRAM), storing the sampled data and transferring them via direct memory access (DMA) into the memory of the digital signal processor (DSP) (see Keller et al. 1996).

Each input channel has its own power supply for the sensors and preamplifiers. In order to meet the safety restrictions in a simple way, the output current of each power supply is limited to 0.5 mA. This requires the use of sensors and preamplifiers with extremely low power consumption (< 500 μA). If the power consumption of a sensor is higher, the sensor has to be equipped with its own power supply and has to be well isolated.

If electromyograms (EMGs) are sampled during electrical stimulation, a large stimulus artifact could jolt the EMG amplifiers out of range for a considerable period of time. To prevent stimulus artifacts, the output stage generates a signal to switch off the EMG amplifiers during the stimulation pulses.

2.2.2 Output stage

The output stage for neuromuscular stimulation via surface electrodes contains 16 output channels, which are controlled by a Siemens SAB 80C167 microcontroller.

The controller provides a Capture/Compare (CAPCOM) unit, which can compare a timer's content with given values and modify output signals in case of a match. Two tables with stimulation parameters are stored in memory. The regular stimulation table contains data for stimulation, which are continuously updated by the DSP or the laboratory PC. The SAB 80C167 microcontroller performs a plausibility check of these stimulation parameters. In case of emergency (e.g., communication line is disturbed) the controller switches to the emergency table, which gives stimulation parameters supporting the anti-gravity muscles. The stimulation parameters (time of each stimulation pulse, pulse width, pulse current amplitude) are transmitted to the output channels via optocouplers and isolation amplifiers.

To prevent cross-current between pairs of electrodes and to allow simultaneous stimulation of different channels, the output channels are galvanically isolated and completely independent of each other. Each output channel receives a limited amount of energy from two linear power limiters (LT1185) in series with a self-limiting DC/DC converter (Fig. 2). Although the average power of each output channel is limited to 0.8 watts, the energy stored in a load capacitor allows an increase of power for short periods of time (about ten stimulation pulses). A regulated current source, which determines the stimulation current amplitude (0-120 mA), is in series with an analog switch determining the pulse width (0-500 μs). Additional measures have been taken to limit the energy of a single stimulation pulse: three Zener-diodes in parallel limit the output voltage; a pulse width limiter (< 1 ms) and two capacitors (3.3 μF) in series limit the pulse energy at the maximal given voltage of 320 V (see Table 1, B and C). To provide a charge-balanced bipolar stimulation, a capacitor is charged during the rectangular positive current pulse (switch S1 closed, S2 open). 20 μs later switch S1 opens and S2 closes. This allows the capacitor to discharge, thus producing an exponential negative charge balance pulse (Mortimer 1981).

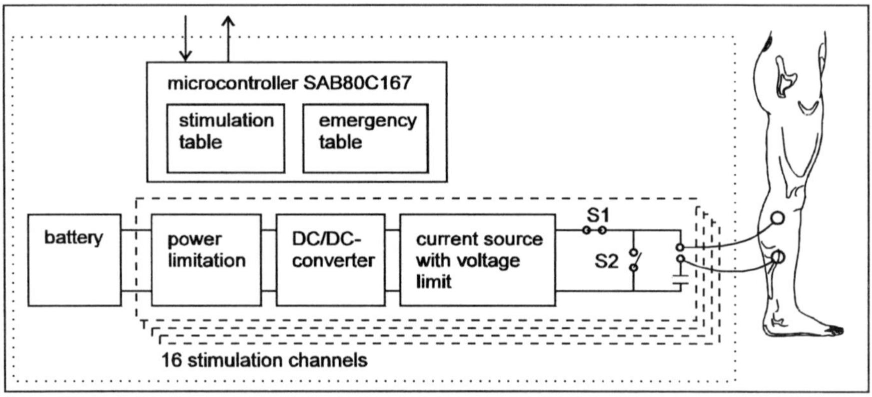

Fig. 2. Output stage

To detect if electrodes become disconnected or if the electrode conductivity worsens, the device monitors the output impedance during stimulation pulses, using an isolation amplifier and the analog-to-digital (A/D) converter of the SAB 80C167 microcontroller. A warning message is given, when the impedance of a specific channel increases or when the absolute maximal value is exceeded.

3 Conclusions

Our project demonstrates that the concept of passive safety can be applied to the design of neurostimulators. Despite the self-limiting design, the performance of the device is sufficient, even for sophisticated FES implementations such as combined pulse-width and frequency modulation or intermittent stimulation with high-frequency bursts. The approving agency, the TÜV Bayern (Technischer Überwachungsverein Bayern, technical surveillance organization of Bavaria), has agreed with this concept of the output stage. We intend to have the complete multi-sensor closed-loop neurostimulator approved for clinical use in countries of the European Union by the end of 1996.

Not all of the safety requirements are defined by the European Norm EN60601-1 and EN60601-2-10; most details of the implementation depend on the internal standards of the approving agency. These internal standards can differ not only between different countries but also between different local agencies in one country. Engineers who develop biomedical devices should contact the responsible agency at an early stage of the project.

Our stimulator can be considered safe with respect to the electrical output parameters (Table 1, A-D). However, even highly detailed design does not eliminate the risk of erroneous software functions and essential component failures. If the device is used for lower extremity applications, these failures may lead to falls of the patient. The patient has to be informed about this remaining risk prior to obtaining his informed consent. The risk of falling has to be reduced by mechanical balance aids and careful patient selection.

References

EN 60601-1 (1991) Medical electrical equipment; general requirements for safety. Deutsche Elektrotechnische Kommission im DIN und VDE, Berlin.

EN 60601-2-10 (1989) Medical electrical equipment; particular requirements for the safety of nerve and muscle stimulators. Deutsche Elektrotechnische Kommission im DIN und VDE, Berlin.

DIN 25424: Fehlerbaumanalyse (German Industry Norm: Fault tree analysis); method and symbols) Normenausschuss Kerntechnik im DIN Deutsches Institut für Normung e.V.

Keller, M., Krauß, P., Hoch, G., Quintern, J. (1996) Design of a multi-sensor closed-loop neurostimulator. Part A: communication unit with wireless data link and digital signal processor. *This volume*, pp. 183-188.

Mortimer, J. T. (1981) Motor prostheses. In: V.B. Brooks (ed.) *The Handbook of Physiology, The Nervous System*, Vol. III, American Physiological Society, Bethesda, pp. 155-187.

A Modular System for Controlled FES and Therapy of Paralyses

R. Rupp, A. Nützel, G. Vossius
Institute of Biomedical Engineering, University of Karlsruhe, Germany

Abstract - The Electrical Stimulation (ES) is not only used for restoring motoric functions of paralysed muscles but also for training of incomplete paralysed muscles and for reduction of spasticity. In these latter cases an objective classification of the success of muscle-training and the level of the spastic activity is very difficult or even impossible. In the following a stand-alone, modular and interactive therapy system for a controlled either functional and therapeutical stimulation is described.

1 Introduction

Soon after the research in the field of the Functional Electro Stimulation (FES) had reached the status of an experimental clinical use, it had become obvious, that due to the huge amount of degrees of freedom of the human motor control system on the one hand a sufficient number of stimulation output channels and on the other hand a comparable number of sensoric input channels had to be provided. In the beginning great efforts have been made to build up FES-systems in an 'open-loop'-mode. The research was therefore concentrated mainly on the development of pure stimulation systems.

Already in 1980 Scholtes et. al. (Scholtes et al. 1980) had designed a processor-controlled stimulation system with the following basic features:

The stimulator hardware was able to produce the specific stimulation patterns in a stand alone operation with a modular structure, i.e. by separating the central unit relatively to hard- and software from the stimulator unit. The central processor unit computed the parameters and the timing for the functional stimulation and was acting as a central control unit for the stimulation modules.

This concept was built up in a 16-channel version with the possibility of implementing more stimulation sub-modules. Furthermore the system included I/O-channels in order to install the features for a 'close-loop'-system by adding a separate processor unit with sensor inputs, which provide sufficient observability.

Based upon this system a special version of a microprocessor-controlled 8-channel system for the FES of walking and standing of paraplegics was developed. It allowed the choice of several implemented movement patterns with the help of simple switch controls. (Belikan et al. 1986) The stimulator provided also the possibility for expansion to a 'closed-loop'-system via 8 inputs for sensory signals. An industrial version of this first kind of a 'walking-computer' for the application of surface electrodes has been made available by Stratec Company. Through this FES of standing and walking has progressed from the experimental status to the use in the clinical and daily routine at home.

Nearly at the same time a battery-supported, portable and voice-controlled FES-system had been developed for quattroplegics. It allowed not only the execution of grip movements but also the programming of the movement by the handicapped himself using simple control words. (Nürnberg et al. 1985)

In 1990 a bi-processor stimulation-system with 16 stimulation-channels was presented, which allowed a wide spektrum of applications in both functional and therapeutical stimulation - even in the case of peripheral paralyses - because of its modular structure and therefore a large versatility of the hard- and software-modules. In this system a 80535-microcontroller was implemented allowing the analysis of sensory-signals and control tasks. On the stimulation-side each sub-system is based on a Z80-processor to control up to 8 stimulation channels. (Guttenberg et al. 1990) This multiprocessor concept allowed the realisation of better observability and controllability.

In the course of the practical tests it became obvious that the speed of the processors was yet too slow for an extended online analysis and classification of the sensory-signals and the implementation of large control-algorithms (Fuzzy-Control, Neuronal Networks, etc.), which proved to be necessary for 'closed-loop' FES. In addition due to our clincal experience it seemed to be advantageous to incorporate also capabilities for the execution of therapeutical ES in the system to cover a wider range of clinical applications. This allows i.e. in a first step the reduction of existing motoric deficits of the handicapped due to the paralysis and from there on the progression to FES.

2 Basic Concept of the Therapy System

Based upon these experiences we designed the following system as a menu-controlled, interactive multi-processor system with a modular structure of its main modules in order to adapt it easily to changing conditions and requirements. Great care has been taken to incorporate sufficient computing power into the system, in order to be able to execute also high level signal analysis and control procedures.The system is divided into three main functional blocks: 1. Sensor-signal measurement and analysis, 2. system supervision and therapy control, and 3. processing, supervision and output of the stimulation patterns.

2.1 Signal measurement and analysis

In the stimulation therapy especially the incorporation of the EMG signal has gained much more importance for control and supervising tasks. This comprises also a complex signal analysis and processing in order to obtain objective EMG-parameters to establish sufficient observability. Basicly we may use the EMG of several muscles and mechanical data from joint angles or force sensors.

For the realisation of a 'closed-loop'-system the online measurement and processing of the signals is necessary, including EMG-recording during ongoing stimulation. The recording of the EMG during stimulation is technically difficult to achieve because of the unfavourable stimulation puls to EMG-signal ratio (> 1000:1), which tends to bring the EMG-amplifier continously to saturation. The long recovery time of the operational amplifiers does not allow the detection of the EMG-signal between two stimulation pulses. To resolve this conflict a special EMG-recording circuit has developed, similar to the one already presented by Holländer et. al. (Holländer 1987). This EMG-amplifier has been working reliably in clinical tests.

Special Digital Signal Processor units (Motorola DSP56001) are implemented, each DSP serving 4 EMG-channels. Different signal analysis procedures may be applied online, i.e. statistical data pre-processing in the time and frequency domain (i.e. the calculation of a 256-point FFT needs 820 µs). This way EMG parameters are extracted real-time.

In addition each DSP board provides 8 input channels. Furthermore there are 8 channels controlled by the main-processor, for instance processing signals from mechanical sensors.

2.2 System supervision and therapy control

The tasks of the main processor (Motorola MC68302) are generally the system management and the control of the therapy via:

- Integration and coordination of the different sub-modules including the transmission of the stimulation parameters to the externally connected stimulators
- Further analysis of the pre-processed sensor data, i.e. classification of the EMG-parameters by Artificial Neuronal Networks
- Implementation of control algorithms as Adaptive, Parameter Identifying or Fuzzy Logic strategies (Vossius 1995)
- Handling of the menu operated, user interactive therapeutic system
- Dokumentation of the therapy via recording of a protocol

All these complex software tasks are supported by a MS-DOS™ compatible operating system specially developed for the minimized hardware environment, which allows the use of the system in a stand-alone or PC-controlled operation mode. Several dedicated software modules developed for each of the hardware modules help to reduce the programming time, when developing future application software, which might be written in a high level language.

2.3 The stimulation unit

Up to 4 stimulator units might be connected to the main unit. Each stimulator unit has 8 stimulation channels controlled via serial ports of the main-processor. The units may also be operated in a stand-alone mode. The frequency of the biphasic-square wave pulses may be varied from 0.5 to 30 Hz, the pulse duration between 20 and 512 μs, and the amplitude up to 102 mA.

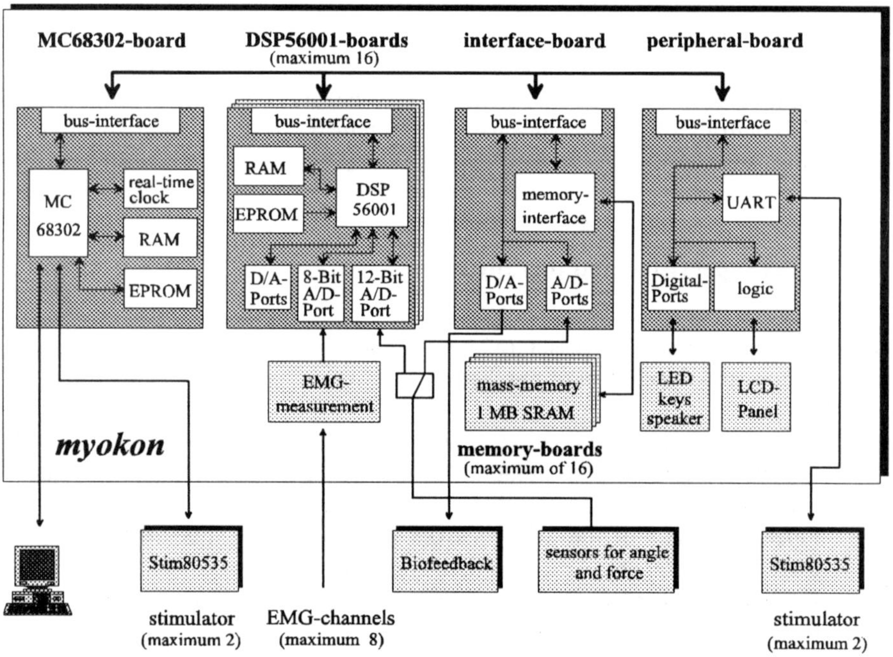

Fig. 1. Overview of the hardware of the therapy system 'myokon'

3 Results

The decribed modular, battery-powered and portable multiprocessor system is a powerful menu operated, user interactive therapeutic and FES closed loop stimulation unit with capabilities for extraction and classification of EMG-parameters during stimulation, including up to 8 low-noise EMG and 32 stimulation channels. In clincal tests it has proved these capabilities in controlling limb movements by FES and in supporting the therapeutist in an interactive way when applying therapeutical ES to the patient.

References

Scholtes, T., Setzer, W., and Vossius, G. (1980) Ein mikroprozessorgesteuertes Stimula-torensystem. In: *Biomedizinische Technik:* Band 25 151-153

Belikan, T., Holländer, H.-J., and Vossius G. (1986) Microprocessor controlled 8-channel stimulator with surface electrodes for FES of gait. In: *2nd Vienna International Workshop on Functional Electrostimulation:* 71-73

Nürnberg, H. G., Eicher, M., and Vossius, G. (1985) Spracheingabe zur programm-gesteuerten Elektrostimulation der Hand. In: *Biomedizinische Technik:* Band 30 76-77

Guttenberg, U., Holländer, H.-J., and Vossius, G. (1990) 16 channel stimulation systems for the use of FES and related applications. In: *Advances in external control of human extremities:* 319-326

Holländer, H.-J., Huber, M., and Vossius G. (1987) An EMG-controlled multichannel stimulator. In: *The Ninth International Symposium on external control of human Extremities:* 291-295

Vossius, G. (1995) Control requirements for executing FES. (*this volume*)

Optimized Experimental Control of FES-Induced Swing Phase of Paraplegic Gait

H. M. Franken[1], P. H. Veltink[1], G. Baardman[2], H. B.K. Boom[1]
[1]Biomedical Technological Institute, University of Twente, Enschede, NL
[2]Roessingh R&D, Enschede, NL

Abstract - Parameterized swing phase of paraplegic gait was obtained by stimulating the main hip flexors, hamstrings, and quadriceps using surface electrodes. The hip flexors were stimulated to generate a desired hip angle range. The hamstrings provided footclearance in the forward swing. The quadriceps were stimulated to acquire knee extension at the end of the swing phase. Stimulation patterns were optimised on the basis of an experimental sensitivity analysis. During open-loop stimulation with the optimized stimulation patterns, the hip angle range varied in time due to the effects of potentiation and muscle fatigue. This time dependent behaviour was succesfully compensated for using a cycle-to-cycle PID controller, which computed the hip flexor stimulation pattern on the basis of the achieved hip angle range in previous cycles.

1 Introduction

Functional Electrical Stimulation (FES) can restore or enhance motor functions, such as walking, in paraplegics (Andrews et al. 1989, Kralj et al. 1983, Marsolais and Kobetic 1987).

Fast fatigue of artificially stimulated muscles limits the time a task, such as walking, can be performed (Franken et al. 1993). Current FES-systems have pre-programmed stimulation patterns which are applied in open-loop. These systems are tuned such that, initially, exaggerated hip joint angles result, in order to provide a margin of safety at the time the subject's muscles become fatigued (Marsolais and Kobetic 1987).

In the current paper, the swing phase of paraplegic gait was parameterized with desired objectives. Subsequently, we derived stimulation patterns for the main swing-phase muscles to achieve these objectives. Parameterization of the swing phase on a cyclic level facilitates adaption of the stimulation patterns from cycle-to-cycle. This cycle-to-cycle control concept was investigated by using a discrete-time PID controller. The controller succesfully maintained the desired swing phase objectives by adjusting the stimulation patterns on the basis of the error between desired and actually obtained swing phase objectives in the previous swing cycles.

2 Methods

2.1 Optimization of stimulation patterns

Swing phase objectives: The consider system with the main swing phase muscles is displayed in Fig. 1. Angle definitions are also shown. The stimulation pattern for the three muscle groups were optimised by observing the motion of the leg on the level of a swing cycle. The generated movement should satisfy the following desired objectives. The *hip angle range* should be approximately 45 deg. corresponding to natural human gait (Inman 1981). The foot clearance in the forward swing should be sufficient (> 1 cm), in order to prevent the subject from stumbling. *Knee extension* was desired at the end of the forward swing to ensure safe body weight bearing during stance phase.

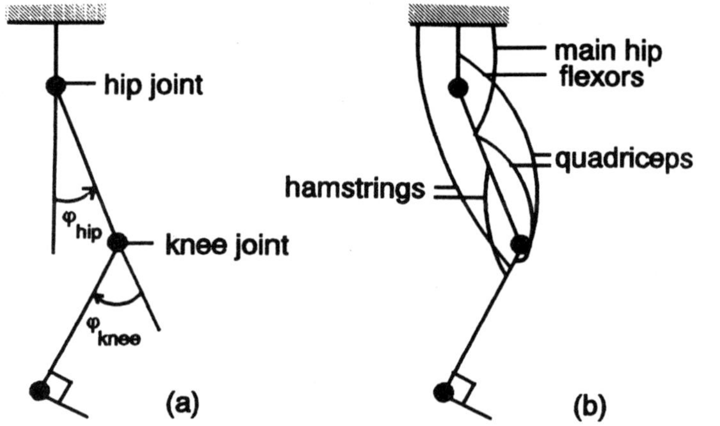

Fig. 1. Schematic of the leg, freely swinging in the sagittal plane. The position of the hip is fixed. Angle definitions are shown in (a) [hip: φ_{hip} and knee: φ_{knee}]. The stimulated muscle groups are shown in (b).

Stimulation timing: Each muscle was stimulated with one burst with constant stimulation frequency (hip flexors: 50 Hz; quadriceps, hamstrings: 25 Hz) at maximal recruitment each swing cycle. The stimulation frequency for the main hip flexors was significantly higher than for the hamstrings and quadriceps. This was necessary to obtain functional movement and to ensure a reasonable control space. The burst times were minimized. Optimization of the timing was performed experimentally in three stages. First, the stimulation burst for the main hip flexors, yielding the desired hip angle range, was found. Subsequenty, the hamstrings were stimulated to obtain foot clearance. Finally, the quadriceps were stimulated to obtain knee extension. Cocontraction was accounted for by minor adjustment of the burst times.

The stimulation onset for the hamstrings and the main hip flexors was triggered on the hip angle passing through a certain threshold angle in the backward swing. The onset for the quadriceps stimulation was triggered on the same threshold angle in the forward swing. This threshold angle was equal to the hip angle when the patient was at rest in the stand set-up. The hip angle always passed through this threshold during a prolonged experiment. Triggering the stimulation in this fashion facilitated easy optimization of onset and burst times. The stimulation burst for each muscle group was timed such that it accelerated the considered limb in the beginning of the movement. The nomenclature for the stimulation parameters is displayed in Fig. 2.

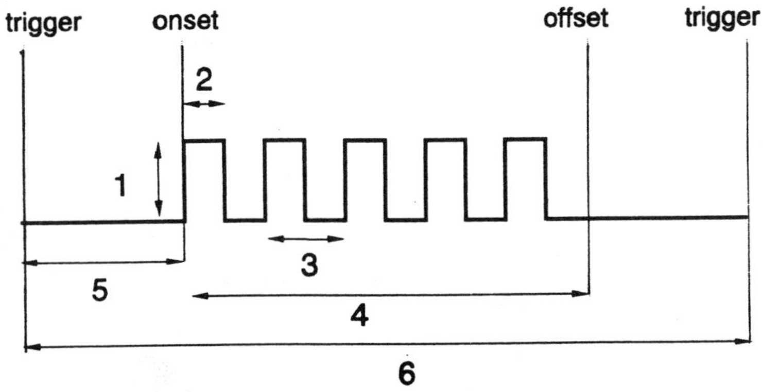

Fig. 2. Stimulation nomenclature: 1 = amplitude, 2 = pulse width, 3 = inter-pulse interval, 4 = burst time, 5 = wait time, 6= cycle time. After being triggered, the onset of the stimulation occurs when the wait time has passed. Offset is determined by the desired burst time.

2.2 Cycle-to-cycle control strategy

A discrete-time PID controller was tuned on the natural frequency of the swinging leg (Veltink 1991). The considered controller adjusted the burst time of the muscle groups on the basis of the error between desired and actually obtained swing phase objectives. It was to maintain the desired swing phase objectives. The obtained objectives in previous swing cycles were compared with the desired values and PID action was undertaken when deviation occured. This concept is displayed for hip flexor burst time in Fig. 3.

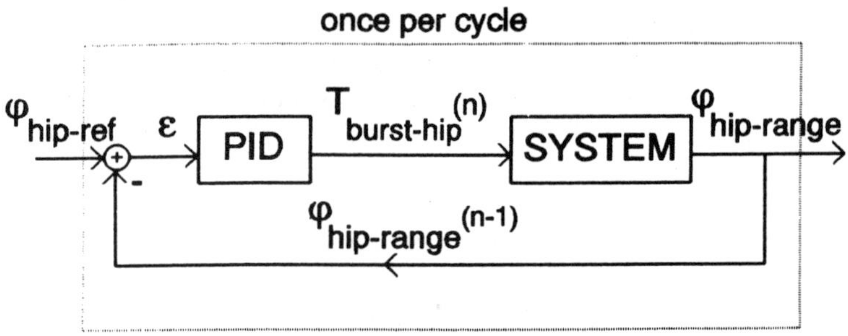

Fig. 3. Schematic of PID controller for adjusting the hip flexor burst time for the next cycle ($T_{burst\text{-}hip}$ (n)) on the basis of the error (ε) between reference ($\varphi_{hip\text{-}ref}$) and the hip angle range obtained in the previous swing ($\varphi_{hip\text{-}range}$ (n-l)).

2.3 Subjects

Two complete T5-T6 level spinal cord injured patients participated. Both had been enrolled in an FES-training program of at least 6 months. Subject 2 exhibited significant active spasm, limiting the funtional effect of the applied stimulation. The training period of subject 2 was also shorter and less intensive than that of subject one.

2.4 Experimental setup

Stand set-up: The subjects were positioned a controlled stand set-up with arm support (see Fig. 4). A self-fitting modular orthosis restricted the motion of the freely swinging leg in the sagittal plane. Hip and knee angle of the standing leg were fixed to zero. The standing leg was elevated by a block. A bicycle sport-saddle provided additional stability in the frontal plane. Hip and knee angle of the swinging leg were measured with goniometers.

Electrode placement and data recording: Adhesive surface electrodes (Pals, Axelgaard Manufacturing co, Ltd. Fallbrook, USA, 9x5 cm^2) were placed in the groin foil for hip flexor stimulation, over the quadriceps (rectus femoris, vastus lateralis/medialis) and over the hamstrings (near knee joint). The gonio signals were sampled at 100 Hz.

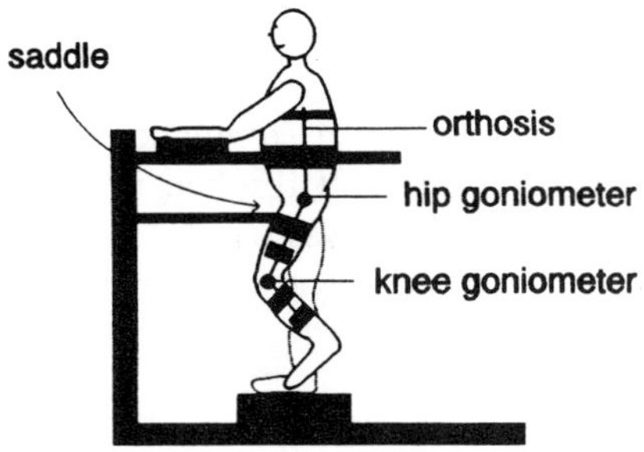

Fig. 4. Schematic drawing of a paraplegic subject in standing position in the stand set-up. The patient wore a self-fitting modular orthosis. This orthosis restricted the motion of the freely swinging leg to the sagittal plane. The standing leg was elevated by a block. The knee and hip angle of the standing leg were fixed by the orthosis to zero degrees.

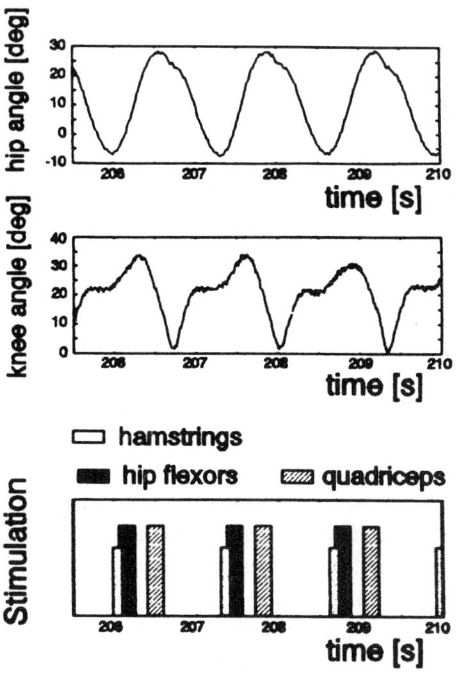

Fig. 5. Hip and knee angle registration with optimized stimulation timing for the main hip flexors, hamstrings and quadriceps in subject 1. The influence of each stimulation site can be detected in the hip and knee angle signal.

3 Results

Swing phase objectives: The optimized stimulation timing of the three muscle groups was similar in both subjects. It resulted in a satisfying swing (Fig. 5), although the achieved hip angle range was smaller in subject 2 (Subject 1: 45 deg; subject 2: 25 deg), due to active spasm and a less intensive training period.

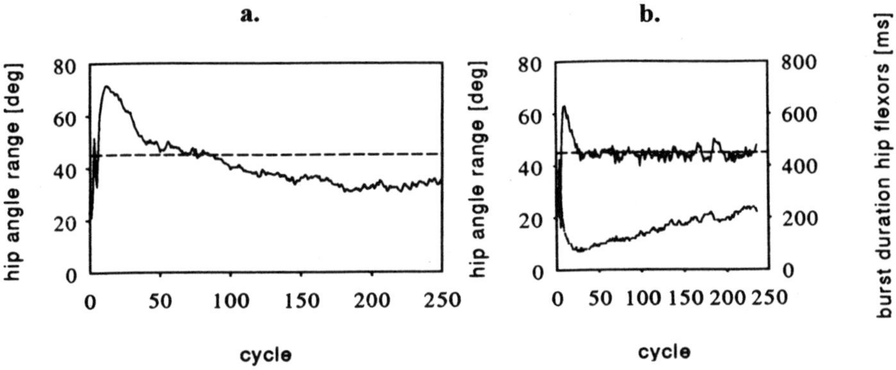

Fig. 6. Hip angle range per swing cycle. During the open-loop control trial (a) the three muscle groups were stimulated with the optimized stimulation patterns each cycle without adaption. During the cycle-to-cycle control trial (b) the burst time for the hipflexors was adapted. The quadriceps and hamstrings were stimulated in open-loop fashion with the optimized patterns.

Open-loop control: During a prolonged period of open-loop stimulation with the optimised stimulation patterns in subject 1, the hip angle range initially increased above the desired value of 45 degrees due to the effect of potentiation in the hip flexors and subsequently decreased below this desired value due to muscle fatigue (Fig. 6a). The mechanical performance of the hamstrings, in maintaining sufficient foot clearance, and the quadriceps, in obtaining knee extension at the end of the forward swing, was relatively unaffected during the open-loop trial.

Cycle-to-cycle control: It was observed during the open-loop experiments that only the hip flexor stimulation needed adaption. The PID controller was able to maintain a constant hip angle range by adapting the hip flexor burst time. Noteworthy, potentiation was adapted for by burst time decrement of the burst time (initial part of Fig 6b). Muscle fatigue was compensated for by burst time increment.

4 Conclusions and Discussion

Stimulation patterns can be derived such that swing phase objectives, characteristic for natural human gait, can be achieved in paraplegics.

Slowly time-varying system characteristics, such as the effects of muscle fatigue and potentiation, were succesfully compensated for using a discrete-time controller acting on the level of a cycle. This controller avoided exaggerated hip joint angles and maintained the desired parameterized swing phase motion when fatigue occured by incrementing the burst time.

A control strategy from cycle-to-cycle seems promising to compensate for slowly changing system characteristics. This controller should be used in combination with an *on-line* (*predictive*) controller in the case that occuring disturbances should be compensated for as well. An alternative controller structure is to compute stimulation timing on the basis of a desired hip and knee angular trajectory in time. This will most likely be problematic due to the large inertial properties of the leg. The controller structure should simultaneously adapt for slowly changing characteristics, such as fatigue, and disturbances.

The experiments showed that the rate of fatigue in hamstrings and quadriceps was much smaller than in the hip flexors. This was most likely caused by the fact that the hip flexors had to accelerate the entire leg (large inertia) while the hamstrings and quadriceps acted on the lower leg only.

Without orthosis, surface stimulation of the main hip flexors generated significant hip ad- and abduction during the forward swing, emphasizing the essential role of the orthosis.

References

Andrews, B. J., Barnett, R. W., Phillips, G. F., and Kirkwood, C. A. (1989) Rule-based control of a hybrid FES orthosis for assisting paraplegic locomotion, *Automedica,* **11**: 175-199

Franken, H. M., Veltink, P. H., Fidder, M., and Boom, H. B. K. (1993) Fatigue of intermittently stimulated paralysed human quadriceps during imposed cyclical lower leg movements, *Int. J. Elec. & Kin.*, **3**: 3-12

Inman, V. T., Ralston, H. J., and Todd, F. (1981) Human Walking, Williams and Wilkins, University of California

Kralj, A., Bajd, T., Turk, R., Krajnik, J., and Benko, H. (1983) Gait restoration in paraplegic paients: a feasibility demonstration using multichannel surface electrode FES. *J. Rehab. Res. Dev.*, **20**: 3-20.

Marsolais, E. B. and Kobetic, R. (1987) Functional electrical stimulation for walking in paraplegia, *J. Bone and Joint Surg.*, **69A**: 728-733

Veltink, P. H. (1991) Control of FES-induced cyclical movements of the lower leg, *Med. Biol. Eng. Comp.*, **27**: NS8-NS12

Development of Control Strategies for FES-Supported Closed-Loop Standing-Up

S. Heinze[1], P.H. Veltink[1], P.L. Jensen[2], R.E. Mayagoitia[1], H.J. Hermens[3], H.F.J.M. Koopman[1], P.A. Huijing[1,4]
[1] Institute of Biomedical Technology, University of Twente, The Netherlands
[2] Centre for Sensory-Motor Interaction, University of Aalborg, Denmark
[3] Roessingh Research and Development bv, Enschede, The Netherlands
[4] Faculty of Human Movement Sciences, Free University, Amsterdam, The Netherlands

Abstract - A two dimensional three-segment biomechanical model with three degrees of freedom has been developed to simulate control strategies for FES-supported standing up.

Preliminary simulation results of the closed-loop control of standing-up using mono-and biarticular muscles are presented. Results indicate that real-time closed loop control is feasible in well trained subjects if angular velocities rather than angles are used. Further developments in control are based on an analysis of the sit-to-stand transfer chosen from the literature, where characteristic phases and events are defined. After definition, control and optimisation criteria can be assigned to each phase. Experimental results of the standing-up transfer with open-loop stimulation of only quadriceps and both quadriceps and hamstrings are presented.

1 Introduction and State of the Art

Spinal cord injury (SCI) is one of the most devastating injuries of the nervous system. The number of SCI subjects is not negligible and half of them are younger than 25 years of age when injured. For Europe the average prevalence rate of SCI has been estimated of 500 per million (Capildeo et al., 1984). Functional electrical stimulation (FES) may offer an alternative to conventional rehabilitation techniques and improve the mobility considerably. The first application of FES to a paraplegic patient was reported in 1963 (Kralj et al., 1989). But the clinical applications as mentioned by Kralj et al. (1995) are rather limited with number of ideas and the investigations, developments and investments performed.

Standing up is a physiologically essential function and an important prerequisite for gait and many everyday activities. It is vital for the proper functioning of many organs, for blood circulation, and it is very important from the psychological point of view.

A well-coordinated standing up requires a good modulation of stimulated muscles acting at the knee and the hip and also at the ankle. During a sit-to-stand transfer it is at least desired to extend knees and hip simultaneously and to develop smooth and precise movements by simultaneous stimulation of an agonist and antagonist muscle pair (Petrofsky et al., 1983). The role of biarticular muscles during standing up is being investigated because they can act as antagonists of the quadriceps at the knee and additionally as agonists at the hip as extensor. Therefore arm force would only be needed for balancing and not for erecting the trunk..

Control of standing up as such has not been studied very extensively. More studies can be found in the field of complex FES walking systems and postural control. Straight forward control strategies to accomplish standing up of paraplegic subjects were applied, although very complex muscular and skeletal models were derived for cat muscles or for single joint muscles in humans (Petrofsky et al., 1983a, 1983b, 1984, 1986). Marsolais et al. (1984) introduced a closed-loop control strategy for standing including a simple open-loop procedure for the actual standing up. Some controllers for external stimulation via quadriceps muscles for the standing-up transfer have been designed (Petrofsky et al., 1983a, Mulder et al., 1987, Mulder et al., 1992). Petrofsky et al. (1986) included additional stimulation of the gluteus maximus to stabilize the hip. The controller designed by Petrofsky et al. (1983a) was a finite state controller using exclusively position feedback of ankle, knee and hip joints. Mulder et al. (1987, 1992) introduced a controller described in state space, including feedback of knee angle and angular velocity.

2 Preliminary Experimental Tests of Open-Loop Controlled Standing-Up

Preliminary results of open-loop control were obtained, where standing-up procedures with quadriceps stimulation and simultaneous quadriceps and hamstrings stimulation were compared. The stand-up tests were performed with three SCI patients. Movements were measured with a VICON motion analysis system, ground reaction forces measured with AMTI force plates and arm forces measured with an instrumented parallel bars like arm support. The effect of redistribution of energy and redirection of the ground reaction force became clear in the stick figure diagram (fig. 1). While stimulating only the quadriceps the moment about the hip is insufficient to erect the trunk and the knees lock with an unnecessary high velocity. The subject has to use arm force to erect the trunk. In the stick figure diagram (fig. 1) the ground reaction force goes behind the centre of mass, so that the body would fall forward if it would not be compensated by the arms. Adding hamstrings stimulation results in a more balanced transfer but also in excessive hip extension. The ground reaction force points in front of the centre of mass, as indicated in the stick figure diagram (fig. 1). This means the body would fall backwards without the compensating arm force.

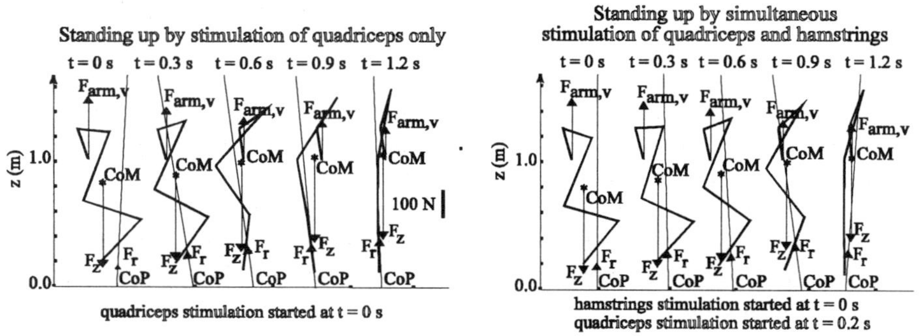

Fig. 1. Standing up with open loop stimulation of one patient (TN), (Veltink et al. 1994). A stimulation amplitude of 80mA for quadriceps and 90mA for hamstrings were applied via adhesive surface electrodes.

From these results, it was concluded that a closed-loop strategy is required to modulate hamstrings stimulation to obtain a well balanced standing up procedure. Apart from improving balance closed-loop control may also reduce high energy consumption and the effect of external disturbances. It may also account for activities of the upper extremities and the nonlinear and time varying properties of the system.

3 Direct Musculo-Skeletal Model

To avoid burdensome experimental tests of several control strategies with SCI subjects a direct biomechanical model is being derived.

To develop a practical model of the system several assumptions have to be made. Only movements in the sagittal plane during standing up are taken into account. The skeletal part of the model of the human body consists of a series of rigid segments with a fixed point mass at its centre. The segments are connected via hinge joints. The equations of motion are derived by Lagrangian dynamics. The muscle model includes two parts: the activation dynamics and the musculotendon dynamics. The activation dynamics are modelled by a first-order process (time constant 30 ms) and the musculotendon dynamics of quadriceps and hamstrings muscles were described by a phenomenological based, lumped-parameter model including force-length dependencies. The force-velocity relationships were not included. The voluntary activity of the upper extremities is modelled by an arm force controller to ensure a constant vertical velocity of the centre of mass. Thereby the horizontal arm force is modelled such that the centre of mass is also transferred above the ankle position.

The developed biomechanical model includes now quadriceps and hamstrings muscles. Model parameters of one subject (JO) were partly identified by measurements and data taken from the literature (Winter, 1990, Yamaguchi et al., 1990). Experimental tests were performed under isometric conditions using a KINCOM dynanometer system. Knee extension moments were measured at several combinations of hip and knee angle to identify the quadriceps muscle parameters. To determine knee and hip angle dependencies of the moment generated by hamstrings muscles, a distinct centre of rotation and a constant position of the hamstrings attachment at the hip joint were assumed according to Brand et al. (1982). On the basis of these measurements and assumptions all the information could be obtained to calculate knee and hip torques dependent on knee and hip angles.

4 Simulation Results

Having identified the model, several simulations have been carried out to develop a suitable control strategy to modulate hamstrings activation.

First a simple closed-loop control strategy was implemented based on a linear relation between knee and hip angle (Kelley et al., 1976). The first control strategy which was simulated the hamstrings muscles were stimulated if hip extension was smaller than knee extension. Three simulations were performed with different strengths of the hamstrings muscles: 1, 2, 3.5 times the hamstrings strength of JO. The muscles of the subject of JO were not sufficiently trained and the strength of 3.5 times was comparable with the strength of a 2nd subject. The simulation indicated that the hip extension moment generated by the hamstrings muscles started too late to influence the movement because of high inertia (see fig. 2).

Cordo et al. (1994) presented results indicating that the Central Nervous System (CNS) extracts and uses proprioceptive information related to both the velocity and the angular position of the joint during movement. That the use of velocities as feedback signals would theoretically provide a better way to control the movements of lower extremities was already suggested but not proved by Petrofsky et al. (1983a), Mulder et al. (1987), van Alste et al. (1987).

Therefore a control strategy including a linear knee/hip velocity relationship was implemented. The tracking of the linear angle relationships was predicted to improve as can be seen in fig. 2.

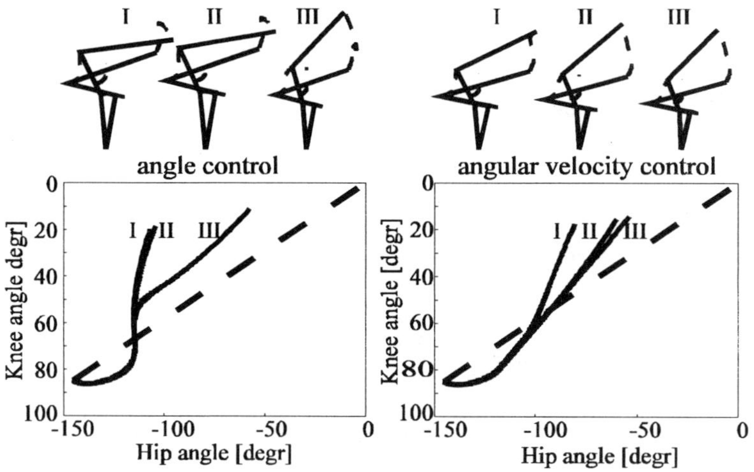

Fig. 2. Real-time feedback control of hamstring stimulation (simulation results).

The control strategies tested until now only considered the ascending phase of standing up: the phase between the seat-off event and the beginning of the actual standing phase. (Knee and hip extension velocities cannot be assumed to be equal because they are dependent on the initial angle configurations.) In order to control the whole standing up procedure the sit-to-stand transfer should be divided in different characteristic phases with well defined start and end events.

5 Definition of Standing-Up in Terms of Finite States

Based on a normative data presentation of standing up in humans according to Kralj et al. (1990) characteristic events and their specific times of occurrence can be defined (see fig. 3). This cycle diagram is comparable to a possible definition of gait in state space and makes it therefore suitable for the development of a general control concept of FES-assisted movements of paraplegics.

The following figure 3 shows the cycle diagram described in terms discrete events or finite states. This model has to be restricted for the development of a robust and practical controller such that every transfer event from one to another state is controlled using an adequate strategy.

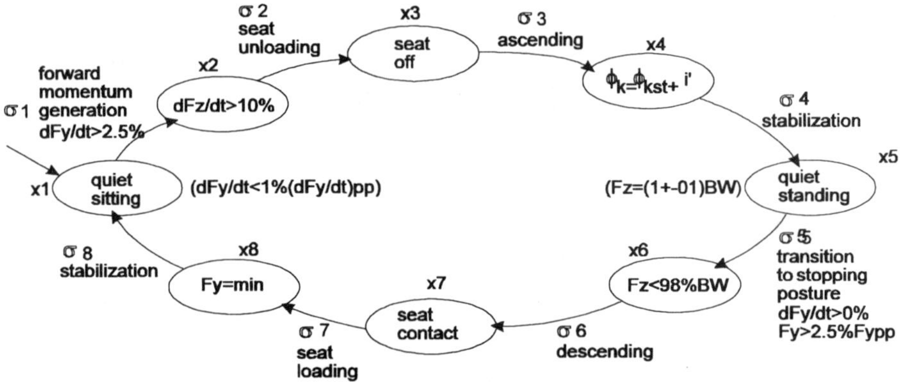

Fig. 3 Finite State Model of the standing-up and sitting down procedure with definition of states (x_1, x_2 ...x_8) and events (σ_1, σ_2...σ_8). Suggested control or optimization (red coloured) are included.
$\vec{F} = (F_x, F_y, F_z)$ ... ground reaction forces, BW ... body weight

6 Discussion

Recent experimental and simulation results indicate that biarticular muscles play an important role in achieving a balanced transfer from sitting to standing (Veltink et al., 1994). While stimulating quadriceps permanently in the ascending phase, hamstrings activation has to be modulated via closed-loop control. To achieve a well balanced standing up movement by using the biarticular nature of the hamstrings the possibility of closed-loop force modulation exists and can replace the usual open-loop control. Under certain conditions hamstrings stimulation should be avoided, e.g. if quadriceps cannot generate sufficient force or if the relation between the forces produced by hamstrings to forces produced by quadriceps is insufficient to achieve standing up. That means that the movement of standing up characterised by knee and hip extension should not be converted such that knees are flexed because quadriceps force is too small to extend the knees. Therefore a monoarticular muscle that extends the hip but does not act at the knee, like the gluteus maximus, may have to be used alternatively and also should also be included in the model for simulations.

Stating the problem in terms of characteristic events defined by different kinetic and kinematic quantities implies the development of event dependent objectives or optimisation criteria. For instance, starting angles, end angles and desired angular velocities and accelerations can be used to define new optimisation criteria. During the actual ascending phase the knee and hip extension velocities dependent on the initial state can be used as control quantities. In addition the transfer from the acceleration to the deceleration phase can be recorded by measuring the acceleration of the centre of mass. Furthermore, in the stability phase balance can be controlled by using the direction of the ground reaction force. Dependent on this, hamstrings stimulation should be turned on and off to keep those vectors in the limited range necessary for stable standing. Instead of using ground reaction forces to control posture it has to be thought about the application of accelerometers.

References

Brand, R.A., Crowninshield, R.D., Wittstock, C.E., Pederson, D.R., Clarck, C.R., Krieken, F.M. (1982), A Model of Lower Extremity Muscular Anatomy. *J. Biomechanical Eng.*, **104**: 304-310.

Capildeo, R., Maxwell, A. (1984), Progress in rehabilitation. *Paraplegia*, Macmillan Press, London, England.

Cordo, P., Carlton, L., Bevan, L., Carlton, M., Kerr, G.K. (1994), Proprioceptive Coordination of Movement sequences: Role of Velocity and Position Information. *J. of Neurophysiology*, **71:** 1848-1861.

Hill, A.V. (1938), The heat of shortening and the dynamic constants of muscle. *Proc. Roy. Soc.*, **B126:** 136-195.

Kelley, D.L., Dainis, A., Wood, G.K. (1976), Mechanics and Muscular Dynamics of Rising from a Seated Position. Biomechanics V-B, Komi V.P. (Ed.), Park Press Baltimore, England.

Kralj, A., Bajd, T. (1989) Functional electrical stimulation: standing and walking after spinal cord injury. CRC Press, Florida, United States.

Kralj, A., Jaeger, R.J., Munih, M. (1990), Analysis of Standing Up and Sitting Down in Humans: Definitions and Normative Data Presentation. *J. Biomechanics*, **23:** 1123-1138.

Kralj, A., Bajd, T., Vodovnik, L. (1995), FES for mobility: The lesson learned in 30 years. *Proc. of the 5th Vienna Int. Workshop on Functional Electrostimulation, Vienna, Austria,* pp.: 13-20.

Marsolais, E.B., Kobetic, R., Chizeck, H., Mansour, J., Borges, G., Rosenthal, J. (1984), Standing of Paraplegics using Closed-Loop Controlled Stimulation. *Proc. of the 8th Int. Symp. on ECHE*, Dubrovnik, pp.: 63-66.

Mulder, A.J., van Alste, J.A., Hermens, H.J., Zilvold, G. (1987), Closed-loop Control of Standing and Standing up. *Proc. of the workshop: "Restoration of Walking aided by Functional Electrical Stimulation"*, Enschede, The Netherlands, pp.: 37-46.

Mulder, A.J., Veltink, P.H., Boom, H.B.K. (1992), On/Off Control in FES-Induced Standing Up: A Model Study and Experiments. *Med. & Biol. Eng. & Comput.*, **30:** 205-212.

Petrofsky, J.S., Phillips, C.A. (1983a), Computer Controlled Walking in the Paralyzed Individual. *The Journal of Neurological and Orthopaedic Surgery*, **4:** 153-164.

Petrofsky, J.S., Phillips, C.A. (1983b), Closed-Loop Control of Movement of Skeletal Muscle. *CRC Critical Rev. BME*, **13:** 35-96.

Petrofsky, J.S., Phillips, C.A., Heaton, H.H. (1984), Feedback Control System for Walking in Man. *Comput. Biol. Med.*, **14:** 135-149.

Petrofsky, J.S., Phillips, C.A., Douglas, R., Larson, P. (1986), A Computer-Controlled Walking System: The Combination of an Orthosis with Functional Electrical Stimulation. *J. of Clinical Eng.*, **11:** 121-133.

Veltink, P.H., Geerdink, B.M., Koopman, H.F.J.M., Huijing, P.A., Boom, H.B.K. (1994), Control of FES-Assisted Standing Up in Paraplegics - The Role of Mono- and Biarticular Muscles. *Proc. of the 16th Ann. Int. Conf. of the IEEE EMBS*, pp.: 444-445.

Winter, D.A. (1990), Biomechanics and Motor Control of Human Movement. John Wiley & Sons, Inc., 2nd edition.

Yamaguchi, G.T., Zajac, F.E. (1990), Restoring Unassisted Natural Gait to Paraplegics via Functional Neuromuscular Stimulation: A Computer Simulation Study. *IEEE Trans. on Biomed. Eng.*, **37:** 886-902.

Unsupported Standing of Paraplegics by Stimulation of the Plantarflexors: some Results from the Wobbler Apparatus

N. de N. Donaldson[1], F. M. D. Barr[1], G. F. Phillips[2], T. A.Perkins[1]
[1]Implanted Devices Group, Deptartment of Medical Physics & Bioengineering, University College London, UK
[2]FES Research Unit, Royal National Orthopaedic Hospital Trust, Stanmore, London, UK

Abstract - It is desirable that FES be used with automatic controllers but success will depend on the type of controller used and how the controller can be tuned for the individual and his pathology. In the analysis and experiments described in this paper, we are studying a servo-type controller for a simplified system, which is the unsupported standing of paraplegics by stimulation of the plantarflexors, with all the joints above the ankles braced. This simplification of the usual biomechanics allows us to investigate whether paraplegic muscles can achieve this realistic task, and, if so, how it can be done. From measurements made on the isometric muscles, linear methods are used to design a robust controller with two nested feedback loops: one for ankle moment and one for ankle angle. An apparatus called the Wobbler is used. Methods for measuring the muscle frequency responses are presented and compared. The ankle stiffness is found to be elastic and small in the frequency range of interest. A controller for ankle joint moment is described and its performance illustrated.

1 Introduction

Experiments in which muscle stimulators are used with feedback from sensors to obtain automatic control of force or position have been performed for over 25 years, since Vodovnik *et al.* (1967). Chizeck (1992) has written an up-to-date review. The advantages of using feedback control are well-known and would be valuable in FES: the system is less affected by changes in the plant (e.g. muscle fatigue) and by external disturbances. Much of the experimental work with feedback controllers has been done on animals, often on single muscles with cuff electrodes on the motor nerve or with intramuscular electrodes, and with the transected tendon attached to a force transducer. Such a preparation avoids cutaneous reflexes and muscle coactivation which may occur when stimulating paralysed human subjects with skin electrodes. Also, experimental animals are healthy with no pathological disorders. To what extent these results indicate that satisfactory performance is possible with paraplegics is unclear. The difficulties, which may occur when stimulating paraplegics with skin electrodes, include coactivation of antagonists, spasticity and spasms. The joints may not move freely, due to contractures and useful muscles may not be excitable due to loss of their lower motor neurones. There may also be interference from the cutaneous or the Hoffman reflexes. Muscles which are stimulated continuously, so as produce near to the maximal possible force, weaken, typically within a few minutes. This loss of force is accompanied by a reduction in the speed of response of the whole muscle, as the fast-acting motor units tire more rapidly. Feedback control has been used with plegic subjects, but only Ewins *et al.* (1990) seems to have a system in routine clinical use. Their system maintains the knee in hyperextension during standing, rather than in the mid-range of the joint, so the controller may not need to be continually active.

Could some paraplegics be given controllers which would provide unsupported standing so that the arms and shoulders were freed from the task of balancing the trunk on the extended legs? There is at present a wide gulf between the supported standing which has been attempted for clinical use (e.g. Ewins *et al.*, 1990), and the modelling of unsupported standing which has been studied by Khang and Zajac (1989). They simulated a 13-muscle model which simultaneously controlled the hip, knee and ankle in the anterior-posterior plane. Our approach to bridging this gulf is to restrict the problem to control of the ankles while the knees hips and trunk are braced. With only one degree of freedom, the controller can be much simpler, but the difficulties, listed above, of working with actual paraplegics remain. We are doing experiments on unsupported standing of paraplegics using the ankle muscles. Experiments with ankle controllers were begun by Bajzac and Jaeger (1987) but they did not report feedback-controlled standing.

Our experiments are based on the hypothesis that despite the paraplegics' ankles, considered as electrically-activated moment motors, being far from the ideal of linear time-invariance, it will be possible to design a satisfactory controller using linear design methods, but with a fixed non-linearity preceding the muscle to correct the recruitment non-linearity.

2 Original Design Concept

2.1 The Inverted Pendulum

Balancing a person upright in the anterior-posterior plane, while only controlling the ankle muscles, can be modelled as a single-link inverted pendulum (Jaeger, 1986) maintained upright by a variable moment at the foot. If this pendulum has mass m, moment of inertia J and its centre of mass is at height l; its equation of motion is

$$M + mgl\theta_o = J\frac{d^2\theta_o}{dt^2} \qquad (1)$$

Where M is the moment at the ankle and θ_o is the inclination to the vertical. The controller of Fig. 1 can be used to control the ankle angle. The control law is

$$-M = G\theta_i - P\theta_o - D\frac{d\theta_o}{dt} \tag{2}$$

where θ_i is the set point for the controller. These equations lead to a closed-loop transfer function of

$$\frac{\theta_o}{\theta_i} = \frac{G}{Js^2 + Ds + (P - mgl)} \tag{3}$$

This transfer function will be stable if P>mgl. For the low frequency gain to be unity, G should be set to equal (P-mgl). The damping is determined by the derivative term D.

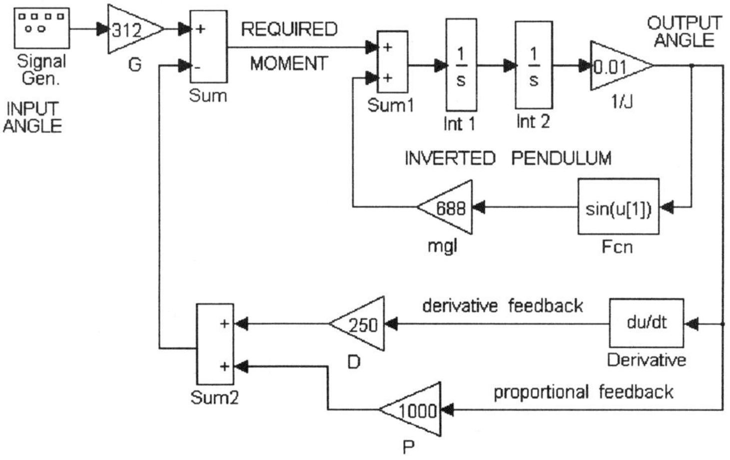

Fig. 1. Controller to maintain an inverted pendulum upright. An ideal moment actuator is assumed.

The fact that the response is dependent on the difference between the proportional term (P) and the weight term (mgl) shows that if the loop gain (i.e. P) were to change, due to fatigue, the pendulum will tend to become unstable. If one attempts to avoid instability by raising the initial gain, the response will, at first, be excessively fast, requiring larger restoring moments which the muscles may not be able to deliver. So, if one placed the muscles directly into this ankle angle control loop, it is probable that either the system would become unstable with fatigue, or, that the muscle would not operate in a linear manner, thus invalidating the method of design.

2.2 Nested Feedback Loops

This difficulty is avoided, and the controller made more robust, if the ankle moments are made available as feedback signals to the controller. This gives a nested structure with moment-control loops inside the angle-control loop of Fig. 1. The inner loop will tend to correct for the changes in the muscles, the imperfect neutralisation of the non-linearity and the muscle stiffness, while the outer loop can be set for the best speed of response of the angle controller without requiring excessive moment from the muscles. The muscle stiffness is modelled as a transfer function which causes additive changes in the ankle moment due to the ankle motion. Fig. 2 shows this system as a continuous-time controller.

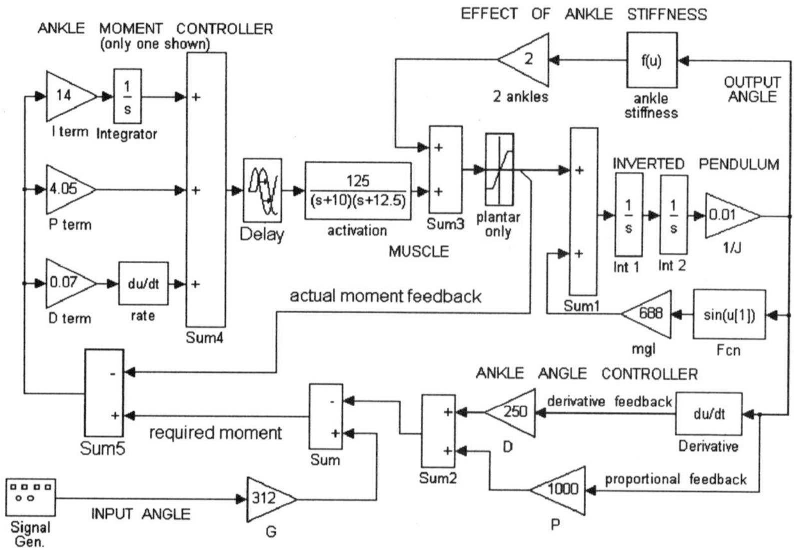

Fig. 2. Only one ankle moment controller is shown, though in practice, two are used. An unknown stiffness function is shown. This stiffness causes ankle moments due to the changing ankle angle.

The inverted pendulum is described by two parameters, the moment of inertia about the ankles (J) and the product of the weight and the height of the centre of gravity (mgl). In the short term, these will be constant, so once measured, the ankle-angle controller (P, D & G) is determined and need not be altered. The muscle properties, represented in the simulation model by the second order lag, change quickly, at least due to fatigue, and so the method used for measuring muscle model is very significant.

2.3 Isometric Moment Controllers

Much work has been done on the parametric model identification of muscle: the idea being that once the model is known, a suitable controller can be designed (Trnkoczy *et al.*, 1978; Allin and Inbar, 1986; Bernotas *et al.*, 1986). However the muscle is not only non-linear but time-varying, so that even the best linear models, obtained after a good deal of work, may not match the muscle very well. If linear design methods are to be used, a simple approach, following Bajzac and Jaeger (1989), is to use Bode Plots of the muscles' frequency response (i.e. non-parametric models), and to design the controllers by setting the open-loop phase margin (Ellis, 1991).

We model the isometric muscle as an static non-linearity (Fig 3), followed by a linear transfer function (the Hammerstein model, Durfee and MacLean, 1989). The transfer function is likely to approximate a second order lag with an additional transport delay of about 20 msec (Trnkoczy *et al.*, 1978; Allin and Inbar, 1986; Durfee and MacLean, 1989). We expect the parameters of the transfer function will change as the muscle fatigues (but see below). A non-parametric description of the isometric muscle will, under these assumptions, be represented by one recruitment curve and a family of Bode Plots, corresponding to the changes in the transfer function with fatigue. The delay appears as part of the phase lag of the frequency function.

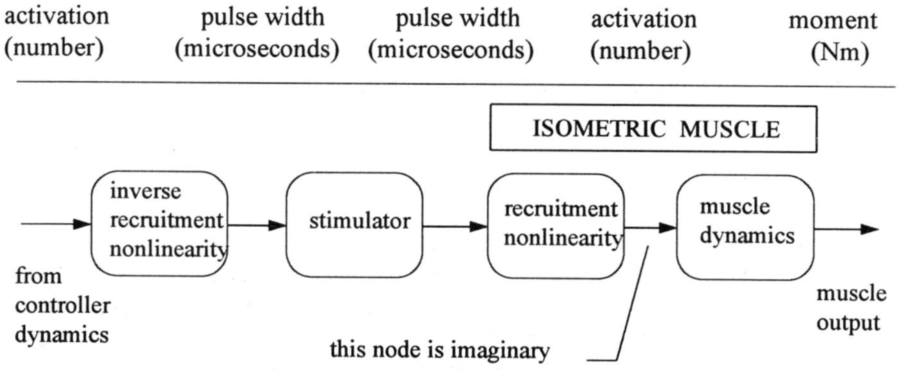

Fig. 3. Neutralising the recruitment nonlinearity.

From the Bode Plots, a controller for moment ("the isometric moment controller") can be designed. This will comprise the inverse non-linearity and the dynamic part of the controller. To minimise the static error due to the stiffness, fatigue and residual nonlinearity, the loop gain should be as large as is practicable.

In the simulator block diagram of Fig. 2, the inner loop contains a PID controller with a closed-loop -3 dB breakpoint at 3 Hz. The outer loop, which stabilises the ankle angle, has a P term, chosen so that moments, following large step changes in input angle, are within the range of the muscles' expected isometric moment range. The derivative term is adjusted to give a slightly over-damped response so that falls will not occur on the "overshoot". The limiter following the activation block represents the extreme isometric moments which the plantarflexors can produce. We originally supposed that a suitable stiffness transfer function may be approximated using data from Weiss *et al.* (1988), Toft *et al.* (1991), Sinkjaer *et al.* (1992), Flaherty *et al.* (1994) or Robinson *et al.* (1994). No source of spasmodic muscle activity is shown.

3 Methods

3.1 Subject and Stimulator

A 32-year old male with a complete T4/5 lesion volunteered to participate in the experiments. He has no complications and had been standing regularly. He was eleven years post-injury at the beginning of a six week bilateral training program of the calf muscles. The tibialis anterior and gastrocnemius muscles were stimulated alternately and isometric contractions were obtained by restraining the ankle with a bespoke orthosis. According to Benton *et al.* (1981), this prevents loss of joint range and increased spasticity. Plantarflexion moments increased from 3 Nm on both sides to 36 on the left and 45 on the right.

During the stimulation experiments, pairs of 75 mm diameter self-adhesive electrodes are placed over the midline of soleus, about 150 mm between centres. The stimulator uses a pre-defined current and produces stimulating pulses in the range 0-500 microseconds with constant increments of 2 microseconds.

3.2 Body Brace

The joints of the knees, hips, trunk and neck are braced so that only the ankles are free. A body brace has been made with vacuum-formed polythene shells for the head, back and legs. These shells are reinforced and joined by steel strips. Measurements of the subjects' weight, moment of inertia and centre of gravity is made while he is wearing this brace. For stimulation experiments, he is strapped into the brace while lying on a tilt-bed; his feet are then inserted into shoes in the Wobbler apparatus, and he then pulls himself upright and is fixed there by rope stays.

3.3 The Wobbler

This apparatus allows several types of experiments to be conducted.

- By fixing the feet at some suitable plantarflexion angle, the isometric plantarflexion moments of both ankles can be measured during stimulation. Closed-loop controllers can be tested while the ankles are not in motion.

- With or without stimulation, the feet can be rocked sinusoidally at frequencies up to 6 Hz. By measuring the angle which is common to both ankles, and the moment in each ankle, the stiffness of both ankles can be measured.
- In "Imitation Standing", the feet are rocked, while the body is fixed. This is analogous to the body swaying in the anterior-posterior plane, about the ankles. Given the fixed transfer function in the ankle angle feedback path (P and D in Fig. 2), the moments which would be required to stabilise the pendulum can be calculated in real time, and fed to the two ankle moment controllers. If, despite the motion and any other effects, the actual ankle moments are close to those required by the angle controller, then artificial balance should be possible.

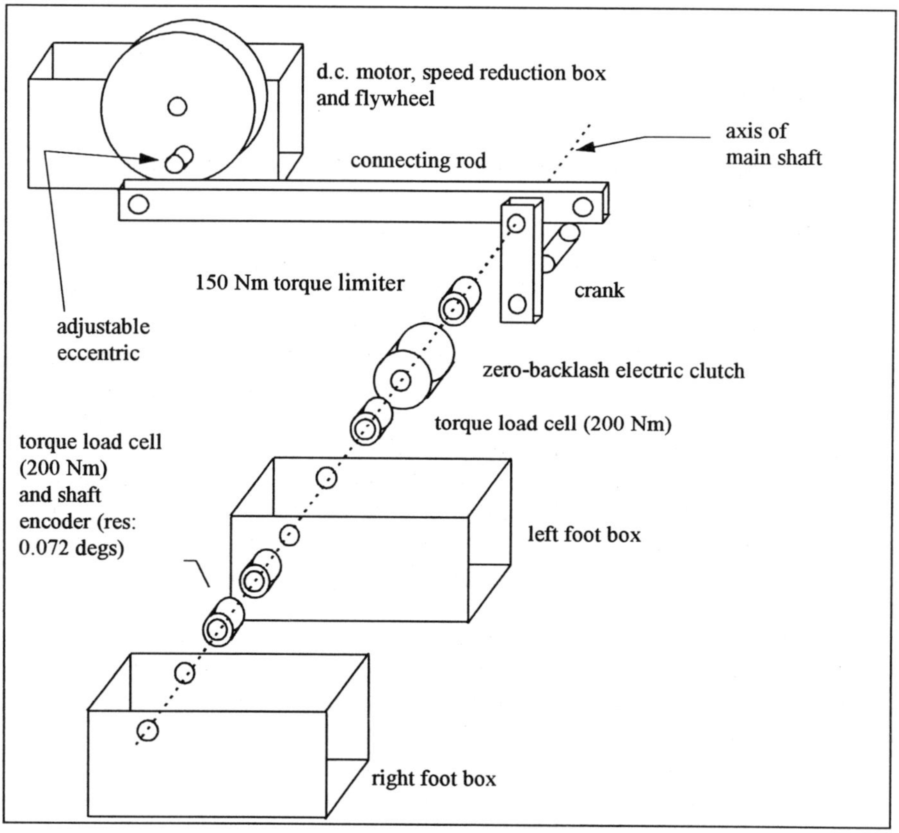

Fig. 4. Exploded view of the Wobbler Apparatus

The shoes are fixed in open-top boxes, in line with a horizontal shaft which is aligned with the transverse axis of the ankle joints. Fig. 4 is an exploded schematic view of the apparatus. The boxes are in the foreground, on a shaft with a rotary encoder and two torque load cells to measure the two moments. The boxes are made of a sandwich of polystyrene foam with a glass-reinforced resin skin, so as to be stiff but with low moment of inertia. The shaft is driven in near-sinusoidal motion by a crank-rocker through an electrically-operated clutch which allows the feet to be rapidly disengaged. The subject's ankles are protected from strain by mechanical stops which are adjusted to limit the travel of the ankles if, by accident, the clutch were to be engaged in the wrong position. If this should happen, a 150 Nm torque-limiter prevents damage to the apparatus. The speed of wobbling is derived from a d.c. motor which drives the crank through a toothed-belt, speed-reduction box. There is also a tachometer on the motor.

4 Some Results

4.1 Measuring the frequency response and the recruitment nonlinearity

Durfee & Maclean (1989) pointed out that a quick way to estimate the recruitment nonlinearity is to use twitch responses to stimulating pulses with a range of intensities. This Impulse Response Method (IRM) can also be used to find the frequency response by taking a Fast Fourier Transform of one twitch response.

In our experiments, we first set the stimulator current so that at maximal pulse width, there was a strong plantarflexion contraction but without provoking spasm of contraction of the dorsiflexors (Test A). In Test B, we applied 50 impulses at intervals of 1.2s, long enough for the response to subside. Ten pulse widths were used, each repeated five times and in a random order. The pulse widths were in the series 50, 100, 150 ....500 microseconds. For each pulse width, the five responses were averaged and displayed as in Fig.5. The recruitment curve is obtained by looking at the height of the peak response versus the pulse width: effectively cutting the surface in the plane of the peaks.

Fig. 6 shows the results of repeating Test B when the muscles had been fatigued by various other tests. The jaggedness is due to the relatively large proportion of noise. Note that although the twitch amplitude is about ten times smaller due to the fatigue, the speed of response is little changed.

Bode Plots are produced by Fourier Transformation of the average twitch response. Transformation gives the shapes of the gain and phase curves but not the magnitude of the response to the steady-frequency tetanic contraction which is to be used. A "calibration" test (Test C) is needed to give this information: a five second burst of stimulation is applied at the tetanic frequency (20 Hz in this case), and the average moment is recorded after the response has settled. This moment, divided by the activation level used during the burst, gives the "low-frequency gain" of the muscle. Our units are Nm/mAct; where 1000 mAct, or 1 Act, corresponds to full activation of the muscle. Thus a low-frequency gain of 0.032 Nm/mAct corresponds to a maximal contraction moment of 32 Nm. The gain-frequency curve, obtained by transformation of the impulse response is rescaled, using the low frequency gain to give tetanic frequency response curves like those in Fig 7 (continuous line graphs). These curves derive from the 350 microsecond pulse response in Fig. 5.

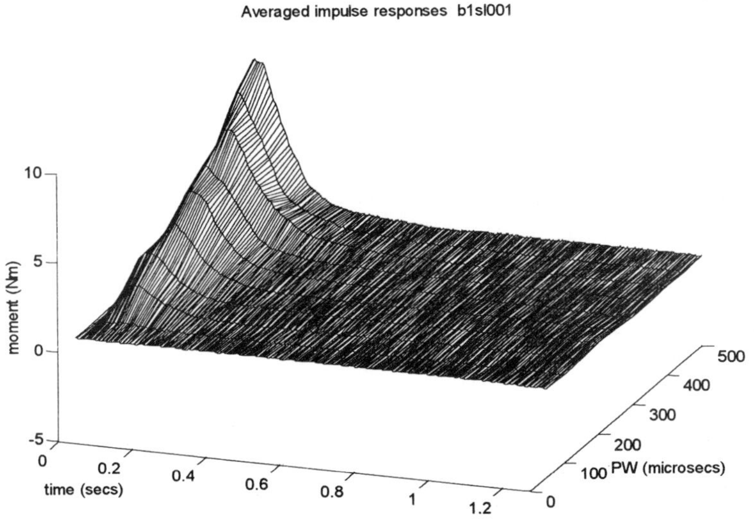

Fig. 5. Averaged twitch responses for fresh muscle.

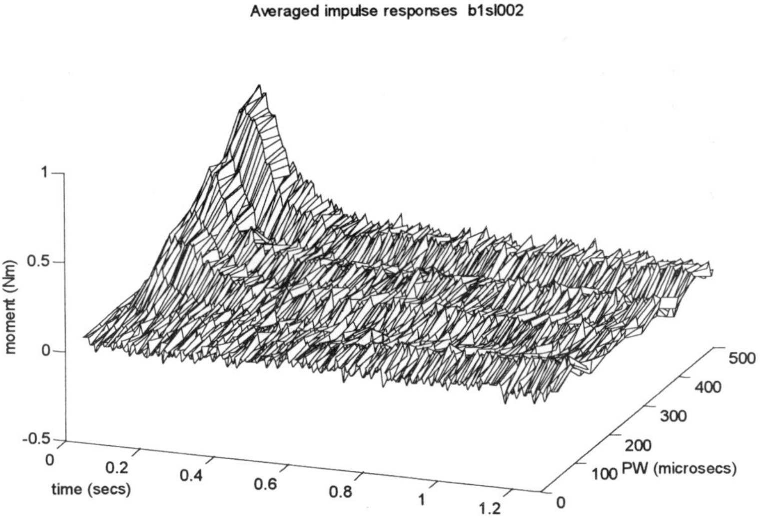

Fig. 6. Averaged twitch responses for fatigued muscle.

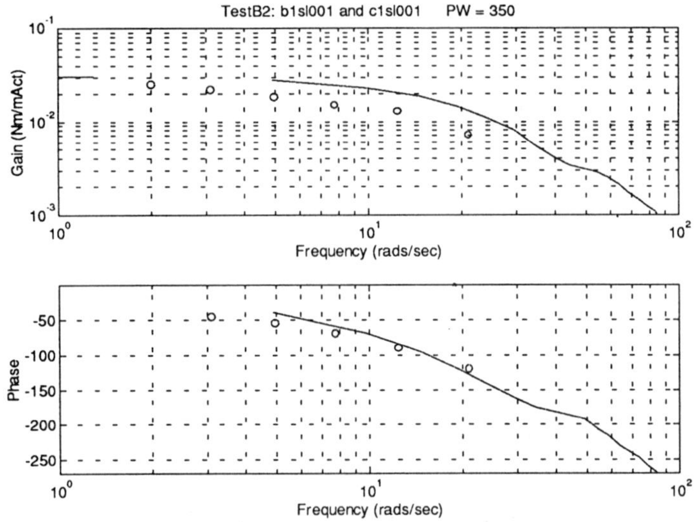

Fig. 7. Bode Plots from Test B, the IRM (line), and Test G (circles).

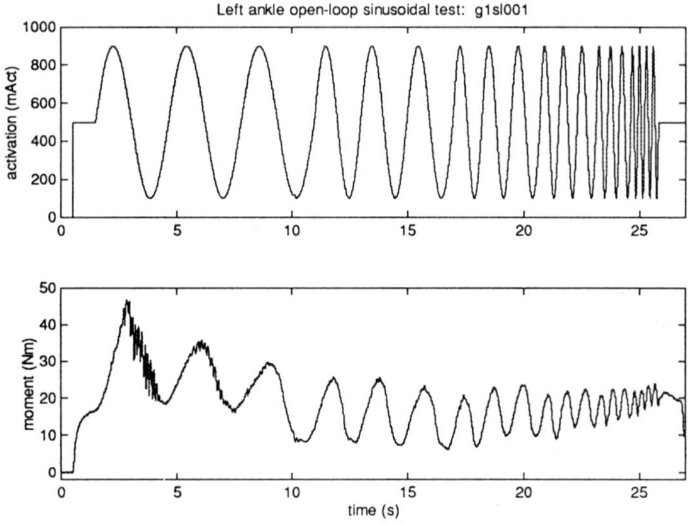

Fig. 8. Sinusoid test (Test G)

4.2 Comparison of the IRM with sinusoidal testing

For comparison, we can test the muscles with a sinusoidally-modulated tetanic stimulus. To minimise the duration of this test (Test G), we apply only a few cycles at each of the frequencies, with abrupt changes in frequency but without discontinuities in the intensity. This test must follow Test B which provides the recruitment curve. After the test, the frequency response is obtained by cross-correlation of the output and the delayed input. This test finds the phase and gain responses, including the low-frequency gain (i.e. it does not require the results of Test C). Fig. 8 shows the activation signal and the moment response from a sinusoid test run shortly after the impulse test of Fig. 5. The gain and phase for the modulation frequencies, found by cross-correlation, are also displayed in Fig. 7. This is a typical comparison of the results of the two tests.

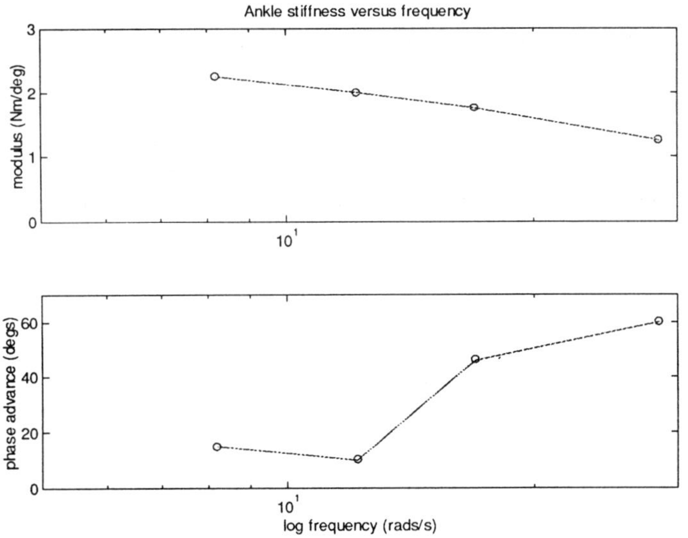

Fig. 9. Stiffness measured by "wobbling" the ankles.

4.3 Joint stiffness versus frequency

The stiffness is measured while the muscles are continuously stimulated at a constant level of activation. In this test (Test H), the wobbling frequency is set manually with an autotransformer. The amplitude is preset by the eccentric on the flywheel. The displacement and ankle moments are measured by the shaft encoder and torque load cells respectively.

Fig.9 shows a series of measurements made at half activation. It can be seen that at low frequencies, the stiffness becomes elastic, because the phase between the displacement and the moment tends to zero. At high freqency, the moment leads the displacement and declines in amplitude. This behaviour is to be expected, according to the biomechanical model described by Flaherty *et al.* (1994): at low frequencies, the stiffness is only the parallel elastic element, representing the surrounding tissue, while at high frequencies, the series elastance of the muscle and the dashpot introduce phase lead. The fall in magnitude is due to the resonance between the mass of the foot/footbox and the ankle elasticity. Because of the low mass of the foot boxes & shoes (0.096 Nms^2), this resonance is above the range of measurement and doesn't interfere with the estimation of joint stiffness at sway frequencies.

Given the weakness of the stimulated muscles compared to the inertia of the inverted pendulum, it is unlikely that the sway frequency will exceed 0.4 Hz or 2.5 rads/s[1]. This result shows that, at the sway frequencies we are trying to control, the stiffness is approximately a pure elasticity.

4.4 Elasticity of the joint as functions of activation and fatigue

Accepting that the stiffness is elastic at low frequencies, we measured the stiffness at one low frequency (1 Hz) as a function of activation and fatigue. These data are shown in Fig. 10. The later measurements were made after intentionally fatiguing the muscles severely by prolonged stimulation.

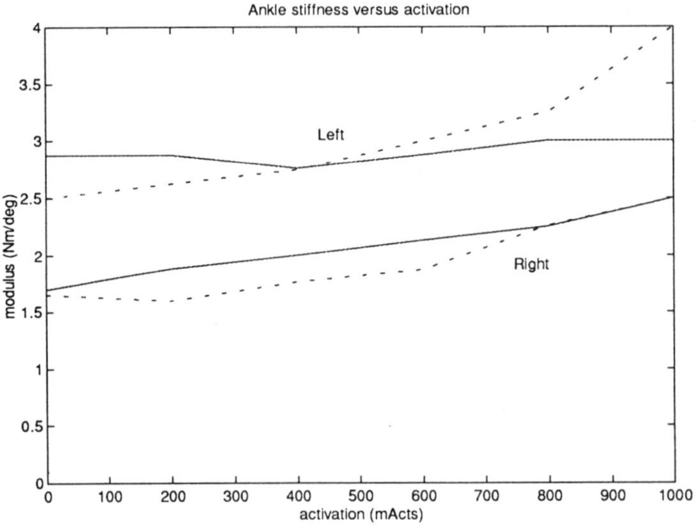

Fig. 10. Stiffness versus activation. Fresh muscles (___); fatigued muscles (- -).

---

[1] If the effective "positive elasticity" (see section 4.4) is raised from the -13 Nm/deg, of the inverted pendulum, to + 10 Nm/deg by feedback action, this will be the natural frequency of the pendulum with a moment of inertia of 95 Nms^2, the measured value.

The significance of the magnitude of these elasticity figures can be assessed by consideration of the inverted pendulum. The elasticity provides a moment which tends to restore the ankle joint to its neutral position; contrariwise, the inverted pendulum has the property that the gravitational moment tending to displace it from the neutral position increases with displacement. The inverted pendulum is like a "negative elasticity". The magnitude of this negative elasticity, for the paraplegic, is 13 Nm/deg. Comparing this with the positive elasticity of the ankles, approximately 2.5 Nm/deg/ankle, we see that their contribution to stability is approximately 38 %. The remainder must be provided by feedback action in the stimulator-controller. We also note that the stabilising effect of the ankle stiffness does not change much with fatigue.

4.5 A Moment Controller with Anti-Windup

The PID controller of Fig. 2 has the disadvantage that step changes in the input cause infinite output in the rate-of-change term. When we implemented a controller with this structure as a discrete-time controller with integrator limits so that the integral term would not "wind up", it responded incorrectly at negative steps, due to the wide bandwidth of the differentiator.

Fig. 11 shows a better controller with anti-windup, 0-1000 limiter inside the integrator loop, and the differentiator in the main feedback path instead of the feedforward path. The blocks in the feedback path may be regarded either as a differentiator with a high-pass filter to limit the bandwidth, or as a phase-advance network.[2]

The controller is tuned using the open-loop Bode Plots so as to achieve some specified phase margin at a chosen frequency. The closed-loop frequency response is then calculated for all frequencies using the open-loop frequency response: if unsatisfactory, other combinations of phase margin and frequency can be tried. The phase-advance network serves to increase the phase margin. Adding phase advance should not occur over a very narrow range of frequency, for good closed-loop response, and an arbitrary constant maximal phase advance of 36 degrees is used (Ellis, p. 96). The centre-frequency of the phase-advance network is always placed at the frequency at which the total open-loop gain is to be unity. The controller constants are calculated by a MATLAB program which also displays the calculated closed loop responses.

The response of the muscle to such closed-loop control (Test M) is shown in Fig. 12. The input is a series of sine waves with increasing frequency.

[2] We are grateful to Dr D. Sbarbaro of the University of Concepcion, Chile, for recommending this form.

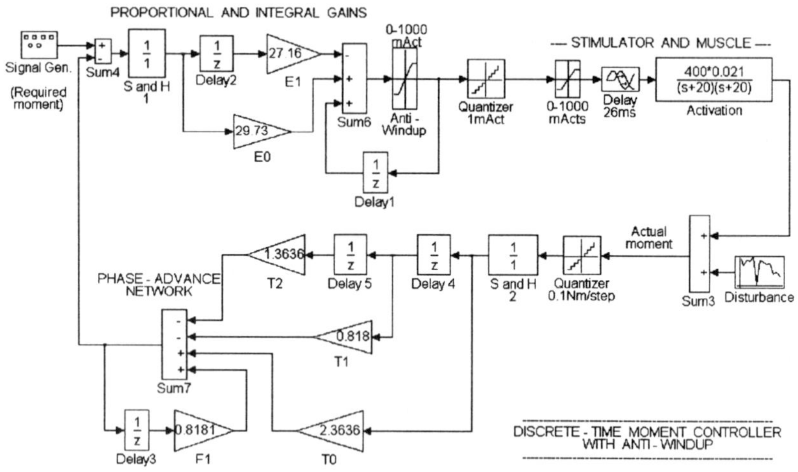

Fig. 11. Block diagram of one moment controller.

5 Conclusions

The Wobbler allows us to measure the ankle joints' stiffness, the open-loop frequency response and test controllers with the ankle fixed; all with paraplegics in a standing posture and with their weight on their feet. These tests should be realistic.

Although both the Impulse Response Test and the Sinusoid Test take about one minute, the IRM finds the recruitment curve as well as the frequency response. Furthermore the IRM is much less fatiguing of the two, and is generally preferred.

We have been surprised to find that the phase-frequency responses and the shape of the gain-frequency responses, so obtained, are very stable, both as the muscle fatigues, and from month to month. Of course the magnitude of the gain itself falls dramatically, during the experiments, by about ten-fold typically, if the stimulation current is maintained constant for all the experiments. This constancy suggests that an adaptive controller would only need to alter the loop gain to compensate for fatigue. It also means that the frequency characteristics of the controller probably can be constant for long periods.

As the ankle stiffness at sway frequencies is elastic and not strongly dependent on activation level or fatigue, its effect can be easily allowed for in the design process by reducing the "negative elasticity" of the pendulum by the approximate positive elasticity contributed by the ankles together. This is simpler than adding the additional feedback pathway for stiffness, shown in Fig.2.

Taking these facts together, and given the relative constancy of the subject's weight, height and moment of inertia, we have found that, on any day, the only unknown which must be measured is the Low Frequency Gain of each ankle. That is not to say that the amount of spasm is not highly significant to success.

What is most unsatisfactory about the moment controllers we have used is their poor phase response, even at low frequencies. This can be seen in Fig. 12. Using feedback control improves the gain-frequency response but does little to improve the phase-frequency. Typically it is possible to obtain a gain response within 3 dB up to 20 rad/s but to find that at upper sway frequency of 2.5 rad/s, the phase lag will be in the region of 45 degrees.

A practical limitation to this work is due to the weakness of the subject's stimulated muscles, compared to the weight and height of the pendulum. With the one subject we have been studying, stimulating by surface electrodes, he could never recover from disturbances beyond 4 cm at his centre of gravity. That is when his muscles are fresh, as they tire during a few minutes of stimulation, this largest disturbance will quickly diminish.

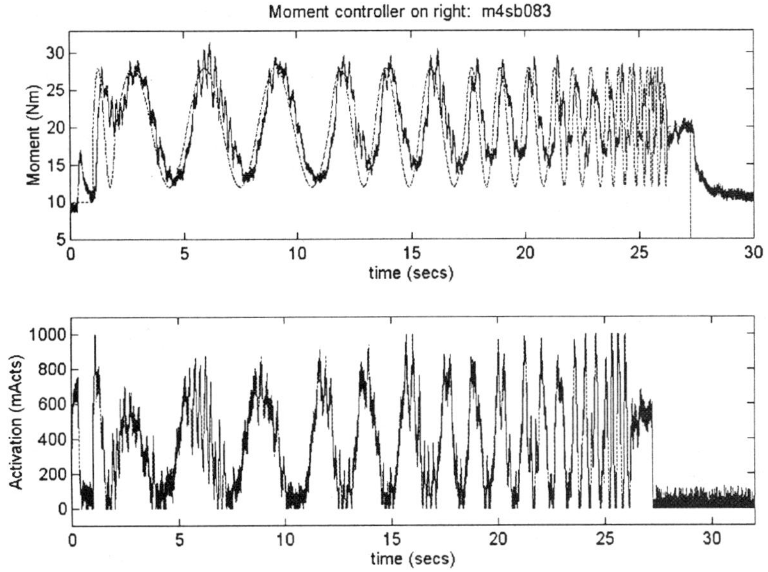

Fig. 12. Typical result from the moment controller with ankle fixed. The upper graph shows the input (required) moment and the actual moment produced.

Acknowledgement

We wish to thank the British Medical Research Council for their support.

References

Vodovnik, L., Crochetiere, W. J., and Reswick, J. B. (1967) Control of skeletal joint by electrical stimulation of antagonists. Med. Biol. Eng., *5*, 97-109.

Chizeck, H.J. (1992) Adaptive and nonlinear control methods for neural prostheses. In: *Neural Prostheses*, eds: Stein R.B., Peckham P.H. & Popovic D.B., Oxford University Press, p. 298.

Ewins, D. J., Taylor, P.N., and Swain, I. D. A functional closed-loop sit/stand system for mid/low thoracic paraplegics. In: *Advances in External Control of Human Extremities, X*, ed: Popovic, Nauka, Belgrade, 261-264, 1990.

Khang, G. and Zajac, F. E., (1989) Paraplegic standing controlled by functional neuromuscular stimulation: part I - Computer model and control system design. IEEE Trans. Biomed. Eng., *36*, 873-894.

Bajzek, T. J. and Jaeger, R. J. (1987) Characterisation and control of muscle response to electrical stimulation. An. Biomed. Eng., *15*, 485-501.

Jaeger, R. J. (1986) Design and simulation of closed-loop electrical stimulation orthoses for restoration of quiet standing in paraplegia. J. Biomech., *19*, 825-835.

Trnkoczy, A., Bajd, T., and Malezic, M. (1978) A dynamic model of the ankle joint under functional electrical stimulation in free movement and isometric conditions. J. Biomech., *9*, 509-519.

Allin, J. and Inbar, G. F. (1986) FNS parameter selection and upper limb characterisation. IEEE Trans. Biomed. Eng., *33*, 809-817.

Bernotas, L., Crago, P.E., and Chizeck, H. J. (1986) A discrete-time model of electrically stimulated muscle. IEEE Trans. Biomed. Eng., *33*, 829-838.

Ellis, G. (1991) Control System Design Guide, Academic Press.

Durfee, W. K. and Maclean, K. E. (1989) Methods for estimating the isometric recruitment curve of electrically stimulated muscle. IEEE Trans. Biomed. Eng., *36*, 654-667.

Bawa, P. and Stein, R. B. (1976) Frequency response of human soleus muscle. J. Neurophysiol., *39*, 788-793.

Weiss, P. L., Hunter, I. W., and Kearney, R. E. (1988) Human ankle joint stiffness over the full range of muscle activation levels. J. Biomech., *21*, 539-544.

Toft, E., Sinkjaer, T., Andreassen, S., and Larsen, K. (1991) Mechanical and electromyographic responses to stretch of the human ankle extensors. J. Neurophysiol., *65*, 1402-1410.

Sinkjaer, T., Gantchev, N., and Arendt-Nielsen, L (1992) Mechanical properties of human ankle extensors after muscle potentiation. Enceph. Clin. Neurophysiol., *85*, 412-418.

Flaherty, B., Robinson, C., and Agarwal G. (1994) Determining appropriate models for joint control using surface electrical stimulation of soleus in spinal cord injury. Medical and Biological Engineering and Computing, **32**, 273-282.

Robinson, C., Flaherty, B., Fehr, L., Agarwal, G. C., Harris, G. F., and Gottlieb G. L. (1994) Biomechanical and reflex responses of joint perturbations during electrical stimulation of muscle: instrumentation and measurement techniques. *Ibid*, **32**, 261-272.

Benton, L. A., Baker, L. L., Bowman, B. R., and Waters, R. L. (1981) *Functional Electrical Stimulation - A practical clinical guide*. Pub. Rancho Los Amigos Rehabilitation Engineering Center. Downey. California.

Biomechanical Simulation of the Lower Extremity for the Development of Control Strategies for FES

R. Riener[1], J. Quintern[2]
[1]Department of Automatic Control Eng., Technical University Munich, Germany
[2]Neurological Clinic, University of Munich, Germany

Abstract - We developed a detailed model of the lower extremity in order to predict FES-generated knee motion during dynamic activation. The lines of action of 13 musculotendon actuators were defined on the basis of their anatomic relationships to 3-D bone surface representations. The model consists of nonlinear musculotendon and nonlinear body-segmental dynamics. Especially muscle fatigue and viscous properties were treated in detail. Model results correspond well with experimental data obtained by stimulating the quadriceps muscle with surface electrodes correspond well. The model can be applied to the design and test of closed-loop control strategies.

1 Introduction

Muscles and tendons control body movement by developing forces and exerting moments about joints. Models of the musculoskeletal system can be used to study how specific actuators and specific neural inputs contribute to movement coordination in able-bodied persons, and also to design FES systems for persons with paralyzed muscles. Modeling of the human musculoskeletal system supports and accelerates the design and test of closed-loop controllers. For example, control parameters can be adjusted and different control strategies tested in the model (Khang and Zajac, 1989 b), thus, avoiding or at least shortening troublesome and time-consuming adjustments in experiments with patients. This is very important, because fatigue causes the stimulated muscle to act differently during the experiment. Furthermore, simulation of the human musculoskeletal system is needed to understand how musculotendon actuators produce force and moment during any static or dynamic task, since only invasive methods allow measurement of many biomechanical quantities *in vivo*. In the present paper we concentrated on FES-generated knee motion. We compared simulation and experiments in order to show that the model can be applied to FES-related predictions of joint angle or joint torque.

2 The Musculoskeletal Model

Our broke down our dynamic model of the human knee into three subsystems (Fig. 1): activation dynamics, contraction dynamics, and body-segmental dynamics. The state variables describing the biomechanics of the system are coupled with each other. The system of equations is solved numerically. We use an interactive graphical interface that allows the user to visualize the computed motion in a 3-D shaded display (see also Riener et al., 1996).

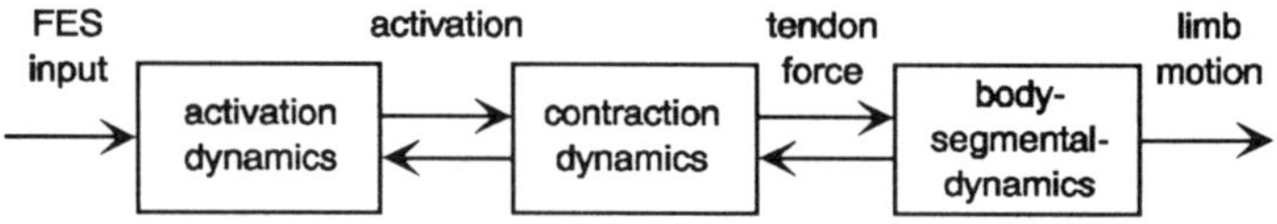

Fig. 1. Block diagram showing the interactions among the major compartments of musculoskeletal model. *Activation dynamics* describes how the muscle activation is related to the FES input (variable pulse width, frequency, and amplitude). *Contraction dynamics* generates tendon force that acts on *body-segmental dynamics* to produce motion of the body segments.

Activation dynamics provides the activation needed by muscles to generate desired force. We expanded on a discrete-time model proposed by Khang and Zajac (1989 a), where muscle force is assumed to be controlled by adjusting pulse width or pulse amplitude (recruitment modulation) and pulse frequency (rate modulation). The discrete-time character of this model allows the user to observe the influence of the stimulation frequency. For example, low frequencies lead to a fidgety dynamic behavior of the simulated system, which may be interesting for the design and test of closed-loop strategies. Unlike Khang and Zajac (1989 a) who applied a piecewise linear recruitment curve, we introduced a more complex, nonlinear recruitment curve (Fig. 2) that yields better agreement between measured and simulated results. The percentage of recruited fibers a_r can be calculated as a function of the pulse width d, applying the following equation:

$$a_r(d) = c_1 \{ (d - d_{thr}) \arctan[\kappa_{thr}(d - d_{thr})] - (d - d_{sat}) \arctan[\kappa_{sat}(d - d_{sat})] \} + c_2, \quad (1)$$

where d_{thr} and d_{sat} denote pulse width values corresponding to threshold and saturation, respectively. The above-cited equation was selected, because the curvatures of the recruitment curve in the area of threshold and saturation can be adjusted by changing κ_{thr} and κ_{sat}, respectively. The recruitment curve is scaled by the constants c_1 and c_2 in order to satisfy the conditions $a_r(0) = 0$ and $a_r(d \to \infty) = 1$.

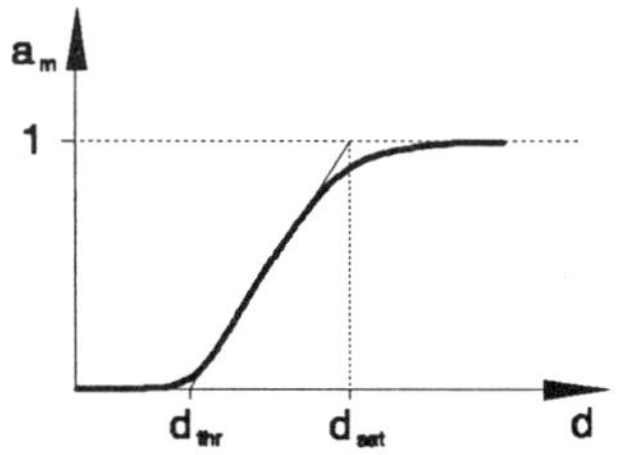

Fig. 2. Schematized recruitment curve. The magnitude of a_m is adjusted by changing the pulse width d. Pulse widths less than threshold d_{thr} produce no activation, and activation is saturated when $d > d_{sat}$.

To describe the effect of muscle fatigue we introduced a fitness value *fit(t)*, which can be expressed by the following first-order relation:

$$\frac{d\,fit(t)}{dt} = \frac{[fit_{\min} - fit(t)]a(t)}{T_{fat}} + \frac{[1 - fit(t)]\,[1 - a(t)]}{T_{rec}} \tag{2}$$

This equation considers the change of fitness due to effects of both fatigue and recovery, where T_{fat} and T_{rec} are the time constants for fatigue and recovery, respectively. Compared to other approaches (Giat *et al.*, 1993) this model can be applied to any shape of stimulation input, an advantage for describing muscle fatigue. There was a good agreement between fatigue in the model and FES experiments.

In the *contraction dynamics* component 13 musculotendon actuators were modeled to span the knee joint as a composition of elements with nonlinear viscoelastic, elastic, and force-generating properties. The force-generating properties of a specific musculotendon actuator are derived by scaling a generic, Hill-based model (Zajac, 1989). The generic model accounts for the static and dynamic properties of both muscle and tendon (Fig. 3). All the actuator properties are modeled by nonlinear characteristics as proposed in the literature. Special attention was paid to the description of the passive viscous property of muscle. The muscle's damping force F_{PV}^M was modeled as a relation between muscle velocity v^M and damping coefficient k_d^M:

$$F_{PV}^M = k_d^M \cdot sign(v^M) \cdot \left|v^M\right|^n \tag{3}$$

For n=1, equation (3) leads to the common linear relation $F_{PV}^M = k_d^M v^M$. We found no report in the literature which treated the PV element as a nonlinear element. However, by selecting n=0.5, we obtained a closer correspondence between simulated and measured passive pendulum tests in both patients and healthy subjects (see Riener et al. 1995, Fig. 2). Since no muscle-specific data exist for the damping coefficients of single muscles, the values of k_d^M were scaled according to the muscle's cross-sectional area.

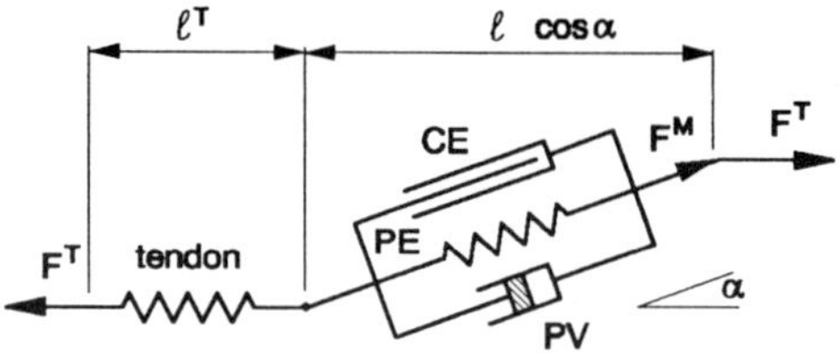

Fig. 3. Hill-type model with tendon in series. The contractile element (CE) accounts for the force-length and force-velocity properties of the muscle, which also depend on the amount of activation of the muscle. The passive properties of muscle are assumed to be viscoelastic (parallel elastic, PE, and parallel viscous element, PV).

To scale the generic model to represent a specific actuator, the user must supply some parameters that are specific to each actuator. This method was proposed in the literature (more details in Delp, 1990).

The mathematical model used to describe *body-segmental dynamics* of the shank is given by a nonlinear, one-degree-of-freedom equation of motion. This equation accounts for joint elasticity and viscosity caused by ligaments, skin, and joint friction. Muscles and tendons control shank motion by developing forces and exerting moments about joints. Multiplying tendon forces by respective moment arms yields the moments that the actuators contribute to the total joint moment. The moment arm is a function of the knee angle, φ, and it can be described as

$$ma = \frac{\partial l^{MT}}{\partial \varphi} \tag{4}$$

To obtain information about the stress in the joint ligaments, we calculated the moment arms not only about the axis of flexion-extension, but also about the axis of rotation and varus-valgus (Riener *et al.*, 1995). Musculotendon length, l^{MT}, is calculated as the sum of the lengths of the line segments that connect the points defining the muscle path. To compute muscle paths we used a detailed kinematic model of the human knee joint that considers patellofemoral and tibiofemoral motion (Yamaguchi and Zajac, 1989) and the lines of action of 13 musculotendon actuators (Delp 1990). For two-joint muscles on the thigh and shank it was necessary to consider also hip and ankle joint angles. We modeled these joints as simple hinges with angles assumed to remain constant during knee motion.

To simulate closed-loop experiments, we implemented a simple PID controller (Fig. 4). In addition, we inserted a noise generator and considered quantization effects caused by an A/D-converter. This allows the user to study the influence of sensor disturbances. Characteristic noise parameters were obtained from spectrum and autocorrelation analysis of the measured data. In the model, then, noise is generated by a Gaussian random generator (σ=1). The influence of external disturbances (e.g., additional weight attached on the foot) can be studied, too. With a well-identified model the control parameters of, for example, an implemented PID controller can be estimated. In addition, other strategies can be tested in order to improve the control behavior of the simulated system.

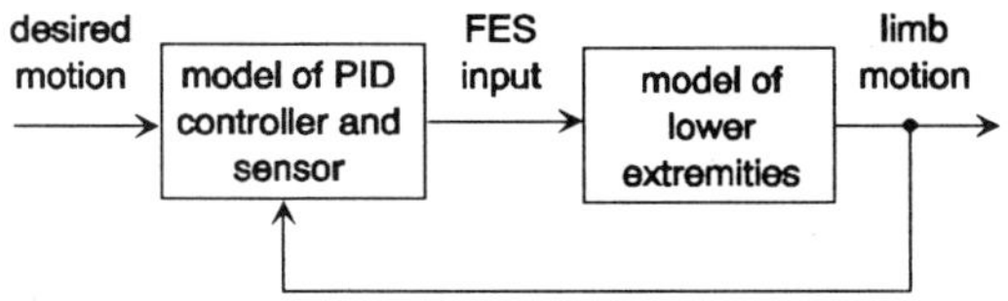

Fig. 4. Model of PID position control.

The model can also be used to simulate FES-induced shank motion or isometric knee flexion/extension moment. The user of the program can in addition decide which muscles should be stimulated in the model. Furthermore, he can prescribe various kinds of stimulation patterns and desired motion trajectories for open and closed-loop control, respectively.

3 Methods

The stimulation experiments were performed in five patients with complete thoracic spinal cord injury. The patients who were lying down with the thigh supported. The quadriceps muscle was stimulated by surface electrodes. Under isometric conditions the shank was fixed at a strain gauge-based torque transducer. The knee joint angle was measured under condition of freely swinging shank using an electrogoniometer. Data were digitized and stored in a computer. Balanced bipolar stimulation pulses were delivered by a computer-driven stimulator. For the experiments described in the present paper only pulse width modulation (rectangular or triangular modulation) with predefined current amplitude and stimulation frequency (20 Hz) was used. For the closed-loop experiments the same PID controller was implemented as applied to the model.

To adapt our model to an individual, patient-specific parameters were identified by specific procedures such as anthropometric measurements, a passive pendulum test, and specific open-loop stimulation experiments (more details in Riener *et al.* 1995). After scaling and validating the model by comparing it with model results and experimental data, we used it to predict optimum control parameters of the applied PID controller.

4 Results

Fig. 5 shows the isometric torque about the knee joint versus pulse width when the quadriceps muscle is stimulated with a triangular stimulation pattern. Due to fatigue the generated moment during the first triangular ramp is higher than during the second. For pulse widths below threshold d_{thr}, only passive elements contribute to muscle force; this yields constant moment levels.

In Fig. 6 FES-induced shank motion is shown for a rectangular modulation of pulse width.

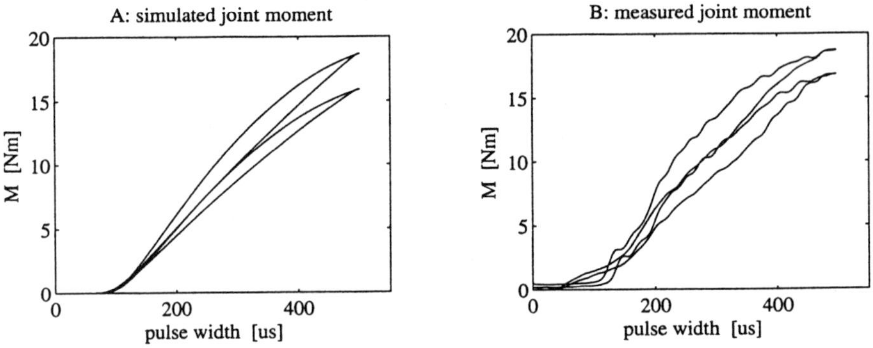

Fig. 5. Joint moment versus pulse width for triangular modulation, simulation (A), and measurement (B) under isometric conditions. The total time (two periods) was 40 s. Note that for t=0, the moment in both graphs was set to zero.The sample rate of the stimulation experiment was too low to measure the ripple appearing at 20 Hz with sufficient resolution. Thus, we smoothed the simulated data for this comparison.

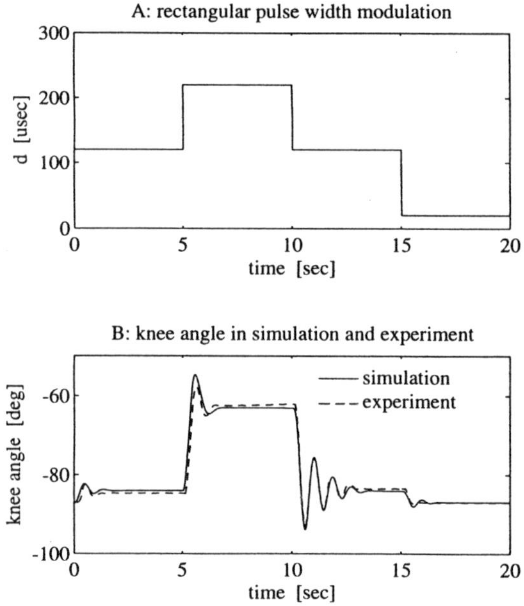

Fig. 6. Comparison of simulated and measured knee flexion angle for rectangular pulse width modulation (open-loop).

Figs. 5 and 6 show the good correspondence between simulation and measurements. In view of this agreement, the model can be used to predict the control parameters required in the experiments to obtain optimum position control behavior (Fig. 7). The control behavior could be significantly improved by adding a feedforward path that concludes inverse model components (Quintern *et al.*, 1996).

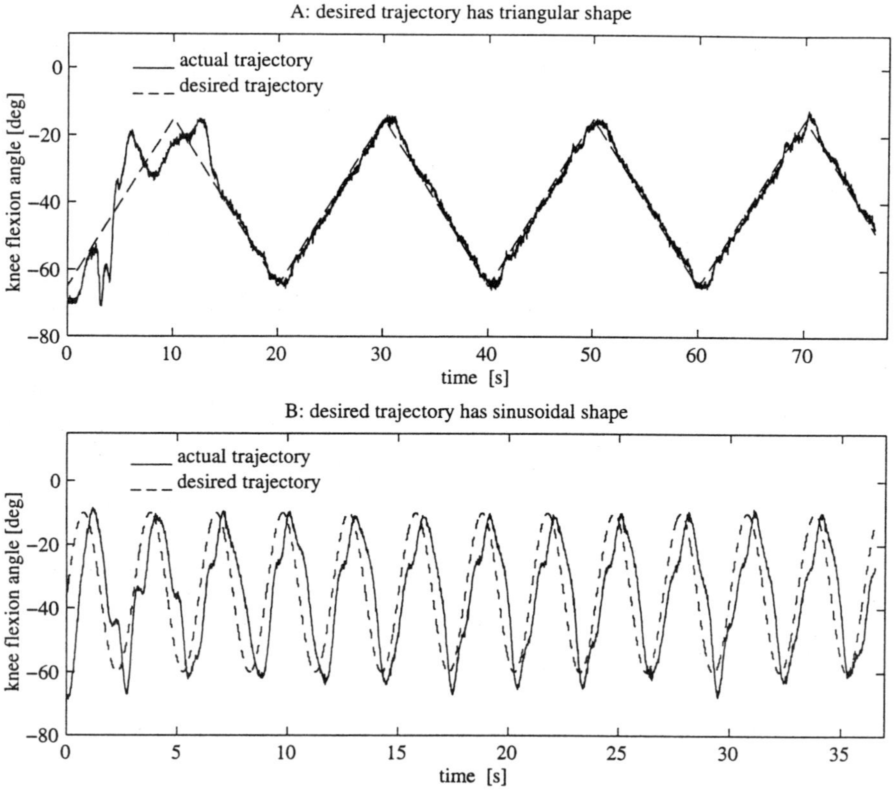

Fig. 7. Closed-loop position control for two different input trajectories. In (A) the oscillations during the first seconds of the experiment are due to spasticity. A delay between desired and actual angle of approximately 0.5 s occurred in both (A) and (B). Adding a feedforward component significantly reduced this delay (Quintern *et al.*, 1996).

Figure 8 shows the resulting knee flexion angle (A) and intermediate biomechanical quantities (C)-(F) for a closed-loop stimulation. The desired trajectory is presented in (A). Only the pulse width is modulated (B). Sensor noise was not considered. Due to discontinuous stimulation (f=20 Hz) the number of recruited muscle fibers changes only every 0.05 s (C). We observed that high pulse frequencies improve the control behavior. Musculotendon forces of rectus femoris, vastus medialis, vastus intermedius, and vastus lateralis are presented in graphs (D) and (E). Note that passive viscoelastic forces act also in muscles that are not stimulated.

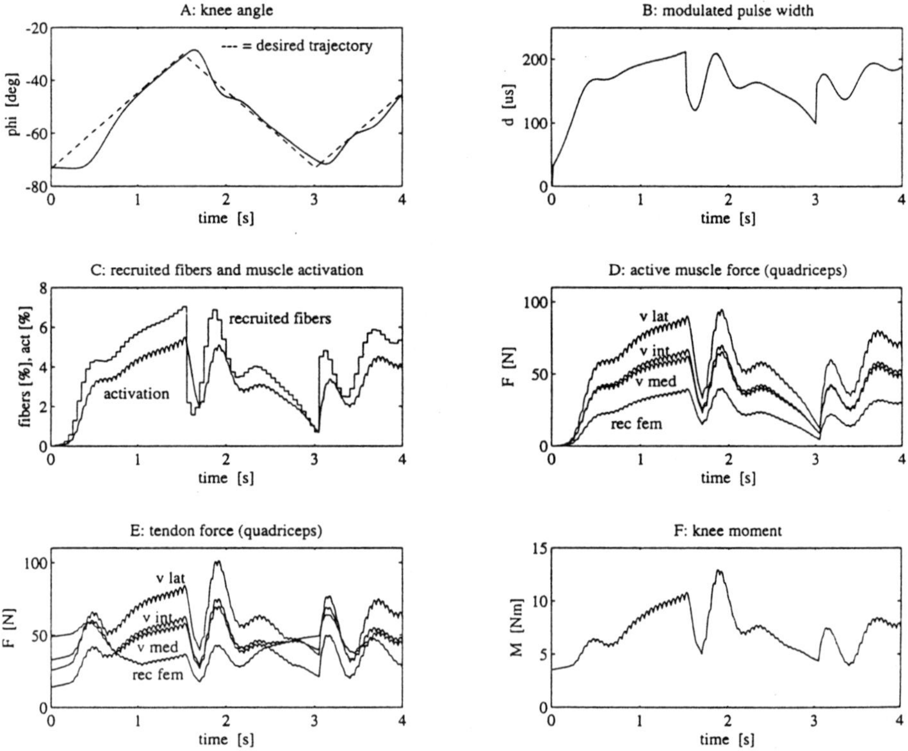

Fig. 8. Knee angle (A) and intermediate biomechanical quantities (C)-(F) for closed-loop position control modulating pulse width (B) with a PID controller. The simulation starts from shank resting position (φ=-73°, trunk in upright position) with initial pulse width $d(t_o)$=0.

5 Discussion

The objective of this study was to develop an experimentally tested biomechanical model of the lower extremity which can be employed to test different control strategies and to predict control parameters required for optimal joint position control in FES experiments.

In contrast to others (Khang and Zajac, 1989 a and b), this model accounts for fatigue and recovery as well as nonlinear muscle viscosity. Both properties are very important for the simulation of FES-related tasks. Muscle fatigue is a significant problem during FES. In some patients FES-induced muscle force drops to half of the initial value within less than a minute. Thus, the performance of a neural prosthesis is strongly affected by muscle fatigue. It is also necessary to model viscosity in musculotendon units (equation 3) in order to characterize the absorption of impact energy, for example during gait when a foot strikes the floor. Without viscosity the active force that has to be developed to compensate for the impact energy would be intolerably high.

A further advantage of our model is the large number of muscles: the user can investigate the stimulation of different combinations of muscles, and thus determine which combination develops minimum varus-valgus and rotational moments and optimum joint loading during FES in order to avoid overstress of joints and ligaments (Riener *et al.*,1996). The model is an effective tool for such investigations, since varus-valgus and rotational moments can hardly be measured noninvasively. A detailed, physiologically based modeling of the musculoskeletal system is also necessary to obtain intermediate quantities and to enable the user to observe the biomechanical consequences after changing model inputs or certain model parameters.

One difficulty of our model appears to be its complexity, which requires many parameters to describe the musculoskeletal system. However, it has been shown that simulation corresponds well with measurements (Figs. 5 and 6). One could argue that it would be easy to fit the simulated and experimental trajectories by iteratively modifying one of the various parameters, arbitrarily, without any physiological basis. This, however, does not hold true in our case, because, on the one hand, patient-independent parameters were taken from the literature (e.g., parameters describing muscle paths, joint kinematics, or musculotendon properties such as the force-length, and force-velocity relations). On the other hand, the remaining parameters for describing viscoelasticity of joints and muscles, fiber recruitment behavior, muscle fatigue, anthropometry, etc., were identified with specific procedures (Riener *et al.*, 1996). Note that the musculoskeletal system contains a number of redundant muscles, which makes it very difficult to determine muscle-specific parameters. Therefore, some specific muscle properties (e.g., muscle damping and elasticity) were derived by scaling generic muscle characteristics (Zajac, 1989). Some of the parameters for scaling a single muscle were taken from the literature (pennation angle, optimal muscle fiber length, and maximum shortening velocity). The remaining musculotendon parameters (tendon slack length, peak isometric muscle force, and muscle damping coefficient) were identified, because they vary considerably among individuals. Especially in paraplegic patients, spastic paresis causes changes in musculotendon lengths. The changes in these values also depend on the preferred posture of the patient. Patients who sit in wheelchairs most of the time may have shortened knee flexors and lengthened knee extensors. This phenomenon was also revealed by our parameter identification experiments.

Parameter identification could be improved further by stimulating single muscles with small surface or wire electrodes in order to identify more specific muscle parameters. Additional data on the viscoelastic properties of two-joint muscles at the knee could be obtained from passive elastic moment experiments also with hip and ankle joints. Anatomical studies (e.g., X-ray images) could provide other parameters for describing the geometry of joints and muscles.

The influence of increased spinal reflexes due to spasticity poses another difficult problem. In many paraplegic patients phasic polysynaptic reflexes, also known as spasms, were occasionally observed during the first seconds after onset of the stimulation (Fig. 7). These reflexes lead to complex movements with considerable variability between subjects. In view of this variability and the occasional occurrence of these reflexes only during the first seconds of stimulation, we did not consider these phasic polysynaptic reflexes in this paper. Tonic stretch reflexes are more predictable than phasic reflexes. The mechanical effect of tonic stretch reflexes is mainly a velocity-dependent increase in muscle force. Therefore, in a future version of the present model tonic stretch reflexes will be modeled as a sort of additional viscous components during muscle stretch.

Despite such difficulties and limitations, we have shown that the simulation model presented satisfactorily describes the input-output relation of the human musculoskeletal system and allows, in addition, access to certain intermediate quantities. This model has been tested to evaluate and optimize open- and closed-loop control strategies for FES. Control parameters predicted by the model led to satisfying tracking control behavior of shank motion induced by stimulating quadriceps muscle. In this study only a conventional PID controller was tested. We expect considerable improvements in the control behavior by testing learning algorithms and adaptive-predictive control strategies, stimulating extensor actuators in combination with flexor actuators, and applying simultaneous recruitment-frequency modulation. From preliminary data we conclude that the modeling of the human musculoskeletal system in the way described here can support and accelerate the development of neural prostheses.

6 Acknowledgement

We are grateful to Dr. L. Scott Delp for providing exact anatomical locations of the reference frames and muscle paths, and the musculotendon parameters. We also thank Stefan Rupprecht and Stefan Volz for their support during the measurements. We thank Prof. Schmidt in particular, for the productive discussions on many aspects of this work.

This work was supported by the German Federal Department of Education and Research (BMBF, 01K094026).

References

Delp, S. L. (1990) Surgery simulation: a computer graphics system to analyze and design musculoskeletal reconstructions of the lower limb. PhD. thesis, Stanford University, Stanford, CA.

Giat, Y., Mizrahi, J., and Levy, M. (1993) A musculotendon model of the fatigue profiles of paralyzed quadriceps muscle under FES. *IEEE Trans. Biomed. Eng.* **40**(7), 664-673.

Khang, G. and Zajac, F. E. (1989 a) Paraplegic standing controlled by functional neuromuscular stimulation: part I. - computer model and control-system design. *IEEE Trans. Biomed. Eng.* **36**(9), 873-884.

Khang, G. and Zajac, F. E. (1989 b) Paraplegic standing controlled by functional neuromuscular stimulation: part II-computer simulation studies. *IEEE Trans. Biomed. Eng.* **36**(9), 885-886.

Quintern, J., Riener, R., Volz, S., and Straube, A. (1996) Inverse models for control of movements (*this volume*).

Riener, R., Villars, S., Quintern, J., and Schmidt, G. (1996) Biomechanical Simulation and Animation of the Lower Extremity for the Design of Neural Prostheses (*this volume*).

Yamaguchi, G. T. and Zajac, F. E. (1989) A planar model of the knee joint to characterize the knee extensor mechanism. *J. Biomechanics* **22**(1), 1-10.

Zajac, F. E. (1989) Muscle and tendon: properties, models, scaling, and application to biomechanics and motor control. In *CRC Crit. Rev. Biomed. Eng.* **17**(4), 359-411.

Biomechanical Modelling in Artificial Control of FES assisted Mobility

P.H. Veltink
Institute for Biomedical Engineering / Faculty of Electrical Engineering
University of Twente, Enschede, the Netherlands

Abstract - Biomechanical modelling is an essential tool in control of FES-assisted movements. It can be used to simulate the performance of alternative control strategies before actual experimental testing. Alternatively, models can be used as parts of control strategies. Finite state models may be used to identify and control movement tasks at a relatively high level. Nonlinear model-based control of joint angle trajectories can be used in the control of relatively slow movements of the upper extremities. The control of lower extremity ballistic movements may benefit from model-based predictive control strategies.

1 Introduction

Biomechanical modelling is an essential tool in the development of control strategies for mobility in paraplegics assisted by Functional Electrical Stimulation (FES) of the neuromuscular system. This modelling may serve several different objectives, requiring rather diverse characteristics of the models. Complex full body biomechanical models may be required for simulating the preformance of alternative control strategies before actual experimental testing in patients (Yamaguchi 1989, Veltink et al. 1992, Veltink et al. 1995b, Heinze et al. 1995). Alternatively, biomechanical models may be part of model-based control strategies for FES supported mobility. The characteristics of the models depend on the hierarchical control level at which they are applied (Andrews et al. 1989, Chizeck et al. 1988). Finite state models are used in the high level task identification and intention detection (Andrews 1989, Veltink 1995a). Specific models of muscle - joint systems are used in low level nonlinear joint angle control (Veltink et al. 1991) or predictive control of balistic movements.

The requirements and characteristics of models for these different objectives will be described in this paper, illustrated by examples from our research.

2 Biomechanical modelling for pre-experimental simulation of control strategies

In the development of control strategies it may be advantageous to predict the performance of alternative strategies by model simulations. Yamaguchi and Zajac (1989) described a computer simulation study of unassisted natural gait in paraplegics using FES. They applied an extensive 3D whole body model for optimization of stimulation patterns. However, they did not verify their predictions experimentally. Mulder et al. (1992), Veltink et al. (1995b) and Heinze et al. (1995) described 2D biomechanical models for simulation of the control of standing-up. The studies were combined with experimental tests of the control principles. Veltink et al. (1992a) described a model of cyclical leg movements from stance, studying strategies for the optimization of stimulation patterns for the swing phase of gait, which were subsequently used by Franken et al. (1995) in an experimental study.

In all of these applications of biomechanical models for pre-experimental simulation of control strategies, the models are complex and contain many parameters which cannot be identified for individual subjects. Normally, average literature values are taken for most model parameters, which may be scaled to the characteristics of the individual subject (e.g. weight and length). Therefore, these model studies only indicate average performances of alternative control strategies in a qualitative way, but should not be expected to yield precise quantitative predictions, which are in exact agreement with subsequent validation results.

3 Model-based control strategies

Apart from the application of biomechanical models in the simulation of alternative control strategies before experimental validation, it may be advantageous to apply the knowledge of the biomechanical system more directly in the control strategies. This can be done by incorporating descriptive finite state models or biomechanical models in these strategies. In contrast to the extensive models used for simulation, descriptive finite state models and biomechanical models applied as part of control strategies should be identifiable, robust and simple. They should be identifiable, because the controller should be optimally tuned for individual subjects. They should be robust, because the model should still give a good description of the biomechanics if the system behaviour is time dependent or variable or when the system is externally disturbed. Finally, they should be of low complexity, since they have to be calculated in a real time scheme. For these reasons, the application of biomechanical models is mainly limited to the low level control of a limited number of muscles acting on one or two joints. Finite-state descriptive models can be used in the high level task identification and user interface part of FES control systems.

Examples of finite state descriptive models for high level control and biomechanical models for low level control will be discussed in the following.

3.1 Finite state models for task identification and control

At a high level, the control of FES-assisted mobility should identify the mobility task the user wants to perform. Veltink et al. (1995a) described an intention detection system for FES assisted mobility in paraplegics, based on a finite state description of tasks to be performed and possible transfers between tasks (figure 2). These transfers were defined in terms of signals from sensors mounted on the assistive orthosis (joint lock switches, inclinometers) and crutches (force sensors). This high level control system enabled automatic control of stimulation for support of standing-up, standing, gait and sitting down without the requirement of explicit user inputs.

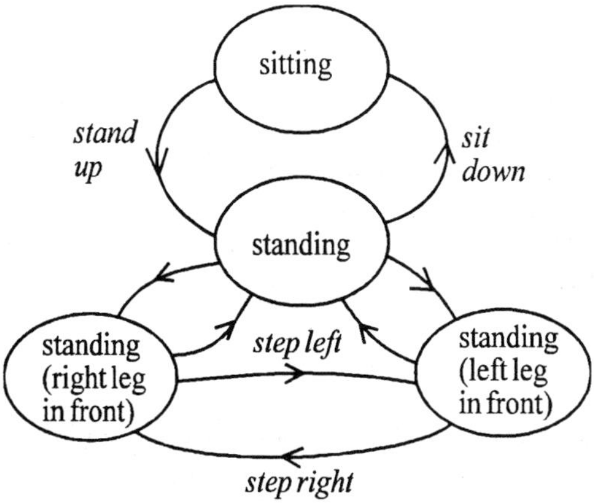

Fig. 1. Finite state model of sitting, standing-up, standing, and gait, used for control of stimulation at a high level, avoiding explicit user input (Veltink et al., 1995a).

3.2 Real-time nonlinear control of joint angle trajectory

Veltink et al. (1989, 1992b) described model-based nonlinear control of joint angle by electrical muscle stimulation, applied at the ankle joint of a cat, loaded with an external second order load. The applied multiplicative model structure is presented in figure 2. Dynamics A, angle dependency f_φ angular velocity dependency $f_{\dot{\varphi}}$ of the muscle were identified from isometric and isokinetic tests.

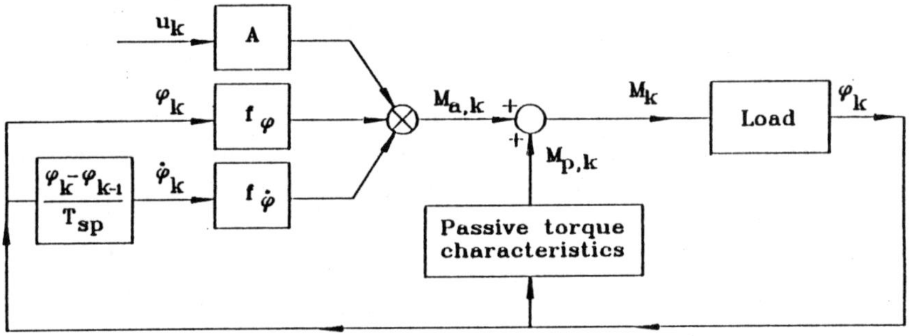

Fig. 2. Discrete-time model structure of the electrically stimulated cat soleus acting on an externally loaded ankle joint (Veltink et al. 1992b). u_k is recruitment input, φ_k is the ankle joint angle, $M_{a,k}$ is the ankle torque actively generated by soleus contraction, $M_{p,k}$ is the ankle torque generated by the passive system, and M_k is the total ankle torque. A represents the activation dynamics, modeled as a second order critically damped system, f_φ the angle dependency and $f_{\dot{\varphi}}$ the angular velocity dependency of ankle torque generated by soleus.

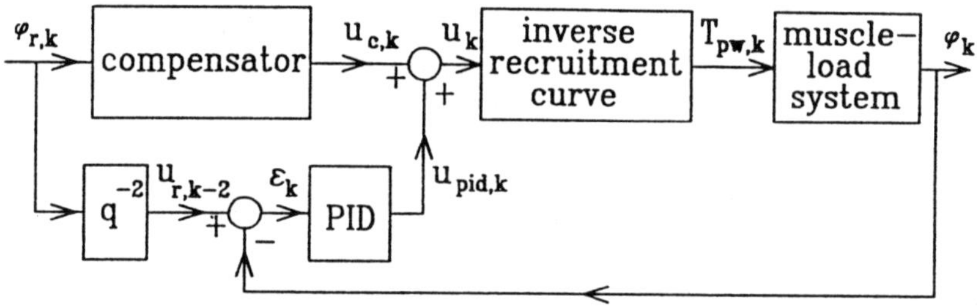

Fig. 3. Combined controller consisting of an open-loop nonlinear compensator and a feedback PID controller (Veltink et al., 1992).

The objective set out in this study was to follow desired joint angle trajectories with minimal error. An open loop nonlinear compensator was compared to a conventional PID controller and a feedforward nonlinear compensator combined with a PID controller. The combined controller is depicted in figure 3. The performance of the open-loop nonlinear compensator appeared to depend strongly on the accuracy of the identified model. Significant steady state errors occured if the model was inaccurate. On average, the performances of the open loop nonlinear compensator and the PID controller were not significantly different.

However, the combination of both controllers performed significantly better, because it combined the error reduction by system knowledge and by feedback. Typical responses of all three controllers are shown in figure 4.

The study also showed that trajectory following by recruitment modulation can only be used for rather slow movements in the presence of low inertia loads. Clamping of the control signal occurs if these conditions are not satisfied. These strategies may therefore be useful in the control of slow movements of the elbow or hand, but are not applicable in the control of lower extremity tasks like walking. For such applications other strategies are required.

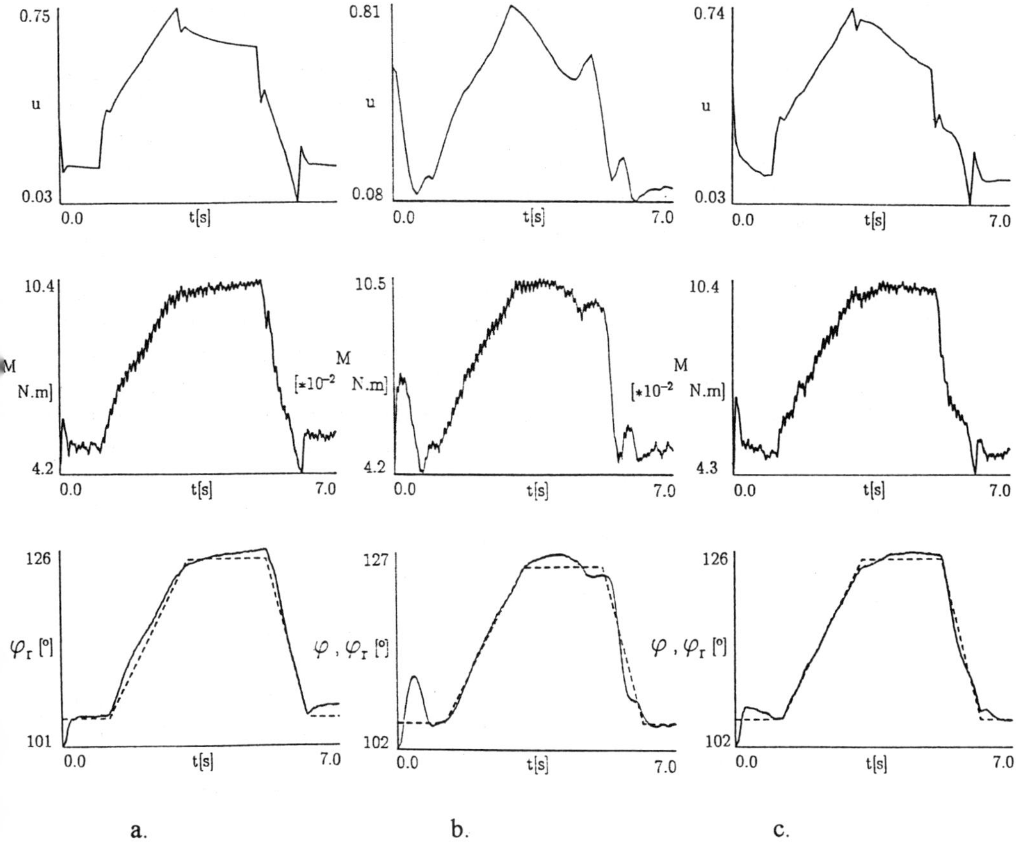

Fig. 4. Typical responses of the open-loop nonlinear compensator (a), the PID controller (b) and the feedforward nonlinear compensator combined with the feedback PID controller (c) (Veltink et al. 1992); *u* is the recruitment level computed by the controller, *M* is the measured ankle torque, φ is measured ankle angle and φ_r the ankle angle reference trajectory.

3.3 Model-based predictive control

Walking involves ballistic movements of the legs and the body, which have high inertias, while the stimulated muscles produce moderate torques. A propulsive movement should be generated, whilst ensuring joint stability and body balance. These criteria cannot directly be translated into trajectories, but rather into movement objectives like step size, foot clearance and knee extension at the end of the swing phase. Body balance may be controlled by the patient using crutches or other walking aids. Based on the before mentioned movement objectives, Veltink (1991) and Franken et al. (1995b) developed strategies for cycle to cycle control, in which stimulation patterns are not adjusted during a cycle, but only between cycles. The adjustments are based on an evaluation of the movements in previous cycles.

We subsequently posed the question whether it would be possible to effectively control the leg movements by adjustment of the stimulation during the cycles. Real time trajectory control can not be expected to be effective, because of the high inertias and rather low strength of the stimulated muscles. However, a model-based predictive control strategy may enable the adjustment of stimulation early in the cycle on the basis of a continuous prediction of the expected errors in realising the movement objectives. This approach was tested in the simplified control problem of cyclical shank movements generated by quadriceps stimulation. Figure 5 describes the model-based control strategy, which was tested. Comparable to the objective of a certain step size in control of gait, the control objective was a maximum knee angle, which should be reached each cycle. In each movement, stimulation started until the biomechanical model predicted that the maximum angle would be reached without further stimulation. Disturbances during the early phase of the movement may be compensated by this approach. Apart from disturbance rejections during the cycle, the control strategy adapts the modeled maximal knee torque generated by the quadriceps in the presence of fatigue.

Before implementing the model-based control strategy the required model structure had to be determined. The same basic structure was used as in the study on nonlinear control of joint angle trajectory (figure 2). Franken et al. (1993, 1995a) evaluated the predictive performance of the full model structure in comparison to reduced structures. It appeared that modeling activation dynamics did not improve predictive performance, because the shank dynamics is dominant. Angle and angular velocity factors however did improve the predictive performance in comparison to a zero order system without these factors. However, in the model-based predictive control study a zero order system without angle and angular velocity factors was used, since quadriceps activation always occured under approximately the same angle and angular velocity conditions.

Figure 6 illustrates the performance of the model-based predictive control strategy in comparison with trajectory following and cycle to cycle control. Only the model-based control strategy was able to compensate for disturbances when they occured early in the movement, as is shown in figure 6. Later disturbances could not be compensated. The model-based and cycle to cycle control strategies were both able to adaptively compensate for muscle fatigue. The trajectory following strategy was not able to effectively compensate for disturbances and fatigue.

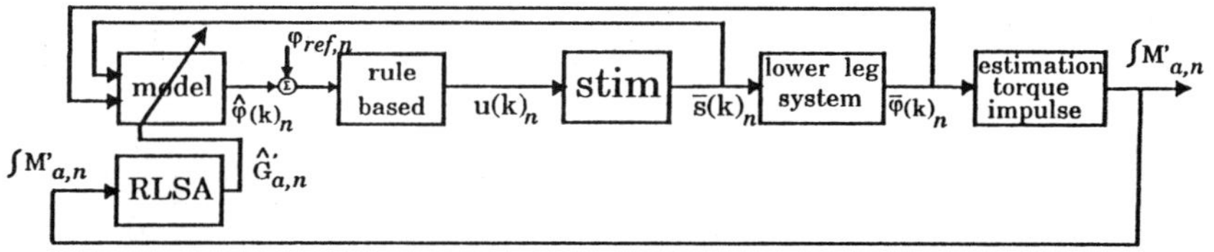

Fig. 5. Block diagram of the adaptive model-based predictive strategy for control of repeated shank movements generated by quadriceps stimulation. During the movement, the biomechanical model of the quadriceps - shank system continuously predicts the maximal knee angle $\hat{\varphi}$, which will be reached if stimulation is stopped. The rule base stops stimulation if the predicted maximal knee angle equals the reference maximal knee angle φ_{ref}; u is the recruitment input, which was set to 0 or 1; $\bar{s}$ is the stimulation parameter vector and $\bar{\varphi}$ the actually measured knee angle, angular velocity and angular acceleration. Both the input and the output of the lower leg system are fed back to the model as input for the predictions. After each movement cycle, the total torque impulse generated by quadriceps are estimated (see Franken et al. 1993). On the basis of this estimate the maximal quadriceps torque is adapted in the model, using a recursive least squares algorithm.

4 Conclusions

Biomechanical and finite state descriptive modelling are important tools in the design of control strategies for FES-assisted mobility. As presented, the application of models may have several objectives. Models can be used to simulate alternative controller performances, but are also applicable as parts of the actual control strategies.

Pre-experimental simulation of control strategies require extensive whole body biomechanical models. These models can normally not be identified fully and therefore do not give an accurate description of the performance for individual subjects. however, such models are useful in the prediction of comparative performances of different control strategies.

Models can be applied in control strategies at several hierarchical levels. High level control requires finite state models of mobility tasks. At a lower level, nonlinear model based control strategies can be used for trajectory following, preferably in combination with feedback control in order to reduce the influence of model inaccuracies. The control of relatively fast ballistic movements may benefit from model-based predictive control. However, disturbances can only be rejected if they occur early in the movement.

a. trajectory following

b. cycle to cycle control

c. model based predictive control

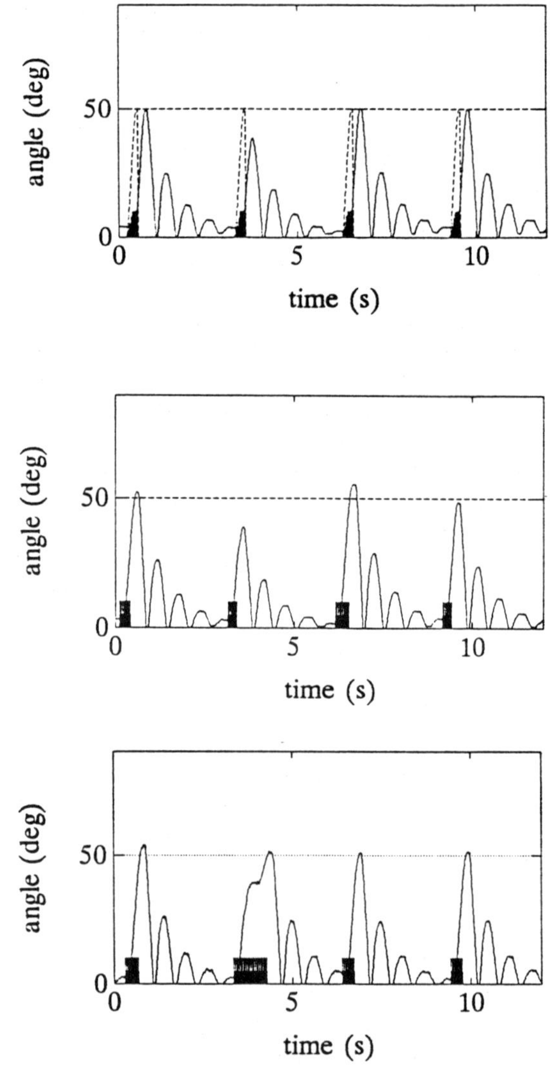

Fig. 6. Example of disturbance rejection response of trajectory following (a), cycle to cycle control (b) and model-based predictive control strategies (c). Knee angles are shown as a function of time. The reference maximal knee angle and the reference knee angle trajectory for the trajectory following strategy are indicated by dashed lines. The shank moves freely when quadriceps are stimulated. After a swing the shank movement is stopped by a cushion, which limits knee flexion. Every 3 s, when the shank is at rest, the stimulation is repeated. In all three displayed tests the movement is disturbed at the second stimulation burst. Only the model-based control strategy was able to compensate for the disturbance in part of the cases. The cycle to cycle control strategy erroneously increases stimulation burst width in the cycle after the disturbed cycle.

References

Andrews, B.J., Barnett, R.W., Phillips, G.F., and Kirkwood, C.A. (1989) Rule-based Control of a Hybrid FES orthosis for Assisted Paraplegic Locomotion, *Automedica*, **11**: 175-199.

Chizeck, H.J., Kobetic, R., Marsolais, E.B., Abbas, J.J., Donner I.H., and Simon, E. (1988) Control of Neuromuscular Stimulation Systems for Standing and Locomotion in Paraplegics, *Proceedings of the IEEE*, **76**: 115-1165.

Franken, H.M., Veltink, P.H., Tijsmans, R., Nijmeijer, H., and Boom, H.B.K. (1993) Identification of Passive Knee Joint and Shank Dynamics in Paraplegics Using Quadriceps Stimulation, *IEEE Transactions on Rehabilitation Engineering*, **1**: 154-164.

Franken, H.M., Veltink, P.H., and Boom, H.B.K. (1994) Restoring Gait in Paraplegics by Functional Electrical Stimulation, *IEEE Engineering in Medicine and Biology Magazine*, **13**: 564-570.

Franken, H.M., Veltink, P.H., Tijsmans, R., Nijmeijer, H., and Boom, H.B.K. (1995a) Identification of Quadriceps - Shank Dynamics Using Randomized Interpulse Interval Stimulation, *IEEE Transactions on Rehabilitation Engineering*, **3**: 182-192.

Franken, H.M., Veltink, P.H., Baardman, G., Redmeijer, R.A., and Boom, H.B.K. (1995b) Cycle-to-Cycle Control of Swing Phase of Paraplegic Gait induced by Surface Electrical Stimulation, *Med. & Biol. Eng. & Comput.*, **33**: 440-451.

Heinze, S., Veltink, P.H., Jensen, P.L., Mayagoitia, R.E., Hermens, H.J., Koopman, H.F.J.M., and Huijing P.A. (1995) Development of Control Strategies for FES-supported Closed-Loop Standing-Up, *Neuroprosthetics - from basic research to clinical applications,* A. Pedotti, M. Ferrarin, J. Quintern, R. Riener (eds.), this publication.

Veltink, P.H. and van Alsté, J.A. (1989) Dynamics and Control of a Muscle-Load System during Electrical Nerve Stimulation, *Automedica*, **11**: 91-98.

Veltink, P.H. (1991) Control of FES-induced Cyclical Leg Movements of the Lower Leg, *Med. & Biol. Eng. & Comput.*, **29**: NS8-NS12.

Veltink, P.H., Franken, H.M., van Alsté, J.A., and Boom, H.B.K. (1992a) Modelling the Optimal Control of Cyclical Leg Movements induced by Functional Electrical Stimulation, *J. Artificial Organs*, **15**: 746-755.

Veltink, P.H., Chizeck, H.J., Crago, P.E., and El-Bialy, A. (1992b) Nonlinear Joint Angle Control for Artificially Stimulated Muscle, *IEEE Transactions on Biomedical Engineering*, **39**: 368-380.

Veltink, P.H., De Vries, W., Baardman, G., Hermens, H.J., Sweeney, P., and Van Riel, W. (1995a) Design of an Intention Detection System for FES Assisted Mobility in Paraplegics, *Proceedings of the 5th Vienna International Workshop on Functional Electrostimulation*, Vienna, pp. 43-46.

Veltink, P.H., Trooster, J.J., Leth Jensen, P., Heinze, S., Koopman, H.F.J.M., and Huijing, P.A. (1995b) Control Strategies for FES-supported Standing Up, *Proceedings of the 5th Vienna International Workshop on Functional Electrostimulation*, Vienna, pp. 31-34.

Yamaguchi, G.T. and Zajac, F.E. (1989) Restoring Unassisted Natural Gait to Paraplegics via Neuromuscular Stimulation: a Computer Simulation Study, *IEEE Transactions on Biomedical Engineering*, **37**: 886-902.

Inverse models for control of movements

J. Quintern[1], R. Riener[2], S. Volz[1], S. Rupprecht[1], A. Straube[1]
[1]Neurological Clinic, Klinikum Grosshadern, University of Munich, Germany
[2]Dept. of Automatic Control Engineering, Technical University, Munich, Germany

Abstract - Inverse dynamic models are one possible way to compensate for non-linearities in the generation of motion induced by functional electrical stimulation (FES). This paper deals with inverse models of the electrodes, the stimulated nerve and the musculoskeletal system in the feedforward control of knee flexion-extension movements in patients with complete spinal cord injury. With a proper identification of the patient-specific parameters a satisfactory performance could be achieved, as long as the muscle did not fatigue. Further improvement could be achieved when inverse feedforward was combined with closed-loop control. With the present model, the sign of the tracking error was always different for shortening (concentric) and lengthening (eccentric) contractions of the spastic muscle. It is assumed, that these differences are due to either tonic stretch reflexes or changes of the muscle properties after upper motor neuron lesions.

1 Introduction

Despite more than thirty years of development, FES for restoration of motor functions has not yet gained wide acceptance among patients and physicians. Especially lower extremity FES for restoration of stance and gait in paraplegic and hemiplegic patients has not yet emerged to a practical aid for use in daily life. Presumably the main reason for the low acceptance of current FES systems is insufficient functional gain for the patients.

Today clinically applied motor neural prostheses are open-loop systems with empirically derived stimulation patterns. Motion induced by these systems usually is inharmonious, not well coordinated and rather inefficient. Fundamental problems of FES-induced motion are the numerous non-linearities in the electrophysiological and biomechanical pathways from electrical stimuli to limb movements (Hatze 1978; Riener et al. 1996), the rapid changes of muscle properties due to fatigue, the limited number of muscles which can be selectively stimulated, and the lack of proprioception and afferent feedback.

Scientists have followed two different kinds of approach to improve motion control with FES: (1) implanted systems and (2) closed-loop control. Implanted FES systems can provide a more selective activation of muscles than systems with surface electrodes. However, implantation of electrodes and stimulators doesn't solve most problems of open-loop FES systems.

Closed-loop control can partly compensate for some of the above mentioned problems (Quintern et al. 1989). Within a certain limit, lead-lag controllers automatically neutralize nonlinearities of the plant (electrode-nerve interface, neuromuscular junction, and musculoskeletal system). Closed-loop controllers also can compensate for changes of muscle force output due to fatigue. Closed-loop control allows to adjust the level of stimulation to the actual requirements and thus helps to prevent early fatigue due to overstimulation of muscles.

Most of the controllers tested so far for FES have been either linear controllers (Crago et al. 1980; Jaeger, 1986; Quintern et al. 1989; Abbas and Chizeck 1991) or finite state controllers (Mulder et al. 1992). However, linear controllers are not the best way to control a highly nonlinear system. They can provide sufficient performance only for force control under isometric conditions, when the limb dynamics can be neglected. When linear controllers such as the popular proportional-integral-derivative (PID) controller are used for control of limb trajectories during unconstrained movements, they cause considerable delays and do not provide robust and accurate control. Therefore, some researchers have introduced nonlinear elements as part of the controller, which should cancel some of the nonlinearities of the plant (Wilhere et al. 1985). However, there have been only few attempts to compensate for nonlinearities in all parts of the neurophysiological and biomechanical chain involved in FES-induced motion. In a recent paper (Veltink et al. 1992) a nonlinear compensator based upon an inverse muscle model was developed and successfully tested in the soleus muscle of anaesthetized, deafferented cats (deafferentation by crunching the sciatic nerve proximal to the stimulation site). However, the situation may be different in patients with upper motor neuron lesions, when the contractile properties of the muscle fibers are altered (Dietz et al. 1981) and stretch reflexes are enhanced.

The aim of the our study was to test, if inverse models of the stimulated nerve and the musculoskeletal system can improve motor control of FES-induced limb movements in patients with complete spinal cord injury. One important question was, if inverse models already provide a satisfactory feedforward prediction of FES-induced unconstrained movements. It should also be tested, if additional feedback control with a conventional linear controller can improve the performance of the system.

2 Methods

2.1 Inverse model

The inverse model of FES-induced knee motion is based on a more detailed direct model of the human knee (Riener et al. 1996; Riener and Quintern 1996). Both models consist of three basic parts: activation dynamics, contraction dynamics and body segmental dynamics. Several simplifications are made to the inverse model to allow real-time calculation even on slow microprocessors. The model considers the human knee joint with the thigh supported and the shank freely swinging. The joint angle is controlled by stimulation of the quadriceps femoris muscle via surface electrodes, the knee flexion moment is provided by gravity. Recruitment modulation with varying pulse width and fixed current amplitude (80 mA) and fixed interpulse interval (50 ms) is assumed. The input to the inverse model is the desired trajectory of knee joint angle, the output is the stimulation pulse width for stimulating the quadriceps muscle. The model is a discrete time model with the time step equal to the interpulse interval. The model consists of the following calculation steps:

- Calculation of the net knee moment, M_{net}, from the desired knee angle, φ, by applying the equations of motion, considering gravity and inertia of the shank and foot.
- Calculation of the active knee moment, M_A, generated by the quadriceps muscle from M_{net} by subtracting the moments M_v and M_e caused by viscous and elastic properties in the joint and muscles. M_e is near zero for the most part of the movement range, there is a steep increase of M_e when the knee angle is close to full extension (Audu and Davy 1985).
- A transfer function which is scaled by three parameters, C_1, C_2, and C_3, relates the active knee moment, M_A, with the activation, A_t, at time t. This transfer function considers the changing lever arm of the quadriceps muscle, force-length relation and the force-velocity relation f_{fv}:

$$f_{fv} = 1 - d\varphi/dt \cdot C_{fv} \tag{1}$$

$$A_t = \frac{M_A - C_3}{f_{fv}\,(C_1 + C_2\varphi)} \tag{2}$$

  C_{fv} depends on the moment arm and the optimal musculotendon length and is assumed to be 0.04 for the quadriceps muscle. The other parameters $C_1..C_3$ are approximated by computer simulations in an iterative procedure.

- The activation dynamics of the muscle were assumed to be a first order differential equation (a_r is the percentage of recruited fibers; T_{act} the time constant for muscle activation):

$$a_r = A_t + T_{act}\,\frac{A_t - A_{t-1}}{\Delta t} \tag{3}$$

- The inverse recruitment curve, approximating stimulation pulse width d by linear interpolation between threshold pulse width, d_{thr}, and saturation pulse width, d_{sat}, for $0 <= a_r <= 1$.

2.2 Parameter identification

The anthropometric parameters (center of gravity, mass, and moment of inertia of the foot and shank) were estimated from external measurements applying regression equations (Zatsiorsky and Seluyanov, 1983). The viscous damping coefficient was identified by a passive pendulum test. The function for nonlinear elastic moments at the knee joint (Audu and Davy 1985) was scaled by measurements of passive moments at different joint angles. The threshold and saturation pulse widths, d_{thr} and d_{sat}, were taken from isometric stimulation tests. The time constant for muscle activation was assumed to be 0.05 s. For the stepwise approximation of the three parameters of the contraction dynamics, C_1, C_2, and C_3 (equation 2), the results of open-loop stimulation experiments with freely swinging shank were compared with the output of a direct model in a standardized iterative procedure.

2.3 Stimulation experiments

Stimulation experiments were performed in two patients with complete thoracic spinal cord injury. The patients lay supine with the thigh supported and the shank hanging down. The quadriceps femoris muscle was stimulated by surface electrodes. For parameter identification the knee torque was measured under isometric condition with a strain-gauge based transducer. Under the condition of freely swinging shank, the knee angle was measured with an electrogoniometer (full knee extension was defined as 180°). Data were digitized and sampled at a rate of 160 Hz. The computer was also used, to produce the modulation waveforms, to apply the control rules, and to control the stimulator. For open-loop experiments without inverse model, the modulation waveforms (sinusoidal and triangular, with constant or varying frequency) were applied to the stimulus pulse width. For experiments with the inverse model and for closed-loop experiments, the modulation waveforms were applied to the desired knee angle trajectory. The inverse model was used only in the feedforward part of the control loop.

In some experiments inverse feedforward was combined with closed-loop control with a PID controller. The input to the PID controller was the error between the measured and the desired knee angle. The output of the controller was added to the pulse width calculated by the inverse model. Prior to the experiment the parameters for the PID controller were optimized in a computer simulation.

3 Results

3.1 Open-loop experiments without inverse model

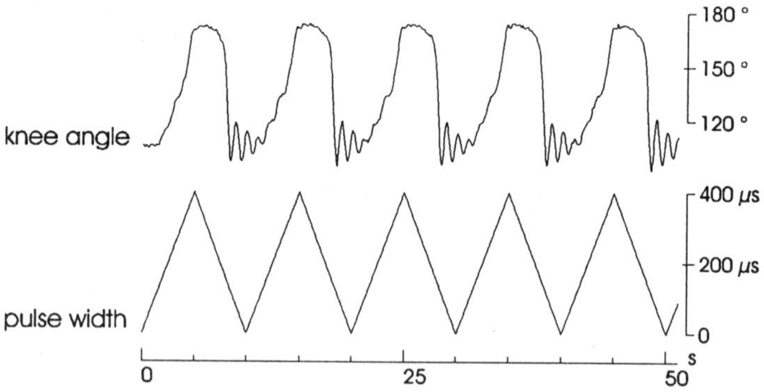

Fig. 1. Open-loop stimulation without inverse model, triangular pulse width modulation

A typical open-loop stimulation experiment without inverse model is shown in fig. 1 and fig. 3A. The nonlinearities, especially the hysteresis between the flexion and the extension phase, and the oscillations at the flexed position were observed in all experiments.

3.2 Open-loop stimulation with inverse model

In these experiments, the desired knee angle was the input to the inverse model. The output of the model, the pulse width, was transferred to the stimulator. When the muscle was not fatigued, the amplitude of the actual knee joint movement agreed well with the desired movement (fig. 2). The inverse model compensated for some of the nonlinearities (fig. 3B) of FES-induced movements. The oscillations at the end of the knee flexion movement (fig. 1) were damped by the inverse model (fig. 2). However, there was still a significant tracking error and a hysteresis between the extension and flexion phase of the movement (fig. 3B). This tracking error could be reduced, when the viscous damping coefficient was arbitrarily increased far above the value which was identified by the passive pendulum test. The movement amplitude decreased considerably and the tracking error increased, when the muscle fatigued.

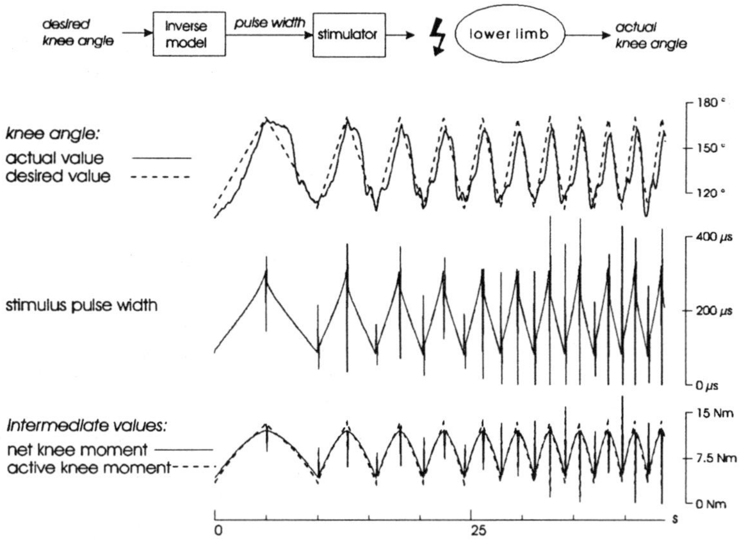

Fig. 2. Feedforward control of knee angle with an inverse model. The experimental arrangement is shown in the *schematic* above the curves. For this experiment the desired trajectory was a triangular waveform (170°-110°) with varying period. *Upper*: superimposed desired and measured (actual) knee angle. *Middle*: stimulus pulse width. The positive and negative peaks of the stimulus pulse width are caused by the high accelerations at the points of inflection. *Lower*: net knee moment, M_{net}, and active knee moment, M_A, are superimposed as an example of intermediate values provided by the inverse model. Please notice, that differences between M_{net} and M_A (equivalent to sum of the passive moments M_v and M_e) are small for this version of the inverse model.

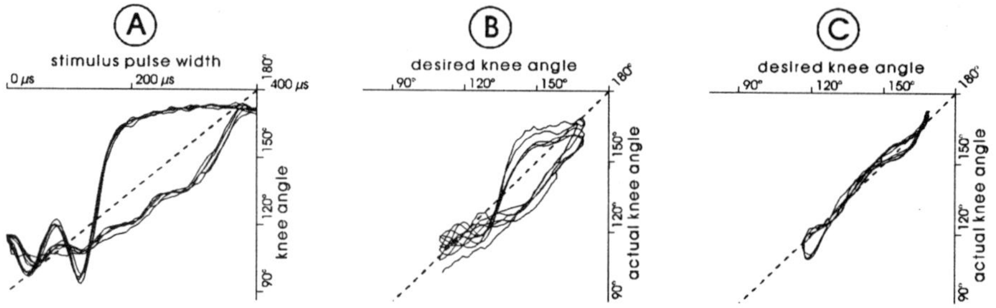

Fig. 3. X/Y plots of stimulation experiments with different control strategies (modulation waveform: triangular). **A**: open-loop stimulation without invers model; the stimulation pulse width (abscissa) is plotted against the resulting knee angle (ordinate). **B**: feedforward control with the inverse model; abscissa: desired knee angle, ordinate: measured knee angle. C: feedforward with the inverse model combined with a PID controller.

3.3 Inverse feedforward combined with a PID controller

When feedforward control with the inverse model was combined with a PID controller, the tracking error could be reduced further. In fig. 3C an almost perfect control of knee joint angle is shown. However, inverse feedforward combined with linear closed-loop did not always provide good results. Although the tracking error usually was smaller than with feedback control alone, the system often got unstable when the muscle fatigued.

4 Conclusions

4.1 Comparison between model prediction and experimental results

Predictive (feedforward) control with inverse models has the potential to compensate for most nonlinearities of FES-induced movements. However, in our application of inverse models in paraplegic patients there was still a considerable tracking error. The sign of this tracking error was different for shortening (concentric) and lengthening (eccentric) contractions. During flexion movement, which was achieved by gravity acting against a gradually decreasing stimulation of knee extensors, the knee remained extended for a longer time than it was predicted by the model. This finding has to be interpreted in such a way that the force exerted by the quadriceps muscle during lengthening contractions is higher than predicted. The most likely explanation for this phenomenon is an improper identification of the model's parameters, especially of the viscous damping coefficient. However, the viscous damping coefficient was carefully identified with the passive pendulum test. Therefore, it must be concluded that the muscle tone is further increased in spastic patients, when the muscle is activated. This hypothesis is consistent with earlier neurophysiological studies (Dietz et al. 1981; Hufschmidt and Mauritz 1985). Another possible explanation for the inaccurate model predictions could be the occurrence of tonic stretch reflexes during eccentric contractions. For further improvement of the inverse model, the resistance of the electrically activated muscle against external loads has to be analyzed.

4.2 Complexity of the model and parameter identification

The major disadvantage of complex physiologically based models is the numerous parameters which are often difficult to be identified separately. Also, physiologically based models need more calculation steps than a "black box approach" with abstract transfer functions. However, physiologically based models have several advantages, which makes them an ideal tool for research on the field of FES: physiologically based models help to understand how the system works, deficiencies of the model can be analyzed and explained on the basis of the knowledge in neurophysiology, parameters can be attributed to physiologic quantities, and the model can be easily adapted to different conditions. Still, in a later stage of development, physiologically based models can be simplified and converted to transfer functions.

4.3 Feedforward versus feedback control of movement

The pure feedforward approach in the control of FES-induced movements has the advantage, that no sensors have to be mounted at the body of the patient. For several types of movements, e.g., the swing phase during level walking, a feedforward control seems to be sufficient. However, there are clear limitations for a pure feedforward approach, especially when the internal parameters of the system change due to fatigue. In these cases, an adaptive control of the inverse model's parameters could be a good solution. When an external load which cannot be exactly predicted is applied to the body, a feedback control of the stimulation parameters themselves becomes necessary. It is difficult to provide an accurate and robust feedback control of such a highly nonlinear system. Since linear controllers do not provide robust control, inverse model components in the feedback loop could enhance the performance of the control system.

4.4 Possible role of inverse models in the control of multijoint movements

Inverse models of a multi-joint system have the potential to synchronize movements at different joints, because they automatically consider the coupling of moments between joints. Although the complexity of these models increases significantly with each degree of freedom, the computational effort required is still below that of artificial neural networks. The multisensor closed-loop neurostimulator developed by our group (Keller et al. 1996) provides enough computational power to realize inverse-models of a multijoint system.

Acknowledgments

This work was supported by the German Federal Department of Education and Research (BMBF, project number 01K0 94026).

References

Abbas, J.J., Chizeck, H.J. (1991) Feedback control of coronal plane hip angle in paraplegic subjects using functional neuromuscular stimulation. *IEEE Trans. Biomed. Eng.*, **38**: 687-698.

Audu, M.L., Davy, D.T. (1985) The influence of muscle model complexity in musculoskeletal motion modeling. *ASME J. Biomech. Eng.*, **107**: 147-157.

Crago, P.E., Mortimer, J.T., and Peckham, P.H. (1980) Closed-loop control of force during electrical stimulation of muscle. *IEEE Trans. Biomed. Eng.*, **27**: 306-312.

Dietz, V., Quintern, J., Berger, W. (1981) Electrophysiological studies of gait in spasticity and rigidity. Evidence that altered mechanical properties of muscle contribute to hypertonia. *Brain,* **104**: 431-449.

Jaeger, R.J. (1986) Design and simulation of closed-loop electrical stimulation orthoses for restoration of quiet standing in paraplegia. *J. Biomechanics,* **19**: 825-835.

Hatze, H. (1978) A general myocybernetic control model of skeletal muscle. *Biol. Cybern.*, **28**: 143-157.

Hufschmidt, A. and Mauritz, K.-H. (1985) Chronic transformation of muscle in spasticity: a peripheral contribution to increased tone. *J. Neurol. Neurosurg. Psych.*, **48**: 676-685.

Keller, M., Krauß, P., Hoch, G., Quintern, J. (1996) Design of a multisensor closed-loop neurostimulator. Part A: Communication unit with wireless data link and digital signal processor. This volume, pp. 183-188.

Mulder, A.J., Veltink, P.H., Boom, H.B.K., Zilvold, G. (1992) Low-level finite state control of knee joint in paraplegic standing. *J. Biomed. Eng.*, **14**: 3-8.

Quintern, J., Minwegen, P., Mauritz, K.-H. (1989) Control mechanism for restoring posture and movements in paraplegics. In: J.H.J Allum, M. Hulliger (eds.) *Progress in Brain Research*, **80**, Elsevier, Amsterdam, pp. 489-502.

Riener, R., Quintern, J. (1996) Biomechanical simulation of the lower extremity for the development of control strategies for FES. This volume, pp. 233-244.

Riener, R., Quintern, J., Schmidt, G. (1996) Biomechanical model of the human knee evaluated by neuromuscular stimulation. *J. Biomechanics,* in press.

Wilhere, G.F., Crago, P.E., Chizeck, H.J. (1985) Design and evaluation of a digital closed-loop controller for the regulation of muscle force by recruitment modulation. *IEEE Trans. Biomed. Eng.*, **32**: 668-676.

Veltink, P. H., Chizeck, H. J., Crago, P. E., El-Bialy, A. (1992,b) Nonlinear joint angle control for artificially stimulated muscle, *IEEE Trans. Biomed. Eng.*, **39**, 368-380.

Zatsiorsky, V. and Seluyanov, V.(1983) The mass and inertia characteristics of the main segments of the human body. In: *Biomechanics VIII-B*, University Park Press, pp. 1152-1159.

Neural Networks for the Control of Posture and Locomotion

W.J. Daunicht
Neurologisches Therapiecentrum an der
Heinrich-Heine-Universität, Düsseldorf, Germany

Abstract - The strategy to develop a control system for the stabilization of stance and gait in paraplegics by means of a closed loop neuroprosthesis is an unresolved problem. Here a unified control concept is proposed, that is based on the notion of attractors and meta-attractors; it is suggested to implement the nonlinear stages of the appropriate controllers by training of artificial neural networks. Designed especially to train the neural network and test the behavior of the neuroprosthesis in closed loop, a comprehensive simulation of the human musculo-skeletal system is presented.

1 Introduction

A closed loop neuroprosthesis for restoration of stance and gait has not only the advantage of compensating disturbances such as external forces, variations of the environment and changes of internal parameters, it also offers the chance to stabilize the body in an upright posture, thereby removing harmful strain from the joints of the upper extremity, so far as the use of crutches can be avoided. However, in the development of a closed loop neuroprosthesis for paraplegics one faces a number of very difficult problems; among other things, one of the most important questions is how to design a development environment, as the control system to be developed has to meet a number of demands simultaneously: it has to be safe, to be handled comfortably, to generate a rich variety of movements and to allow being actually implemented in miniaturized electronics. The designer also has to take into account, that for any portable processor there are severe limitations to physical size and energy consumption. Given these limitations present day microprocessors are not very well suited to process a large number of signals in real time. Even the capacity of today's most powerful single processor is barely comparable to that of a fly (Heemskerk 1995). In view of these technical limitations it seems crucial to optimize the control system design.

Concepts for the artificial control of posture and locomotion have mainly been based on the use of (nested) servo loops. Control of posture has been studied using servo loops with an input for an explicit trajectory signal representing the desired movement; for a review see (Beckmann 1994). In this concept the generation of the movement is usually considered to be carried out by a separate mechanism and possibly just recalled from a storage. On the other hand, control of locomotion has been treated using coupled (neural) oscillators (Taga 95); the output of the oscillators is then being used as input for servo loops. In this concept the problem is still open, how to start and stop the periodic behavior. Also, combinations of posture and locomotion control are difficult to envisage.

In the following I will propose a novel unified concept that does not only allow to control posture and locomotion in the same framework, but also solves the problem of transitions between different activities. As it relies on meta-attractors realized with artificial neural networks, it may also - if implemented in dedicated massively parallel hardware - eliminate the real time problem of closed loop control.

2 The Meta-Attractor Concept

An attractor is the subset of states which describe the long term behavior of a system, when system parameters remain unchanged and no disturbance is present. The simplest attractor is a (0-dimensional) fixpoint; it is a single state (point in the phase space) that is approached asymptotically by the system. Another attractor, the limit cycle, forms a closed (1-dimensional) curve in the phase space and describes a periodic behavior of a system. However, it must not be confused with a fixpoint describing a circular trajectory: a limit cycle attractor does not require an oscillator that drives the periodic bahavior.Therefore the period of a limit cycle attractor can change due to external disturbances, while the period of a periodically moving fixpoint cannot. There exist also attractors with a fractional dimension (>1), which can also be used for stabilizing purposes; they are called chaotic attractors.In fact, limit cycle attractors are typical for relatively simple systems, and it is highly probable, that because of its complexity the human body can only be stabilized by a chaotic attractor.An attractor is characterized by its basin of attraction. Such a basin comprises all initial points which lead to the same given attractor. An other words, within these limits the state of the system moves predictably to a given goal independent of the initial state.

A meta-attractor is here defined as that subset of attractors of a system with variable parameters, which describes the behavior of the system, when no disturbance is present. The basin of a meta-attractor is the set of all attractors, which lead to the same given subset of attractors.

Attractors have already been used for control; conventional control aims - given constant inputs - at the stabilization of a system in a fixpoint. In contrast, the central idea of concept proposed here is - given constant commands - to stabilize the system by way of a meta-attractor. For example, if a closed loop system with variable parameters can produce both a fixpoint and a limit cycle, and the meta-attractor (selected by command) is the limit cycle, then the system will tend towards those parameters which destabilize the system in the fixpoint and stabilize it in the limit cycle.

The application of the meta-attractor concept to the design of a neuroprosthetic controller for posture and locomotion has a number of implications. On one hand, if the concept is successfully implemented, high levels of safety can be ensured by covering all essential ranges of the state space with even redundant attractor basins. Also, if disturbances are strong enough to push the system over the border of the current attractor, in this concept different attractor is to be generatedautonomously to keep the system stable in a global sense.Further, transitions from one activity to the other, in particular from locomotion to stance and back, are generated autonomously. Finally, command input can be very comfortable, as it may consist merely of a selection from a small set of meta-attractors. On the other hand, while for the creation of fixpoints the techniques of conventional control theory suffice, the creation of more complex attractors requires new techniques involving nonlinear dynamics.

3 Realization of the Meta-Attractor Concept with Neural Networks

According to our experience a three-stage nonlinear system has been sufficient to create the attractors required for a closed loop neuroprosthesis: the first and third stage consist of multivariate linear filters, while the second stage consists of a multivariate nonlinear static function.

The problem can thus be broken up into several subproblems; one of them is the creation of the appropriate nonlinear function by the second stage.To solve that problem the use of artificial neural networks seems to be optimal.Neural networks can approximate continuous nonlinear functions with arbitrary accuracy, they can be trained by examples or by a critique, and they are intrinsically parallel, so that an implementation in dedicated hardware may solve the real time problem.

For the development of a closed loop controller in general and for the training of neural networks in particular, it is an unescapable prerequisite to have a comprehensive and realistic model of the process to be controlled. In case of a neuroprosthesis training by means of a computer model is all the more important, as the safe operation of the system has to be demonstrated, before it can be used, and no user would perform endless iterations to train a system, before it provides the first benefit, anyway. The crucial part of such an environment for the development of a closed loop controller (Fig. 1) is a fully 3-dimensional model of muscle stimulation, muscle dynamics, musculo-skeletal biomechanics, interaction with the environment, various sensor classes and the function of the remaining nervous system.

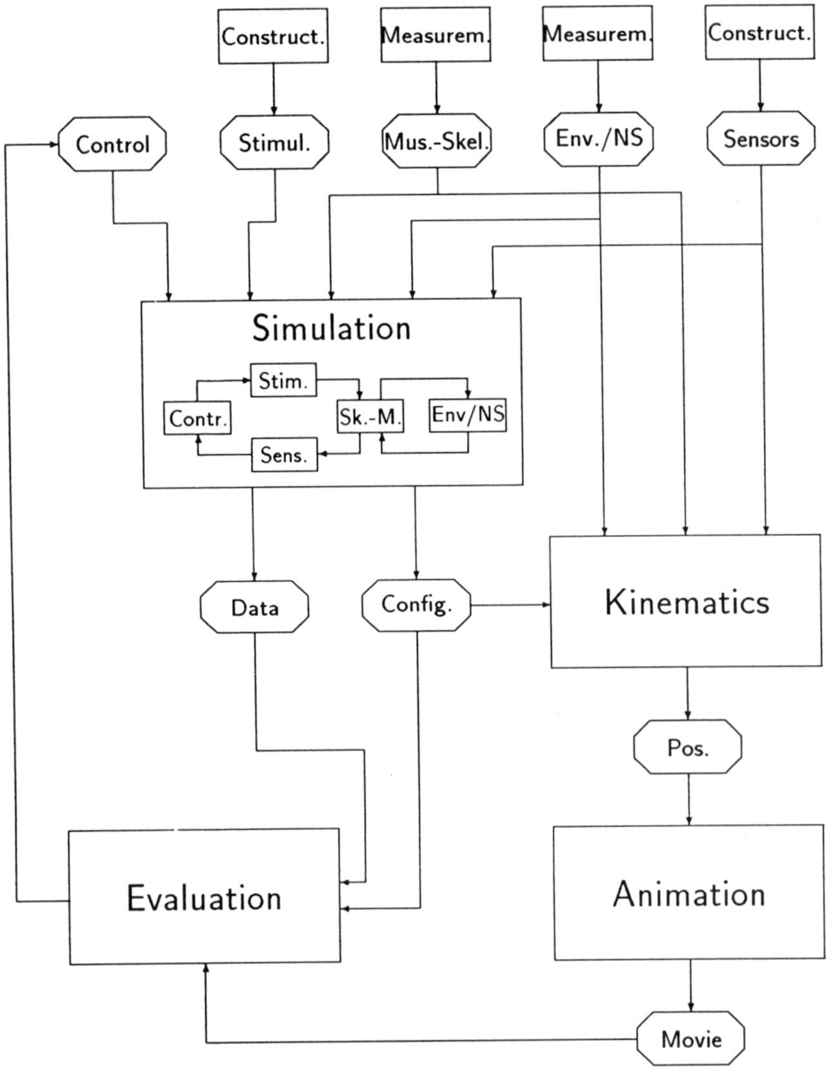

Fig. 1. Scheme of the software environment at the NTC. Large rectangulars denote algorithms, octogons denote parameter and data files, and small rectangulars denote sources of knowledge.

When a model has been established and the general controller structure has been selected, the crucial procedure is the evaluation of the resulting movements. Following the meta-attractor concept, the evaluation is performed in two phases. In the first phase, a number of attractors attributed to the essential activities like sitting, standing, walking etc. is trained to the network. In the second phase the meta-attractors are established. In both phases the size and shape of the basins of attraction can be used as a measure of quality to adapt the parameters of the neural network.

4 Results

In order to design a software environment for the training of neural networks we started out by composing a biomechanical model that comprises the necessary components to develop and test a controller for a neuroprosthesis (Daunicht et al. 1995). Parameters for the simulation of muscle stimulator and sensors were taken from the technical construction, while parameters describing a malemusculo-skeletal system were obtained from adapted from different experimental sources and were estimated, if experimental data were not available.

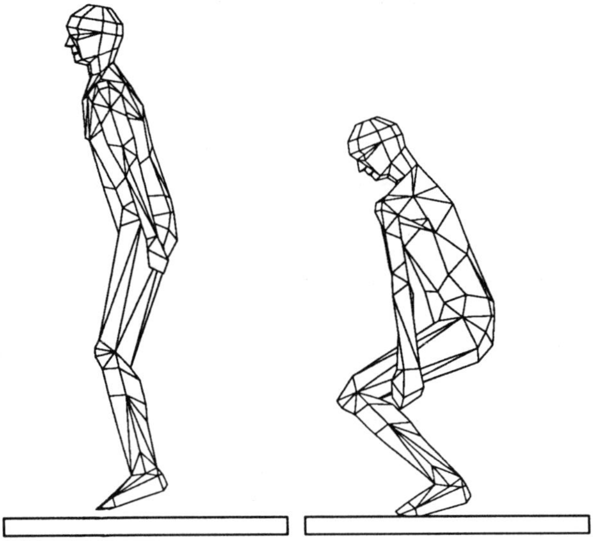

Fig. 2. Simulation of the interaction with the ground during passive collapse of the model. The lifting of the heel is due to simulated ankle joint properties.

The general model of the musculo-skeletal system is based on the 3-dimensional dynamics of up to 19 rigid bodies with up to 42 degrees of freedom; its complexity can be scaled up and down relatively comfortably (Hatze 1981, Wittenburg 1977). The simulation also includes a representation of the ground as a hard surface (Steiner and Daunicht 1993). The interaction between the biomechanical system and the ground allows to predict the reaction forces, which are propagated through the whole model (Fig. 2).

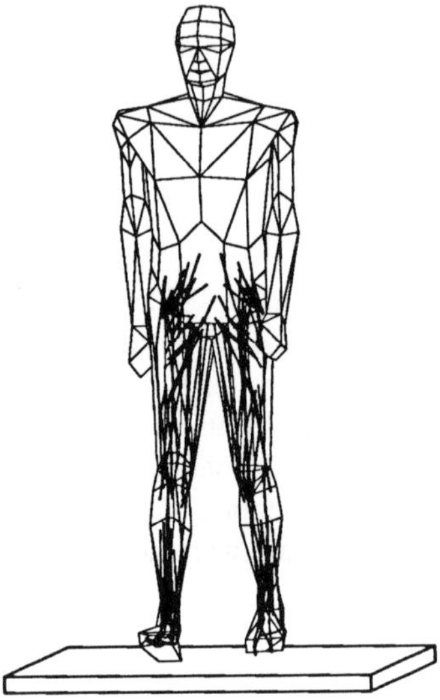

Fig. 3. Geometry of 86 leg muscle paths.

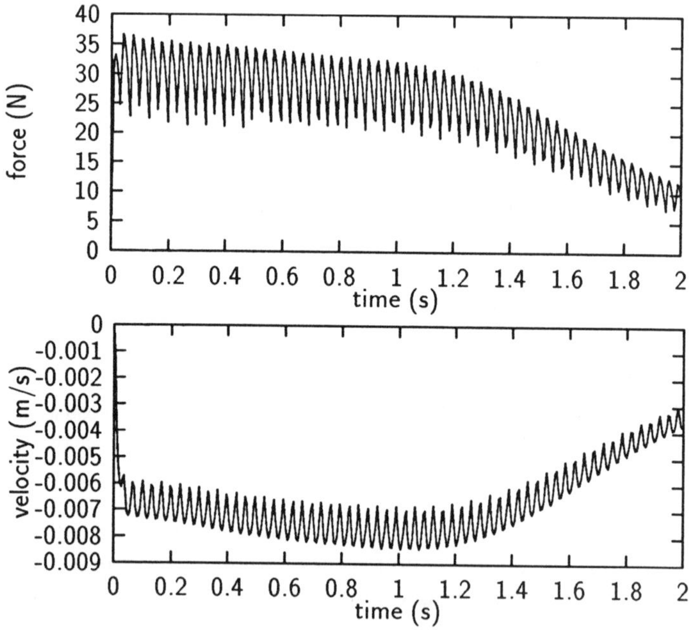

Fig. 4. Simulation of muscle force (upper part) and contraction velocity (lower part) of one of the mm. gemelli during symmetrical constant activation of the mm. gemelli.

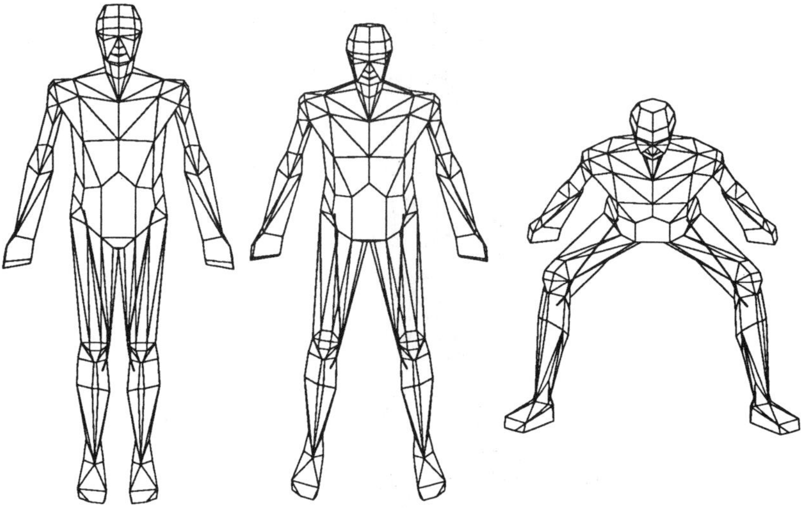

Fig. 5. Simulation of a movement due to symmetrical constant activation of mm. sartorii in the absence of gravitational effects.

The muscle model simulates geometrical as well as dynamical properties (Zajac 1989, Delp 1990) and includes currently 86 muscles (Fig. 3). Based on the integration of the muscles into the model, it is possible to calculate the time course of variables characterizing the state of the muscle, while the muscle length is changing due to its own direct and indirect action on the whole body (Fig. 4). Since many leg muscles act on more than one joint, the resulting movement may be rather complex; we have used real time animations check the results for plausibility (Fig. 5).

Another important component is the simulation of sensors. With a portable neuroprosthesis in mind, we restricted our simulations to sensors which can actually be worn on the body. Systems which determine the positions of markers with reference to an external coordinate system can be simulated easily, but were not considered as appropriate for a neuroprosthesis. For our simulations we chose three kinds of sensors, which are already commercially available: capacitive ground reaction force sensors, piezoresistive accelerometers and goniometers based on strain gauge technique. This choice was supported by our experience with a variety of control scenarios (see below). Simulation parameters are not only the technical data such as sensitivity and frequency response of the individual sensors, but also the location and orientation of sensors (Fig. 6). It must be expected that these parameters are not always exactly known or may change and that the actual choice may be redundant with respect to the system state, therefore these effects have to be accounted for in the design of a controller. The simulated sensor signals were obtained as a result of simulated body movements (Fig. 7).

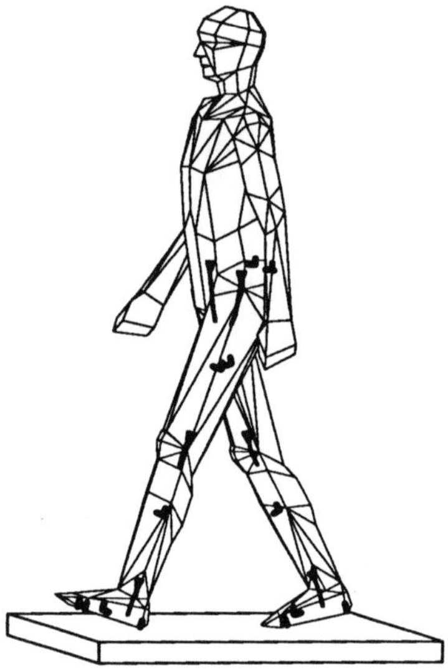

Fig. 6. Spatial placement of 2x3 goniometers, 2x4x3 accelerometers and 2x3 ground reaction force sensors.

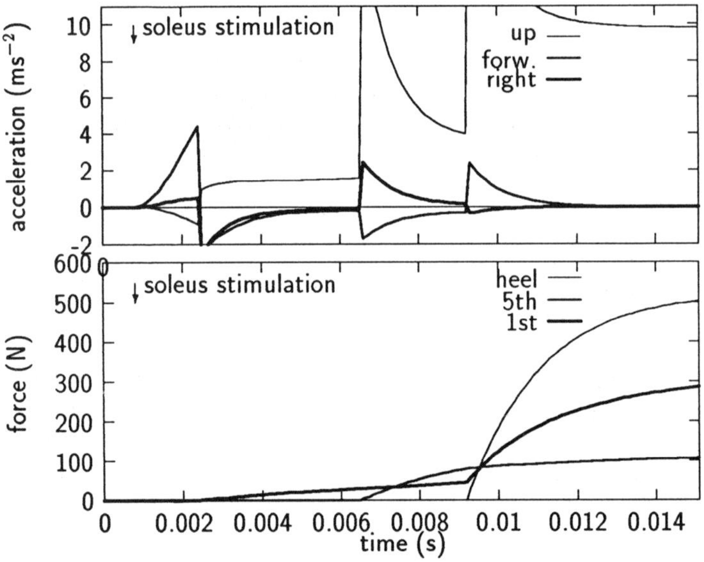

Fig. 7. Simulated signals of 3 orthogonal accelerometers placed on the left foot and 3 reaction force sensors under the sole. After a short period of free fall the stimulation of the soleus is picked up by all accelerometers, but not by the reaction force sensors. Contact with the ground leads to three peaks of acceleration. With full contact, only the vertical sensor measures the gravitational acceleration, while the reaction force sensors pick up a changing distribution of forces.

To study the performance of closed loop controllers we have developed several scenarios. In the first case we have studied the control of various changes of postures using nonlinear fixpoint control.The model used for that study was reduced to 6 degrees of freedom with planar dynamics, including a detailed model for 6 muscles and sensors for angles, acceleration and reaction force. The structure of the controller was consistent with the concept proposed hereand consisted of two stages of linear filters with a static nonlinear stage in between. The results indicated that closed loop control of posture changes like sitting down, standing up (Fig. 8) and squatting were considerably improved by appropriate nonlinearities implemented in a neural network compared to a completely linear control system (Beckmann et al. 1993).

In a second scenario we have studied the control of the dynamic balance in the frontal plane as well as initiating and finishing of walking by different attractors. The model used was reduced to 4 degrees of freedom with 2-dimensional architecture of the controller had the same three-stage structure, in particular it did not include any central oscillators. Within this scheme it was possible to demonstrate that fixpoint and limit attractors could be generated by only minor modifications of parameters in the static stage. It could be shown that periodic behavior with different frequencies and stable against external disturbances could be generated without oscillators. Disturbances of long duration were compensated not only be the generation of counteracting forces but also by considerable changes of the period.These experiments demonstrated the feasibility of control by an attractor different from a fixpoint, here a limit cycle (Fig. 9) (Steiner et al. 1995).

In a third scenario we have studied the control of walking with different velocities in 3-dimensional space. Here the model had 8 degrees of freedom with 3-dimensional dynamics, again the degrees of freedom at the ankle joints were unpowered. The architecture of the controller had a similar three-stage structure as above. The results showed, that by implementing the attractor behavior it is not only possible to maintain dynamic stability in space, but also to achieve different walking speeds. It should be noted that the model could also be stabilized with zero mean velocity, i.e. stabilization was achieved by small compensating steps rather than by torques in the ankle joints.

The reduced systems studied so far have a rather low complexity, in particular, the number of sensors and actuators could be kept relatively small. Therefore the nonlinear stage of the controllers had a low complexity, too, and required only small feedforward neural networks. To control the human musculo-skeletal system or a model of it with the full complexity as outlined above, it will be necessary to use much larger neural networks. Unfortunately the training time of large networks with iterative methods is a serious problem, as it increases more than linear with the number of synaptic weights and training by analof values must be terminated with some error level left. If the development is carried out as usually in emulations with sequential computers, the power of the increase of training times is even higher than 2.

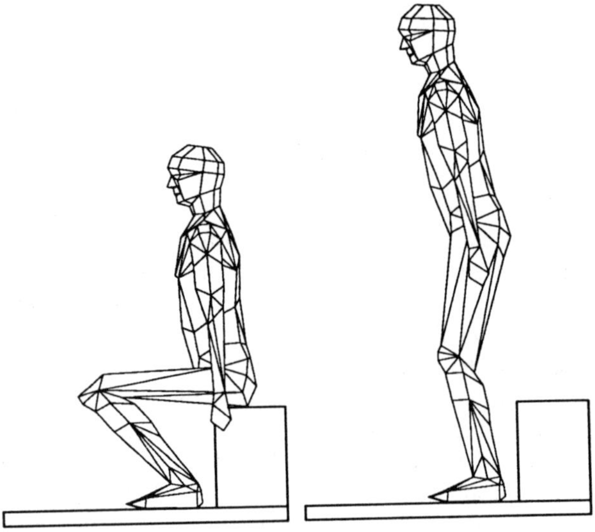

Fig. 8. Standing up under feedback control using neural networks (Beckmann and Daunicht, unpubl.).

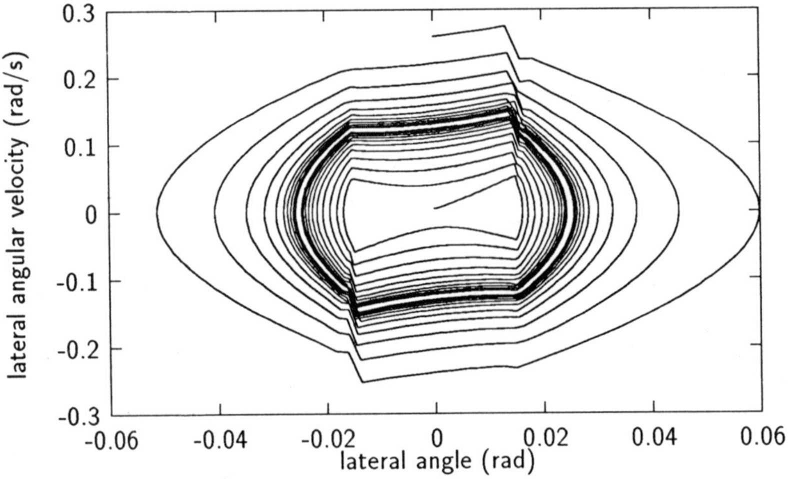

Fig. 9. Phase diagram of lateral dynamic balance of a biped. Two trajectories starting from outside and inside approach asymptotically a limit cycle attractor; rapid changes of velocity result from ground contact (Steiner and Daunicht, unpubl.).

That problem may be solved by using networks the synaptic weights of which can be calculated from the desired values rather than trained. For a DEFAnet, which has been developed particularly for the usage in sensorimotor signal processing (Daunicht 1991, Daunicht 1993), there exist such fast and accurate algorithms and they can be implemented very effectively. The calculation time of the fastest algorithm for a DEFAnet increases only linearly with the number of synapses simulated on sequential computer.The remaining error even for analog training examples is zero. Therefore we consider the DEFAnet calculus as an essential component of the software environment for the development of a neuroprosthesis.

5 Conclusion

Attractors required for control, such as limit cycles and chaotic attractors, can be constructed using filters, nonlinear static functions and human biomechanics, i.e. without central oscillators or other explicit function generators.

A consistent 3-dimensional model of the complete closed loop system required to develop sophisticated nonlinear controllers, in particular neural network based ones, is doable. Training of neural networks can be a time consuming process, but there exist procedures to cut this process short.

Meta-attractor control allows to integrate control of posture and locomotion into one framework and to initiate and finish walking by autonomous generation of stable transitions.

Autonomous reactions to disturbances may be very flexible with meta-attractors. For example, quiet stance could be controlled by a fixpoint attractor; when the system state leaves the attractor basin (due to a strong push), the meta-attractor may invoke a chaotic attractor, which initiates one or more compensating steps, until the state returns to the basin of the fixpoint attractor, and may then invoke the fixpoint attractor again. Thus safety of a given activity, e.g. quiet standing, is improved due to a meta-attractor structure.

When a task is identified with a meta-attractor, the command input is rather comfortable, as it is reduced to the selection of an item from a small menu, while a manifold of purposeful movements is generated autonomously in a reproducible way.

As neural networks are intrinsic parallel processing structures an implementation in dedicated hardware will result in real time responses of the controller.

6 Acknowledgements

This project was supported by Deutsche Forschungsgemeinschaft.

References

Beckmann, J. (1994) *Neuronale Netzwerke zur Kontrolle funktioneller elektrischer Stimulation bei Querschnittspatienten* Verlag Shaker.

Beckmann, J., Daunicht, W., and Hömberg, V. (1993) Functional electrical stimulation with neural network controlled state feedback. In: S. Gielen and B: Kappen (eds.) *ICANN '93; Proceeding of the International Conference on Artificial Neural Networks*, Springer, London, p. 869.

Daunicht, W. (1991) DEFAnet-deterministic neural network concept for function approximation. *Neural Networks*, **4**: 839-845.

Daunicht, W., (1993) DEFAnet2 - advancements of a deterministic function approximation. In: S. Gielen and B. Kappen (eds.) *ICANN '93; Proceeding of the International Conference on Artificial Neural Networks*, Springer, London, p. 510.

Daunicht, W., Swoboda, S., Steiner, R., and Hömberg, V. (1995) Software environement for the development and test of neuroprotheses to restore free stance and stepping in paraplegics. *XVth Congress ISB*, Jyväskylä, pp. 198-199.

Delp, S. (1990) *Surgery simulation: A computer graphics system to analyze and design musculoskeletal reconstructions of the lower limb,* PhD thesis Stanford University.

Hatze, H. (1981) A comprehensive model for the human motion simulation and its application to the take-off phase of the long jump. *J. Biomechanics*, **14**: 135-142.

Heemskerk, J. (1995) Overview of neural hardware. Unit of Experimental and Theoretical Psychology Leiden University, ftp.mrc-apu.cam.ac.uk/pub/nn.

Steiner, R. and Daunicht, W. (1993) Spatial simulation of human body motions during collisions and contact with hard surfaces. *I.S.B XIVth Congress Abstr.* **II**, pp. 1286-1287.

Steiner, R., Chini, G, and Daunicht, W. (1995) Stable control of periodic motion without a pescribed trajectory. *XVth Congress ISB*, Jyväskylä, pp. 880-881.

Taga, G. (1995) A model of the neuro-musculo-skeletal system for human locomotion. *Biol. Cybern.*, **73**: 97-111.

Wittenburg, J. (1977) *Dynamics of systems of rigid bodies.* Teubner Stuttgart.

Zajac, F. (1989) Muscle and tendon: properties, models, scaling, and application to biomechanics and motor control. *Crit. Rev. Biomed. Eng.*, **17**: 359-411.

Self Tuning Control in FES with Compensation of Nonlinear Recruitment Characteristics by Artificial Neural Networks

J. Schultheiss[1], T. Keller[2]
[1]Automatic Control Laboratory, Swiss Federal Institute of Technology,
[2]Paraplegic Centre Clinic Balgrist, Zürich, Switzerland

Abstract - An adaptive control system with nonlinear compensation of muscle recruitment characteristics is presented. The nonlinear compensation is accomplished by artificial neural networks. A self tuning regulator with a linear forgetting algorithm is implemented and tuning is switched according to changes in the controlled output to avoid wrong parameter estimates in the absence of suitable excitation. Experimental results for the control of the free swinging shank of able bodied persons are shown.

1 Introduction

Functional electrical stimulation is a well-known technique to restore muscle movements in paraplegics. In recent years, applied researchers have become increasingly interested in using closed-loop control to cope with time- and subject-varying aspects of electrical stimulation. Most controllers developed so far assume that the electrically stimulated muscle can be modeled with the so-called Hammerstein model (Bernotas *et al.* 1986, Hatwell *et al.* 1991, del Re *et al.* 1994). These Hammerstein type models consist of a static input nonlinearity followed by a linear, possibly time-varying transfer function, usually of second order.

In the present work the nonlinear compensation of the muscle recruitment characteristics is accomplished with neural networks.

In Section 2, we show how the artificial neural network is set up and trained; in Section 3, the adaptive controller is discussed; and in Section 4, experimental results are presented. Finally, the results are discussed in Section 5 and an outlook for future research is given.

2 Muscle Modeling

Neural networks are known to be particularly good in finding nonlinear mappings. A common danger however is to over-parameterize the network by choosing an excessively large network structure. Another drawback in neural networks is that the resulting weights are often difficult to interpret. For that reason, a rather simple network structure has been chosen to model muscle behavior due to electrical stimulation (see Fig. 1). Note that the output function of the last neuron in Fig. 1 is a linear transfer function.

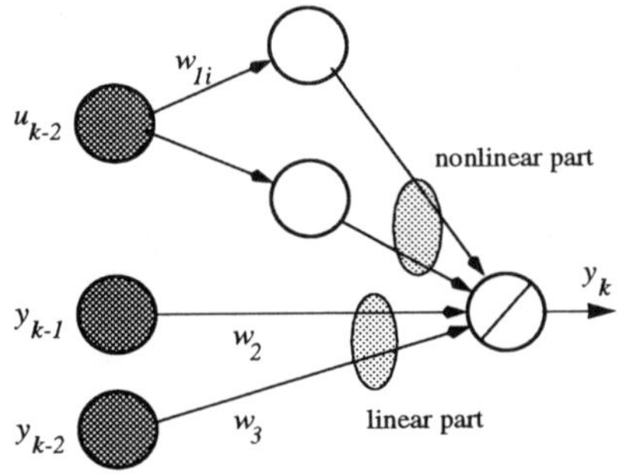

Fig. 1. Neural network structure

The *one step ahead* predictor equation of the artificial neural network in Fig. 1 is

$$\hat{y}_k = f(u_{k-2}) + w_2\, y_{k-1} + w_3\, y_{k-2} \tag{1}$$

where y_k is the normalized knee angle at time step k. The *nonlinear* part in Fig. 1 should replicate the input nonlinearity whereas the weights w_2 and w_3 should be comparable to the results of the linear identification using ARX models.

The training data set has been obtained from an open-loop experiment with an equally distributed random input signal. Prior to the experiment, a normalization procedure has been carried out which scales stimulus intensity (*i.e.* pulse width) so that the normalized pulse width of one corresponds to the fully stretched leg ($\doteq$ knee angle one).

The network has been trained with an error back propagation method, which is the so-called Levenberg-Marquardt algorithm.

3 Adaptive Controller

The advantage of Hammerstein models is the possibility of linear controller design. In order to obtain this possibility one has to premultiply the controller output with the inverse of the estimated input nonlinearity. In the present work the inverse input nonlinearity is estimated directly from input-output data. The network structure to accomplish this task is shown in Fig. 2.

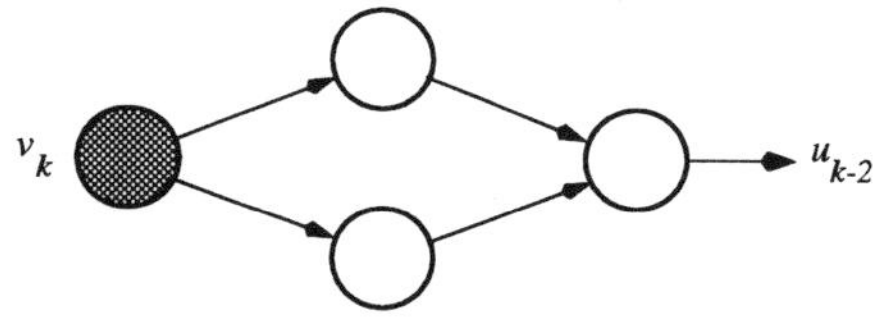

Fig. 2. Network structure to estimate inverse recruitment characteristics

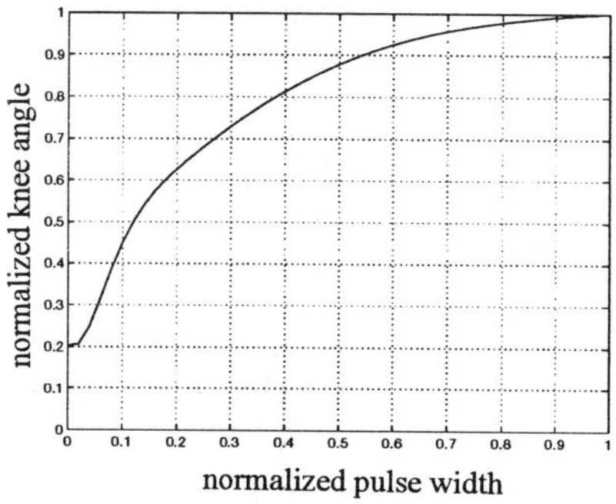

Fig. 3 Estimated inverse recruitment characteristics

The network input v_k is a filtered output sequence, namely

$$v_k = y_k - w_2\, y_{k-1} - w_3\, y_{k-2} \tag{2}$$

where the values for w_2 and w_3 are taken from the previous network in Figure 1.

The network (in Fig. 2) was trained with the same input-output data and the same training algorithm as the previous one. The estimated inverse recruitment characteristic is shown in Fig. 3.

The control scheme of the self tuning controller is shown in Figure 4. The controller design is based on a pole-zero placement approach and basically remained the same as in del Re *et al.* (1994) where it has been described in detail.

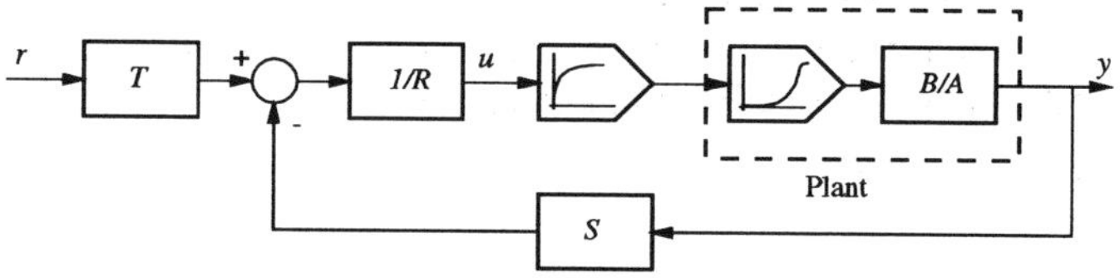

Fig. 4. Control scheme of self tuning regulator

4 Results

In Fig. 5, different time signals are shown. The dotted curve represents the reference input, the dash-dotted line is the uncompensated controller output, whereas the dashed line in Fig. 5 stands for the compensated controller output. Finally, the normalized knee angle is displayed in solid.

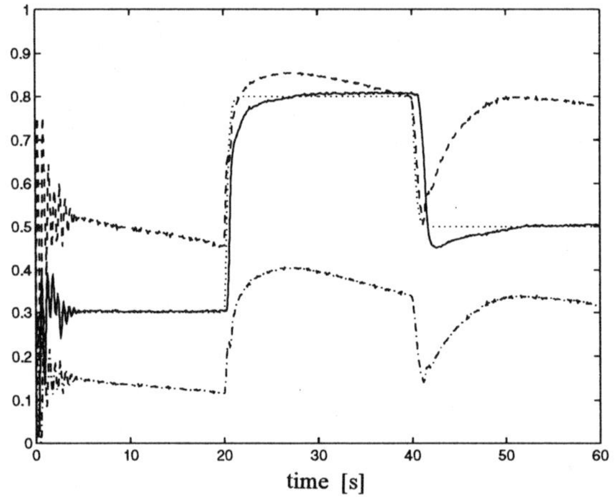

Fig. 5. Controlled plant

The reference signal has been chosen in such a way that the muscle is controlled at different operating points.

5 Discussion

As one can see in Fig. 5, the controller has difficulties in tracking the reference signal during the first 5 seconds. This is due to the fact that very low stimulus intensity which is close to the dead zone of the input nonlinearity is needed to achieve the desired knee angle. For knee angles, where higher stimulus intensity is needed, the controller works satisfactory.

In our future research we would like to extend the network structure to cope with hysteresis effects of electrically stimulated muscle.

References

Bernotas, L. A., Crago, P. E. and Chizeck, H. J. (1986). A discrete-time model of electrically stimulated muscle. *IEEE Trans. Biomed. Eng.* **33**(9), 829-838.

del Re, L., Kraus, F., Schultheiss, J., and Gerber, H. (1994). Self-tuning PID controller for lower limb FES with nonlinear compensation. In: *Proceedings of the 1994 American Control Conference*. Vol.2. pp.2015-19.

Hatwell, M. S., Oderkerk, B. J., Sacher, C. A., and Inbar, G. F. (1991). The development of a model reference adaptive control for the knee joint of paraplegics. *IEEE Trans Automatic Control* **36**, 683-691.

Chapter 4

Biomechanics Applied to Neuroprosthetics

Biomechanical Simulation and Animation of the Lower Extremity for the Design of Neural Prostheses

R. Riener[1], S. Villars[1], J. Quintern[2], G. Schmidt[1]
[1]Department of Automatic Control Eng., Technical University Munich, Germany
[2]Neurological Clinic, University of Munich, Germany

Abstract - A detailed model of the lower extremity is being developed in order to predict lower limb motion induced by Functional Electrical Stimulation (FES) during dynamic activation of selected muscles. The simulation is supported by an interactive graphic interface with a realistic 3-D display.

1 Introduction

The simulation of the human musculoskeletal system can help us understand how musculotendon actuators produce force and moment and how specific actuators and specific neural inputs contribute to movement coordination without resorting to invasive methods. Such a model can be used to design and test stimulation patterns as well as feedback control strategies (Khang and Zajac, 1989). This reduces the number of experiments in humans and, thus, accelerates the development of neural prostheses.

2 Methods

2.1 Model

The musculoskeletal model consists of three major parts:

Activation Dynamics provides the activation needed by muscles to generate desired force. A dynamic-time model (modified from Hatze, 1978) that relates the FES input (pulse width, amplitude or frequency) to the muscle activation is used (Riener *et al.*, 1995 b). A fitness function *fit(t)* takes muscle fatigue and recovery into consideration.

Contraction Dynamics generate tendon force to produce motion of the body segments. All relevant musculotendon actuators of the lower extremity are defined based on their anatomical relationships to 3-D bone surface representations (Delp, 1990). Each muscle is modeled as a composition of elements with nonlinear properties (Fig. 1).

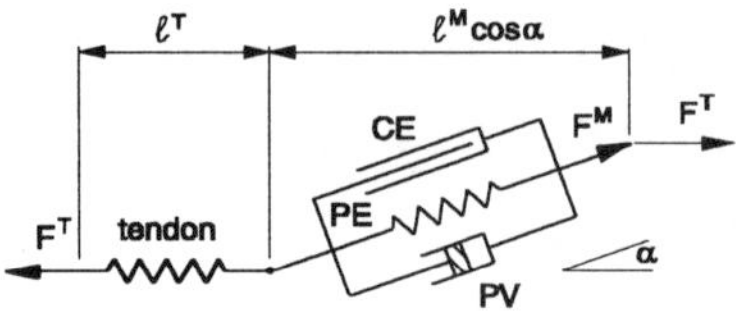

Fig. 1. Muscle contraction dynamics. The contractile element (CE) accounts for the force-length and force-velocity property of the muscle, which also depends on the amount of activation of the muscle. PE is the parallel elastic and PV the parallel viscous element. The forces in CE, PE, PV, and tendon are nonlinear functions of tendon length l^T, muscle length l^M, and muscle velocity v^M.

Body Segmental Dynamics determine the moment arms by muscle paths and joint geometry during limb motion. A 2-D kinematic model of the knee was taken from the literature (Yamaguchi and Zajac, 1989) and modified. The hip is simply modeled as a ball and socket joint, the ankle is modeled as double-hinge with non-orthogonal axes. The mathematical model used to describe the dynamics of foot, shank, and thigh, is given by a nonlinear, 6 DOF differential equation of motion. The computed motion is visualized by the interactive graphic interface AnySIM (IFP, Dornach, Germany), which allows to observe the kinematic consequences immediately after changing model input or model parameters.

2.2 Parameter Identification

Patient-specific model parameters such as peak isometric muscle force, recruitment, and fatigue parameters are identified by isometric stimulation experiments (Fig. 2 A). Regression equations (Zatsiorsky and Seluyanov, 1983) are used to determine anthropometric parameters. Passive viscous properties of muscle are identified by passive pendulum tests at hip, knee and ankle joint (Fig. 2 B). Additional passive pendulum tests and measurements of passive joint moments at different joint angles provide tendon slack lengths.

Patient-independent parameters, which were not changed during the studies, are optimal muscle fibre lengths, pennation angle, maximum shortening velocity, contraction/relaxation time constants, and parameters describing joint viscoelasticity, joint geometry, and muscle paths.

3 Preliminary Results

We investigated different stimulation patterns under isometric condition as well as under condition of freely swinging shank and obtained good agreement between motions generated in the simulation model and motions traced in FES experiments with paraplegic patients (Riener *et al.*, 1995 a). Since we have modeled all relevant muscles of the lower extremity, the user can optimize the choice of muscles to be stimulated. We observed that the joint moments about the

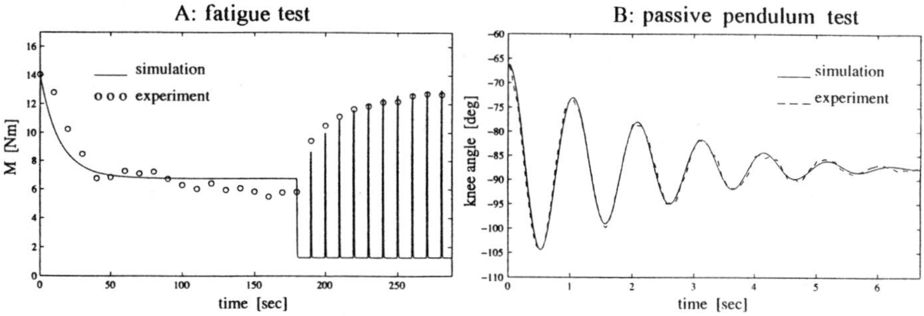

Fig. 2. Parameter identification, A: Effect of muscle fatigue and recovery on isometric knee moment during stimulation of the quadriceps muscle (f=20 Hz, d=320 μs). During recovery, the muscle was stimulated only in short intervals of 0.5 sec. B: Simulated and measured passive pendulum test of the shank after parameter adjustment.

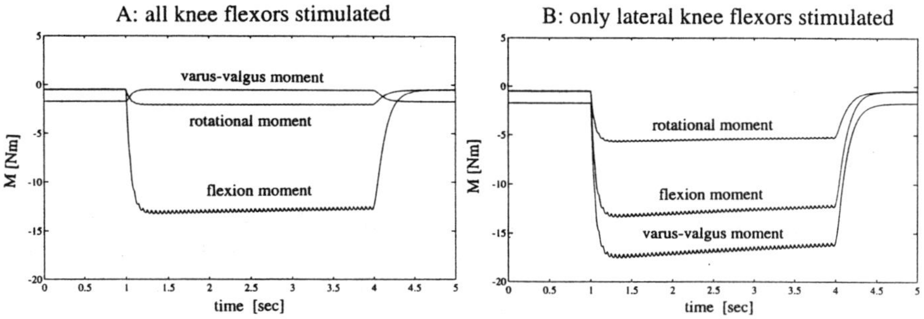

Fig. 3. Simulation results: flexion, varus-valgus, and rotational moment for two different sets of isometrically stimulated knee flexor muscles. The knee is flexed 30°, while the hip is fully extended. A: All flexors are stimulated at the same intensity. B: An unfavorable combination of muscles stimulated (in this example only lateral ones) yields high varus-valgus and rotational moment.

varus-valgus and rotational axes of the knee strongly increase when, for example, only lateral knee flexor muscles are stimulated instead of all flexor muscles together (Fig. 3).

4 Discussion

The objective of this study is to develop an experimentally tested biomechanical model of the human lower extremity which can be employed to predict FES-generated lower limb motion during dynamic activation of selected muscles. The presented simulation accounts for muscle fatigue and recovery which makes it possible to optimize muscle stimulation patterns so as to allow only minimum fatigue. It is also necessary to model nonlinear viscosity in musculotendon units in order to characterize the absorption of impact energy, for example during gait when a foot strikes the floor. Because of the large number of muscles taken into consideration, the simulation allows to optimize the choice of muscles to be stimulated to obtain desired motion while minimizing joint load.

One difficulty of the model is its complexity, and the high number of parameters needed to describe the musculoskeletal system. However, patient-independent parameters are taken from the literature, and the remaining ones are identified with specific experimental procedures. To simplify the identification of the numerous muscle parameters we applied a scaling procedure as proposed by Zajac (1989). Identification could be improved further by stimulating single muscles with small surface or wire electrodes to identify more specific muscle parameters.

The presented simulation model satisfactorily describes the input-output relation of the human musculoskeletal system and allows, in addition, access to certain intermediate quantities. It can be used to evaluate and optimize open- and closed-loop control strategies for FES. From preliminary data we conclude that the modeling of the human musculoskeletal system in the way described can support and accelerate the development of neural prostheses.

References

Delp, S. L. (1990) Surgery simulation: a computer graphics system to analyze and design musculoskeletal reconstructions of the lower limb. PhD thesis, Stanford University, CA.

Hatze, H. (1978) A general myocybernetic control model of skeletal muscle. *Biol. Cybern.* **28**, 143-157.

Khang, G. and Zajac, F. E. (1989) Paraplegic standing controlled by functional neuromuscular stimulation: part I: computer model and control-system design. *IEEE Trans. Biomed. Eng.* **36**(9), 873-884.

Riener, R., Quintern, J., Volz, S. (1995 a) Comparison of simulation and experiments of different closed-loop strategies for FES. Part1: simulation model. In: Proc. of the Vth Vienna International Workshop on Functional Electrostimulation (IFESS). Vienna, August 1995, 251-254.

Riener, R., Quintern, J., Psaier, E., Schmidt, G. (1995 b) Physiologically-Based Multi-Input Model of Muscle Activation (*in this volume*).

Yamaguchi, G. T. and Zajac, F. E. (1989) A planar model of the knee joint to characterize the knee extensor mechanism. *J. Biomechanics* **22**(1), 1-10.

Zajac, F. E. (1989) Muscle and tendon: properties, models, scaling, and application to biomechanics and motor control. In *CRC Crit. Rev. Biomed. Eng.* **17**(4), 359-411.

Zatsiorsky, V. and Seluyanov, V. (1983) The mass and inertia characteristics of the main segments of the human body. *Biomechanics VIII-B*, University Park Press, 1152-1159.

Optimal Trajectory Generation for a Paraplegic Patient Rising from a Chair by means of FES

F. Bahrami, R. Riener, M. Buss, G. Schmidt
Department of Automatic Control Engineering;
Technical University of Munich, Munich, Germany

Abstract - Based on a planar model of the human body with three degrees-of-freedom (DOF), an algorithm was developed which generates optimal joint angle trajectories during rising from a chair. Optimality is defined with respect to the exerted joint torques and torque changes calculated for a rigid body dynamic model. The results of the investigation may be useful for generating FES induced movements in paraplegic patients.

1 Introduction

One possibility of controlling the movement of a paraplegic patient by means of Functional Electrical Stimulation (FES) is to use a tracking control approach (Khang *et al.,* 1989). Joint torques induced by FES are limited compared with joint torques in healthy subjects. Moreover, FES causes greater muscle fatigue than does natural stimulation (Boom *et al.,* 1993, Rabischong *et al.,* 1993). Hence, application of trajectories recorded from healthy subjects may be inappropriate references for motion control of patients stimulated by FES. We developed an algorithm based on a 3-DOF model to generate optimal trajectories under constraints induced by physical limitations when rising from a seated position. To validate the resulting trajectories, we have considered the motion of healthy subjects. The algorithm presented in this paper can be used to compute the joint trajectories for movements induced by FES in paraplegic patients.

2 Methods

2.1 Mathematical Description

Assuming symmetrical planar motion, the human body is described as a three-segment dynamical model (3-DOF) including shanks, thighs, and upper body (head, arms, and trunk) with frictionless joints:

$$M(\underline{q}) \cdot \underline{\ddot{q}} + C(\underline{q}, \underline{\dot{q}}) + G(\underline{q}) = J_\tau \cdot \underline{\tau}, \tag{1}$$

where $\underline{q}, \dot{\underline{q}}, \ddot{\underline{q}}$ are joint angular displacement, velocity, and acceleration vectors, respectively. M is the inertia matrix, C represents the coriolis and centrifugal, and G the gravitational terms acting on the body segments. $\underline{\tau}$ is the total joint torque vector composed of two components. One is induced by muscles and the other by passive elastic and viscous properties due to connective tissue. J_τ is the Jacobian matrix mapping torque input to joint space.

2.2 Model Validation

To validate the model, joint positions and ground reaction loads of two healthy subjects were recorded simultaneously by a motion analyser (ELITE, BTS, Milan) and a Kistler force platform, respectively (Fig. 1). The dynamic model (eq. 1) and the measured kinematic and anthropometric data were used to calculate joint torques $\underline{\tau}$, horizontal and vertical components of ground reaction forces $F=(F_X, F_Y)^T$, mass center of body (MCB), and center of pressure (COP). Computed vertical ground reaction force shows good agreement with experimental measurements when the body is not in contact with the chair (Fig. 2).

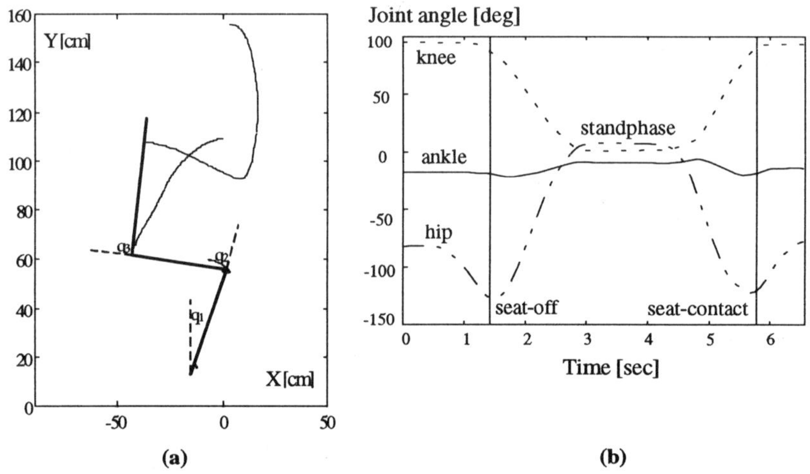

Fig. 1. a) Trajectories of knee, hip, and shoulder joints in the sagittal plane when rising from a chair. The subjects sat with their arms folded across their chest. During movement two CCD cameras recorded the Cartesian coordinates of four infrared-reflecting markers placed on one side of the body, at the ankle, knee, hip, and shoulder (sampling rate: 100 Hz). b) Computed joint angles for normal rising after low-pass filtering of the kinematic data with a 9th-order Butterworth filter (f_{cut}=3 Hz).

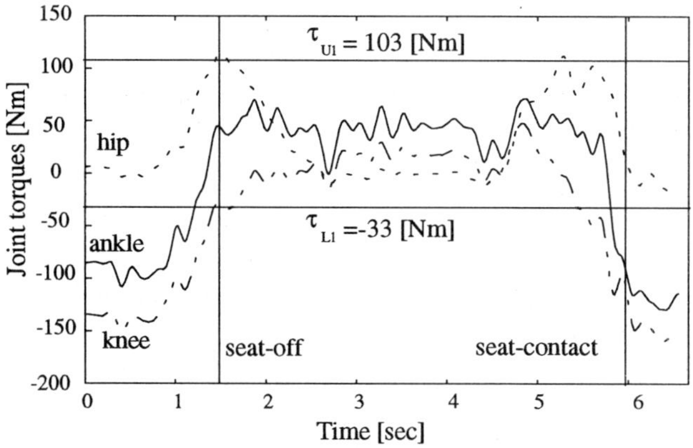

(a)

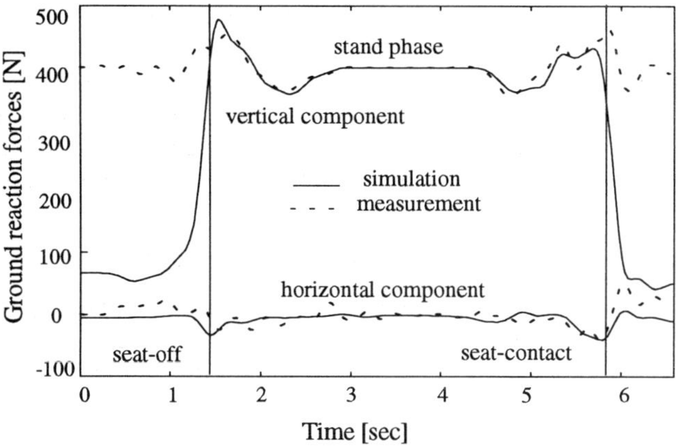

(b)

Fig. 2.a) Knee, hip, and ankle joint torques. The ankle joint torque remains between the upper and lower limits. These limits correspond to maximum and minimum static ankle torque allowed before tipping over. b) Simulated and measured ground reaction forces. The seat-off instant was obtained by measuring the chair reaction force for one leg. A peak in F_X appears at the instance of seat-off (also observed by Roebroeck *et al.*, 1994).

2.3 Optimal Trajectory Problem

Taking the limitations of human body movement in healthy as well as paraplegic subjects into consideration, we developed an optimization algorithm to generate joint angle trajectories when rising from a seated position. Optimality here is defined with respect to the performance measure c_τ:

$$c_\tau = \frac{1}{t_f - t_0} \int_{t_0}^{t_f} (\underline{\tau}^T(\underline{q}, t) \cdot W_M \cdot \underline{\tau}(\underline{q}, t) + \dot{\underline{\tau}}^T \cdot W_V \cdot \dot{\underline{\tau}}) dt \tag{2}$$

where the first term in c_τ penalizes excessive torques and the second term, torque changes. The weight matrices W_M and W_V allow specification of their respective importance. The optimization problem is to minimize c_τ, giving initial and final conditions for $\underline{q}, \dot{\underline{q}}, \ddot{\underline{q}}$ subjected to constraints, e.g.,

- *friction limits* at feet (Coulomb's friction law: $\mu \cdot |F_Y| > |F_X|$);
- *limited joint torques* ($\tau_{Li} < \tau_i < \tau_{Ui}$) or the similar constraint *limited joint angular accelerations* ($|\ddot{q}_i| \le a_i$);
- *COP condition* ($x_{heel} < x_{COP} < x_{toe}$), which indicates the dynamic stability of movement;
- *MCB condition* ($x_{heel} < x_{MCB} < x_{toe}$), describing static stability of movement;
- *geometric constraints* ($Y_{hip} > h_{chair}$).

To summarize: the problem is to find joint trajectories $\underline{q}(t)$ that minimize c_τ subjected to eq. (1) and a set of given constraints.

This optimization task is inherently infinite dimensional, since the search space is a space of continuous trajectories. To solve the problem, we parametrized the trajectories. For further simplification, we assumed a fixed start and end time for the movement between seat-off, t_0, and standing, t_f. The proposed algorithm is as follows:

- specification of start and final body states $(\underline{q}(t_0), \dot{\underline{q}}(t_0), \ddot{\underline{q}}(t_0), \underline{q}(t_f), \dot{\underline{q}}(t_f), \ddot{\underline{q}}(t_f))$;
- discretization of trajectories q_i with n equally spaced control points at time instances t_k (Fig. 3). The trajectories at time t, $t_k < t < t_{k+1}$, are reconstructed using quintic splines, which yield smooth torque trajectories. The first and n^{th}

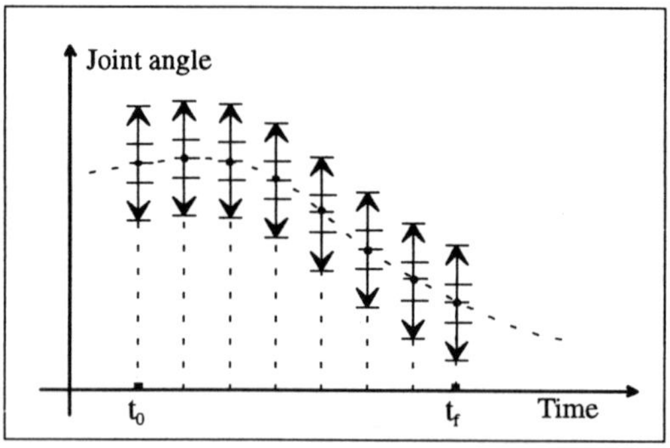

Fig. 3. The initial values of control points at discrete time instants t_k ($t_k \in [t_0, t_f]$, $k=1...n$, $t_{k+1}-t_k = \Delta t$) and discretized joint angle.

control points are fixed due to the start and final conditions, and 3(n-2) control points are used as optimization parameters; the search space is therefore 3(n-2)-dimensional;

- minimization of c_τ over the 3(n-2) control points under the defined constraints using a Quasi-Newton method from the MATLAB optimization toolbox.

3 Results and Discussion

To implement the optimization algorithm we chose three different motions categorized according to the speed after seat-off (fast, normal, and slow). n, the number of control points and their distance (Δt), depended on the time duration between instant of seat-off and standing. In each case t_f-t_0 was defined by measurements. The values of joint angles and their corresponding angular velocities and accelerations of the starting control points at t_0 and the joint angles at t_f were also determined from measurements. Angular velocities and accelerations at t_f were defined to be zero (standing position). The initial values of the other control points were either calculated from measurements or they were chosen on the partially linear curves connecting the start and final points of joint trajectories. With healthy subjects, we first defined only the friction and COP conditions as inequality constraints. The friction constant μ = 0.5, and the limits for COP-condition X_{heel}= -7 cm and X_{toe}= 22 cm were chosen.

To investigate the optimal trajectories three cases were considered:

1. W_M=0 and W_V=I, which correspond to minimum torque change criterion;
2. W_M=I and W_V=0, which describe the minimum torque criterion; and
3. W_M=λ_1I and W_V=λ_2I,

where I denotes the unity matrix. Considering the numerical values of min(c_τ) in the first and second case, the values of λ_1 and λ_2 in the third case were defined by choosing $\lambda_1 \cong [\min(c_{\tau1})/\min(c_{\tau2})]\lambda_2$.

We observed that, under the two defined inequality constraints and in comparison with measurements, minimization of *total torque change* (case 1) yields a smoother movement than minimizing the *total joint torque* (Fig. 4-a,b). In the third case, which is a weighted combination of two previous performance measures, some improvement can be observed (Fig. 4-c). Furthermore, there is a weak agreement in case 2 between optimized and measured ankle trajectories. This difference makes the movement in case 2 different.

As regards the minimization of *total joint torque,* we observed the followings:

- when the maximum joint accelerations (as an additional constraint) were limited, the optimization algorithm yielded a smoother movement than otherwise (Fig. 4-b). To limit the joint accelerations we used the results of actual measurements. According to the optimized trajectories, the highest acceleration occures earlier than in the case of measurements. In fact minimizing total joint torque means a faster movement (high acceleration) at the beginning which is followed by a slower movement (Fig. 4-b, joint angle trajectories). During the

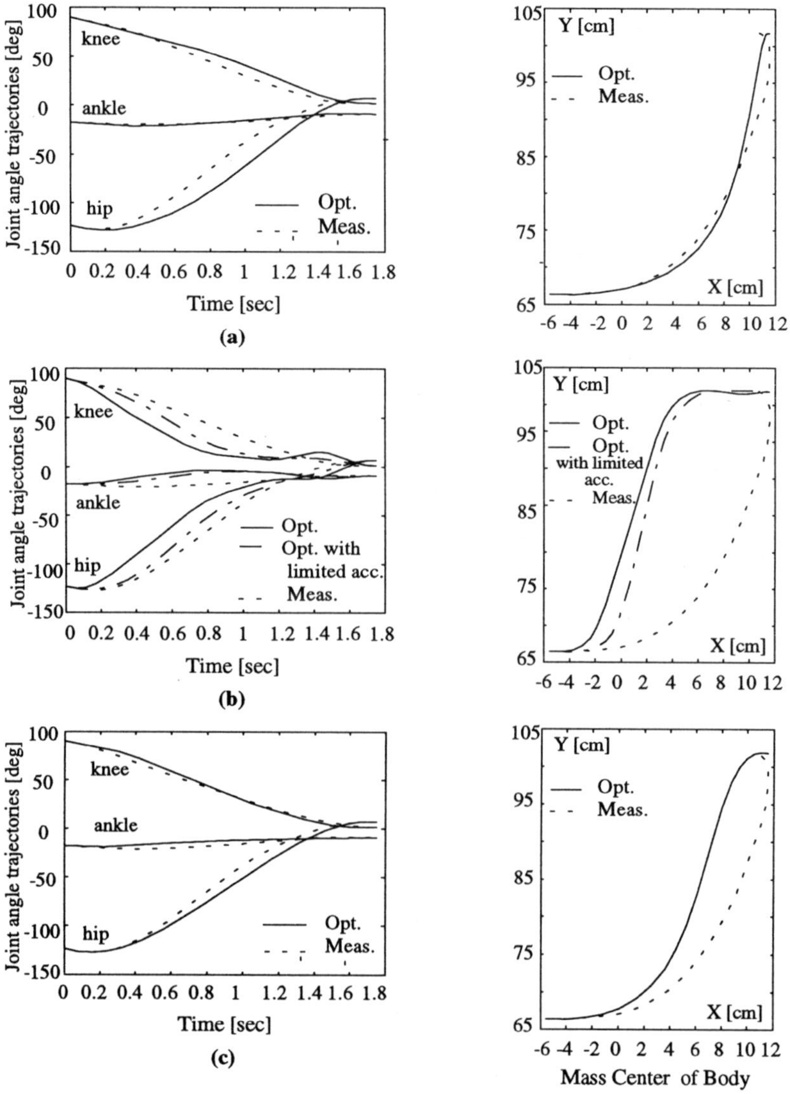

Fig. 4. Optimal trajectories for different weigth matrices in the performance measure. a) Trajectories calculated by minimizing the *total torque changes* (W_M=0, W_V=I). b) Trajectories obtained by minimizing *total joint torque* (WM=I, W_V=0). Results are for optimization with and without limited joint accelerations. c) Optimal trajectories after minimizing c_τ ($W_M=\lambda_1 I$, $W_V=\lambda_2 I$, $\lambda_1/\lambda_2 \cong [\min(c_{\tau 1})/\min(c_{\tau 2})]$).

fast part of motion, almost all of the vertical displacement and also a part of the horizontal displacement of MCB is achived. Through the slow part, the rest of horizontal displacement takes place (Fig. 4-b, MCB trajectory);

- when the final control point was also defined as an optimization parameter rather than as a fixed point, the optimal trajectories always had zero final values, which means ideal standing. The same observation was also made for the third case, which has a component of *minimum torque* criterion in the performance measure. Minimizing the *total torque change,* one must define the final values of control points.

The starting time t_0 can affect the agreement between measured and optimized trajectories. This means that the history of the optimized trajectories is always almost the same, and is relatively independent of the history of the initial trajectories (which were chosen from measurements). Changing t_0 can cause better agreement between the results of measurements and optimization without effecting a big change in the optimized trajectories.

Table 1 summarizes the numerical considerations and results for different cases. Termination tolerance of the algorithm for the performance measure was set to 0.1 and for optimization variables 0.05 (rad). The algorithm always converged.

Table 1: The numerical results for different motions and performance measures. The initial control points are chosen on the measured trajectories.

motion	Δt [s]	n	case 1 iterations	case 1 min ($c_{\tau 1}$)	case 2 iterations	case 2 min ($c_{\tau 2}$)	case 3 iterations	case 3 min ($c_{\tau 3}$)
fast	0.16	6	476	20.9	673	12474.6	482	49.21
normal	0.25	8	517	2.33	808	4856.21	526	5.52
slow	0.35	13	711	0.29	1428	4122.24	740	0.92

4 Conclusion

An algorithm was developed to find the optimum trajectories when rising from a chair. To reduce high computational efforts resulting from infinite dimensionality of search space, we parametrized the problem. The performance criterion which was the weighted combination of total joint torque and joint torque changes yielded optimal joint trajectories, which were in satisfactory agreement with experimental measurements. In view of our preliminary results, it seems probable that the central nervous system applies a combination of minimum torque change and minimum joint torque strategy during the process of rising from a seated position. To obtain more rigorous results in the future we plan to model the effect of chair contact, include other physiological criteria in the performance measure (e.g., minimum muscle force), and therefore improve the model, optimize the duration of the motion, and consider the limitations due to FES such as limited muscle forces and increased muscle fatigue.

References

Boom, H.B.K., Mulder, A.J., and Veltink, P.H. (1993) Fatigue during functional neuromuscular stimulation, *Progress in Brain Research*, Vol. 97, Elsevier Science Publication, Ch. 36, pp 409-419.

Khang, G.and Zajac, F.E. (1989) Paraplegic standing controlled by functional neuromuscular stimulation: part I computer model and control-system design, *IEEE Trans. Biomed. Eng.*, Vol. 36, No. 9, September, pp 873-884.

Rabischong, E. and Guiraud, D. (1993) Determination of fatigue in the electrically stimulated quadriceps muscle and relative effect of ischaemia, *J. Biomed.*, Vol. 15, November, pp 443-450.

Roebroeck, M.E., Doorenbosch, C.A.M., Harlaar, J., Jacobs, R., and Lankhorst, G.J. (1994) Biomechanics and muscular activity during sit-to-stand transfer, *Clin. Biomech.*, No. 4, September, pp 235-244.

Crutch Assisted FES Gait and Upright Stability Assessment

T.Karčnik, A.Kralj, T.Bajd
Faculty of Electrical and Computer Engineering
University of Ljubljana, Ljubljana, Slovenia

Abstract - FES assisted gait of paraplegic patients is inferior compared to a healthy subject. The difference can be observed in terms of speed, up-right balance, biomechanical energy consumption and generation of propulsion forces in the direction of walking. The biomechanical structure is the same as in normal, however the mode of walking differs significantly because of the reduced number of activated muscles and primitive control. The healthy subject is utilizing two-point semidynamically stable gait. The paraplegic patient is employing 4-channels of FES and utilizing a four-point statically stable gait. We believe that FES gait can be improved if converted into a semi-dynamically or dynamically stable gait. The gait is considered statically stable if the center of gravity (COG) projection on the ground (PCOG) is inside the supporting area. In quadruped this is only possible if it is utilizing creeping crawl gait. In this paper the relationship between PCOG and the supporting area are discussed as a criterion for dynamic stability assessment. Results are shown for three different modes of two-point and four-point gaits.

1 Introduction

In selected spinal cord injured patients the restoration of biped gait can be realized by means of functional electrical stimulation FES (Kralj and Bajd, 1989). The patients are using 4-channel surface FES. Swing phase is realized through afferent FES provoking flexion reflex resulting in simultaneous flexion of hip and knee and ankle dorsiflexion and thus providing clearance of the foot from the ground. Stance phase is achieved by stimulating bilaterally knee extensors enabling sufficient support to the patient utilizing crutches for balance and partial support. Such FES assisted gait of paraplegic patients is in terms of biomechanics significantly inferior to a healthy subject gait. The main drawbacks are:

- Velocity is considerably lower. Average speed achieved by a paraplegic is about 0.15 m/s. A healthy person walks at about 1.5 m/s (Kralj and Bajd, 1989).

- Energy inefficiency is resulting in high energy consumption, which is about 14 J/kg m for paraplegic walking at 0.15 m/s. A healthy subject gait at 1.5 m/s requires only 3.3 J/kg m (Kralj and Bajd, 1989).
- Insufficient horizontal propulsion impulse in the direction of walking is clearly demonstrated from the amplitude ratios of propulsion forces in paraplegic (40 N) and healthy subject (200 N) (Bajd *et al.*, 1993).
- Up-right balance is adjusted mainly by hands provided forces.

In addition, there are also other factors. It is evidently that all of the factors are interrelated in a complex manner.

Owing to it the gait cannot be improved on a subjective way or by simply copying a normal biped gait. In both gaits we are dealing with the same biomechanical structure consisting of segments and rotational joints but with FES performing a different gait mode. The FES gait is a quadrupedal gait because the subject is utilizing the crutches for balance, partial propulsion and support. As it is unlikely for the balance problem to be solved in the near future, the FES enabled gait will remain quadrupedal and therefore we are dealing with the problem of how to improve the existing four-point FES gait (Kralj *et al.*, 1994; Bajd *et al.*, 1995). To clearly distinguish and evaluate different types of gait, a universal stability index has to be developed. This can be used in biofeedback loops to indicate either dangerous or good posture and movement. Such feedback loops have already been proven to be successful in gait enhancement (Erzin *et al.*, 1993).

The basic theoretical approach of multilegged gait analysis is derived from robotics, where several walking and running machines have already been constructed. The whole analysis is performed for walking on the flat, hard, level surface. Here, several new terms are introduced into the analysis.

2 Methods

2.1 Theoretical background

The supporting area in a certain phase of gait is defined as the minimum convex point set in the ground plane such that all the leg contact points are contained (McGhee and Frank, 1968). The center of gravity location (COG) is defined as the first normalized moment. In human walking the COG is, because of its difficult assessment, often replaced with the center of body (COB), which is defined as a fixed anatomical quantity: the center of the cross-section at the height of the second sacral vertebra. Mathematically is COB calculated as the location of the COG in quiet standing. Though such replacement could introduce significant errors - mainly in non gait activities, it is often used because of its simple application. Another important parameter is the vertical projection of COG on the ground level (PCOG). Similar vertical projection of the COB on the ground plane is marked as PCOB. The parameters are explained in depth in (Karcnik *et al.*, 1995). The sum of the ground reaction forces (GRF) is calculated as a vector sum of forces under each supporting leg/crutch. GRF is a vector quantity and is always pointing from the point on the ground level, called center of pressure (COP), towards the COG. Therefore COP can be defined as the point projected on the ground along the direction of the resultant reaction force acting to the COG. Ground reaction forces are related by Newton's 2nd law to the acceleration of COG. An important conclusion is that the COP is always inside the supporting area, while this is not true for PCOG.

A statically stable gait is a gait pattern (McGhee and Frank, 1968), when the PCOG is during the whole gait cycle inside the supporting area. There are 5040 nonsingular gait patterns (McGhee and Frank, 1968) out of which only three can be statically stable. Out of these three creeping patterns (McGhee and Frank, 1968) the crawl gait offers superior static stability properties. This type of gait is adopted by four-legged animals for a slow walking and intuitively also by FES assisted paraplegic subjects. The main characteristic of statically stable gait is that a system, in our case the paraplegic subject, can maintain its posture in any gait phase for an arbitrary amount of time. Such a gait must and can be as slow as desired, but is consequently at the higher velocities not feasible.

Quite opposite a healthy person is utilizing semidynamically stable gait. This is a gait mode with both statically stable and statically unstable phases. The statically unstable states in the gait cycle occur, when PCOG is outside the supporting area. When the gait cycle consists of only statically unstable states the gait is truly dynamically stable, e.g running. The movement assures the stability of the system in statically unstable phases. If the system stops, it falls. In statically unstable gait phases the dynamics of the mechanism together with the propulsion forces determines the gait velocity. As the statically unstable phases are mandatory gravity and inertia driven, the gait cannot be arbitrary slow. Thus developing a FES assisted (semi)dynamically stable gait would doubtlessly lead into faster and more efficient gait.

2.2 Stability criteria

So far no quantity or index has been proposed to enable a quantitative analysis or description and to be universally valid for both static and dynamic gait stability. Therefore numerous approximations have been introduced. When measuring system (in)stability, the first approximation is to use the simple relationship between PCOG and the supporting area as a stability measure. This approach neglects all inertial and propulsive forces. Therefore, it is suitable only for a very slow statically stable gait. It is a reliable indicator whether certain gait phases are statically unstable or not. In statically unstable phases of the gait, a system is mandatory gravity/inertia driven what reduces the energy consumption.

For assessment of system (in)stability in faster but still statically stable gait the COP compared to the supporting area can be used instead of PCOG vs. supporting area relationship (Lin and Song, 1993). COP position depends not only on system posture but also on system inertial or ground reaction forces. In faster statically stable gait the static stability margin is smaller as compared to a slower gait modes. This means that the control system needs to react faster, specially when static stability margin is small. The COP can come close to the supporting area edge not only because the mechanism is actually close to the static stability edge or transition to an unstable phase, but also because of the high propulsion/breaking forces. The COP to supporting area relationship cannot be used in (semi)dynamically stable gait, because there is no information, whether a system is statically stable or not.

The only useful parameter in (semi)dynamically stable gait is the PCOG compared to the supporting area, while the COP is always inside the supporting area and is therefore useless. PCOG determines whether the mechanism is in certain moment statically stable or not.

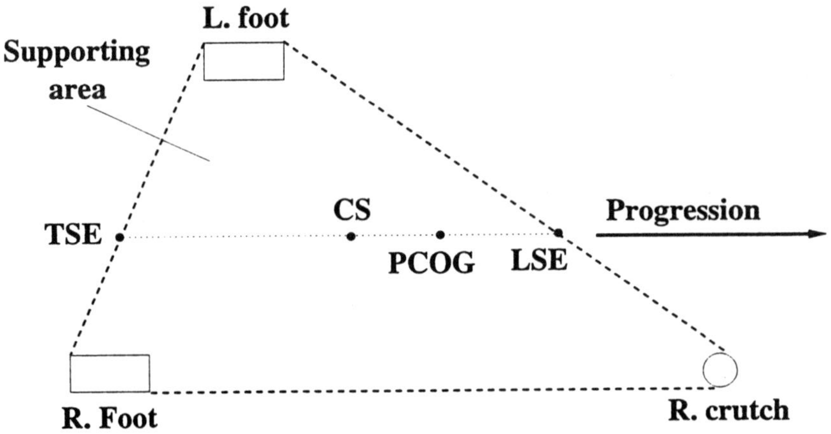

Fig. 1. Parameters for the definition of static stability index

To understand these basic stability criteria we have measured the static stability index in heathy subject biped gait, healthy subject forced four-point gait, in a below knee amputee and in an incomplete paraplegic. Dimensionless relative static stability index (SSI) is defined in eq.(1):

(1)

Leading stability edge point (LSE) is the intersection point of the supporting area leading edge and the line through the PCOG in the direction of the instantaneous COG velocity. Trailing stability edge point (TSE) is the equivalent point at the trailing supporting area edge. Center of stability area (CS) is the midpoint between LSE and TSE. Figure 1 graphically explains the parameters used in the definition of SSI.

When SSI is positive, a mechanism is statically stable. The negativity of SSI increases if the mechanism static unstability increases. Theoretically there is no lower limit on SSI as the denominator in eq. (1) can be arbitrary small. The SSI equals one if PCOG is projected exactly into CS. To assess the SSI index only the knowledge of COG positi on and motion and supporting area geometry is required.

3 Results

3.1 Measurement protocol and stability assessment

We used the OPTOTRAK contactless motion analysis system to determine both the COG position/motion and supporting area. Due to easier assessment, we measured the motion of the COB instead of the COG. The foot-floor contact model has been characterized by three different types: heel contact only, toe contact only and foot flat. The first two contacts were modeled as irregular triangles, while the latter one included a rectangular support area in between the triangles. The dimensions of modeled foot-floor contact were assessed individually for each tested subject. The supporting area was modeled as polygon and the actual shape and dimensions were assessed for each recorded data frame independently. The crutch-floor contact was modeled as point contact. MATLAB$^{@}$ was used for numeric data processing and visualization.

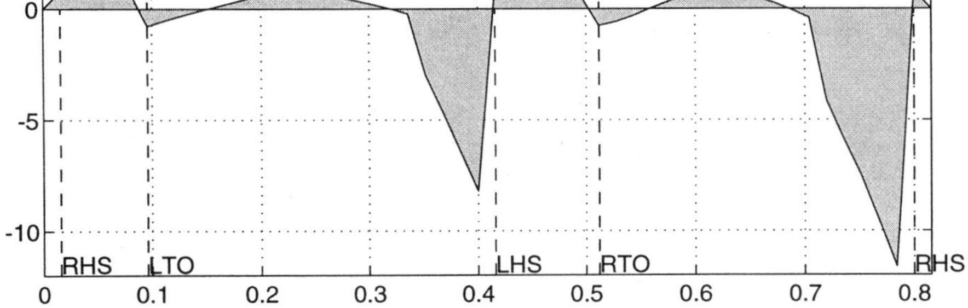

Fig. 2. SSI assessed in a healthy person biped gait; RHS: right heel strike, LHS: left heel strike, LTO: left toe off, RTO: right toe off

Figure 2 shows the SSI for a healthy subject biped free gait. As expected there are two statically unstable gait phases: initial and final part of the single support phase. The variance of SSI in the final part of the single support phase before the heel strike is due to small foot-floor contact area. So even a small variation from step to step causes significant changes in SSI. The distance between PCOG and CS rarely exceeds 10 cm, which is only about 12% if compared to the vertical distance from COG to the floor. So even a small swing of COG around its vertical position enables semi-dynamically stable gait.

Figure 3 shows the SSI for a healthy subject four-point gait in slow pace. As expected the minimum value of SSI is higher than in biped gait. However, the gait is still semidynamically stable. The variance of SSI is higher.

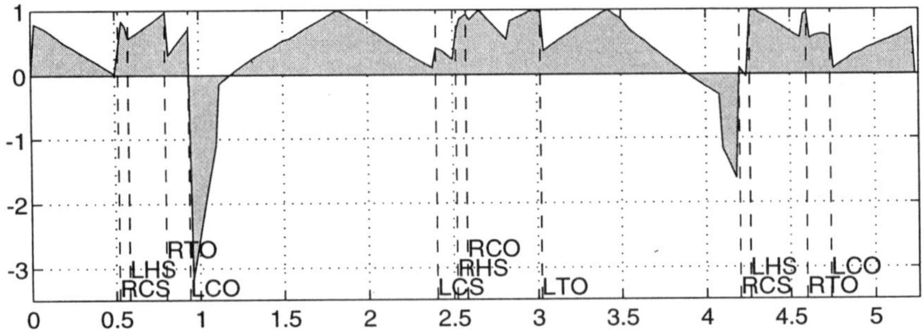

Fig. 3. SSI in a healthy subject forced four point gait; RHS: right heel strike, LHS: left heel strike, LTO: left toe off, RTO: right toe off; LCO: left crutch off, RCO: right crutch off, LCS: left crutch stike, RCS: right crutch strike

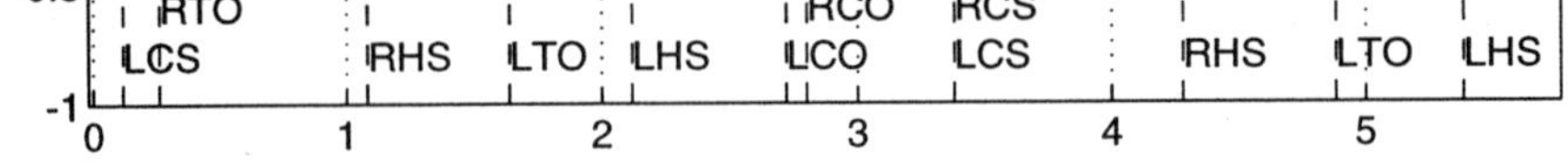

Fig. 4. SSI in C6-7 incomplete paraplegic; RHS: right heel strike, LHS: left heel strike, LTO: left toe off, RTO: right toe off; LCO: left crutch off, RCO: right crutch off, LCS: left crutch stike, RCS: right crutch strike

Figure 4 shows the SSI for a an incomplete C6-7 male paraplegic free gait. His left leg is nearly normal while his right leg is almost completely paralyzed. We used two stimulation channels both on the paralyzed leg: the first one was used for knee extensors to enable the leg support and the second was used to elicit the flexion reflex to enable the swing. The subject was unable to walk without FES. This particular subject was, unlike most of the others, utilizing a gait pattern where both crutches were transferred forward nearly simultaneously during the healthy leg support phase. This kind of gait is specific for the patients who have one leg intact. This is also neither creeping nor crawl gait. It is rather surprising that the SSI is almost always positive. This means that the subject is statically unstable only for a very short period of time at the beginning of the healthy leg swing phase.

4 Conclusions

We hypothesize that the introduction of the unstable states into the paraplegic gait can improve its efficiency and increase the average speed (Bajd *et al.*, 1995). Because it is impossible for an FES walker to utilize a normal-like gait, we are forced to copy other four-point gaits, which already incorporate unstable states. Above/below knee amputees walking by crutches are good four-point walkers as shown in our previous work (Karcnik *et al.*, 1995). They serve as a model for paraplegic FES gait. Still an important difference exist. Amputees heavily utilize hip flexors and extensors, which are difficult to stimulate by surface electrodes and are not used in here described FES gait. We showed here that statically unstable phases do not occur regularly even in an incomplete paraplegic with one leg virtually intac. Such gait is not truly semidynamically stable. In our future work we will try to find out, if semidynamically or dynamically stable FES gait in complete paraplegic is possible at all and if it is possible, we will try to synthesize it.

To quantitatively assess the dynamic stability a new criterion needs to be established which will include the mechanism kinetic energy as well. SSI doesn't suffice for assessing the dynamic stability. Namely, even if the mechanism is statically unstable, e.g. biped walking at the beginning of the single support phase, it can recover into a statically stable posture, e.g. mid single support phase, without any propulsion forces. The reverse is also true: a mechanism can slip out of statically stable state just because of its kinetic energy, e.g. transfer from mid to end of single support phase. This kind of phenomena occur in faster multilegged gaits as well. Therefore, the understanding of dynamic stability control is essential particular for the synthesis of semidynamically stable FES and crutch assisted gait and for biofeedback purposes as well.

References

Bajd, T., Kralj, A., Karcnik, T., Savrin, P., and Obreza, P. (1993) Importance of FES Assisted Terminal Stance Phase, Proc. of the Ljubljana FES conference, pp. 57-60, Ljubljana.

Bajd, T., Zefran, M., and Kralj, A. (1995) Timing and Kinematics of Quadrupedal Walking Pattern, Proc. IROS '95 IEEE/RSJ Inter. Conf. on Intelligent Robots and Systems, Pittsburgh, pp. 303-307.

Erzin, R., Bajd, T., Kralj, A., and Benko, H. (1993) Influence of Sensory Biofeedback on FES assisted Walking, Proc. of the Ljubljana FES conference, pp. 89-92, Ljubljana.

Karcnik, T., Kralj, A., and Bajd, T. (1995) Stability and energy critera in healthy and paraplegic subjects gait, Proc. of the 5th Int. Vienna Workshop on Functional Electrostimulation, pp. 87-90, Vienna.

Kralj, A. and Bajd, T. (1989) Functional Electrical Stimulation: Standing and Walking after Spinal Cord Injury, CRC Press, Inc. Boca Raton, Florida.

Kralj, A., Bajd, T., Karcnik, T., and Munih, M. (1994) Robotic Aspects of Four-Point FES Gait Synthesis, Workshop of RAFT: Control of Ambulation using FES, Entschede, pp. 15-18.

Lin, B. S. and Song, S. M. (1993) Dynamic Modeling, Stability and Energy Efficiency of a Quadrupedal Walking Machine, Proc. IEEE Conf. on Robotics and Automation, Atlanta, pp. 367-373.

McGhee, R. B.and Frank, A. A. (1968) On the Stability Properties of Quadruped Creeping Gaits, Math. Biosci., Vol. 3, pp. 331-351.

Sensor Staircase for the Measurement of Ground Reaction Loads: Preliminary Results

R. Riener[1], J. Quintern[2], H. Boedrich[1], T. Barner[1], F. Freyberger[1], G. Schmidt[1]
[1]Department of Automatic Control Eng., Technical University Munich, Germany
[2]Neurological Clinic, University of Munich, Germany

Abstract - A multi-sensor staircase was developed to measure ground reaction forces and moments during stair climbing. A new approach to sensor arrangement permits accurate recording, especially of ankle joint moments and the center of pressure. In this paper the design of the staircase and preliminary measurements with a single step are presented.

1 Introduction

Stairs appear to be unsurmountable obstacles for paraplegic patients. Functional Electrical Stimulation (FES) has the potential of enabling the patients to ascend and descend stairs, thus enhancing the quality of their life. However, ascending and descending stairs has not yet been solved satisfactorily with conventional FES approaches. One reason for this is that going up and especially down stairs requires highly coordinative efforts of the artificial control system.

The recording and analysis of gait patterns such as ground reaction loads of normal and FES-induced motions can support the development of neural prostheses. On the one hand measured load signals can serve as additional sensor input to the feedback control-loop during stair climbing. On the other hand the recorded signal can be used together with kinematic data of the motion to assess the gait of a healthy subject or artificially stimulated patient.

2 Design

The whole system consists of a staircase with four sensor steps, one platform at the upper end of the staircase, and banisters on both sides (Fig.1). All components are characterized by a robust design which minimizes vibrations. The steepness of the staircase can be readily adjusted (20.0°-42.0°). During adjustment, the weight of the staircase is supported by two gas springs. Since the staircase is employed together with kinematic motion analysis, it has been designed so that no part hides the foot.

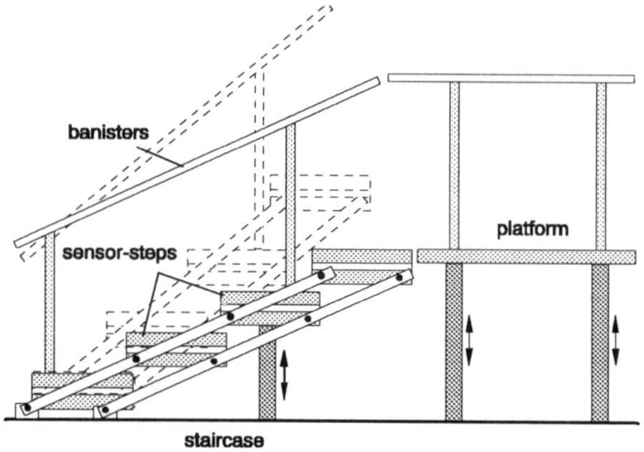

Fig. 1. Schematic drawing of staircase, platform, and banisters. Height of staircase and platform can be readily adjusted.

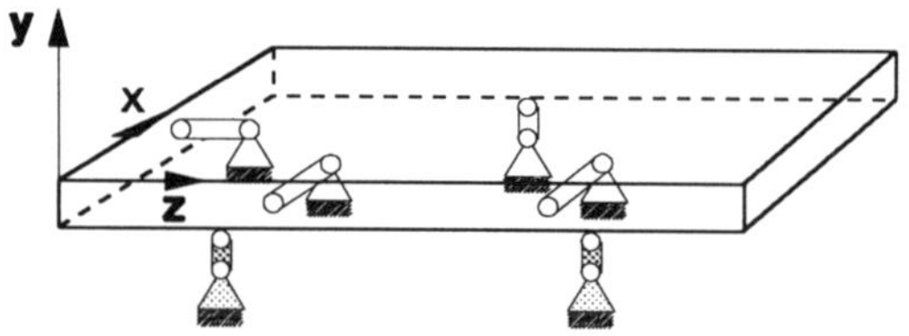

Fig. 2. Drawing of a single stair with the positions of the bearings. Three vertical and three horizontal one-component force transducers record the load acting between foot and ground.

There are six components that act between foot and ground at each step. They are measured by six strain-gauge-based force transducers (AST, Dresden GmbH, Germany) included in the bearings. Unlike most existing forceplates (Bobbert and Schamhardt, 1990; Sanchez-Lacuesta *et al.*, 1992), the upper part of the step is connected with the lower part by a statically determined arrangement of bearings (Fig. 2). The measured signals are amplified directly at the transducers to minimize noise and are sampled by a 12-bit A/D card.

3 Results and Conclusion

One single sensor step has been built and evaluated. We made measurements of level walking and stair climbing (Figs. 3 and 4). Forces and moments can be computed for the ankle joint, providing that its position has been obtained by kinematic measurements. An off-line program was written which computes x, y, z forces and x, y, z moments (e.g., at the ankle joint), the center of pressure COP (Fig. 4), the vector diagram of ground reaction force, and the torsional moment at the COP.

The small error occurring during static measurements was reproducible. This suggests that a static error correction function could be applied, for example, a polynomial interpolation algorithm, which would compensate for the occurring error (Press *et al.*, 1994). Note that the error is a function of the estimated COP location and the vertical force.

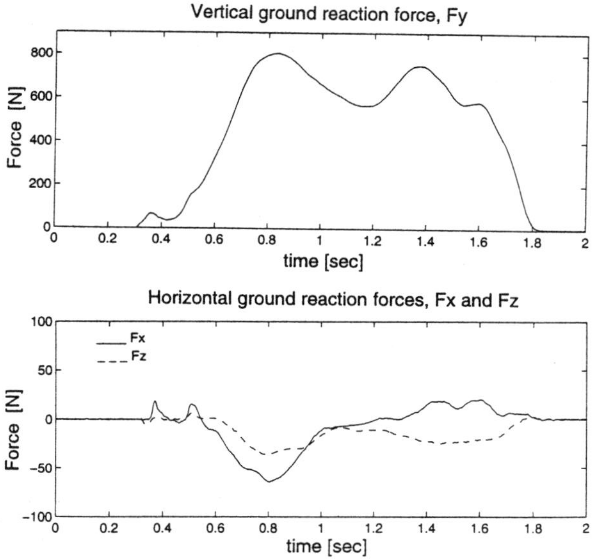

Fig. 3. Data recorded during ascent of stairs. Upper diagram: vertical ground reaction force F_y supported by the right leg. Below: horizontal forces F_x and F_z. The subject walked in positive x-direction.

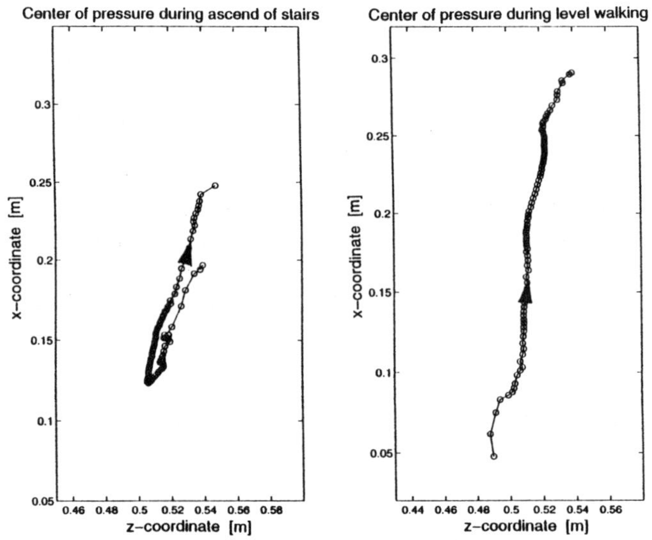

Fig. 4. Center of pressure trajectories during ascent of stairs (left graph) and level walking (right graph). Note that during ascent of stairs the trajectory changes its direction, because the subject's toes touch the ground before the heel does.

During dynamic measurements small hysteresis effects due to friction and slight vibrations due to free play in the bearings have been observed. To avoid these effects we suggest preloading the upper part of the step with very stiff elastic springs.

Advantages of the sensor step over other sensor platforms are that moments and COP are measured with high accuracy due to the statically determined bearing-concept (compare Collins and DeLuca, 1993; McCaw and DeVita, 1995), there is no drift during long-term measurements, and the geometry of a single step is adapted for a staircase which is adjustable in step height and depth. In addition, the presented device is less expensive than platforms available commercially.

Technical data of a single step:		
Size:	l_x, l_y, l_z	0.34 x 0.19 x 0.8 m
Range:	F_x, F_z	-1500 ... +1500 N
	F_y	0 ... +3000 N
Calibrated partial range:	F_x, F_z	-1000 ... +1000 N
	F_y	0 ... +2000 N
Overload:	F_x, F_z	-3000 / +3000 N
	F_y	6000 N
Resolution:	F_x, F_z	0.5 N
	F_y	1 N
Linearity:		< 0.1 %
Accuracy:		< 0.5 % (without error correction)
Cross talk:	$F_y \Rightarrow F_x, F_z$	< 1.5 % of F_y (without error correction)
Natural frequency:		> 40 Hz (without improvement of bearings)
Error center of pressure (COP):		< 2 mm (without error correction)

References

Bobbert, M. F. and Schamhardt H. C. (1990) Accuracy of determining the point of force application with piezoelectric force plates, *J. Biomechanics*, **23**, 705-710.

Collins, J. J. and DeLuca, C. J. (1993) Open-loop and closed-loop control of posture: a random-walk analysis of center-of-pressure trajectories, *Exp. Brain Res.*, **95**, 308-318.

McCaw, S.T. and DeVita P. (1995) Errors in alignment of Center of Pressure and foot coordinates affect predicted lower extremity torques. *J. Biomechanics*, **8**, 985-988.

Press, W., Teukolsky, S. A., Vetterling, W. T., and Flannery, B. P. (1992) Numerical Recipes, The Art of Scientific Computing, 2nd Ed., Cambridge University Press.

Sanchez-Lacuesta, J., et al. (1992) New forceplate design for the analysis of musculo-skeletal and neurological diseases. Preliminary experience. In: Europäisches Symposium über klinische Ganganalyse, ETH Zürich, April 1992, Schlieren Verlag.

Modeling of Joint-Rotations during Line Tracking Arm Movements

J. Laczko[1], J. Quintern[2], S. Krafczyk[2]
[1]Research Inst. for Measurement and Computing Technics, Budapest, Hungary
[2]Neurological Clinic, Klinikum Grosshadern, University of Munich, Germany

Abstract - For human limb-movements, a required displacement of the endpoint of the limb may be the result of different combinations of rotations of individual joints and different combinations of activities of muscles. The Cartesian coordinates of an intended displacement of the endpoint can be transformed into joint-rotations in infinite different ways. We study such transformations experimentally and theoretically. We recorded target tracking human arm movements using the ELITE movement analyzing system and studied the change of the angles in the joints of normal subjects during the movements. On the other hand we developed a mathematical model and computer program to give a prediction for a possible time course of the angular changes in the joints of the multi-segmental system of the trunk and arm. The input of the model was the initial position of the joints and the trajectory of a moving target. First we assumed a certain direction of the angular velocity vector (rotational axis) in each joint. These directions were changing during the movement depending on the configuration of the arm. In the next step the error between the actual finger and target position was transformed into rotations around these axes. Considering three rotating joints (shoulder, elbow, wrist) and the fact that in each joint the axis of rotation can be choosen at many different ways, there are many possibilities for selecting a set of rotational angles. We considered the minimization of the weighted sum of the squares of the rotational angles. The weights were related to joint-stiffnesses. Comparing the measured and predicted movement patterns we investigated how the choice of the angular velocity effect movement execution and which choice provides a better alignment with expected movement patterns.

1 Introduction

In order to control movements of musculoskeletal structures, the central nervous system (CNS) solves the computational problem of coordinating a redundant set of joints and muscles. Our task in the RAFT project is to study such coordination and develope and test models of control strategies for human upper limb movements. These models must deal with rotational kinematic properties of the controlled structure In principle the angular position of the arm or the direction of the instantaneous rotational axis in each joint can be choosen at many different ways. For pointing and for throwing movements it was shown that the angular postions of the arm were confined to a 2-dimensional surface. (Hore et al., 1992, 1994). It is still unknown whether during natural movements the direction of the instantaneous rotational axis in a rotating joint is also choosen from a special subset of the 3-dimensional (3-D) space. In this paper we study whether the angular velocity vectors of each arm segment during pursuit movements are chosen from a 2-D plane or surface. The angular velocity is a vector which has a direction and a magnitude. Its direction alignes with the instantaneous axis of rotation and its magnitude is the time derivative of the rotational angle. The sensory information of joint angles and rotational axes of all of the rotating joints must be combined by the CNS to have proper intrinsic representation of the spatial orientation and configuration of a limb. Using this information a particular set of rotations and translations in the joints are generated to produce a planned arm movement. Point to point movements of the human arm are executed in a straight line fashion (Flash and Hogan 1985). This observation led to a number of hypotheses about how the CNS plans arm movements. Several models are known that provide a trajectory of the end effector (hand) between two points. For instance the minimum torque change model and the minimum jerk model. They propose a trajectory which minimizes the integral of the sum of the squares of the joint torques (Uno et al., 1989) or the square of the jerk of the end effector (Flash, 1985). The equlibrium point hypothesis minimizes the change of potential energy (Mussa-Ivaldi, 1988). In the case of these pointing movements the CNS plans the trajectory of the finger. When target tracking arm movements are considered then the trajectory is given by the moving target that has to be followed by the finger. The given trajectory has to be reconstructed by angular changes in the joints. Our model transforms intended finger trajectories into angular changes of the joints. We study how an instantaneous direction of the finger's movement can be reconstructed in joint-space and how might the angular velocity vectors in the joints be chosen to generate a displacement of the finger into the intended direction. We suppose that the instantaneous angular velocity vectors depend on the configuration of the multi-joint system and the direction of the mevement of the finger. Choosing appropriate angular velocities and rotating the neighbouring segments around appropriate axes, the movement will be executed more efficiently.

2 Methods

2.1 Experiments

Normal subject's arm movements were measured experimentally at the department of Neurology at Klinikum Grosshadern in Munich. The subject sat in front of a transparent window onto which a laser beam was projected. We changed the position of the laserpoint along a straight line with a sinusoidal velocity profile (40cm amplitude and 0.2 Hz.). The subject was asked to track the laserpoint with the finger keeping the trunk fixed. Reflecting markers were placed at anatomical landmarks of the sternum (manubrium sterni), the shoulder (processus coracoideus), the elbow (olecranon), the wrist (processus styloideus radii), and the finger. Each movement was recorded and analyzed off-line using a motion analysis system (ELITE, BTS). The sampling rate was 100 Hz. The data of two cameras were used to calculate the trajectories of the marker positions in a 3-dimensional Cartesian coordinate system. A stickfigure representation was generated and the spatial angles between the segments of the stickfigure were computed and the time course of these angles was graphically represented.

2.2 Theoretical methods: Definition of rotational axes and natural coordinate systems

We studied the geometric properties of line tracking human arm movements. The following ill-posed computational problem arose: the coordinates of the trajectory of a target (that has to be followed by the finger) must be transformed

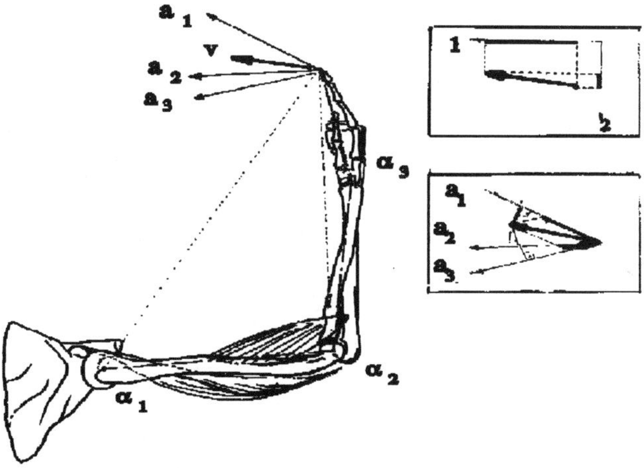

Fig. 1. The human arm and a natural joint-coordinate-system defined by the joints of the human arm. Each joint defines a coordinate axis that is orthogonal to the line that connects the joint and the finger and also orthogonal to the axis of rotation. (in the case of planar movements the axis of rotation is orthogonal to the plane of the page). Small rotations in the shoulder (α_1), elbow (α_2) or wrist (α_3) moves the finger along the corresponding axis (a_1,a_2,a_3). On the right side an external 2-dimensional orthogonal corrdinatesystem and a natural 3-dimensional joint coordinatesystem is shown.

from external "world coordinates" into intrinsic "body-coordinates". The time dependent 3-D vector that connects the actual finger and target position must be expressed by rotations in the joints. There are an infinity of different ways of representing this 3-D displacement vector by ordered sets of angular changes in the joints. We assume that the instantaneous rotational axis (direction of the angular velocity vector) in each joint is chosen at a special way and this choice helps to define natural joint-coordinate systems. If all of the joints remain in the same plane during the movement and the trajectory that has to be traced lies also in this plane then the axis of rotation in each joint is orthogonal to this plane. The axes of rotations are fixed and the values of the rotational angles determines the displacement of the finger (Fig 1.).

Thus in the 2-D case, the size of the rotational angles in the joints determines the displacement of the finger. The 3-D case is more complicated. In 3-D cases we have many choices for the rotational axes in each joint. The size of the rotational angles do not specify a unique displacement of the finger. To compute the change of the finger position, the direction of the rotational axes also have to be specified in each joint. The rotational axes are different in different joints and changing in time so both the rotational axis and the rotational angle must be given in each joint to determine the change of the hand position. From a mathematical point of view this means that not only the magnitude but also the direction of the angular velocities in the joints are changing. The question is how to choose one particular set of angular velocity vectors to move the hand in a given direction: how to define the direction of the angular velocity vector (rotational axes) in each joint and how to decompose a small intended displacement of the finger into joint-rotations around these axes. In robotics, fixed and moving coordinate-systems are used to describe the kinematics of the parts of a robot arm. This approach is also widely used in describing the movements of the human arm. Body fixed and bone fixed coordinate systems are used and the relation between the different bone fixed coordinate sytems is given by transformation matrices (Karlsson, 1992). The coordinate axes are usually perpendicular to each other and a desired rotation is given by consecutive rotations around these orthogonal axes. This is a numerical method for computing the change of the coordinates of the end effector (hand) but tell us nothing about the direction of the angular velocity vectors (instantaneous rotational axis) that are applied by the CNS during human movements.

Let us consider the next geometric task: move the hand from one position to another by a rotation in the shoulder. (The hand will move on a ball whose center is the shoulder and radius is the distance between the sholuder and the hand). The same displacement of the hand on this ball can be implemented by different rotations. The rotational axis must always be in the plane that is orthogonal to the line connecting the initial and final handposition. Any of the lines of this plane can be used as the rotational axis. The size of the rotational angle depends on the chosen line. This made us thinking about a rotational axis which might be preferably used during arm movements.

We developed a mathematical model and computer simulation to predict the change of the angles in the joints of multijoint systems during line tracking movements. Using the simulation we study how the movement would be executed by applying a certain set of the instantaneous rotational axes. The output of the computer simulation is the time course of the external 3-D coordinates of the joints. From this output the time course of the spatial angles between neighbouring segments can also be computed.

The joints have many degrees of freedom e.g. the shoulder joint is supposed to be a ball joint, thus, in principle the arm can be rotated around any axes in the shoulder. The question arises whether there exist a special subset of the set of the 3-D vectors, e.g. a 2-D plane, to which any natural rotational axis must belong.

2.3 Computer simulation

Our simulation is a further development of a former computer modeling technique (Laczko et al., 1987, 1988, 1994). Our present simulation computes movement parameters of planned 3-dimensional movements of multi-joint sytems. This type of computer simulation is used mostly for testing control strategies in human movement control. The advantage of the mathematical and computer simulation is that not only the resulting output of the sytem but also the internal processes and internal parameters can be tested (Quintern, 1989). We developed the simulation on a Macintosh computer using the "Mathematica " computer language. The input was the initial configuration of the arm and the trajectory of a moving target. The configuration of the arm was given by the 3-D world-coordinates of the markers at the sternum, shoulder, elbow, wrist and the finger as they were recorded by the ELITE system at the start of the movement. The path of a target was generated, like the path of the laserpoint in our experiments. We devided the whole movement for small steps and we redefined the joint angular velocity vectors (and the corresponding joint-coordinatesystems) in each step along the path. In each step the error between the actual finger and target position was decomposed into rotations around the instantaneous rotational axes. Then the rotations were generated and the new configuration of the arm was computed. In the next step the rotational axes were redefined according to the new configuration and further rotations were calculated towards the new target position. Figure 2. shows the block diagram of the algorithm. This algorithm can be applied for a multijoint system of n joints (n is an arbitrary positive integer variable). The function f that we minimized in the simulation, was the sum of the squares of the weighted rotational angles in each cycle of the algorithm.

$$f=\Sigma (s_i*\alpha_i*r_i)^2 \qquad (1)$$

s_i is the stiffness of the ith joint, r_i is the distance of the ith joint from the end effector. We assumed a high stiffness of the trunk and thus the trunk rotation was not significant. The stiffness is the force F which is required for unit angular change,

$$s_i = F_i/\alpha_i \qquad (2)$$

thus from (1) and (2) follows

$$f=\Sigma\,(F_i * r_i)^2 \qquad (3)$$

so that our optimization criteria is compatible to the minimum torque change model

In our closed-loop control algorithm, where the feedback parameters are the position and orientation of the body segments. It is known that joint receptors detect changes of limb position and signal the position of the joint and the movement's direction (Brandt, 1977). These parameters are used as feedback parameters in our model. We compute these parameters during the simulation and determine how to continue the movement's execution.

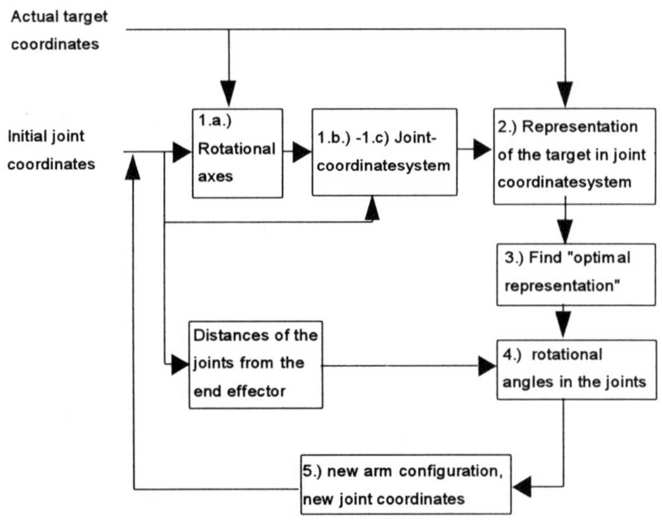

Fig. 2. The block diagram of the computer simulation. The subroutines which implement step 1 and step 3 can be replaced by other routines. Thus it is possible to define the joint coordinate systems in different ways or to use different optimization criteria. The computer simulation provides a frame to test the effect of the change of rotational axes, intrinsic coordinate systems, and optimization criteria.

4 Results: Comparison of Measured and Predicted Data

We compared the measured and the predicted (simulated) movement patterns. On the basis of the above experiments and simulation we found that the predicted and measured relative size of the changes of the joint angles were the same. We found the largest angular change to be in the shoulder, and the smallest in the wrist. This was true for both the measured and simulated movement patterns.

Studying experimentally measured angular changes, in the elbow we found a double period: one large and a smaller maximum in each cycle. (Fig 3.) The mean values of the joint angles were the same in the predicted and in the measured case. For the shoulder the difference between the minimum and maximum angle was larger in the predicted case than in the measurements. The difference between the smallest and largest shoulder angle was about 20° in the measurements and 30° in the prediction.

In the predictive mathematical model (Laczko, 1995) we defined one rotational axis in each joint and generated movement patterns supposing that:

a) the rotational axis in any joint was orthogonal to the plane spanned by the joint, the finger, and the target (Fig 4.a).

b) the rotational axis in the shoulder and the wrist was defined as above in a), and in the elbow the rotational axis was orthogonal to the plane spanned by the shoulder, elbow and wrist joint (Fig 4.b).

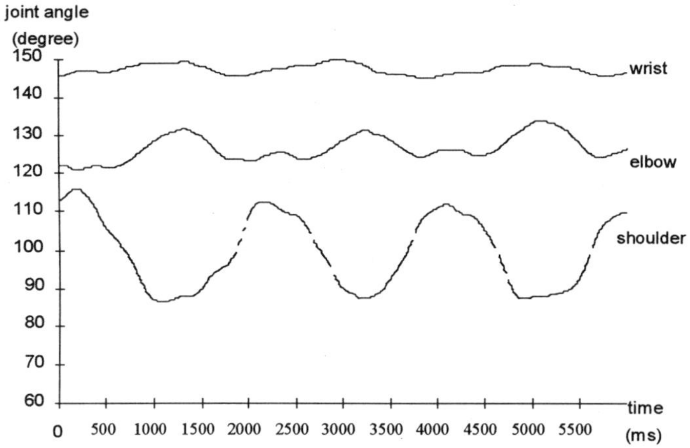

Fig. 3. Experimentally measured change of joint angles during 6 second while the finger followed a target that moved on a straight horizontal line with sinusoidal velocity profile

We gained the best match between measured and predicted patterns in case b. This suggests that the rotation in the shoulder has no torsional component around the line that connects the shoulder and the finger and similarily there is no torsion around the line that connects the wrist and the finger. In the elbow joint there is no torsion around the line that connects the elbow and the wrist.

We expect better alignment by changing the stiffness of the joints in the simulation. In our optimization criteria we have considered that the stiffnesses of the joints were different and the stiffness was the largest in the trunk. This implies that the simulated trunk rotation was very small.

The difference between the measured and predicted data may depend on the stiffness of the joints. The alignment could also be improved by applying another definition for the rotational axes. However we found the best alignment by applying the above defined rotational axes.

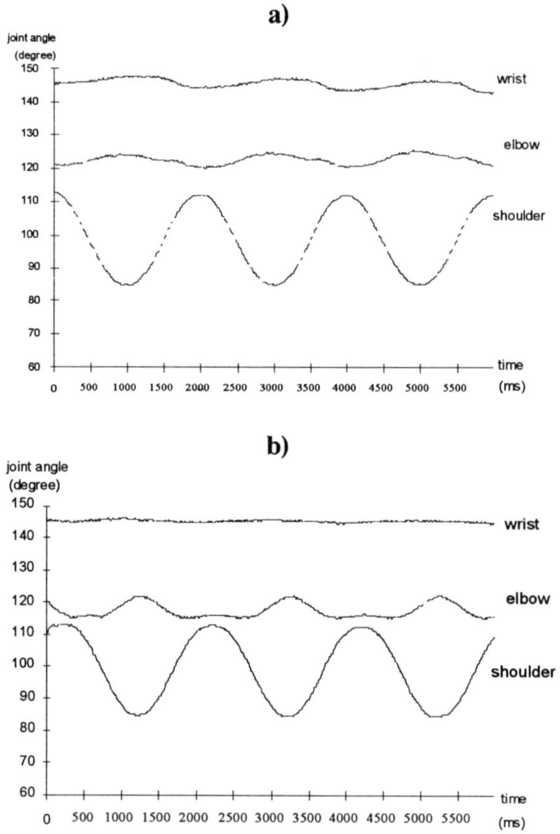

Fig. 4. Theoretically predicted angular changes assuming that a) the rotational axis in any joint is orthogonal to the plane of the joint, the finger and the target. b) the rotational axis in the shoulder and wrist is the sane as in a.) but the elbow's axis is orthogonal to the plane of the shoulder, elbow and wrist.

Conclusion

Our computer simulation shows that movement execution depends on the choice of the rotational axes in the joints. In our model of smooth pursuit arm movements we applied one rotational axis for each joint. We used this approach because we suppose that the CNS does not use consecutive rotations around orthogonal axes in the joints when executing a desired movement of the arm. It rotates arm segments simultaneously around the direction of the instantaneous angular velocity vector in each joint. It is still an open question how the angular velocity vector in a joint is generated by the CNS. Comparing the result of our simulation with experiments we found that the angular velocity in the shoulder and the wrist may depend on the shoulder, wrist and target position but in the elbow it depends on the configuration of the shoulder-elbow-wrist system and there is a tendency to minimize the torsional component around certain axes and choose the angular velocity vector from a certain plane. Thus the number of degrees of freedom can be decreased. Predicted movement pattern was most similar to the natural one when the rotational axes in these joints were chosen on that way that the rotation moved the endpoint of the limb into the direction of the target using the smallest possible rotational angle. This means a tendency to minimize the net joint torque.

Ultimately, the movement of the endpoint of a limb has to be transformed into rotations around rotational axes defined by the muscles contribute to the movement. Each muscle that articulates a joint may rotate that joint around a different axis and this axis can be computed using the data available about muscle attachments. We studied how a planned movement will be executed if the arm's segments are rotated around a certain set of rotational axes. Since each muscle rotates the segments around a certain time dependent axis, it is important to study that around which axes the joints has to be rotated and by which muscle's activation a natural movement pattern can be reached. The simulation is being extended to study which rotations and, consequently, which muscles yield the most natural movement patterns during functional electrical stimulation.

References

Brandt, T., Buechele, W., and Arnold F. (1977) Arthrokinetic nystagmus and ego motion sensation. *Exp. Brain Research*, 30: 331-338.

Flash, T. and Hogan, N. (1985) The coordination of arm movements: An experimentally confirmed mathematical model. *The Journal of Neuroscie.* 5: 1688-1703.

Hore, J., Watts, S., and Tweed, D. (1994) Arm position constraints when throwing in three dimensions. *J. Neurophysiol.* 72: 1171-1180.

Hore, J., Watts, S., and Vilis, T. (1992) Constraints on arm position when pointing in three dimensions: Donders' law and the Fick gimbal strategy. *J. Neurophys.* 68: 374-382.

Karlsson, D. and Peterson, B. (1992) Towards a model for force predictions in the human shoulder. *J. Biomech.* 25.

Laczko, J. (1995) Implications of rotational kinematics on patterns of line tracking arm movements. In: Control of Ambulation using Functional Electrical Stimulation. Ed. PH Veltnik, ,B. Boom, 65-70.

Laczko, J., Quintern, J., Glasauer, S. (1994) Implications of rotational axes for patterns of pursuit arm movements using a predictive geometric model. *Soc. Neurosci.* Abstr 20: 853

Laczko, J., Pellionisz, A., Jongen, H., and Gielen, C. (1988) Computer modeling of human forelimb muscle activation in multidimensional intrinsic coordinate frames. *Soc. Neurosci.* Absts. 14: 955

Laczko, J., Pellionisz, A., Peterson, B. W., and Buchmann, T. S. (1987): Multidimensional sensorimotor patterns arising from a graphics-based tensorial model of the neck-motor *Soc. for Neoroscience, Absts.* 13: 372.

Mussa-Ivaldi, F., Morasso, P., and Zaccaria, R. (1988) Kinematic Networks: A Distributed model for representing and regularizing motor redundancy. *Biol. Cyb.* 60: 1-16.

Pellionisz, A. (1984) Coordination: A Vector-Matrix Description of Transformations of Overcomplete CNS Coordinates and a Tensorial Solution Using the Moore-Penrose Inverse. *J. Theor Biol.* 110: 353-375

Quintern, J., Minwegen, P., and Mauritz, K.-H. (1989) control mechanisms for restoring posture and movements in paraplegics. *Progress in Brain Res.* 80: 489-502.

Uno, Y., Kawato, M., and Suzuki, R. (1989) Formation and control of optimal trajectory in human arm movement -minmum torque- change model. *Biol. Cyb.* 61: 89-101.

Chapter 5

Artificial and Natural Sensors

3D Movement Analysis Using Accelerometry - Theoretical Concepts

P. H. Veltink, H. B. K. Boom
Institute for Biomedical Technology, Faculty of Electrical Engineering, University of Twente, Enschede, The Netherlands

Abstract - Accelerometers have a high potential for use in ambulatory 3D movement analysis systems: they are small, do not need an attachment to a reference and provide a "rich" signal, incorporating acceleration and inclination information. However, the analysis of movements from accelerometer data is not straightforward in general, because the information components of the signal can not be distinguished. In this paper the methods for analysing movements using accelerometers are reviewed.

1 Introduction

In many clinical and biomechanical applications the analysis of unconstrained movements in a natural environment for relatively long observations times (several hours) may open new perspectives: e.g. a rehabilitation treatment can be assessed by evaluating the activities of daily living (ADL) before and after a rehabilitation treatment (Bussmann et al., 1994). These activities may be monitored by an ambulatory movement analysis system (Veltink et al., 1994). Also, when assessing the severity of heart disorders it is clinically relevant to measure blood pressure and ECG simultaneously with movement activities in a 24 hour period under ADL circumstances (Tulen et al., 1994). Some other clinical applications requiring kinematic measurements of unconstrained movements include spasticity assessment by combining long-term ambulatory EMG measurement (Kleissen et al., 1991) with mobility activity monitoring (Bussmann et al., 1994) during daily living, real time control of Functional Electrical Stimulation of paralyzed muscles for restoration of motor functions (Franken et al, 1994), ergonomic analysis of the work place (Leskinen et al, 1983; Dolan and Adams, 1993), and instability and fall detection in elderly. In biomechanics, an inverse dynamic analysis, yielding joint torques and contact forces, requires a full 3D analysis of human movements, currently only possible with expensive laboratory bound optokinetic systems.

Prerequisites for the development of ambulatory 3D movement analysis systems is the availability of powerful ambulatory recorder systems, adequate sensors and adequate movement analysis methods and algorithms. Recent developments of powerful ambulatory recorder systems based on low power and high performance microprocessor technology fulfills the first prerequisite. Several types of small, leight-weight, low power kinematic sensors, which can be mounted on the body with low interference with body activities are also available. Accelerometers preferably satisfy these requirements: they are small, do not need an attachment to a reference and provide a "rich" signal, incorporating acceleration and inclination information (Willemsen, 1990, 1991). Other alternatives include inclinometers and gyroscopes. Inclinometers provide body segment inclinations for slow movements, equivalent to low-pass filtered accelerometer signals. Vibrating gyroscopes sense angular velocity through the Coriolis effect (Söderkvist, 1994), but do not directly provide acceleration and inclination information. The third requirement for ambulatory 3D-movement analysis systems, adequate movement analysis methods and algorithms, have not been investigated sufficiently. The feasibility of developing such methods and algorithms depend on the type of kinematic sensors to be used.

We are currently investigating whether a full 3D ambulatory analysis of human movements can be obtained using body mounted kinematic sensors linked to an ambulatory recorder system. Especially, we investigate the potential of accelerometers, which provide a "rich" kinematic signal, incorporating acceleration as well as inclination information.

The three-dimensional kinematic and dynamic analysis methods based on accelerometer signals reported sofar only considered the movement of one single rigid segment. No analysis has yet been described of the full 3D kinematic and dynamic analysis of multi-segment systems on the basis of accelerometry. Morris (1973) and Padgaonkar et al. (1995) proposed a three-dimensional analysis of kinematics of a single rigid body using a minimum of three three-axial accelerometers per segment. Van den Bogert and Read (1994) showed the possibility of 3D dynamic analysis using four sets of three-axial accelerometers on the trunk to estimate torque at the hip joint of the weight bearing leg during alpine skiing. They assumed torques and forces only to exist at one joint. Methods for 2D kinematic analysis of human leg movements have been described by Willemsen et al. (1990), requiring two two-axial accelerometers per leg segment. This method enables the online calculation of joint angles without integration by expressing the extrapolated accelerometer signal at the joint in the body-fixed coordinate systems of both segments connected by the joint. This method can however only calculate joint angles. Absolute segment angles can only be determined if a reference body with known orientation is present

It is the objective of this paper to describe a theoretical phramework for 3D movement analysis of multi-segment bodies using accelerometry. This may lead to the development of ambulatory 3D movement analysis systems to be used outside of the laboratory.

2 Theoretical Concepts

The accelerometer signal is a "rich" signal, providing acceleration as well as inclination information. It has several *properties*, which can be used in 3D movement analysis. On the basis of these properties, several *movement analysis methods* follow that can be used in the analysis of the 3D kinematics of the human body, consisting of many segments.

2.1 Properties of the accelerometer signals

Property 1:

A triaxial accelerometer signal consists of an actual acceleration component and a gravitational acceleration component, which can be distinguished in special cases (e.g. static situations), but in general, are provided indistinguishably together in one signal:

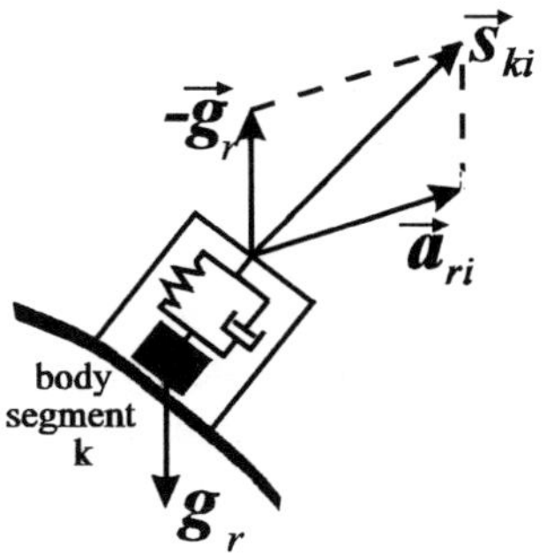

Fig. 1. The accelerometer signal s_{ki} measured on position i of a rigid body segment k is the summation of the acceleration a_{ri} and the gravitational acceleration $-g_r$, expressed in the body fixed coordinate system of rigid body segment k.

A triaxial accelerometer (figure 1) attached on a position i on a rigid body k measures a 3D signal s_{ki} in the coordinate system of body k, being the summation of the acceleration a_{ri} of the accelerometer and the gravitational field g_r in vertical direction, both expressed in inertial reference coordinates (index r):

$$s_{ki} = T_k^{-1}(a_{ri} - g_r) \tag{1}$$

With T_k being the transformation matrix from body fixed to reference coordinates.

<u>Property 2:</u>

The angular acceleration vector and the square of the angular velocity vector can be determined from the measurement of minimally three triaxial accelerometer signals per rigid segment (Morris, 1973; Padgaonkar et al., 1975):

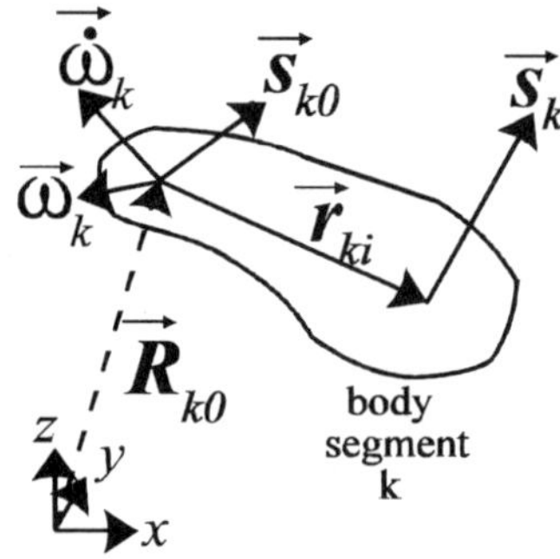

Fig. 2: The accelerometer signal s_{ki} at position i is related to the accelerometer signal on a reference position 0 via equation (2), taking into account the angular velocity vector ω_k and the angular acceleration vector $\dot{\omega}_k$ of segment k.

If several triaxial accelerometers (index i) are mounted on the rigid body k on distance r_{ki} from a reference point, indicated with index $i=0$ the signal s_{ki} can be expressed in the body fixed coordinate system of body k (Morris, 1973; Padgaonkar, 1975; Willemsen, 1990; van den Bogert and Read, 1994):

$$\mathbf{s}_{ki} = \mathbf{s}_{k0} + \dot{\omega}_k \times \mathbf{r}_{ki} + \omega_k \times (\omega_k \times \mathbf{r}_{ki}) \tag{2}$$

ω_k being the angular velocity vector of body k (figure 2). The vectors ω_k, $\dot{\omega}_k$ and s_{k0} can in principle be solved from the nonlinear equations (2) for this rigid body k when using three triaxial accelerometers (Padgaonkar et al., 1975). Van den Bogert and Read (1994) used four triaxial accelerometers in order to avoid singularities. If equation (2) is treated as a differential equation, only two triaxial accelerometers are required, and ω_k is solved by integration (Morris, 1973).

<u>Property 3:</u>

The 3D accelerometer signal vector in any position on a rigid segment can be calculated by a linear combination of the 3D accelerometer signal vectors measured at three positions on the segment:

This follows from solving ω_k, $\dot{\omega}_k$ and s_{k0} from the nonlinear equations (2) for three triaxial accelerometers, as was pointed out above. It also follows directly from the geometric relations between points on the same rigid body: The position vector $\boldsymbol{r}_{ki}$ of any point in a rigid body, expressed in an orthonormal body fixed coordinate system, can alternatively be expressed as a vector $(x_1, x_2, x_3)^T$ on a base of three independent position vectors $\boldsymbol{r}_{k1}$, $\boldsymbol{r}_{k2}$ and $\boldsymbol{r}_{k3}$:

$$\boldsymbol{r}_{ki} = \sum_{j=1}^{3} x_j \boldsymbol{r}_{kj} \tag{3}$$

The coordinates of the vector $(x_1, x_2, x_3)^T$ can be found by application of Cramer's rule:

$$x_1 = \frac{|\boldsymbol{r}_{ki}\boldsymbol{r}_{k2}\boldsymbol{r}_{k3}|}{|\boldsymbol{r}_{k1}\boldsymbol{r}_{k2}\boldsymbol{r}_{k3}|};\, x_2 = \frac{|\boldsymbol{r}_{k1}\boldsymbol{r}_{ki}\boldsymbol{r}_{k3}|}{|\boldsymbol{r}_{k1}\boldsymbol{r}_{k2}\boldsymbol{r}_{k3}|};\, x_1 = \frac{|\boldsymbol{r}_{k1}\boldsymbol{r}_{k2}\boldsymbol{r}_{ki}|}{|\boldsymbol{r}_{k1}\boldsymbol{r}_{k2}\boldsymbol{r}_{k3}|} \tag{4}$$

Since the acceleration vector $\boldsymbol{a}_{ki}$, expressed in the orthonormal body fixed coordinate system of body k, is the second derivative of the position vector $\boldsymbol{r}_{ki}$ of the same point, this acceleration vector can be expressed in the same coordinates with respect to the acceleration vectors $\boldsymbol{a}_{k1}$, $\boldsymbol{a}_{k2}$ and $\boldsymbol{a}_{k3}$ at the positions $\boldsymbol{r}_{k1}$, $\boldsymbol{r}_{k2}$ and $\boldsymbol{r}_{k3}$:

$$\boldsymbol{a}_{ki} = \sum_{j=1}^{3} x_j \boldsymbol{a}_{kj} \tag{5}$$

A prerequisite is that the acceleration vectors $\boldsymbol{a}_{k1}$, $\boldsymbol{a}_{k2}$ and $\boldsymbol{a}_{k3}$ are also independent, so they can form a base. Since the gravity acceleration $\boldsymbol{g}_r$, expressed in the orthonormal body fixed coordinate system of body k, is independent of position, the accelerometer signals $\boldsymbol{s}_{ki}$ can also be expressed with the same coordinates as the position vector $\boldsymbol{r}_{ki}$ and the acceleration vector $\boldsymbol{a}_{ki}$ with respect to the accelerometer signal vectors $\boldsymbol{s}_{k1}$, $\boldsymbol{s}_{k2}$ and $\boldsymbol{s}_{k3}$ at the positions $\boldsymbol{r}_{k1}$, $\boldsymbol{r}_{k2}$ and $\boldsymbol{r}_{k3}$:

$$\boldsymbol{s}_{ki} = \sum_{j=1}^{3} x_j \boldsymbol{s}_{kj} \tag{6}$$

Again, a prerequisite is that the accelerometer signal vectors $\boldsymbol{s}_{k1}$, $\boldsymbol{s}_{k2}$ and $\boldsymbol{s}_{k3}$ are independent, so they can form a base. In order to avoid situations (singular point) in which this prerequisite is not fulfilled it can be necessary to measure accelerometer signal vectors at 4 positions, so there will always be three independent accelerometer signal vectors. Also, using more than 3 measurement points may improve the accuracy with which the accelerometer signals in other points can be estimated by using least squares methods.

2.2 Methods for 3D movement analysis of multi-body systems

On the basis of the described properties of accelerometer signals several movement analysis methods follow that can be used in the analysis of the 3D kinematics of the human body, consisting of several segments.

Method 1:

In static situations the triaxial accelerometer gives the direction of the gravitation relative to the segment on which it is mounted (property 1):

In static situations the acceleration vector **a** is zero. In such a case equation (1) yields:

$$\boldsymbol{s}_{ki} = \boldsymbol{T}_k^{-1}(-\boldsymbol{g}_r) \qquad (7)$$

Since the direction and modulus of the gravity acceleration vector in reference coordinates is known, the orientation of the body (described by the transformation matrix $\boldsymbol{T}_k$) directly follows from the signal vector $\boldsymbol{s}_{ki}$, which is measured.

Method 2:

In dynamic situations, the orientation of body segments can be calculated in inertial reference coordinates from the accelerometer signals measured on three positions on the rigid segment if the acceleration of a reference point of the segment is known in the reference coordinate system.

The accelerometer signal $\boldsymbol{s}_{k0}$ in the reference point can be calculated in body-fixed coordinates using property 3 (equation (6)). If the acceleration vector at this reference point $\boldsymbol{a}_{r0}$ is known in coordinates of the reference coordinate system, the transformation matrix $\boldsymbol{T}_k$ can be determined using formula (1), since the other vectors $\boldsymbol{s}_{k0}$ and $\boldsymbol{g}_r$ are known. This transformation matrix fully describes the orientation of the body *k*. De Vries et al. (1994) used this property for the two-dimensional case.

Method 3:

Joint angles (relative angles between segments) can be determined by using property 3:

Consider two bodies *k* and *l*, connected via a ball hinge joint, with orientation vectors φ_k and φ_l respectively. The transformation matrices $\boldsymbol{T}_k$ and $\boldsymbol{T}_l$ (equation (1)) from body fixed to inertial coordinates are nonlinear functions of these orientation vectors. The accelerometer signals at the joint expressed in the body fixed coordinate system of both bodies *k* and *l* ($\boldsymbol{s}_{k0}$ and $\boldsymbol{s}_{l0}$) can be determined using *property 3* (equation (6)). After applying the transformation matrices $\boldsymbol{T}_k$ and $\boldsymbol{T}_l$ from body fixed to inertial coordinates to the accelerometer signals estimated at the joint the results should be equal, since both signals have been determined at the same position:

$$\boldsymbol{T}_k(\boldsymbol{s}_{ki}) = \boldsymbol{T}_l(\boldsymbol{s}_{li}) \tag{8}$$

In principle a vector expressing the angle between two body fixed lines, one line defined in each body, and the orientation of the plane parallel to both lines can be determined by implicit solution of these three nonlinear equations.

In general, method 3 does not provide absolute segment orientations. Only if the orientation of one segment is known (e.g. a foot on the ground), the orientations of the other linked segments can be determined using the estimated joint angles

Method 4:

Segment angles can be determined by integration from the angular acceleration vectors and angular velocity vectors determined on the basis of property 2.

As presented above, the angular velocity ω_k and angular acceleration vectors $\dot{\omega}_k$ of a rigid body k can be determined from the accelerometer signal vectors $\boldsymbol{s}_{ki}$ measured at at least three positions of the body, using equation (2).

3 Discussion

The question remains whether the described methods will result in a comprehensive ambulatory 3D movement analysis system based on accelerometry. Each of the methods described has a limited scope or is only valid under certain conditions. Combinations of the described methods may lead to a versatile ambulatory 3D movement analysis system: e.g. The integration drift encountered in the integration method 4 can be rejected when combining with method 1, applied for static phases in a registration.

Several extensive numerical problems need to be addressed when implementing the presented methods into actual algorithms. For example, integration drift can be reduced and offset angles determined when dynamic periods are preceeded and/or followed by static periods: method 1 gives the offset angle during the static periods and the required offsets for minimal drift, since integration should result in zero angular velocity and constant angle in these static periods. Furthermore, applying methods 2 or 3 for determining joint angles can be combined with the integration method (method 4), to reduce integration drift in the calculation of the segment orientations, because it gives an additional relation between segment orientations. Also, it may reduce high frequency noise, which is encountered when computing joint angles using methods 2 or 3 (Willemsen et al., 1990, 1991), while maintaining the advantage of determining absolute joint angles. Willemsen et al. (1990, 1991) suggested to use method 3 for resetting integration drift errors during the stance phase of gait, because the foot contacts the floor, which has a known orientation. De Vries et al. (1994) however showed that this does not yield an adequate estimation of shank angle during the stance phase, because the contact between foot and floor constantly changes and therefore cannot be considered as a simple hinge joint.

The influence of several sources of errors on the validity and accuracy of the calculated body movements has to be evaluated. Errors may result from inaccurate values of required geometrical parameters, non-ideal segment and joints properties (the segments may not be sufficiently rigid and the joint may not be perfect hinge or ball joints)

Method 2 provides the orientation of a rigid body segment without integration under another condition than in method 3: With method 3, the orientation of a rigid segment can be determined if the orientation of another body to which it is connected by a hinge is known. Method 2 needs the acceleration of one point of the segment in reference coordinates. Both methods need the 3D accelerometer signals at three points on the segment. The conditions in both methods can be met if the rigid segment is linked in a chain of coupled rigid segments, of which one has a constant and known velocity and orientation (e.g. foot on floor).

It may be fruitful to combine different types of kinematic sensors for the analysis of body movements. Especially the combination of accelerometers and gyroscopes have a high potential. If triaxial accelerometers and triaxial gyroscopes would be combined in composite sensors, the number of required sensor positions for a full 3D kinematic analysis may be reduced: The angular velocity vector ω_k of a segment k in equation (2) may than be determined by a 3D gyroscope at one position of the segment, which can be the same position as one of the triaxial accelerometers. Only minimally one additional triaxial accelerometer is then required for a full determination of the vectors ω_k, $\dot{\omega}_k$ and $\boldsymbol{s}_{k0}$ of the rigid segment k. This means minimally two in stead of three sensor positions.

Further analysis and experimental evaluation are required to assess the applicability of the described movement analysis methods for ambulatory gait analysis.

References

Bogert, A. J van den, and Read, L. (1994) A Method for Inverse Dynamics Analysis using Accelerometry. *in: Veltink PH and Van Lummel RC (eds.), Dynamic Analysis using Body Fixed Sensors - Second World Congress of Biomechanics*, The Hague, ISBN 90-9007328-2, pp. 59-64.

Bussmann, J. B. J., Veltink, P. H., Koelma, F., Van Lummel, R. C., and Stam, H. J. (1994) Ambulatory Monitoring of Mobility-Related Activities: the Initial Phase of the Development of an Activity Monitor. *European Journal of Physical Medicine and Rehabiltation*, accepted.

Dolan, P., Adams, M. A. (1993) The relationship between EMG Activity and Extensor Moment Generation in the Erector Spinae Muscles during Bending and Lifting Activities. *J. Biomech.*, 26: 513-522.

Franken, H. M., Veltink, P. H., and Boom, H. B. K. (1994) Restoring Gait in Paraplegics by Functional Electrical Stimulation. *IEEE Eng. in Medicine and Biology*, 13: 564-570.

Kleissen, R. F. M., Baardman, G., Hermens, H. J., and Adolfsen-Schlecht, M. C. (1991) Long-term Ambulatory Recording of Surface EMG in the Assessment of Spasticity. *in: Anderson PA, Hobart DJ and Danoff JV (eds), Proc. 8th Congress of the International Society of Electrophysiological Kinesiology*, Baltimore, 45-52.

Leskinen, T. P. J., Stälhammer, H. R., and Kuorinka, I. A. A. (1983) A Dynamic Analysis of Spinal Compression with Different Lifting Techniques. *Ergonomics*, 26: 595-604.

Morris, J. R. W. (1973) Accelerometry - a Technique for the Measurement of Human Body Movements. *J. Biomech.*, 6: 729-736.

Padgaonkar, A. J., Krieger, A. W., and King, A. I. (1975) Measurement of Angular Acceleration of a Rigid Body using Linear Accelerometers, *J. Appl. Mech.*, 42: 729-736.

Söderkvist, J. (1994) Micromachined Gyroscopes, *Sensors and Actuators, A,* 43: 65-71.

Tulen, J. H. M., Van den Meiracker, A. H., and Man in 't Veld, A. J. (1994) Hemodynamic Variability and Locomotor Activity: Clinical Applications. *in: Veltink PH and Van Lummel RC (eds.), Dynamic Analysis using Body Fixed Sensors - Second World Congress of Biomechanics*, The Hague, pp. 73-77.

Veltink, P. H., Bussmann, H. B. J., De Vries, W., Martens, W. L. J., and Van Lummel, R. C. (1994) Discrimination of Dynamic Activities using Accelerometry. *in: Veltink PH and Van Lummel RC (eds.), Dynamic Analysis using Body Fixed Sensors - Second World Congress of Biomechanics*, The Hague, pp. 3-7.

Vries, W. de, Veltink, P. H., Koper, M. K., and Koopman, B. F. J. M (1994) Calculation of Segment and Joint Angles of the Lower Extremities during Gait using Accelerometers. *in:* Veltink PH and Van Lummel RC (eds.), Dynamic Analysis using Body Fixed Sensors - Second World Congress of Biomechanics, The Hague, pp. 43-50.

Willemsen, A. Th. M., Van Alsté, J. A., and Boom H. B. K. (1990) Real-time Gait Assessment Uitlizing a New Way of Accelerometry, *J. Biomech.*, 23: 859-863.

Willemsen, A. Th. M., Frigo, C., and Boom H. B. K. (1991) Lower Extremity Angle Measurement with Accelerometers - Error and Sensitivity Analysis. *IEEE Trans. Biomed. Eng.*, 38: 1186-1193.

Restoration of Lateral Hand Grasp Using Natural Sensors

A. Lickel, M. Haugland, J. Haase and T. Sinkjær
Center for Sensory Motor Interaction (SMI), Aalborg University
Fredrik Bajers Vej 7D, 9220 Aalborg Øst, Denmark

Abstract - A closed loop control system for controlling the lateral grasp of a C6 tetraplegic patient was developed. Natural sensors served as the source of the feedback signal. The neural signals from cutaneous receptors were picked up by an implanted cuff electrode placed around the radial branch of the median nerve innervating the lateral part of the index finger. Applied mechanical stress to the skin, like pressure and slips, resulted in an increase in amplitude of the recorded neural signal. The goal of the study was to show that the recorded neural signals are able to indicate a slip of an object during lateral grasp, and based on this information to prevent the object from further sliding, by increasing the applied grasp force through functional electrical stimulation of the thumb adductor and flexor. Here we report on our preliminary investigations.

1 Introduction

Spinal cord injuries at the C5 and C6 level cause severe loss of voluntary movement and sensation in the upper extremity. Hand neuroprostheses based on the technique of Functional Electrical Stimulation (FES) have been developed to provide patients with some degree of hand function in daily life. (Crago 1991; Handa 1989).

All systems, that can be used in the daily life, are pure open loop systems, meaning that the output of the system (grasp force or finger position) only depends on the command signal generated by the user. The advantages are the rather simple design and the stability of the system. The trade-off is the required permanent attention of the user to compensate for changes in muscle properties (like muscle potentiation and fatigue and the non-linear relationship between command signals and active muscle force) (Crago 1986). A more advanced approach is to use a feedback signal, derived from artificial position and/or force sensors, to compensate for changes in muscle force. Experiments showed that closed loop control of hand grasp neuroprostheses is feasible, but they also displayed the limitations of the artificial sensors. Difficulties in mounting the sensors on the skin, electrical drift, nonlinearities and breakage are some of the disadvantages that appeared during the experiments (Crago 1986). Those problems raised the idea of substituting the artificial sensors by natural sensors; cutaneous receptors in the foot (Hoffer 1986; Sinkjær 1994), proprioceptors in the joints, etc., since they are already in the body and their functionality often is not affected by the spinal cord injury. The goal is to extract relevant information from the recorded nerve signal and use it as a feedback signal. It has been shown in cat and human experiments (Haugland 1992; Haugland 1994b), that it is very difficult to conclude from the recorded nerve signal on the mechanical event (like magnitude of the applied force on the skin). This is caused in part by temporal adaptation of the cutaneous receptors together with a large increase of the nerve signal during both the onset and removal of a perpendicular force. However, the previous studies have shown that it is possible to extract information about slips across the skin from the nerve signal. This information may be useful for controlling FES system for hand grasp by means of an “event-driven” controller (Haugland 1994a). In this paper we describe the initial results from a study aimed at implementing such a controller in a 'hand grasp system' for a tetraplegic patient.

2 Methods

2.1 Subject

The study was performed on a 27 year old male C6 level tetraplegic patient (8 years post-injury), and was approved by the local ethical committee. This patient had good control of shoulder motion, elbow flexion and some wrist extension, but had no voluntary control over his hand muscles. He had sensation in his forearm and to some extent in his thumb and index finger.

In May 1994, the left hand of the subject was instrumented in a surgical procedure with a tripolar cuff electrode around the digital branch of the palmar nerve innervating the lateral part of the index finger. The cuff electrode was an insulating silicone-tube (Dow Corning), 20 mm long and 2 mm inner diameter with 3 circumferential electrodes inside the cuff (Hoffer 1990). The wires of the cuff electrode (Cooner wire, AS634) were routed subcutaneously to an exit site on the volar side of the forearm, where they were attached to a small external connector. During a short stay in Cleveland, Ohio, in August 1994, 11 percutaneous electrodes (type 316L stainless steel with Teflon coating (Memberg 1993)) were implanted in several hand and forearm muscles to provide him with a lateral grasp (key grip). The involved muscles were FPL (thumb flexor, 1 electrode), EPL (thumb extensor, 2 electrodes), AbPB (thumb abductor, 2 electrodes), FDS (finger flexor, 2 electrodes) and EDC (finger extensor, 2 electrodes). Since the AdP (thumb adductor) was very close to the implanted cuff electrode, insertion of an electrode into the AdP muscle risked damaging the cuff or its leads. Thus it was decided to activate the AdP through stimulation of the ulnar nerve at the wrist (2 electrodes). The implantation of the percutaneous electrodes was done with a hypodermic needle under local anaesthesia.

Finger flexors and thumb adductor (FDS and AdP) were conditioned via the percutaneous electrodes (approx. 4 hours per day, using cyclic stimulation, 2 sec on, 2 sec off), since the patient did not tolerate surface stimulation.

2.2 Experimental set-up

The feedforward path of the system consisted of the controller and a five channel stimulator (only 5 of the 11 electrodes were used at any time). The output signal of the controller (defined to be in the range 0 - 100 %) was assigned to 5 different muscles involved in the lateral grasp by using a lookup-table for the activation of the muscles (grasp template), where 0% corresponded to 'open hand' with full thumb extension, and 100% corresponded to 'maximal force generation' with full thumb flexion and adduction. The stimulator produced current-controlled, biphasic, charge balanced pulses (20 mA negative pulse followed by 5 mA positive pulse) at a fixed rate of 20 Hz. The stimulus intensity was varied by modulating the pulse duration between 0 and 255 μs. The stimulation pulses for the different muscles were delivered sequentially with a temporal spacing between the pulses of 1 ms. The order of muscle stimulation was FPL, EPL, AbPB, AdP and FDS.

In the feedback path, the nerve signal was amplified with a battery powered amplifier (MicroProbe, gain of 100,000) and passed through an isolation amplifier. The signal was then bandpass filtered (4th order Krohn-Hite) with a lower cut-off frequency of 1000 Hz (to remove EMG contamination) and a higher cut-off frequency of 4 kHz, and then sampled at 10 kHz (i.e. 500 samples of the nerve signal between 2 stimuli). A digital signal processor (TMS 320C25) digitally rectified and bin-integrated the sampled nerve signal (to produce the envelope of the nerve signal and remove stimulation artifacts as will be described later) and sent the resulting values every 50 ms (20 Hz) to a PC.

A simple peak detection algorithm was applied on the processed nerve signal to detect occurred slips. This algorithm was similar to the algorithm used in cat experiments (Haugland 1994). The background activity of the rectified and bin-integrated (rbin) nerve signal was removed by subtracting a lowpass filtered (0.7 Hz) and delayed (200 ms) version of the rbin signal (fig. 1B) from the original rbin signal (fig. 1A). This modified 'slip signal' was then presented to a peak detection algorithm with a fixed detection threshold (fig. 1C).

2.3 Experimental protocol

To date two sets of experiments have been performed to investigate the feasibility of using natural sensors as a source of feedback signals.

The first experiment was to study the influence of electrical stimulation of the hand muscles on the recorded nerve signal and to examine the possibility of detecting slip events during a functional grasp.

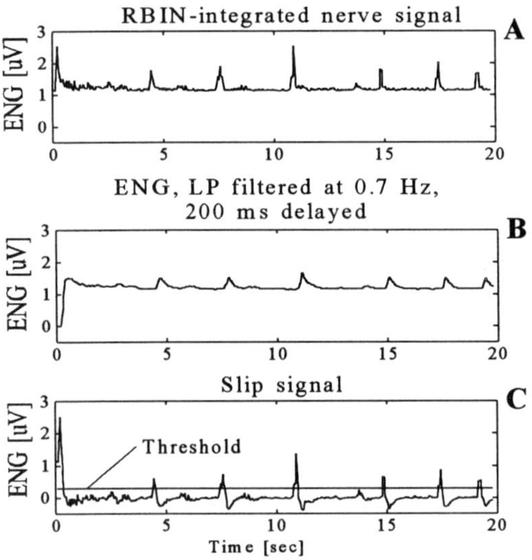

Fig. 1. Removing the background activity from the rectified and integrated signal pronounces the peaks in the nerve signal and makes it easier to set a threshold. **A**: rectified and bin-integrated nerve signal. **B**: background nerve signal, low-pass filtered at a cut-off frequency of 0.7 Hz and delayed for 200 ms. **C**: Nerve signal with removed background activity, the threshold value was set to 0.2 µV.

Mechanical stimuli were applied manually via a force probe that terminated in a plate with a diameter of 20 mm. This probe measured both the lateral and perpendicular forces. It was placed manually on the skin of the index finger with a certain perpendicular force; the lateral force was then increased until it exceeded the friction force and the probe slipped out. We wanted to determine if those events (applied perpendicular force and slip) could be detected in the recorded nerve signal while the hand muscles were electrically stimulated.

In a second experiment we investigated if the system was capable of reacting to small slips of the object with respect to the skin of the index finger, so that the grasp force could be increased. For this purpose we instrumented a rectangular object (80 x 60 x 20 mm) with a force sensor to measure the grasp force.

The experiment was performed by initially stimulating the muscle to produce a secure grip. The grip was then slowly released by reducing the stimulation intensity at a slow constant rate until a slip occurred. If the slip was detected by the computer monitoring the nerve signal as described above, a reaction was initiated to seize the object and secure the grip. This was done by increasing the command level to 100% for a single pulse and afterwards settling at a command level slightly higher than the one right before the slip occurred. The process of slowly decreasing the command level was then resumed.

3 Results

The nerve signal was recorded while each muscle involved in the key grip was stimulated individually. The stimulator generated pulses for all muscles, but only one electrode was connected to the stimulator at the time. Idle outputs were connected to ground. This procedure allowed us to determine the timing and origin of each of the artifacts present in the nerve signal. It was expected that muscles located close to the nerve cuff electrode (AdP, AbPB) would create larger artifacts than muscles further away from the cuff (FPL).

Figure 2 shows the recorded nerve signal during electrical stimulation of the FPL (trace A) and the ulnar nerve which innervates AdP (trace B). The pulse duration was 66 μs for FPL and 192 μs for AdP.

The stimulation caused large stimulation artifacts in the nerve signal, lasting up to about 8 ms after the stimulation. Smaller artifacts occurred when pulses were sent to the four channels not involved in the stimulation. This was attributed to crosstalk between the grounded channels and the active channel. These direct artifacts from the stimulator were not problematic because of their relatively short duration. Blanking the first 13 ms of each interpulse interval (50 ms between 2 stimuli) reduced interference from all five channels significantly and left plenty of artifact free nerve signal to be recorded. However, during stimulation of the ulnar nerve, additional artifacts were picked up. Since the nerve cuff electrode was adjacent to the stimulated thumb adductor (AdP), the M-wave of this muscle, about 7 ms after the stimulation, contaminated the nerve signal. Another artifact was picked up about 35 ms after the stimulation, presumably an F-wave or H-reflex in the adductor. A possible explanation for this can be the stimulation of the ulnar nerve rather than the AdP directly. Even after high-pass filtering at 1000 Hz, as described in Methods, these artifacts created significant interference in the range from 7 ms to 15 ms and from 32 ms to 42 ms (figure 2B).

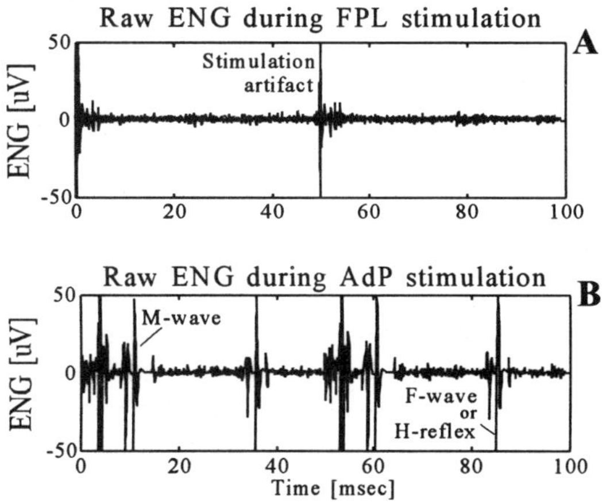

Fig.2: Stimulation artifacts, picked up by the nerve cuff electrode. During a 20 Hz FPL stimulation (trace **A**), the artifact disappeared after 8 ms and left a clear nerve signal. Contrary to that, stimulation of the ulnar nerve caused additional artifacts, which resulted in a restriction of the useful nerve signal (from 15 to 32 ms, trace **B**).

To remove the influence of the artifacts on the processed nerve signal, only samples 150 to 320 (i.e. from 15 ms to 32 ms after first stimulus) were used in the bin-integration, since that period was apparently artifact-free during stimulation of all the involved hand muscles.

Figure 3 shows the recorded nerve signal during the stimulation of AdP. The stimulation intensity was increased from the activation threshold (PW=100 μs) to the maximum pulsewidth of 200 μs. This produced an artifact that increased in both amplitude and duration during the trial, but this was not reflected as an increase of the amplitude in the rbin-signal (trace D). For us it was a proof that we had removed all the artifacts before we calculated the rbin signal.

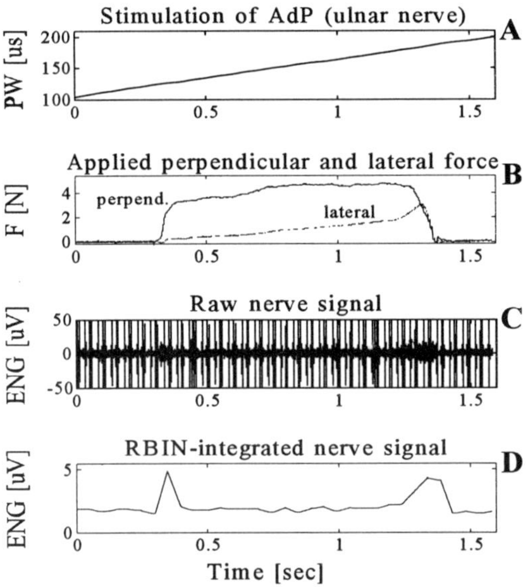

Fig. 3: Slip detection when applying mechanical stress on the skin. While the electrical stimulus intensity was increased (**A**), the force probe was pushed against the lateral part of the index finger (perpendicular and lateral force shown in **B**). This resulted in an increase of the nerve signal (**C**, **D** after 0.35 sec), which could easily be detected in the rbin nerve signal. A second peak appeared when the lateral force overcame the friction and the probe slipped (**C**, **D** after 1.35 sec). Note that the raw nerve signal was strongly contaminated with artifacts (**C**), whereas the rbin-integrated nerve signal (**D**) was apparently unaffected by the increase in stimulation intensity.

Several broken stimulation electrodes caused some difficulties during our experiments. We could not activate FPL, and the AdP showed a very weak response to the electrical stimulation. The elicited force during maximum stimulation seemed not to be sufficient to stop a slipping object. Instead we investigated how well the system detected a slip of the object and reacted to it. An appropriate threshold value for a reliable slip detection was determined from a few test runs and set to a value of 1 μV. The subject held the object in lateral grasp with a given force. Then, the object was pulled by the experimenter and the resulting slip was detected and resulted in an increase of the stimulation intensity.

It was also of interest to know if hand or forearm movement could impair the slip detection and then wrongly be identified as a slip. We asked our subject to supinate and pronate several times, while the thumb was strapped away from the index finger to avoid skin contact (the pronator was not under voluntary control, but by moving his shoulder the subject was able to produce forearm pronation). These forearm movements caused an increase in the recorded nerve signal, and we were not able to distinguish between these movements and real slips, which resulted in a number of false detection of slips.

4 Discussion

The obtained results during the two sets of experiments were encouraging. Slips of an object across the index finger could be detected in the recorded nerve signal. This detection was used as a trigger in the closed loop control system to increase the lateral grasp force. The generated force was not sufficient to stop an eventually slipping object, but it showed that our approach of using a slip signal to control our system was feasible.

However, there were also a number of problems apparent. Our biggest problem was the high number of broken percutaneous electrodes. Three months after their implantation there were only 6 out of 11 electrodes functioning. One explanation of the high breakage rate can be the very active lifestyle of our participating patient. The stimulation of the ulnar nerve rather than the thumb adductor muscle (AdP) itself caused artifacts, that reduced the useful nerve signal between 2 stimuli to only 17 ms.

Forearm movement (like supination and pronation) caused an increase in the recorded nerve signal, which was incorrectly detected as a slip event. Although this was not a very substantial error, since it just triggered the stimulator to increase the grasp force, it was still not desirable. A unnecessarily high grasp force results in an earlier muscle fatigue, which we tried to avoid with our system. Further investigations will be necessary to develop methods to distinguish between forearm movement and real slip events and make the slip detection more reliable.

5 Conclusion

This paper shows the possibility of detecting slips of a grasped object across the lateral surface of the index finger, even during stimulation of adjacent muscle groups. Blanking and filtering is an effective method to eliminate the influence of stimulus artifacts and EMG contamination on the recorded nerve signal during a control process. The system can detect slips and react with an increase of muscle force to stop an occurred slip.

6 Acknowledgement

The authors would like to thank a number of people who gave their contribution to this project. Inger Lauge Jensen for helping us with the selection of the patient. Ron Riso and Peter Slot who worked on the characterisation of the skin receptors, and the group in Cleveland, Ohio, with Hunter Peckham, Pat Crago and Mike Keith for the implantation of the percutaneous electrodes and for numerous helpful suggestions. This project was supported by the Danish National Research Foundation.

References

Crago, P., Chizeck, H., Neuman, M., and Hambrecht, f. (1986) Sensors for use with Functional Neuromuscular stimulation; IEEE Trans. Biomed. Engineering, 33, pp 256-268

Crago, P., Nakai, R., Chizeck, H. (1991): Feedback Regulation of Hand Grasp Opening and Contact Force during Stimulation of Paralysed Muscle; IEEE Trans. Biomed. Engineering, 38-1 pp 17-28

Handa, Y., Ohkubo, K., and Hoshimiya, N. (1989) A portable multi-channel FES system for restoration of motor function of the paralysed extremities, Automedia, pp 221-231

Haugland, M., Sinkjær, T., and Haase, J. (1992): Force Information in Whole Human Sensory Nerve Recordings; 4th Vienna Workshop on FES

Haugland, M., Hoffer, J.A., and Sinkjær, T. (1994) Skin contact force information in sensory nerve signals recorded by implanted cuff electrodes; IEEE Trans. Rehabilitation Engineering, 2-1, pp. 18-28

Haugland, M., and Hoffer, A. (1994) Slip Information provided by Nerve Cuff Signals: Application in Closed-Loop Control of Functional Electrical Stimulation; IEEE Trans. Rehab. Engineering, 2-1, pp 29-36

Hoffer, A., and Sinkjær, T. (1986) A natural 'force sensor' suitable for closed-loop control of functional neuromuscular stimulation; in Proc. 2nd Vienna Int. Workshop on Functional Electrostimulation, pp 47-50

Hoffer, J.A (1990) Techniques to Study Spinal-Cord Peripheral Nerve, and Muscle Activity in Freely Moving Animals; From Neuromethods, Vol.15: Neurophysiological Techniques: Applications to Neural Systems, The Humana Press Inc., Clifton, N.J., pp 65-145

Hoffer, A., and Haugland, M. (1992) Signals from tactile sensors in glabrous skin suitable for restoring motor functions in paralysed humans; in R.B. Stein, H.P. Peckham, D. Popovic, Eds., Neural Prostheses: Replacing Motor Functions after Disease or Disability. New York: Oxford Univ. Press, pp 99-125

Hoshimiya, N. (1989) A master-slave type multi-channel FES system for the control of the paralysed upper extremities; Automedia, pp 209-220

Memberg, W., Peckham, P., Thrope, G., Keith, M., and Kicher, T. (1993) An Analysis of the Reliability of Percutaneous Electrodes in Upper Extremity FNS Applications; IEEE Trans. Rehab. Engineering, 1-2, pp126-132

Riso, R., Haugland, M., Slot, P., Haase, J., and Sinkjær, T. (1994): Characterisation of sensory nerve responses to mechanical skin stimulation recorded by chronically implanted cuff electrodes in man; in Society for Neuroscience, 24th Annual Meeting, Florida, November 1994

Sinkjær, T., Haugland, M., and Haase, J. (1994) Natural neural sensing and artificial muscle control in man; Exp. Brain Research, 98:542-545

Extraction of Slip Information from Digital Nerve Signals in Man

A. Lickel, M. Haugland
Center for Sensory Motor Interaction (SMI), Aalborg University
Fredrik Bajers Vej 7D, 9220 Aalborg Øst, Denmark

Abstract - A cuff electrode implanted on a peripheral nerve has been used to record sensory information from the mechanoreceptors in the index finger of a tetraplegic person. The nerve signal contained clear responses to slip events, and it was our intention to use this information to control an FES stimulator to produce hand grasp. To extract the information about slips reliably from the raw nerve signal, four different methods were suggested and optimized based on experimental data

1 Introduction

Natural sensors (e.g. mechanoreceptors in the skin) in man are often not affected by a spinal cord injury and thus still react on mechanical stress with an increased neural activity (Thomas et. al. 1992). This electrical signal can be recorded with a whole nerve cuff electrode placed on the peripheral nerve carrying the signal. It has been shown, that pressure applied on the skin can be detected in chronically recorded nerve signals in man (Haugland et. al. 1994) and (Sinkjær et. al. 1994). This signal has been used as a substitute for a heel switch in neuroprostheses for drop foot patients (Haugland et. al. 1995) and (Upshaw and Sinkjær 1995). Recording from a multifascicular nerve with a cuff electrode makes it however difficult to extract a clear nerve signal from a single fascicle. In order to use a recorded nerve signal for feedback, it is necessary to develop methods to extract the relevant information, such as a neural response when an object slips across the finger during lateral grasp. In this paper four methods are evaluated to receive a 'reliable' slip information from a whole nerve signal. This slip information can then be applied in closed loop control hand neuroprostheses (Haugland et. al. 1995).

2 Methods

A 27 year old male C6 tetraplegic patient (8 years post injury) volunteered to participate in this research project. The patient gave his informed consent and the study was approved by the local ethical committee. In a surgical procedure, a tripolar nerve cuff electrode was implanted around the digital branch of the palmar nerve innervating the lateral part of the index finger of his left hand. Percutaneous stimulation electrodes were implanted in the FDS (finger flexor) and EDC (finger extensor) as well as in the FPL (thumb flexor), EPL (thumb extensor) and AbP (thumb abductor) to provide him with lateral grasp ('key grip'). AdP (thumb adductor) was stimulated through a percutaneous electrode located in proximity to the ulnar nerve at the wrist.

The muscles were stimulated with biphasic and charge balanced electrical pulses at a rate of 20 Hz. The pulses had a constant amplitude of 20 mA for the cathodic phase and 5 mA for the anodic phase, and the pulse duration was varied between 0 and 255 μs. The nerve signal was amplified (Micro Probe preamplifier) and filtered with a 4th order bandpass filter (Krohn Hite). The lower cut-off frequency was 1 kHz and removed most of the EMG contamination from adjacent stimulated muscles, the upper filter frequency was set to 4 kHz to avoid aliasing artifacts when sampling the signal at a rate of 10 kHz. The sampling of the nerve signal and the stimulation was controlled by an IBM-compatible PC.

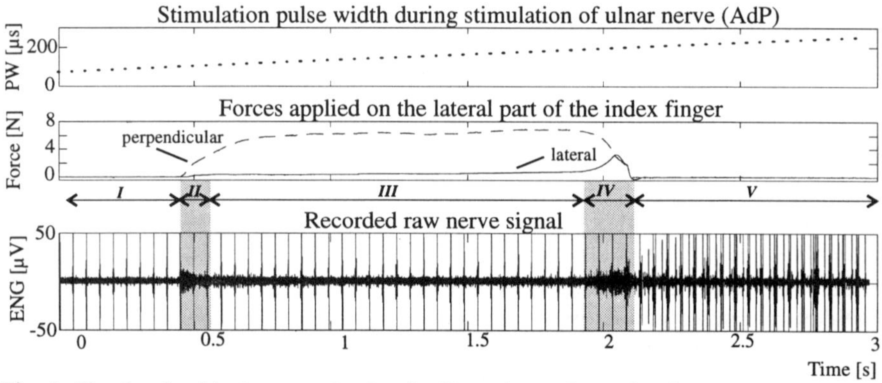

Fig. 1: The thumb adductor was stimulated with an increasing pulse duration and a constant frequency of 20 Hz during a 3 seconds trial. At some arbitrary time, a probe was pressed against the lateral part of the index finger (trace 2, **II** & **III**) and then slipped (trace 2, **IV**). The recorded nerve signal (trace 3) showed an increase in amplitude during the force onset and the slip event (shaded period).

The nerve signal was recorded during electrical stimulation of forearm and hand muscles involved in the lateral grasp. Slip events were generated by a probe, that was pressed on the index finger of the patient and then pushed to the side until it slipped off the finger (fig.1, trace 2). This probe was instrumented with strain gauges to measure the lateral and the perpendicular component of the applied force.

Force onset (fig.1, trace 2, II) and slip (trace 2, IV) were clearly reflected as an increase of the amplitude in the recorded nerve signal (fig.1, trace 3, shaded area). Electrical stimulation of adjacent muscles caused artifacts in the recorded nerve signal, however, a useful, artifact free nerve signal of 17 ms out of approximately 50 ms between two stimuli were left. All the following considerations refer to this artifact-free window between two stimulation pulses.

The recorded nerve signal was divided into five parts:

- *Background 1:* nerve signal before the probe touched the skin
- *Force onset:* the probe touched the skin and the perpendicular force was increased
- *Applied force:* period when the probe touched the skin with a rather constant lateral and perpendicular force
- *Slip event:* the lateral component of the applied force increased and the probe slipped out and was removed
- *Background 2:* nerve signal after the probe was removed from the skin

We developed four different methods to detect slip events and optimized them based on our experimental data. Three methods analyzed the nerve signal in the time domain and one in the frequency domain.

2.1 Signal analysis in the time domain

The nerve signal was digitally rectified and bin-integrated (***rbin-signal***) to produce the envelope of the neural signal, and then sampled at 20 Hz. This signal was then processed with three different algorithms to evaluate each of them against the others:

a) A peak detection algorithm was applied on the rbin-signal. This algorithm reported a slip when the rbin-signal exceeded a predefined threshold. The threshold level was adjusted until all slip events in the experimental trials were detected (no true negative errors).

b) We applied a 2nd order bandpass filter on the rbin-signal to remove slow changes in the signal caused by changing noise level and background activity and to dampen the high frequency variation. This filtered signal was then presented to a peak detection algorithm as described in a). To find the optimal filter, we compared the performance of filters with varying characteristics, i.e. we varied the lower and the higher cutoff frequency (F_1 and F_2) between 0.5 Hz and 10 Hz.

c) Finally, we applied a filter as shown in (Fig.2), on the rbin-signal, before it was evaluated. The rbin-signal was applied to two different lowpass filters with cutoff frequencies F_1 and F_2. Signal S_1 was then delayed for a certain time Delay_time (n samples) before it was subtracted from signal S_2. The resulting slip signal showed only the peak, while the background signal was removed.

The optimal filter configuration was determined by varying F_1 and F_2 between 0.5 and 10 Hz and the Delay_time between 0 and 300 ms.

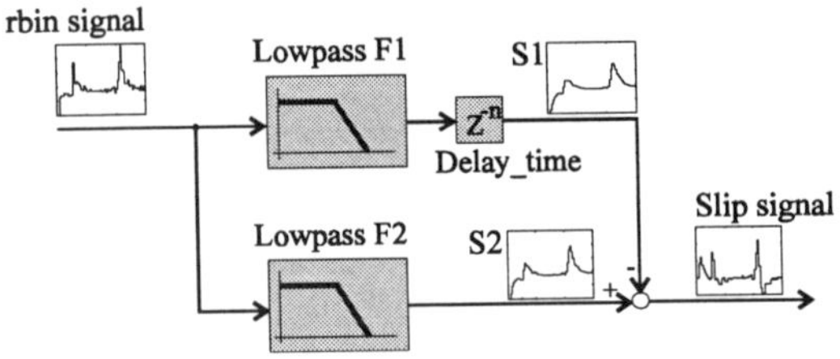

Fig. 2: The rectified and bin-integrated nerve signal (rbin-signal) was applied to two lowpass filters with cut-off frequencies F_1 and F_2. The signal S_1, filtered at frequency F_1, was then delayed for a number of samples before it was subtracted from the signal S_2. The resulting slip signal was then applied to the threshold detection algorithm.

2.2 Analysis in the frequency domain

Mechanoreceptors in the skin react on slips of objects crossing the skin with an increase in their firing rate. This contribution to the recorded compound raw nerve signal was expected to be reflected as an increase in amplitude of the nerve signal at a certain frequency.

The recorded raw nerve signal was piecewise fourier transformed by using the artifact free nerve signal between two electrical stimuli (170 samples) and the spectral power of the signal was estimated (Welch algorithm). This resulted in 60 individual power spectra for every experimental trial (total of 60 stimuli), each spectrum contained 86 frequency bands with a frequency resolution of about 59 Hz. Big variations within each spectrum made it necessary to apply a smoothing window (hanning window). The spectral power at one frequency in the smoothed spectrum was used to describe the transformed nerve signal, resulting in a signal (***spec-signal***) with 60 values, which was further analyzed (see also fig. 3). A peak detection algorithm, as described in section 2.1, was applied on this low frequency signal. 28 slip events were compared, and the one showing the lowest spectral power was chosen as the reference slip signal and used as the threshold level in the peak detection algorithm. Both the size of the smoothing hanning window and the examined frequency were varied to optimize the slip detection.

3 Results

The quality of a slip detection algorithm was described by 3 parameters:

- E_C: number of critical error: a critical error is defined as a detection of a slip although there is no slip. The misdetections were counted during constant applied force and before the probe touched the skin and after it was removed.
- E_T: total number of errors: total number of misdetections of the nerve signal as a slip (false positive error).
- S_M: Safety margin of the threshold: the range in which the threshold could be changed without increasing E_C.

Note: The threshold was set to a value that allowed us to detect all slip events, so the number of true-negative errors was zero in all our experiments.

3.1 Analysis in the time domain

a) The number of critical errors E_C was zero when we applied a peak detection algorithm on the rbin signal. However, when we counted the false alarms during the force onset event as well, the total number of errors (E_T) was 9. The highest possible threshold level was 3.93 μV and could be reduced by 12% (S_M=12%) before we obtained the first critical error .

b) We applied a 2nd order bandpass filter on the rbin-signal and presented the filtered signal to the peak detection algorithm. The optimal filter configuration was evaluated by varying both the lower and the higher cutoff frequency (F_1 and F_2) between 0.5 Hz and 10 Hz. Filtering did not improve the quality of the slip detection at all. The best result was obtained when F_1=0.5 Hz and F_2=10 Hz, thus basically the whole frequency range could pass the filter. In this case, E_C=2 and E_T increased to 20, the optimal threshold was 1.02 μV with a safety margin S_M of 9%.

c) A filter as shown in (Fig.2) was employed on the rbin signal before it was presented to the peak detection algorithm. We adjusted the parameters F_1, F_2 and Delay_time for an optimal result with respect to the number of occurred errors and the safety margin. The best performance was obtained when F_1 and F_2 were 1.5 Hz, and S_1 was delayed by 100 ms before subtracted from S_2 (Delay_time=100 ms). For this configuration, E_C was 2, E_T = 24 and the threshold was 0.76 μV with a safety margin S_M of 11%.

3.2 Analysis in the frequency domain

We considered only the frequencies between 1000 Hz and 4000 Hz, since the raw nerve signal was already bandpass filtered within this range. The high variation in the obtained power spectra made it necessary to apply a smoothing window before the power for one certain frequency was evaluated (fig. 3). The size of the smoothing hanning window was gradually increased from 1 to 86. For every single experimental trial, we varied both the window size and frequency and calculated a set of output signals (spec signal), each with 60 values, which were presented to a threshold detection algorithm. After analyzing all different combinations of window sizes and frequency bands, we noticed, that for certain smoothing window sizes and frequencies the slip events could be detected with no critical error. For some combinations, the number of total errors (E_T) could be reduced to 9. Further, E_C was always zero when E_T reached the minimum of 9, thus, it was sufficient to use the E_T as an evaluation criteria (fig. 4).

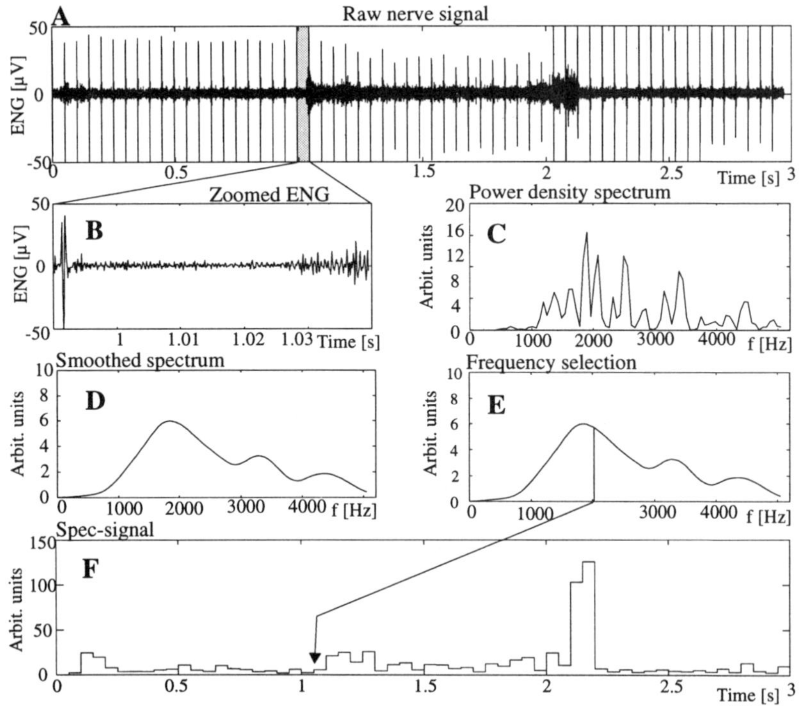

Fig.3: Calculation of the spec signal. The raw nerve signal (A) was splitted into intervals (nerve signal between 2 stimuli, B), the artifact free part of each interval was fourier transformed and its spectral power density was estimated (C). The obtained spectrum was smoothed (D) and the spectral power at one frequency was chosen (E) to represent the transformed interval in the spec signal (F).

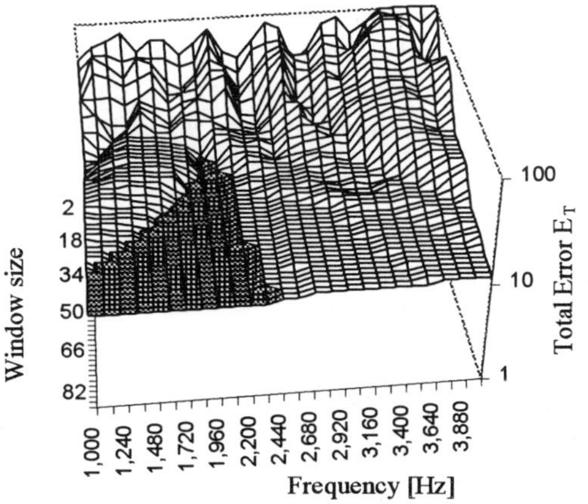

Fig. 4: Different spec-signals were calculated by varying the smoothing window size from 1 to 86 and the analyzed frequency from 1000 to 4000 Hz. The signals were then presented to a peak detection algorithm. The threshold was chosen to be low enough so that no slip was missed. The total number of errors E_T was minimal (E_T=9, dark shaded area) for frequencies between 1000 Hz and 2375 Hz and a window size from 23 to 86.

Both E_C and E_T were minimal for frequencies between 1000 Hz and 2375 Hz and a window size ranging from 23 to 86. The third criteria to describe the performance of the slip detection was the safety margin of the threshold value, which apparently grew with the size of the smoothing window (Fig. 5).

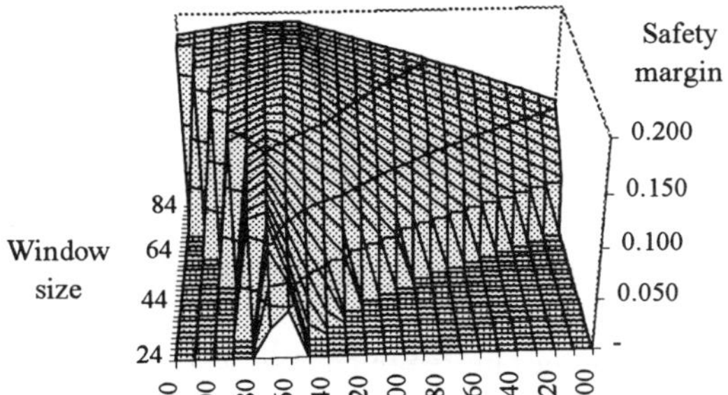

Fig.5: Several combinations of smoothing window size and analyzed frequencies resulted in a total error E_T of 9. The safety margin S_M of the threshold value was used to determine the optimal configuration. S_M was maximal for a frequency of 2080 Hz and a window size of 86.

The best result with respect to the parameters E_C, E_T and S_M was achieved when using the spectral power at 2080 Hz with a smoothing hanning window of size 86. The safety margin in this case was 19 %, meaning that the threshold value could be reduced to 81 % of the highest valid threshold without causing a critical error.

We then investigated if the peak and the median frequency of the spectrum would change during slip events with respect to the other events. We compared all spectra of the five different events (total of 1740 spectra) by calculating both the mean values and the standard deviations. The result was, that the changes in both the peak and the median frequency were insignificant, the differences between mean values were smaller than their standard deviation (Fig. 6). We concluded that neither the peak frequency nor the median frequency of the frequency spectrum could be used as a parameter to distinguish between the different events.

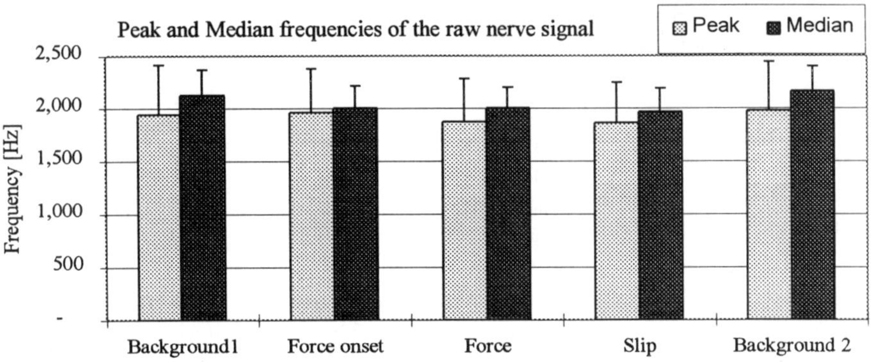

Fig. 6: Both the peak and the median frequencies of the nerve signal during different events were analyzed. The difference in the mean frequencies during different events were smaller than their standard deviation, which led us to the conclusion that both the peak and the median frequency were not useful indicators for an occurred slip.

4 Discussion

We employed different algorithms on the recorded nerve signal to obtain slip information, analyzing the nerve signal in the time and the frequency domain. We considered 28 experimental trials in our study, one trial was excluded because of artifacts in the nerve signal that could not be removed. We were able to detect all slips correctly with no critical error (E_C=0) when the rbin-signal was presented to a peak detection algorithm. The number of total errors E_T in this case was 9, and the safety margin of the threshold level was 12 %. Presenting a filtered version of that rbin-signal to the peak detection algorithm did not improve the slip detection. The filter parameters were optimized to minimize the number of errors, but the lowest number of critical errors E_C we could obtain was 2, and E_T was 20 in case of the bandpass filter and 24 in the other case, which made it useless for our purpose. The results of the spectral analysis of the recorded raw nerve signal showed that the quality of the slip detection did not only depend on the choice of the analyzed frequency, but also on the correct choice of a smoothing window. The best result was obtained when the spectra were smoothed with a hanning window of size 86, before the spectral power at 2080 Hz was evaluated. For this configuration, no critical error occurred (E_C=0), E_T was 9 and the safety margin of the threshold value was 19 %. The advantage of the latter method over the slip detection on the rbin signal was the greater safety margin of the threshold level, that made the slip detection more robust. The tradeoff was the higher computational effort to elicit the same number of errors as for the relatively simple threshold detection on the rbin signal.

We analyzed the data off-line, but none of the described methods would be too complex that it could not be done in a real-time application.

5 Acknowledgments

The authors would like to thank Drs. Jens Haase and Michael Keith for implanting the cuff electrode and the percutaneous stimulation electrodes and Hans Struijk for all the fruitful discussions regarding the technique of signal processing itself. We would also like to thank our subject for participating in our experiments. This work was supported by the Danish National Research Foundation.

6 References

Haugland, M., and Lickel, A., et. al. (1995) Restoration of Lateral Hand Grasp using Natural Sensors; Proc. 5th Vienna Int. Workshop on FES

Haugland, M., and Hoffer, A. (1994) Slip Information provided by Nerve Cuff Signals: Application in Closed-Loop Control of Functional Electrical Stimulation; IEEE Trans. Rehab. Eng., **2**, 1, pp. 29-36

Haugland, M., and Sinkjær, T. (1995) Cutaneous whole nerve recordings used for correction of footdrop in hemiplegic man, IEEE Trans. Rehab. Eng., **3**, 4

Sinkjær, T., Haugland, M., and Haase, J. (1994) Natural neural sensing and artificial muscle control in man; Exp. Brain Research, **98**, pp. 542-545

Thomas, C.K., and Westling, G. (1992): Tactile afferent function after human cervical spinal cord injury; Proc. Soc. for Neuroscience, **22**nd Annual Meeting, Vol. 18

Upshaw, B., and Sinkjær, T. (1995) Natural vs. Artificial sensors applied in peroneal nerve stimulation; Proc. **5**th Vienna Int. Workshop on FES, pp. 239-242

Characterization of the ENG Activity from a Digital Nerve for Feedback Control in Grasp Neuroprostheses

R. R. Riso and P. J. Slot
Center for Sensory-Motor Interaction
Department of Medical Informatics and Image Analysis
Aalborg University, Aalborg Denmark

Abstract - The electroneurogram (ENG) from a branch of the palmer digital nerve innervating the skin of the index finger in a quadriplegic volunteer subject was recorded using an implanted nerve cuff. ENG responses were obtained during precise mechanical stimulation of digital skin to determine if information regarding the mechanical events could be extracted from the evoked neural activity and if such information would be useful for feedback control of neuroprosthetic grasp. The responses to skin stretch were shown to be linearly related to the rate of stretch applied. The responses to slippage of a contact surface over the skin showed an initial decline in nerve activity as the pre-stretched skin recoiled backward under the contactor at the start of the slippage. This was followed by a period of modest activity as the contactor slid along the skin surface; and occasionally episodes of intense neural activity were seen, which corresponded to events when the contactor momentarily stretched the skin before sliding resumed. The utility of signals derived from natural sensors and the possibilities for information extraction from these signals are discussed.

1 Introduction

Electrical activation of forearm muscles is useful in providing grasp function in individuals with C5 and C6 level quadriplegia (Kilgore et al. 1989). Plans for future clinically deployable systems include the incorporation of closed-loop feedback which has been shown in laboratory studies to improve the system controllability and functionality (Chizeck et al. 1990; Crago et al. 1991). Although, wearable transducers to sense object slippage and skin forces during grasping are essential for this effort, their development has remained an elusive goal. An alternative approach is to obtain signals from 'Natural Sensors' such as the mechanoreceptors within the skin (Haugland et al. 1994;1995; Johnson et al. 1995; Riso et al. 1995;). This paper describes some of the response properties of cutaneous mechanoreceptors during controlled mechanical stimulation applied to the index finger and discusses the implications of the findings for neuroprostheses grasp control.

1.1 Control Strategies for Normal and Neuroprosthetic Grasp

Behavioral studies in which normal subjects grasped an object that could be pulled away unexpectedly, showed that a natural servo regulation operates in which the grasp force is increased or relaxed so as to maintain only a modest safety margin to prevent the object from slipping. This regulation acts to preserve a linear relationship between the magnitude of the pulling and grasp forces. Moreover, the constant of proportionality for this relationship is adapted for the friction between the fingers and the grasped object. This concept is illustrated in the cartoon in Figure 1, while actual data obtained from a human subject is presented in Figure 2. It has also been shown that the magnitude of the grip force increase that is evoked by a perturbing increase in the pulling force is graded with the rate of application of the perturbation but is independent of the pre-existing level of the grip force. Details of this sensory-motor behavior can be found in the reports by Johansson and his colleagues (1992 a,b).

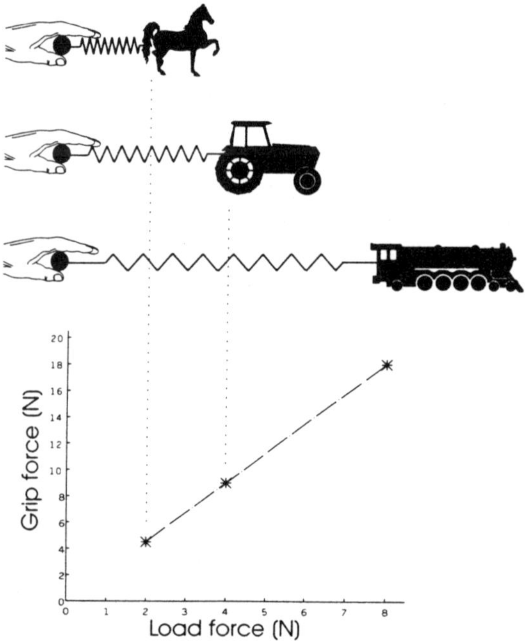

Fig. 1. Illustrating the behavior of the natural grasp strategy that is based on sensing the stretch forces imposed on the skin by a pulling load. As the stretch force is increased (shown in the figure by pulling the spring out to a greater length), the magnitude of the grip force is automatically increased in a proportional manner. The proportionality constant depends on the friction between the skin and the object and on individual personal preferences.

A second mode of natural grasp control is based on automatic increases of the grasp effort that are triggered by small slips between the object and the fingers.

This paper describes the responses of the whole nerve to mechanical perturbations of skin stretch and of slippage of a contactor across the digital skin to determine to what extent the ENG signal can be used in an artificial 'reflex' grasp control strategy that is based on the principals of the natural grasp regulation.

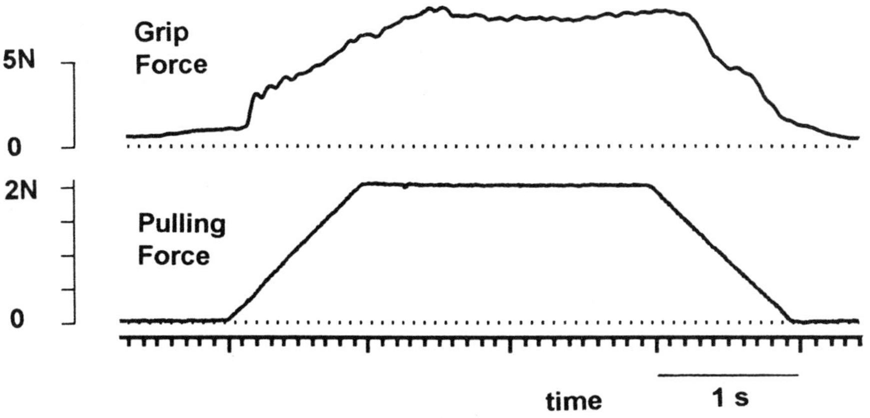

Fig. 2. Depicting the relationship between the grasp force and a pulling load when a normal individual was asked to restrain an object using the precision grip between the index finger and the thumb. A modest level of grip force (ca. 0.7N) was present initially to maintain contact of the fingers with the object. The pulling force was applied at an unannounced time and consisted of a linear ramp increase that applied a shear load to the fingers. As the pulling force increased, the grasp force continually increased in a manner that tracked the demands of the pulling force. The repetitive increases in the grip force during "tracking" reflect an automatic motor control program that is mediated sub-cortically and has a period which is typically between 8 and 15 Hz.

2 Methods

2.1 Location of the Recording Cuff

The ENG was obtained using a tri-polar neural recording cuff (similar to that described in Hoffer et al. 1990) placed around the radial branch of the common digital nerve that innervates the lateral border of the index finger. This nerve branch was selected because its 'receptive field' territory at this position is appropriate to register grasping events during prehension tasks involving 'key grip'.

2.2 Apparatus for Mechanically Stimulating the Skin

2.2.1 Skin Stretch - The experiments involving skin stretch were performed in a laboratory using the dual axis servo apparatus shown in Figure 3. To increase the range of stretch (shear) forces that could be studied at a minimal level of contact force, the contactor was covered with double faced tape. The contactor was then lowered to just make contact with the skin and the contact force was regulated to be equal to 0 N. Activation of the torque motor caused lateral movement of the contactor which imposed a stretching force on the skin. This force was measured and used as a feedback control signal to the torque motor which was programmed to produce trapezoidal force profiles. Our intention was to study the nerve response to stretch without the confounding influence of normal directed (contact) forces as much as possible. A series of stimulus profiles was used during separate trials that consisted of five different rates (1, 2, 4, 8 and 16 N/s) and five different amplitudes (0.5, 1, 1.5, 2, 2.5 N). At least ten trials were tested at each rate and amplitude combination, and the results for identical stimulus trials were studied individually as well as ensemble averaged.

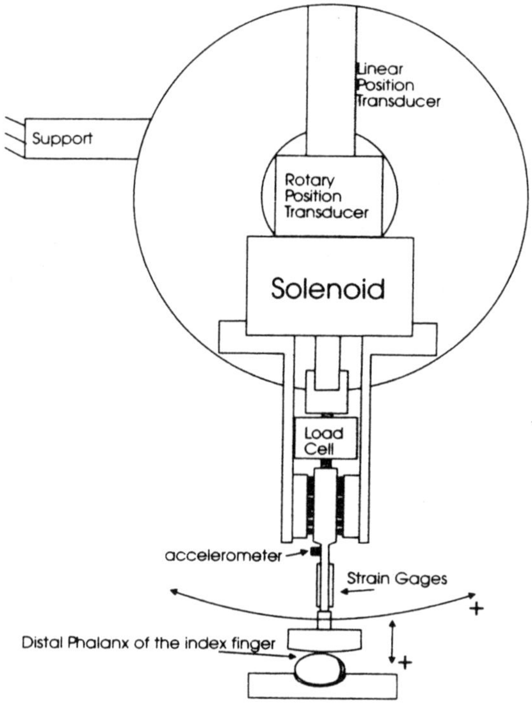

Fig. 3. Dual-axis servo system for mechanical stimulation of the finger. The apparatus consists of two independent motors. The solenoid provides arbitrary levels of contact force. Activation of the torque motor causes a lateral motion of the contactor that can be used to stretch the skin or to simulate slippage of a grasped object. Sensors register the contact and lateral forces and the vertical and horizontal contactor positions. Additionally, an accelerometer provides an indication of slippage events.

2.2.2 Studies of Slippage - The neural response to slippage was investigated by lowering the contactor to the skin and applying a prescribed contact force through servo regulation of the solenoid motor. The contactor was then moved at constant velocity by activation of the torque motor at one of several rates (5, 10, 15, 25 and 35 mm/s). Once the shear force exceeded the frictional force, the contactor began to slide over the skin.

2.3 Neural Recording and Signal Processing

The signal from the nerve was differentially amplified, band pass filtered (800 - 5kHz), digitally sampled at 12,800 Hz, and stored on magnetic disk for off-line analysis. During the analysis, the ENG was full wave rectified and integrated using a sliding window averager (typically 23 ms window). Mechanical signals that were recorded included the shear and normal (contact) forces; the lateral and vertical positions of the contactor, and the output from an accelerometer which aided in detecting slippage events. All of the mechanical signals were sampled at 400 Hz.

3 Results

3.1 Responses to Skin Stretch

The sensory capacity of the digital skin is very sensitive to stretch. A typical example of the response to a ramp stretch is shown in Figure 4. After a minimal level of stretch is exceeded, the magnitude of the integrated nerve response is seen to grow as the stretch force increases. At least two factors may be assumed to contribute to this behavior - For mechanoreceptor afferent units whose receptive fields lie behind the contactor, more and more nerve fibers begin discharging as their thresholds are exceeded by the increasing skin stretch. In addition, once these afferents begin to discharge, their firing rates increase with additional increase in the stretch magnitude. At the same time, but in opposition to these effects, there is a decreasing influence from afferents whose receptive fields lie ahead of the contactor as follows: In unperturbed skin there are always some residual stresses present that cause a percentage of stretch sensitive afferents to be tonically active. To some degree, the forward movement of the contactor acts to 'unload' these inherent stresses in the skin ahead of the direction of movement causing some of these normally discharging receptors to now become silent. Such behavior can be inferred on the basis of the reported results of microneurographic studies of the directional selectivity of stretch sensitive afferents from the digital skin in man (Johansson 1976) and from the interpreted findings of other researchers who studied the mechanics of the glabrous skin (see Pubols et al. 1987 for further discussion and Srinivasan et al. 1990).

The effect of increasing the rate of the skin stretch is to evoke a more rigorous discharge from the nerve. This can be seen in Figure 6 which presents averaged data from stretch trials at rates of 2,4,8 and 16N/s. Measurement of the integrated nerve activity 50 ms after the start of the ramp stretch, yields an approximately linear function with the rate of stretch. (Riso et al. 1994)

This result is encouraging for the use of the nerve signal in grasp regulation, because it suggests that an adaptive control strategy could be employed. Thus, a faster rate of skin stretch implies more rapid build up of shear force and a more imminent possibility for object slippage. This can be anticipated to some degree by detecting the more robust increase in nerve activity evoked by the faster rate of stretch. Such information can then be used to elicit a greater increase in grip force.

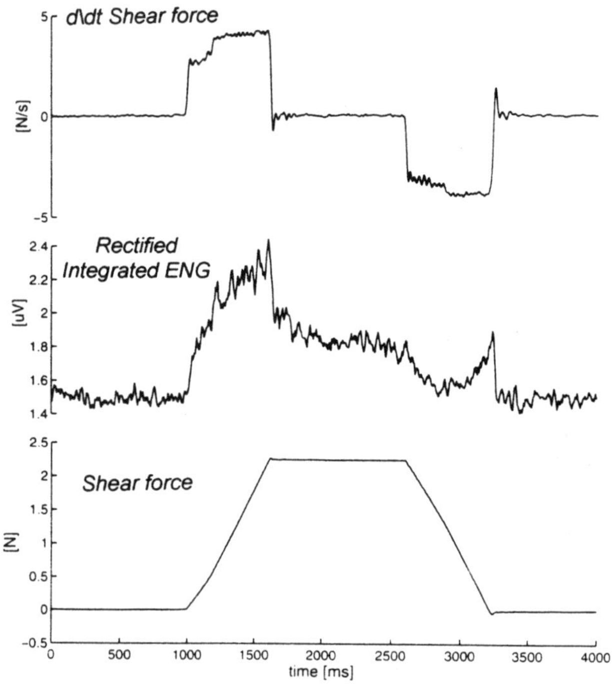

Fig. 4. ENG response of the digital skin to stretch. ENG activity is seen to increase as the magnitude of the applied stretch rises. As soon as the static phase of the stimulus is reached there is an appreciable decline in the activity to a plateau level that is a function of the stretch magnitude.

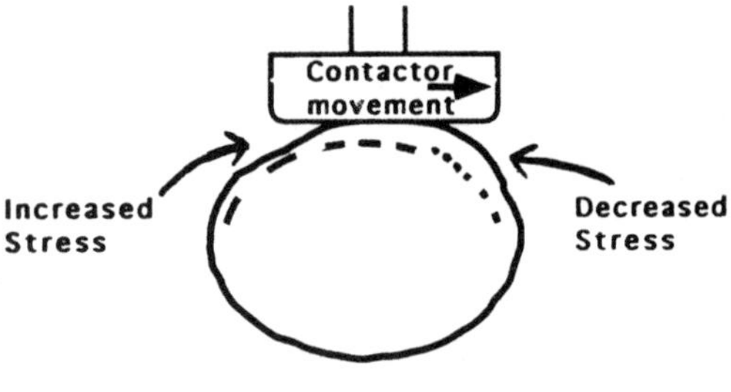

Fig. 5. Depicting the action of the advancing contactor as it stretches the skin. The index finger is shown in end view and with the contactor positioned over the radial aspect of the distal phalange. Movement of the contactor to the right causes the skin behind of the direction of motion to have increased stress while the skin ahead of the contactor motion undergoes a reduction of inherent skin stress. This is illustrated by the use of elongated and fore-shortened dashed lines to the left and right of the contactor, respectively.

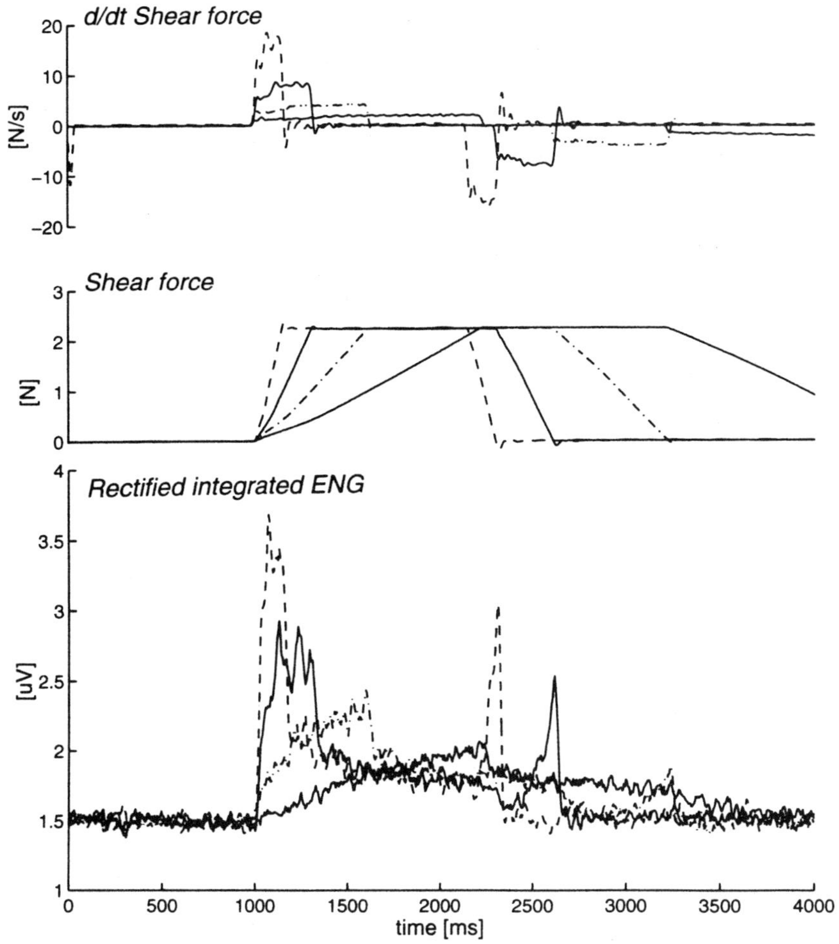

Fig. 6. Effect of rate of stretch on the ENG response. Increasing the rate of stretch results in an increased ENG response which has a shorter latency following the stretch onset. Each trace represents the superimposed average of ten independent test trials at arbitrary velocities of 2, 4, 8 and 16 N/s.

3.2. Responses to Contactor Slippage

While it would be desirable to study the neural responses to pure isolated slippage events, this is not possible to achieve in practice. Slippage involves a series of sequella as follows: Initially, there must be skin contact and this implies the presence of a normal contact force. Secondly, slippage requires that there be a position change of the contactor relative to the skin. Since a contact force is present and there is movement of the contactor surface, then the frictional forces (even if sliding friction) cause the skin to be stretched to some extent so that stretch responses are superimposed with the slippage. Finally, the contact with the skin is upset and replaced with an abrupt partial release of the frictional force, followed by a chattering or bumping of the object along the surface. The salient characteristic of slippage then can actually be a series of stretch and release actions on the skin. Such features are illustrated in Figure 7.

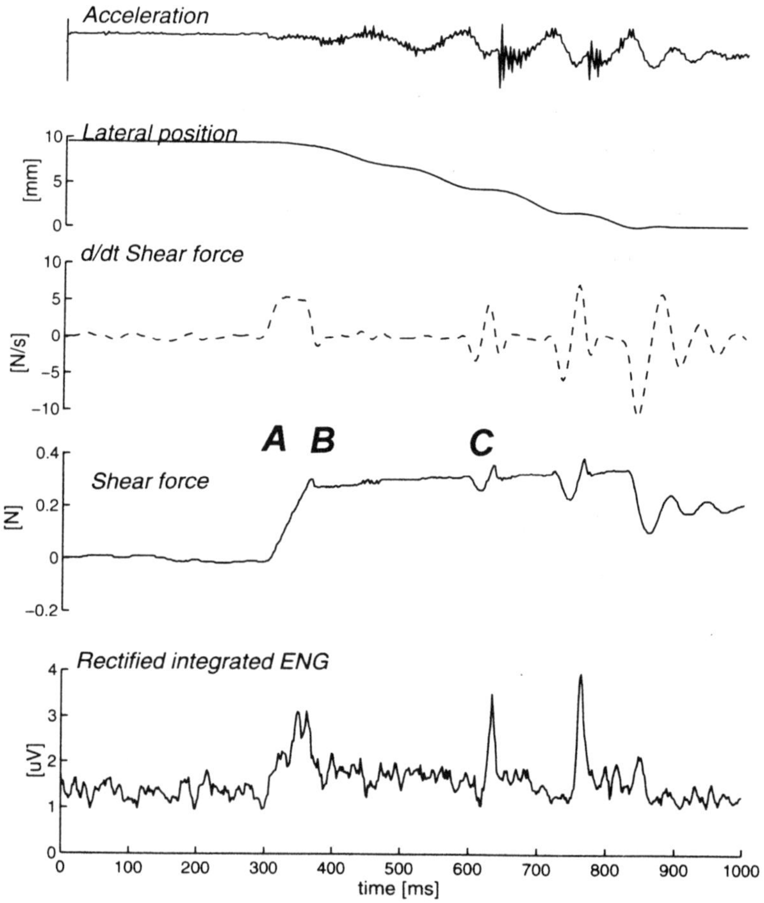

Fig. 7. Depicting a typical ENG response during a slippage test trial. A silk covered contactor was moved at 20mm/s over the skin of the lateral side of the index finger. The contact force was 0.7N throughout the trial. Details see text.

During ***'A'*** the skin is being stretched as verified by the increased shear force that parallels the contactor position change. At ***'B'*** there is an abrupt and partial release of the shear force, and this results in a decrease in the neural activity. An epoch of sliding is seen next as inferred from the rather flat (constant) shape of the shear force trace. In this example the nerve activity for the sliding phase is less than during the stretch phase but greater then the background activity. A dramatic increase in neural activity occurs at ***'C'***, however, when the friction increases abruptly and the skin is suddenly subjected to an increase in stretch. This region deserves some discussion, because it was previously interpreted as the hallmark of a slippage event.

Present efforts to detect the event such as found at ***'C'*** consist of differentiating the integrated nerve activity and passing the resultant signal through a threshold level detector algorithm as was described by Hoffer and Haugland (1992) for the cat toe pad and more recently for application in control of neuroprosthetic key grip (Lickel et al. 1995). Such an algorithm might not detect slips in a reliable manner, however, since the event at ***'C'*** may occur much later then the actual onset of slippage ***'B'***, or the event ***'C'*** might not occur at all despite the presence of prior continual slippage.

It will be important for the controller to react to the stretch response at ***'A'*** by increasing the grip force and hence avoid the slip condition at ***'B'*** altogether. This wouldn't always be possible, however, because the response to the stretch would be very minimal if the stretch is applied at a slow rate. Much work is needed to define a reliable technique to identify slow changes in shear forces and the onset of event ***'B'*** if slippage does occur. To this end it might be useful to search for changes in the frequency spectral components associated with the skin stretch phase ***'A'*** versus the release event ***'B'*** and sliding (Slot and Riso 1995).

An additional analysis that might prove helpful could include the variability in neuronal firing rates during the different mechanical (skin) conditions. The rational behind this speculation derives from the behavior of the tonic SAII (stretch sensitive) mechanoreceptors which normally have a regular discharge rate versus the highly phasic (and less regular) discharge associated with FAI and FAII mechanoreceptors (Vallbo and Johansson 1978).

3.3 Other Characteristics of Slippage Responses

Preliminary studies reveal several additional properties of the afferent activity during slippage. A comparison of the ENG activity during sliding when a more slippery surface is used showed that there are fewer neural discharges for the more slippery surface. This predicts that it will be more difficult to detect slippage for a more slippery surface, and this is just opposite to the relationship that we would like to have for the controller. That is, it is a disadvantage that the slippery surface, which implies an inherently greater risk of object lose by slippage, will evoke a slip signal that will be less easily detected.

The effect of slip rate, however, is more encouraging since the ENG evoked during sliding at a higher rate was observed to increase in comparison to a slower rate. As was previously discussed for the rate sensitivity of the ENG in response to skin stretch, one can experiment with an adaptive control strategy where the neuroprosthetic grasp effort is increased by a greater increment when the magnitude of the response during slippage is greater.

4 Discussion

The use of the whole nerve ENG for feedback control of neuroprosthetic grasp presents some substantial challenges. Such simplistic information such as object contact and release would seem to be readily obtained from the ENG, especially when the user's intention to close or to open the hand is anticipated: Contact is then a transition from background activity to an abrupt increase in activity, and release is a return of the activity to the background level. A problem arises, however, when the finger bends during hand closure (before contacting the object) since this elicits afferent neuronal activity from the finger joint receptors and from the skin that is stretched around the joints. Such nerve activity appears similar on gross examination to that obtained during true object contact. The neural prosthesis controller may simply have to ignor the nerve feedback signal during the object acquisition phase of the grasping function if means can not be developed to distinguish between finger movement and object contact.

More ambitious signal extraction tasks include obtaining information about the magnitude of the grasp force; the magnitude and direction of any shear forces present; the occurrence and magnitude of slippage events and an assessment of the current frictional properties of the grasped object. All of this information is available from the mechanoreceptors during the control of grasp in the intact individual. What makes recovering this information from the ENG difficult is the use of the nerve recording cuff itself which integrates and effectively scrambles the modality specific information provided by the four classes of mechanoreceptors present within the digital skin (i.e. those roughly specialized to register contact, sustained force, stretch and vibration, respectively).

Realizing this, it would seem advantageous to record the afferent information on a single fiber level so that the modality specificity of the various mechanoreceptors is preserved. There are some substantial issues to resolve, however, before a 'single fiber' recording approach can be effectively utilized. The first issue concerns the development of a stable, high channel capacity neural interface. Silicon micromachined electrodes, 'microprobes', are being fabricated and tested in many laboratories and offer channel densities on the order of several dozen for planar arrays and this can be increased to one hundred or more for three dimensional structures (Bement et al.1986; Edell et al. 1992). The biggest problems with using these devices have to do with their stability within the nerve tissue, and the need to maintain the integrity of the lead wires that must connect to the probes. Although the probes can be fabricated with feature sizes of the same order as the neural elements themselves, the smallest movements can bring a given set of recording electrode sites into contact with an entirely different nerve fiber. This could be catastrophic for a controller since the replacement fiber might have a different receptive field territory on the skin or it might subserve a different tactile modality (stretch versus vibration, for example). Impressive achievements such as the production of micro-ribbon cables that are the thickness of a human hair and contain 8 or more conductive vias (Hetke et al. 1990); together with the incorporation of 'on-board' channel multiplexing circuitry may eventually help to solve these problems (Najafi et al. 1985).

In the meantime, nerve cuff technology seems much closer at hand. Implanted cuffs have been deployed clinically for several decades for phrenic nerve activation in respiratory assists (Glen and Phelps 1985) and in other nerve stimulation applications (most notably for bladder control following spinal cord injury) (Brindley 1994). Moreover, initial experiences with chronically implanted recording cuffs in Aalborg have been encouraging (Haugland et al. 1992; Sinkjaer et al. 1994).

It should be useful to continue to explore the limits of the information that can be obtained with the nerve recording cuff approach while making some refinements and innovations in cuff design to improve their safety/biocompatibility and immunity to the pick up of electrical artifacts. A further avenue for cuff development is the possibly to selectively record from different fascicles within the cuffed nerve. Cuffs that contain multiple small electrode facets distributed circumferentially around the nerve (Veraart et al. 1994) may be useful in this regard, and there are efforts underway as well (Tyler and Durand 1993), to design a cuff that contains electrodes that are under moderate spring pressure when installed so that they alter the morphology of the underlying compound nerve by slowly insinuating themselves among its fascicles.

5 Acknowledgments

The authors wish to acknowledge the contributions of several individuals during the preparation and data collection phases of much of the research reported in this article. In particular, Dr. Morton Haugland fabricated the nerve recording cuff that was implanted; Dr. Jens Haase performed the surgical cuff implantation; and Dr. Thomas Sinkjaer provided technical advice and help with coordinating the studies. A large measure of gratitude is extended to Mr. Mads Bendt who was the volunteer subject. We would also like to thank the Danish National Research Foundation and the COWI Foundation for their financial support of the research and the Human Capital and Mobility Program of the EU for providing salary support for Mr. Peter Slot.

References

Bement, S., Wise, K., Anderson, D., Najafi, K., and Drake, K. (1986) Solid-state electrodes for multichannel multiplexed intracortical neuronal recording., IEEE Trans. Biomed. Eng., **33**:230-241.

Brindley, G. (1994) The first 500 patients with sacral anterior root stimulator implants: general description. Paraplegia, **32**:795-805.

Chizeck, H, Lan, L. Streeter-Palmieri, and Crago, P. (1991) Feedback control of electrically stimulated muscle using simultaneous pulse width and stimulus period modulation. IEEE Trans. BME **38**:1224-1234.

Crago, P., Nakai, R., and Chizeck, H. (1991) Feedback regulation of hand grasp opening and contact force during stimulation of paralyzed muscle. IEEE Trans BME **38**: 17-28.

Edell, D, Toi, V., McNeil, V., and Clark, D. (1992) Factors influencing the biocompatibility of insertable silicon microshafts in cerebral cortex.

Glenn, W. and Phelps, M. (1985) Diaphragm pacing by electrical stimulation of the phrenic nerve. Neurosurgery, **17**:974-984.

Haugland, M. Hoffer, J., and Sinkjaer, T. (1994) Skin contact force information in sensory nerve signals recorded by implanted cuff electrodes, IEEE Trans. Rehabilitation Engr. **2**:18-28.

Haugland, M., Lickel, A., Riso, R., Adamczyk, M., Keith, M. Jensen, I, Haase, J., and Sinkjaer, T. (1995) Restoration of lateral hand grasp using natural sensors. Proc. 5th Vienna Intl. Workshop on Functional Electrical Stimulation. 335-338.

Hetke, J., Najafi, K., and Wise, K. (1990) Flexible miniature ribbon cables for long-term connection to implantable sensors. Sensors and Actuators, **A21-A23**:999-1002.

Hoffer, J.A. and Haugland, M. (1992) Signals from tactile sensors in glabrous skin suitable for restoring motor functions in paralyzed humans. In: Stein, R.B., Peckham, P., Popovivic, D. (Eds) Neural Prostheses: replacing motor function after disease or disability. Oxford University Press, New York, 99-25.

Johnson, K.O., Popovic, D., Riso, R., Koris, M, Van Doren, C., and Kantor, K. (1995) Perspectives on the role of afferent signals in the control of motor neuroprostheses. Medical Engineering and Computing. (In press).

Johansson, R.S. (1976) Skin mechanoreceptors in the human hand: receptive field characteristics. In *Sensory Functions of the Skin of Primates* (ed. Zotterman) 159-170. Oxford

Johansson, R.S., Riso, R., Hager, C., and Backstrom, L. (1992a) Somatosensory control of precision grip during unpredictable pulling loads. I. Changes in load force amplitude. Exp. Brain Res **89**: 181-191.

Johansson, R.S., Hager, C., and Riso, R. (1992b) Somatosensory control of precision grip during unpredictable pulling loads. II. Changes in load force rate. Exp. Brain Res **89**: 192-203.

Kilgore K., Peckham, H, Keith, M, Thrope, G., and Gallaher-Stone, K. (1989) Synthesis of hand grasp using functional neuromuscular stimulation. IEEE Trans. BME **36**:761-770.

Lickel, A. , Haugland, M., and Sinkjaer, T.S. (1996) Extraction of slip information from digital nerve signals in man. (This volume).

Najafi, K. Wise, K., and Mochizuki, T. (1985) A high-yield IC-compatible multichannel recording array. IEEE Trans. on Electron Devices **32**:1206-1211.

Pubols, B. Jr. (1987) Effect of mechanical stimulus spread across glabrous skin of raccoon and squirrel monkey hand on tactile primary afferent fiber discharge. Somatosensory Research, **4**:273-308.

Riso, R., Slot, P., Haugland, M., and Sinkjaer, T. (1995) Characterization of cutaneous nerve responses for control of neuromotor prostheses. Proc. 5th Vienna Intl. Workshop on Functional Electrical Stimulation. p 335-338.

Sinkjaer, T., Haugland, M., and Haase , J. (1994) Natural neural sensing and artificial muscle control in man. Exp. Brain Res., **98**:542-545.

Slot, P. and Riso, R. (1995) Spectral analysis of cutaneous mechanoreceptor ENG activity recorded from a digital nerve in man. Abstracts of the Society for Neurosciences 25th Annual Meeting, San Diego, CA.

Srinivasan, M., Whitehouse, J., and LaMotte, R. (1990) Tactile detection of slip: Surface microgeometry and peripheral neural codes. J. Neurophysiology **63**:1323-1332.

Tyler, D., and Durand, D. (1993) Design and acute test of a radially penetrating interfascicular nerve electrode. Proceedings of the 9th Annual IEEE/EMBS Conference on Biomedical Engineering 1247-1248.

Vallbo, Å-B, and Johansson, R.S. (1978) The tactile sensory innervation of the glabrous skin of the human hand. In *Active Touch* (ed. G. Gordon) 29-54. Oxford

Veraart, C., Grill, W., and Mortimer, T. (1993) Selective control of muscle activation with a multipolar nerve cuff electrode. IEEE Trans BME **40**:640-653.

Selective Intraneural Sensing for Neuroprosthetics

L. C. W. Rutten[1] and H. J. Meier[2]
[1]Institute for BioMedical Technology, University of Twente, Enschede, NL
[2]Biotronik, Friedrich-Alexander-University, Erlangen, Germany

Abstract - A brief overview on the possible use of natural sensor signals for control of motion opens this contribution. A model for the calculation of extracellular action potentials inside a rat peroneal nerve, as recorded by intraneural electrodes, is presented. This one-fascicle nerve has the dimensions and conductivities of the rat peroneal nerve branch, which serves as our animal model for human fascicles. The model results show a wide variety of wave shapes to be measured, depending on the position of the intraneural electrode with respect to the fibre axis and to the nodes of Ranvier and depending on the presence of an isolating medium around the nerve. Action potential shapes may range from the 'classical' quasi-biphasic one, to more triphasic, or even more complicated in the case of an isolating cuff being present around the nerve. Results on selectivity measures, based on the same model, are presented also. Finally, preliminary recordings of action potentials made with Tungsten micro electrodes in rat peroneal nerve are presented and compared to model results.

1 Introduction

Forward stimulation of muscle by intraneural electrodes would evolve into local closed loop control of muscle force if supplemented by feedback information, recorded from muscle and tendon afferent (small groups of) fibers.
One of the options for the recording is to consider the use of the intraneural 128-micro-electrode system (figure 1), currently being developed at the University of Twente (BMTI/ MESA institutes) using silicon micromachining technology (Rutten et al, 1995).

The following aspects, among many others, then have to be addressed and worked upon:

1. Is enough known about the way information from natural muscle and tendon sensors is organized and used in the intact system for *control of motion* ? Has tactile information to be added, or is tactile (skin) information even the most important ? Do we know the clues for proximal or distal positioning of implanted systems (for stimulation and recording) along peripheral nerves?
2. Given a single versus a large number of electrodes, how selective can information be extracted? How does the contact spacing between electrode and nerve fibers influence *selective recording*?

This contribution addresses these two aspects, with emphasis mainly on the second, selective intraneural recording aspect.

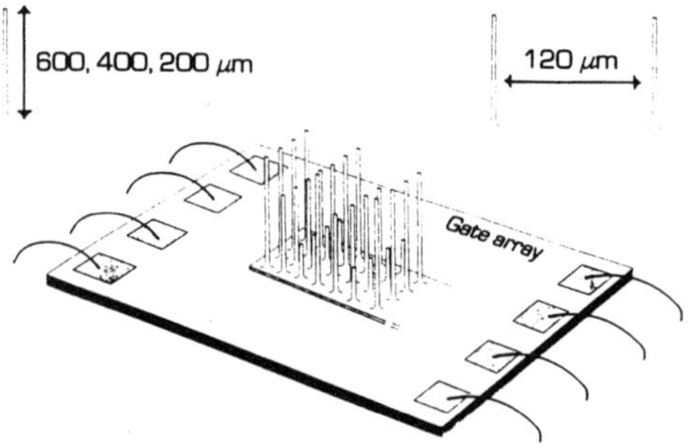

Fig. 1. Schematic drawing of the completely assembled 3D silicon multi-micro-electrode, mounted on the electronic circuitry gate array chip. For clarity, only a portion of the 4 x 32 arrangement of 128 electrodes has been sketched. The circuitry contains multiplexers for electrode selection, current sources for stimulation and amplifiers for recording.

2 Control of Motion

In the classical view, neuromuscular control is proposed to take place by reflexes (Brown, Sherrington, 1911-1924), more specifically by spinal rhythm generators, triggered by sensory signals.

Later this century it was observed that decerebrated cats can walk, trot and gallop on a treadmill by simple electrical stimulation of the locomotor region in what is left from the brainstem.

Modern research (Grillner et al., 1985) basically confirms Brown's proposal: rhythm generators in the spinal cord control each leg of the cat, they continue to do so after eliminating leg-sensory input (this does not mean that sensory input has no use: it may alter the movement pattern).

In most modern research (see Prochazka, 1993, for an overview) the idea is that open loop motor programs do certain tasks; finite-state control, of which the state-transitions are controlled by sensory vectors, performs other tasks.

The problem is, however, that the sensory vectors are almost still unknown, so we do not yet understand the role of physiological sensors. Sensors probably determine the transition to the next state of motor programs; while motor programs may be spinally based; transition decisions are higher brain functions. How the brain interprets the *ASSEMBLIES* of sensory information, is still largely unknown.

Accordingly, the question: *IS THERE A NEED TO USE PHYSIOLOGICAL SENSORS for (closed loop) artificial control?* can in fact not be answered properly. Tentatively, the answer is: maybe there is a need for simple tasks;

probably there is for complicated tasks (but there is a lack of understanding how). For simple tasks, artificial sensors may be preferred (Prochazka, 1993).

Then, if needed: *WHICH PHYSIOLOGICAL SENSORS are to be used?* Again, no clear answer is available, but choices could be: skin sensors (contact, avoidance), muscle spindles sensors (length, velocity); tendon organ sensors (force). Joint sensors ?

Another *BASIC ISSUE*: Can the neural output of physiological sensors, or, more generally, can nerves or (small groups of) fibers be 'contacted' *SELECTIVELY*? For example, for sensing of afferents in restoration of neuromuscular function in FES. Or, for sensing of efferent activity, in case of control of a powered amputee's prosthesis.

This relates directly to the level of selectivity, which should be chosen carefully: is the recording of whole nerve compound action potential bursts (use of neural cuffs) most appropiate ? Or, more selectively, fascicle's CAP bursts (use of fascicular cuffs) are a better choice? Or, utmost selective, do intrafascicular CAP's (use of multi electrode arrays) deserve preference? Although the choice may depend on many practical aspects, we want to stress that the choice must always be subordinate to *Neuroanatomical/Bioelectric/(Micro)Technological boundaries of selective recording.*

3 Selective Recording

3.1 The Model and Model Results

3.1.1 Introduction to the Model

It has been shown that in case of electrical stimulation the highest degree of selectivity will be achieved with dense 3-dimensional "lattices" of electrodes, placed inside the fascicles (Meier et al 1992a, Rutten et al 1991) These intraneural stimulation electrodes, however, can also be used to monitor nerve signals.

One may expect that in a typical fascicle, with diameter of 0.5 mm and a typical fiber diameter of 10 μm, there will be a large influence of the position of the electrode with respect to the nodes of Ranvier and to the fascicle boundary, as the typical node spacing of a 10 μm, fiber is 1 millimeter giving a fasicle radius-to-node- spacing ratio of only 0.5! Therefore, for proper processing the signals (monopolar or bipolar, filtering, averaging) it is of importance to know how the ap-waveshape and amplitude vary with position of the electrode and conductivity of surrounding media.

It will give clues also for the amount of selectivity that can be reached with multi-electrode device configurations.

An algorithm is developed for the calculation of the extracellular potential field of an active myelinated nerve fibre inside a fibre bundle and it is shown how these signals depend on the position of the electrode relative to the fibre and its active nodes. Also the effect of an insulator (cuff) around the nerve is calculated.

3.1.2 The Model

3.1.2.1 Calculation of Extracellular Potential Field of an Active Nerve fibre

For the fibre bundle and its surroundings a simplified conductor model is used and an analytical expression is derived for the potential field of a point current source placed arbitrarily inside this bundle. The active nerve fibre is modeled as a number of point current sources and its potential field is calculated as a linear summation of the fields of these separate sources.

The nerve - A nerve is modeled that contains only one fascicle. It is idealized as two coaxial, homogeneous, infinitely extending cylinders (Fig. 2). The inner cylinder represents the fascicle and has a radius a, a radial conductivity σ_ρ and a longitudinal conductivity σ_z. The outer cylindrical cell represents the epineurium and has a radius b and an isotropic conductivity σ_o.

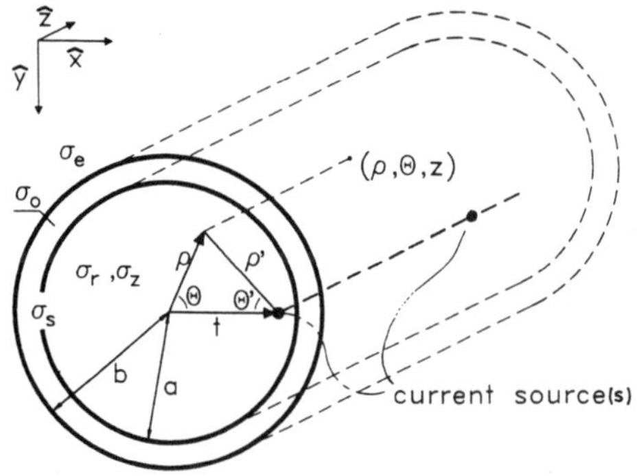

Fig. 2. The volume conduction model of the nerve and its surroundings. Longitudinal and radial conductivity inside the fascicle are σ_Z and σ_r, respectively. Perineural sheath conductivity σ_S; epineural conductvity σ_O and extraneural conductivity σ_e. For parameter values, see Table 1.

σ_ρ=*0.1* $\Omega^{-1}m^{-1}$ *,conductivity of the fascicle in radial direction*
σ_z = *0.5* $\Omega^{-1}m^{-1}$, *and longitudinal direction*
σ_s = *2000* $\Omega^{-1}m^{-1}$, *conductivity of the perineural sheath*
σ_o = *0.1* $\Omega^{-1}m^{-1}$, *conductivity of epineurium*
σ_e = *10/ 0.1/ 0.001* $\Omega^{-1}m^{-1}$, *conductivity of the extraneurium*
a = *250* μm, *radius of the fascicle*
b = *320* μm, *radius of the nerve*
r = *200* μm, *radial position of the fibre*
λ = *1000* μm, *internode length*
v = *57.1 m/s, propagation velocity*

Table 1. Parameter Values

Between the cylinders a sheath, with sheet-conductivity σ_s, represents the thin perineurium. The nerve is immersed in a homogeneous and infinite medium with conductivity σ_e. In Meier (1992b) the calculation of the potential field due to a point current source placed eccentrically inside the inner cylinder is presented in detail (solving Laplace's equation under boundary conditions, using Bessel functions and the appropiate discretization and Fourier transforms).

The conductivities of the different tissues are given realistic values (for a detailed discussion on the conductivities see Meier et al 1992a). The radii of the fascicle and the epineurium are given values as measured in histological sections of rat peroneal nerve. Table 1 lists the parameter values chosen.

The active nerve fibre - The active fibre is simulated as an array of active point current sources along the fibre bundle. Each source represents a node of Ranvier. In the simulation results shown in this paper a nodal distance λ of 1000 μm is chosen. Current values correspond to the nodal currents of an active fibre of 10 μm diameter at one instant of time. These nodal currents are calculated using the simulation model for myelinated nerve fibres developed by Struijk et al (1992), see Fig. 3. The latter model calculates the membrane currents of a myelinated nerve fibre using the kinetics as described by Chiu et al (1979). These kinetics are valid at a temperature of 14 °C. The authors adopted the corrections of Struijk et al (1992) for a temperature of 37 °C.

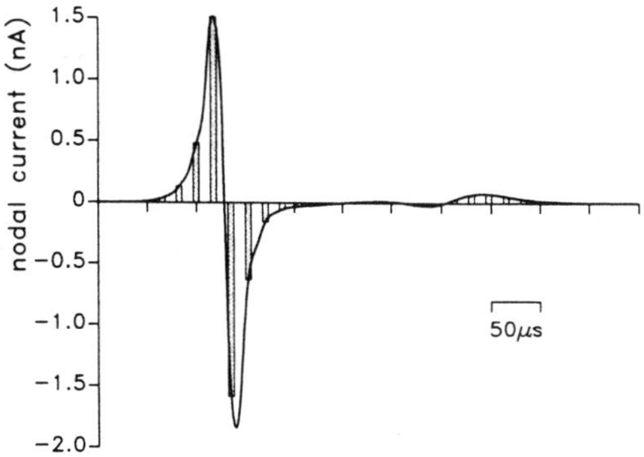

Fig. 3. Nodal currents as a function of time (continuous line) and currents of active nodes at one instant of time (bars), as used as source in the simulations.

3.1.2.2 Calculation of the Signals to be Measured with Intrafascicular Electrodes

The potential φ at a point electrode at position (x_e, y_e, z_e) due to N active nodes of Ranvier can be written as:

$$\varphi(x_e, y_e, z_e, t) = \sum_{j=1}^{N} \left\{ \psi_{x_e, y_e, z_e}(x_j, y_j, z_j) I_j(t) \right\} \tag{1}$$

where $\Psi(x_j, y_j, z_j)$ and $I_j(t)$ are the position and the current of the node indexed by j. According to the reciprocity principle the "lead field" of the electrode, $\Psi_{x_e, y_e, z_e}(x, y, z)$ is equal to the potential field that would be generated by a point source at position (x_e, y_e, z_e) divided by the source current I_e. It can thus be calculated with the same equations as used to calculate the potential field. If only one nerve fibre is active, Eq. 1 can be rewritten as

$$\sum_{n=-\infty}^{\infty} \left\{ \psi_{x_e, y_e, z_e}(x_0, y_0, z_0) I_0 \left(t - \frac{n\lambda}{v}\right) \right\} \tag{2a}$$

or

$$\sum_{n=-\infty}^{\infty} \left\{ \psi_{x_0, y_0, z_0}(x_e, y_e, z_e) I_0 \left(t - \frac{n\lambda}{v}\right) \right\} \tag{2b}$$

where (x_o, y_o, z_o) is the position of the nearest node of the active fibre, $I_o(t)$ the current at this node (see Fig. 3), v the propagation velocity and λ the internodal distance.

3.1.3 Model Results

3.1.3.1 Single Fibre Signals Measured with Intrafascicular Electrodes

Eq. 2 is an expression for the single fibre action potential that is measured at position (x_e, y_e, z_e). This signal is computed for a central active nerve fibre within nerves, surrounded by media of various conductivities. The position of the electrode is varied as shown in Fig. 4. The corresponding single fibre signals are plotted in Fig. 5.

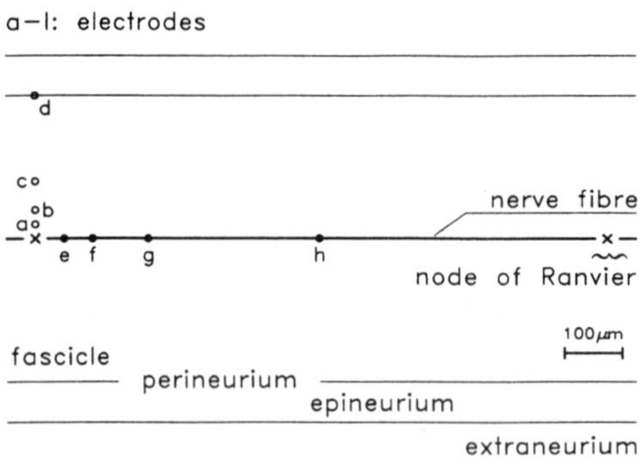

Fig. 4. Positions of electrodes and nerve fibre as used to calculate the single fibre signals shown in figure 5.

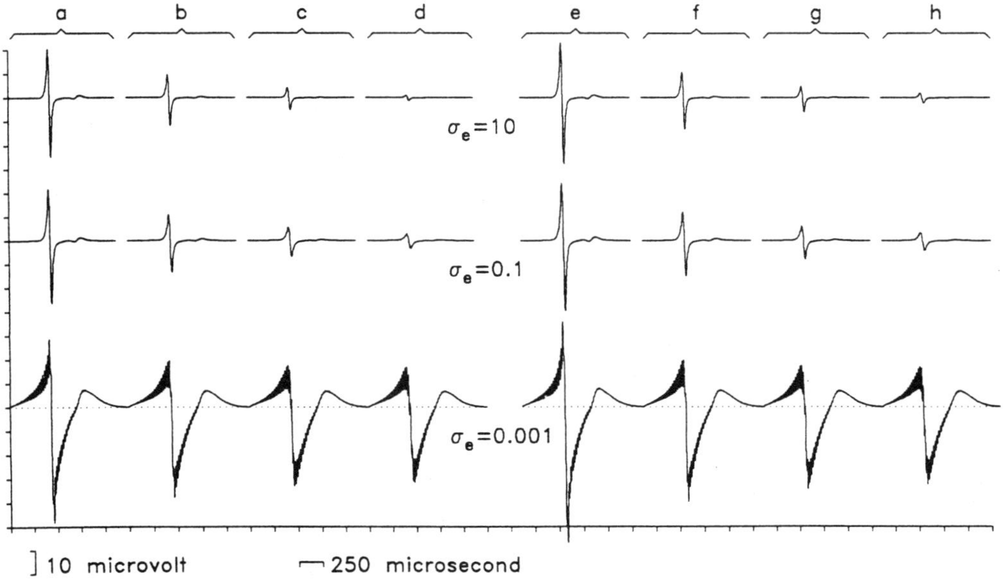

Fig. 5. The action potentials of a central nerve fibre as calculated for various values of the extraneural conductivity at the electrode positions shown in figure 4.

The fibre signals calculated for extraneural conductivities of 10 and 0.1 $\Omega^{-1}m^{-1}$ are predominantly bi-phasic. Their shapes are very similar to the shape of the nodal current as shown in Fig. 3. Their amplitudes decrease not only with the radial distance between fibre and electrode but also with the longitudinal distance between the electrode and the nearest node of Ranvier. Also, most notable at larger distances from the nodes of Ranvier, the amplitudes increase with a decreasing extraneural conductivity.

In case of a low extraneural conductivity of 0.001 $\Omega^{-1}m^{-1}$ the fibre signals not only have increased further but also became three-phasic. Their shape no longer resembles that of the nodal current. The reason is that the field due to the current of the nearest node no longer dominates. Each active node generates a homogeneous field throughout whole the bundle and therefore contributes to the signals measured at any place within.

The signals are also strongly rippled which reflects the saltatory conduction of the action potential. For a node of Ranvier the transition from large positive currents to large negative currents (from phase one to phase two, Fig. 3) takes less time then the action potential to travel one nodal distance. The phase-transition "jumps" from node to node and due to the insulation, its effect is seen on the fibre signal even if the recording electrode is at a large distance.

3.1.3.2 The Effect of a Nerve Cuff on the Single Fibre Signals

In Fig. 6 a nerve is shown that is surrounded by a nerve cuff. The fibre bundle contains an active fibre with a node of Ranvier positioned at the centre at the cuff. Near this node an electrode is placed at a position as indicated by **c** in Fig. 4. Also shown are two electrodes, placed near the two neighbouring nodes, to measure bipolar signals. The various parameter values are unchanged. The signals to be measured with the electrodes are shown in Fig. 7 for various cuff lengths.

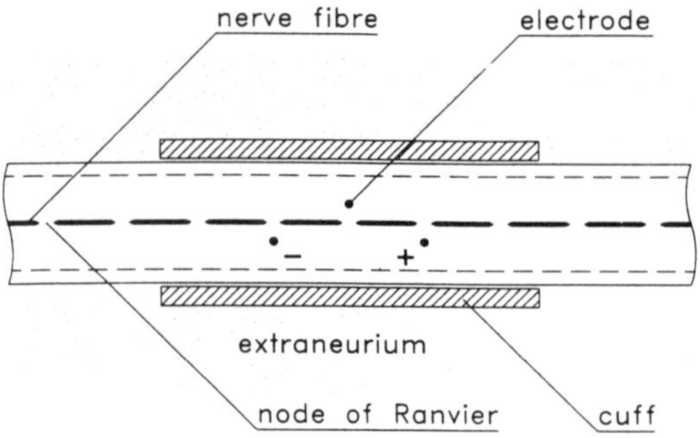

Fig. 6. A schematic view of a nerve surrounded by an isolating cuff. three electrodes are placed inside the fibre bundle to measure the signal of a central nerve fibre. The whole system is embedded in a homogeneous conductive medium; the extraneurium.

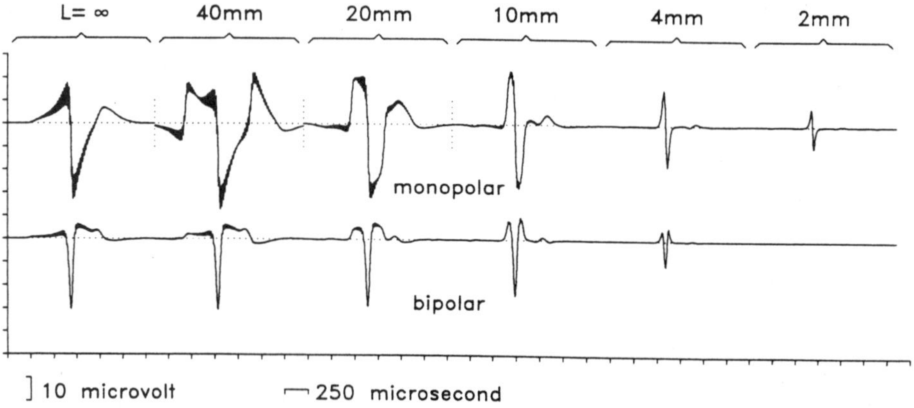

Fig. 7. The signal of a central nerve fibre for a monopolar intrafascicular electrode and for two differential electrodes 2 mm (= 2λ) aprt, at positions as indicated by c in fig. 4. The nerve is surrounded by nerve cuffs with lengths of ∞, 40, 20, 10, 4 and 2 mm. Opposite ends of the cuff are externally shunted. Axially, the electrodes lie in the middle of the cuff.

The monopolar fibre signals calculated for a relatively long cuff of 40 mm is relatively complex and contains five phases. For shorter cuffs the number of phases decreases until the signal is predominantly bi-phasic.

The bipolar fibre signals are all predominantly tri-phasic with a strong second phase, flanked by two small phases of opposite sign. The duration of these small phases decreases with decreasing cuff length.

For both monopolar and tripolar recording the signals amplitude decrease with cuff lengths below 10 mm.

3.1.4 Selectivity of Recording

3.1.4.1 Lead Field Model

Figure 8 shows the lead field for a monopolar electrode. The horizontal axis is the axial direction of the nerve. The lead field indicates for every point in the fascicle how strong a fiber is 'seen' at the electrode when a node of the fiber is positioned at that point. Figure 8 shows the case for realistic fibers in which 20 active nodes carry the action potential. The internode distance is 1 mm (corresponding to a fiber with 10 μm diameter), the fascicle diameter is 0.5 mm. Figure 8 shows one elementary section of a periodical function (periodicity is 1 mm, i.e. the internode distance). See the previous sections for the volume conduction model of the nerve and parameters (Table 1).

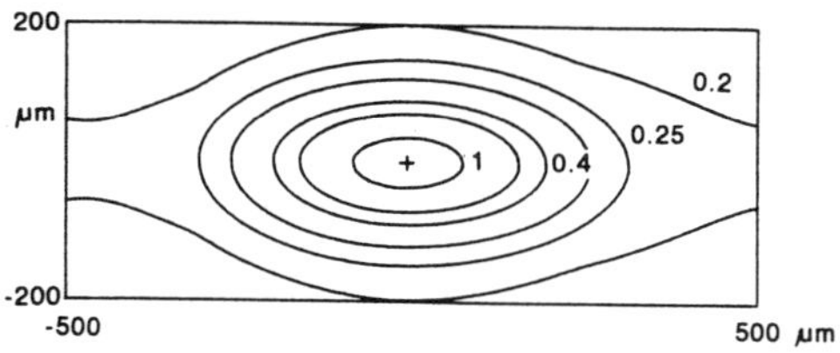

Fig. 8. Lead field (relative) equipotential contours in a cross sectional plane through the axis of the nerve (axial direction: horizontally, radial direction: vertically). The electrode is indicated by the '+' symbol. The active fibers have 20 active nodes, which produce together the action potential. See text for interpretation.

Figure 8 indicates, for example, that the selectivity ratio S (S is by definition the ratio of amplitudes V_1 and V_2 of action potentials belonging to two fibers) is two for one node of one fiber at the innermost contour and another node -of a second fiber- at the next contour, which is radially 33 μm away. It shows that with a discrimation limit of S = 2 the two fibers must be separated more than 33 μm radially, with the first fiber at the central contour. Conversely, two electrodes separated by a radial distance of 33 μm, at the most central and the second contour, would measure the signal of a central fiber with an amplitude ratio of two.

3.1.4.2 Probability Model

The next step is the calculation of the probability P that S equals or exceeds a certain threshold S_{th} (e.g 1.1,1.5 or 2) for an electrode at an arbitrary place in the bundle of nerve fibers. The calculations were done in a 'Monte Carlo' way. One electrode was placed at the center of the nerve. Fourty or hundred fibers were distributed randomly over the nerve cross section, with random node position (but fixed internode distance along each fiber). This was repeated to yield 5000 realisations. For every realisation the ratio S of the two strongest action potentials (usually those nearest to the electrode), was calculated, using the lead fields. The probability P ($S > S_{th}$) is the fraction of realisations for which $S > S_{th}$.

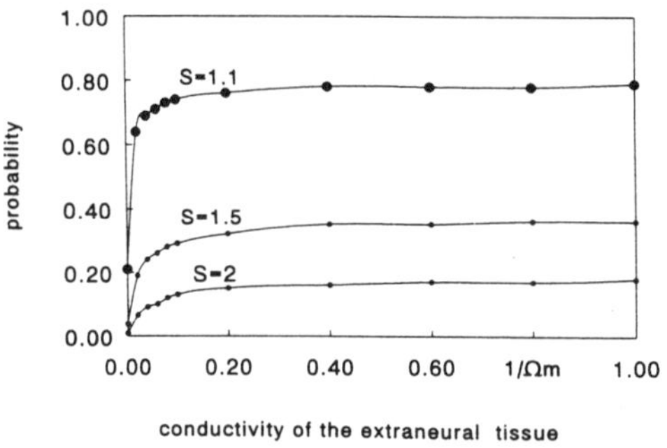

Fig. 9. The probability P ($S \geq S_{threshold}$) that the measured action potentials from those two fibres which are nearest to a central monopolar electrode have an amplitude ratio $S \geq 1.1$, 1.5 or 2, as a function of the conductivity of the extraneural tissue. The nerve has 40 active fibers (20 active nodes each).

Figure 9 shows this probability as a function of the extraneural conductivity (electrode in the center of the nerve), for selectivity thresholds S =1.1, 1.5 and 2, with 40 active fibers. A dramatic decrease in the ability to discriminate two trains is seen when the nerve is insulated from its surrounding tissue, i.e. for zero extraneural conductivity. The curves saturate to the respective limiting values S^{-3}, which is the value that is to be expected in an analytical Poisson-model calculation (infinite space, isotropic conductivity, Rutten et al. 1991, Clark et al. 1987).

From Monte Carlo simulations with 250 afferent fibers it can be derived that a central electrode has a volume with a radius of 40 μm around it, inside which the probability is 0.99 that the fiber with the largest signal at the electrode lies inthere, such that the amplitude ratio to the second largest signal (lying anywhere) $S > 2$. For $S > 1.1$ this radius is 75 μm.

These outcomes suggest that multi electrode devices should have inter electrode distances of 80 μm and 150 μm ($S \geq 2$ and $S \geq 1.1$, respectively), and that the use of insulating cuffs around the nerve should be avoided. However, it should be noted that the calculations assume a distribution of fibers over the total crossection of the fascicle, while in the rat the fibers may be clustered in subsections of the fascicle.

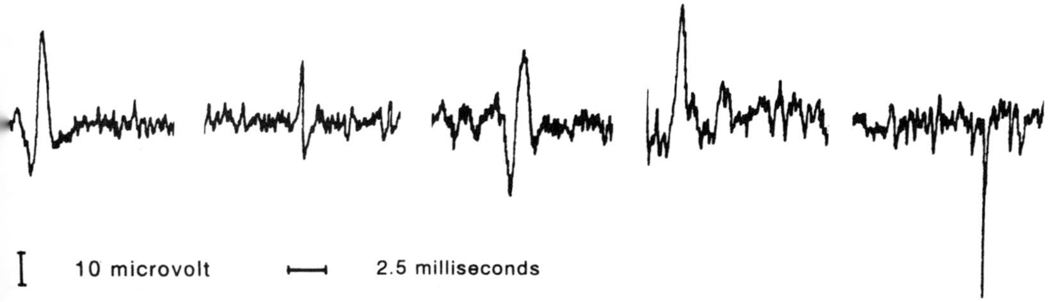

Fig. 10. Five examples of recorded ap-shapes in the five classes triphasic (- + -), biphasic (+ - or - +) and monophasic (+ or -).

3.2 Recordings with Tungsten Micro Electrodes

Tungsten wire microneurography needle electrodes were used to record monopolarly extracellular action potentials from rat peroneal (and some form sural) nerve. The animal was anaesthetised, the hind leg being prepared as to expose the peroneal nerve EDL and tibial muscle and surrounding tissue. The nerve was kept moist, animal, nerve and muscles were held at 39 Celsius. The muscles were attached to a force actuator. The electrode signal was filtered between 300 Hz and 5000 or 10000 Hz; the average noise level was 4 μV rms.
In preliminary experiments the hit rate of recording afferent nerve fibre signals in response to stretch pulses of EDL and tibial muscle was very low. Therefore another method was applied: by pinching the toes of the rat a moderate (reflex) reaction of the nervous system was evoked, resulting in appreciable nerve activity in the peroneal nerve.

By pulsatile forwarding the electrode into the nerve, several fibres were 'contacted' during one track.

Also, spontaneous activity was recorded.

This way, samples of nerve activity were taken at various, random, spots in the nerve.

Figure. 10 shows five examples, one of each class of ap wave shapes; they are taken from the results of one experiment, one animal, in which a total number of 54 ap's were recorded.

The shape classes are triphasic (- + -, 26%), biphasic (+ -, 26% and - +, 20%) and monophasic (+ , 15% and - , 13%). Table 2 gives statistics of the amplitude of each phase, and the total ap-width.

Ap-shape	*Amplitude* (μV)			*Width* (*ms*)	*N*
Triphasic					
- / + / -	*17.5*	*26*	*8.85*	*3.34*	*14*
	(7.3)	*(4.2)*	*(1.96)*	*(0.61)*	
Biphasic					
+ / -	*19.7*	*11.9*		*1.46*	*14*
	(13.3)	*(3.72)*		*(0.82)*	
- / +					
	16.6	*20.6*		*1.9*	*11*
	(5.1)	*(3.44)*		*(0.46)*	
Monophasic					
+	*18.6*			*0.66*	*8*
	(5.9)			*(0.46)*	
-	*56.4*			*0.44*	*7*
	(0.44)			*(0.04)*	

Table 2. Recorded action potentials (N = 54). *Means* and *(sample standard deviations)*

4 Comparision of Recorded and Calculated Potentials

All recordings were monopolar; the extraneural tissue conductivity is not known, it may vary between well conducting and almost isolating (the exposed nerve is lying on a support and is kept moist by saturated air). Comparison of figure 10 with figures 5 and 7 leads to the following preliminary conclusions:

- the threephasic type - + - and the biphasic type - + are not predicted, as well as the monophasic + type and the monophasic - type (although the triphasic - well-conducting case- type may appear as biphasic, when the weak third phase is hidden in the noise).
- amplitudes lie in the predicted range of biphasic shapes (positions b,c,f,g in two top rows of figure 5), and monophasic shapes (bottom row of figure 5, top left row of figure 7, second phase amplitude).
- ap-widths of all five types of recorded shapes are larger than every corresponding calculated shape. While calculation predicts triphasic widths of about 1.25 ms and biphasic widths of 0.2 ms, the corresponding experimental widths are about 3.4 ms, and 1.5/1.9 ms, i.e a factor of about 2 to 10 broader.

5 Discussion

5.1 Action Potential Shape

It has been reported that the presence of a microneurography electrode close to a nerve fiber may block the propagation of the ap (Calancie and Stein, 1988). In that case, the third phase of a triphasic ap disappears and this may explain how the calculated triphasic shape (lower series of figure 5) shows up experimentally as a biphasic +/- shape (second class from left in figure 10), or possibly even as a monophasic + shape, i.e when the second phase disappears in the noise (fourth class in fig. 10).

It may also happen that irritation of a fiber membrane by the electrode locally evokes the start of an ap. In that case the ap recorded by the electrode 'lacks the first phase' of a triphasic shape . This implies that the calculated shapes of the upper two rows of fig 5 (which are triphasic, but with a very weak third phase) would not possess the first phase and appear possibly as the monophasic class in the experiments (utmost right class in figure 10). That leaves us with classes no. 1 and no. 4 as unexplained with regard to shape.

Of course the above arguments apply only to shape aspects, disregarding the width and amplitude aspect.

5.2 Action Potential Width and Amplitude

A minor part of the observed discrepancy in width between calculation and experiment may be caused by the experimental filtering (high-pass at 300 Hz, low-pass at 5000 Hz).

The main part is possibly due to the fact that not single fiber ap's are observed, but that several fibres' contributions add up to a compound ap. In that case it is to be explained that cap-amplitudes lie in the same range as the single fiber ap's, that the width increases and that ap-shape does not change essentially (i.e. triphasic ap's add up to a triphasic cap etc).

By simulation of ap-convolution we tried to clarify these issues. The variables in ap-addition are the 'unit ap-shape' and the distribution of fiber conduction velocities (which are directly proportional to fiber diameters). By convolution of these two a cap can be synthesized.

As basic unit-ap shapes we took the two shapes of figure 5 (upper two rows versus lower row).

The fiber distribution was determined histologically from normal peroneal rat nerve cross sections.

Prelimary results of cap-synthesis are promising, they show that by such a realistic convolved addition of ap's: 1) shapes are unaltered (triphasic ap's add up to triphasic cap, biphasic to biphasic) 2) resulting cap-amplitude is of the same order as the constituing ap-amplitudes 3) cap widths may be a factor two or more broader than the constituing ap widths, depending on how much fibers take part.

References

Calancie, B. M. and Stein, R. B. (1988) Microneurography for the recording and selective stimulation of afferents: an assesment, Muscle & Nerve, vol. 11, pp. 638-644.

Chiu, S. Y., Ritchie, J. M., Rogart, R. B., and Stagg, D. (1979) A quantitative description of membrane currents in rabbit myelinated nerve, J. Physiol., vol. 292, 149-166.

Clark Jr., L. D. and Edell, D. J. (1989) A probabilistic approach to the design of microelectrode layouts for neural signal transducers, IEEE/11th Ann. Conf. of the Eng. in Med. and Bio. Soc., pp. 1-2.

Grillner, S. and Wallen, P. (1985) Central pattern generators for locomotion, with special reference to vertebrates", Ann. Rev. Neurosci., vol. 8, 233-261.

Meier, J. H. (1992b) Selectivity and design of neuro-electronic interfaces, Ph.D. Thesis, University of Twente, Enschede, Netherlands.

Meier, J. H., Rutten, W L. C., Zoutman, A. E., Boom, H. B. K., and Bergveld, P. (1992a) Simulation of multipolar fibre selective neural stimulation using intrafascicular electrodes," IEEE Trans. Biomed. Eng., vol. 39, 122-134.

Prochȧzka, A. (1993)Comparison of natural and artificial control of movement", IEEE Trans. Rehab. Eng., vol 1, 7-17.

Rutten, W. L. C., van Wier, H. J., and Put, J. H. M. (1991) Sensitivity and selectivity of intraneural stimulation using a silicon electrode array," IEEE Trans. Biomed. Eng., vol. 38, 192-198.

Rutten, W. L. C., Frieswijk, T. A., Smit, J. P. A., Rozijn, T. H., and Meier, J. H. (1995) 3D Neuro-electronic interface devices for neuromuscular control: Design studies and realisation steps, Biosensors & Bioelectronics, vol. 10, 141-153.

Struijk, J. J., Holsheimer, J., van der Heide, G. G., and Boom, H. B. K. (1992) Recruitment of dorsal column fibers in spinal cord stimulation: influence of collateral branching," IEEE Trans. Biomed. Eng., vol. 39(9), 903-912.

Myoelectric Signals from Paretic Wrist Extensor Controlling Electrical Stimulation of the Same Muscle

R.Thorsen[1,3], F.Biering-Sørensen[2], S.D.Hansen[3], O.T.Andersen[3]
[1]ASAH Medico A/S, Denmark
[2]Centre for Spinal Cord Injured, The National University Hospital, Denmark
[3]Electronics Institute, Technical University of Denmark, Denmark

Abstract - A device for enhancement of the grip in C5/6 spinal cord lesioned tetraplegics is under development. It uses the myoelectric signals from the paretic wrist extensor for control of functional electrical stimulation of the same muscle. The tetraplegics shall with the device be able to obtain a passive grip between the thumb and the index finger by extension of the wrist. Surface electrodes are used for myoelectric recording and stimulation. Main problems are filtering of the recorded signal and stimulation. Solutions to these problems are addressed and discussed.

1 Introduction

The possibility of using the myoelectric signal from a paretic muscle to control transcutaneous electric stimulation of the same muscle has been proved feasible with the use of surface electrodes (Haxthausen 1992). Others have used implanted electrodes for restoration of the hand function controlled by myoelectric signals from different muscles e.g. the shoulder (Peckham et al.1980) or by position transducers (Hines et al.1992).

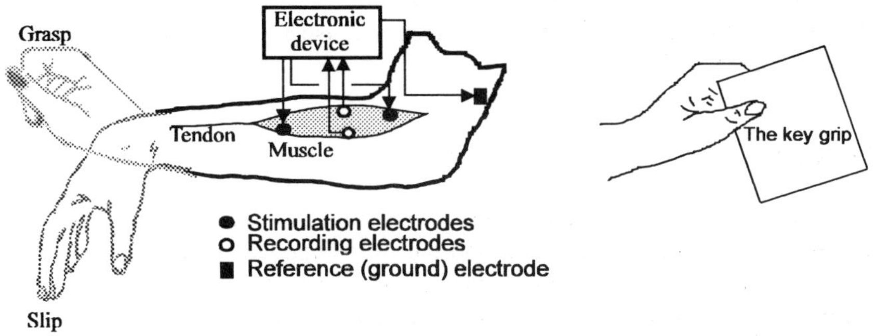

Fig. 1. Enhancement of the key grip using the tenodesis function.

It is obvious that the system must function reliably, so that the patient will gain maximum benefit from the device. This implies the solution to a wide range of problems.

The Voluntary MyoElectric Signal (VMES) from a paretic muscle contains less information than a corresponding normal muscle, because the number of motor units under voluntary control are fewer. This makes accurate estimation of the control signal more critical. Some different techniques for estimating the control signal have been considered e.g. autoregressive models (Hefftner et al. 1988) or the use of neural networks (Costa and Gander 1993). To reduce computation complexity, more simple methods based on the energy of the VMES have been chosen in the initial phase of the present project.

The recorded signal consists of the VMES and noise from different sources. The sources are: Stimulation response, mechanical actions, hum from mains and spontaneous activity. The stimulation response includes the compound motor unit action potentials, artifacts arising from the stimulation and possibly the H-reflex (Tarkka 1986) and F-wave (Stålberg et al. 1993). This is mainly a periodic deterministic signal but it also contains stochastic elements, such as the possible F-wave (Stålberg et al. 1993). In the first instance the stimulation response is the major problem, because it is many times larger than the VMES. In the raw recorded signal, the signal/noise ratio (SNR) is far below one. The mechanical actions including movement artifacts are mainly due to changes in the half cell potential between electrodes and skin. This is an ultra low frequency signal. Spontaneous activity is observed in the presence of single or groups of motor unit action potentials in the electromyogram from the relaxed muscle.

When stimulating the motor nerve of the muscle, the voluntary nerve signals can be blocked by the antidromic impulses caused by the stimulation. This means that the VMES may decrease by increased stimulation, and this must be corrected for, either by the user or by the electronics.

The stimulation of the muscle must be selective so that only the extensor carpi radialis muscles are stimulated, in order to obtain the best possible tenodesis grip. In addition it must create maximum mechanical response in the muscle with the use of minimum electric power. The disturbance of the myoelectric recording in terms of stimulation artifacts etc. must be minimized.

The stimulation-output force relation of a muscle is known to be strongly nonlinear (Hines et al. 1992).

2 Methods

The orthosis will apply five electrodes to the skin. Two for stimulation, two for recording of the myoelectric signal and one reference electrode for reduction of noise. Stimulation and recording electrodes are placed on the skin over the wrist extensor muscle in an arrangement that reduces stimulation artifacts (Fig.1).

From the recording electrodes the signal is fed to the electronic device, which will estimate the voluntary activity in the muscle. This estimate controls the amplitude of a stimulation signal which is fed to the stimulation electrodes.

The non paralyzed parts of the muscle will in this way control innervated but paralyzed parts of the same muscle resulting in an overall increase of muscle strength.

The stimulator contains two balanced current output stages that can deliver ±40mA, limited to 200V to prevent skin damages. True charge balanced biphasic bipolar stimulation is used to minimize stimulation artifacts. The stimulation frequency is chosen as low as possible to minimize the influence of stimulation response and antidromic nerve blocking on the recording of the VMES. A stimulation frequency of 20Hz has proven adequate.

The recording electrodes are connected to a specially designed differential amplifier with a gain of 80-88dB. It has a common mode rejection ratio of at least 100dB. To enhance common mode rejection, the common mode signal is inverted and fed back to the reference electrode on the user. This suppresses effectively the hum from mains. The bandwidth of the amplifier is 20Hz-500Hz based upon a special high pass filter. This allows fast recovery from saturation caused by the stimulation pulse or change of electrode half cell potential.

A digital signal processor performs the real time signal processing of the recorded signal and controls the stimulator. Control and user interfacing are also managed by the digital signal processor. The recorded signal is filtered by a comb filter with band stops at all the harmonics of the stimulation frequency. This eliminates the deterministic components of the noise. The comb filter is a transformed high pass filter that can be either a Finite Impulse Response filter (FIR-filter) or an Infinite Impulse Response filter (IIR-filter).

Three different types of estimation of the control signal are implemented: The average rectified value, the root mean square and the count of band pass filtered samples exceeding a certain threshold.

The value of the estimated control signal changes between consecutive stimulation intervals and is therefore low pass filtered to obtain a smooth movement. The stimulation amplitude is proportional to the filtered signal.

3 Results and Discussion

Preliminarily the system has been tested on a normal subject and a few tetraplegics. No objective evaluation has been done yet but is planned. The system seems to work on one tetraplegic and not on another. One tetraplegic with muscle strength 3 in extensor carpi radialis showed extended force during testing of the device. On another tetraplegic with a somewhat stronger muscle, the stimulation response disturbed the recording to a degree where no VMES could be detected. The latter had to be stimulated twice as strongly as the former. At this point there are still problems to be solved and some training of the user to obtain good control of wrist movement may be required.

Different types of linear comb filters based on fundamentally third order IIR-filters and first and third order FIR-filters have been tested. This has shown that a simple first order FIR-filter is the most efficient of stationary filters. SNR after filtering is still poor. 15mA stimulation on a muscle with muscleforce 2-3 leaves a SNR after filtering of 1-2 using average rectified value or root mean square.

The electronic concept is a low weight, small size and low power battery operated system. The power consumption will depend on the required stimulation amplitude and duration of stimulation. Once incorporated in an orthosis it is expected that it will provide the user with at least a useful key grip. It should be for everyday use in the home and in rehabilitation. It is expected that the user will be able to donn and doff the orthosis without external assistance.

References

Costa, J.D. and Gander, R.E. (1993) Classification of muscle contraction levels with an artificial neural network. Proc. of the 15th Ann. Int. Conf. IEEE Eng. in Med. and Biol. Soc.d Injury Conference 15,1:259-260.

Haxthausen E-U. (1992) Restoration of wrist extension using functional electrical stimulation controlled by the remaining voluntary EMG from the stimulated muscles. Ph.D. Thesis, Electronics Institute, Technical University of Denmark.

Hefftner, G., Zucchini, W., and Jaros, G.G. (1988) The electromyogram (EMG) as a control signal for functional neuromuscular stimulation. Part I-II. IEEE Trans.Biomed.Eng. 35:230-242.

Hines, A.E., Owens, N.E., and Crago, P.E. (1992) Assessment of input-output properties and control of neuroprosthetic hand grasp. IEEE Trans.Biomed.Eng. 39: 610-623.

Peckham, P.H., Marsolais, E.B., and Mortimer, J.T. (1980) Restoration of key grip and release in the C6 tetraplegic patient through functional electrical stimulation. Journal of Hand Surgery - St Louis 5:462-469.

Stålberg E. and Falck B. (1993) Clinical Motor Nerve Conduction Studies. Methods in Clinical Neurophys. 4:pp61-80

Tarkka I.M. (1986) Short and long latency reflexes in human muscles following electrical and mechanical stimulation. Acta Phys. Scand. Supplementum 557.

Study of Methods for Decomposition of Superimposed Signals with Application to Electromyograms

D. Zazula, D. Korže, A. Šoštarič, D. Korošec
Faculty of Electrical Engineering and Computer Science
Smetanova 17, 62000 Maribor, Slovenia

Abstract - The paper presents three deterministic and one statistical procedure for a possible decomposition of superimposed signals modelled as multichannel, linear, time-invariant system outputs. A brief theoretical background is given for short-time cepstral analysis, wavelet transform, iterative parametric search, and higher-order statistics approach. The methods are evaluated according to the results obtained on a synthetic electromyogram (EMG). Their performances are compared and enlightened from the standpoint of an application to the real EMG decomposition.

1 Introduction

Many recent signal processing implementations deal with the problem of multichannel signal separation. Diverse approaches have been proposed in the fields of speech processing, data communication, sonar array processing, seismic exploration, and in the analysis of biological systems. All of them model superimposed signals with multichannel systems whose channels characterize the superimposed signal components. Consequently, recognition and separation of these components is turned over to identification of the model channel characteristics. The methods developed may be considered deterministic and statistical, the latter mostly applicable to deterministic observations too.

One of well known multichannel models is so called convolutional model (Ziolkowski 1984), having been widely used in echo cancellation (Oppenheim et al. 1989), speech analysis, and seismic exploration (Hsueh et al. 1985). Its application relies on homomorphic deconvolution (Oppenheim et al. 1968) that treats signal superimpositions as a result of a basic waveform convolution by a pulse train. Thus, such a model introduces identical channels, which, unfortunately, restricts its relatively simple blind deconvolution solution to a smaller class of problems. However, extensions of the convolutional model have been studied in order to establish necessary conditions for the blind homomorphic deconvolution approach in the case of two different waveforms overlapping (Korze et al. 1992).

Another possibility of signal decomposition emerges from the signals with the superimposed components being repeated in arbitrary long sequences. In such a case, statistical approach extracts the superimposed components with no need of any a priori knowledge, except the type of statistics of the repetition events of individual components. Also stationarity, or at least cyclo-stationarity, of the signal processed is presumed. A variety of system identification methods have been developed based on higher-order statistics (Mendel 1991). They introduce a possible framework for decomposition of superimposed signals. Complexity of such approaches usually forces authors to more or less severe constraints, although a general theory has been stated and proved (Giannakis et al. 1989, Swami et al. 1990, Yau et al. 1992, Yellin et al. 1994).

The signal decomposition methods mentioned so far do not depend on the knowledge about the system channel characteristics, or the exact system channel excitation, i.e., they work "blindly". If, however, some of these elements may be recognized a priori, a large class of iterative algebraic reconstruction techniques copes with the identification problem (Mendel et al. 1991).

Similarly, when dealing with signals strictly localized as well in time as in frequency, time-frequency presentations mean a useful tool in a decomposition procedure (Wood et al.1994). Such a presentation may be obtained by wavelet transform (Rioul et al. 1991), which could be additinally fruitful if wavelets resemble either channel characteristics or excitation inputs of the system whose output signal is to be decomposed.

We studied several signal decomposition approaches, with a special interest in the electromyograms (EMGs). Our main goal was to investigate resolutions of superimpositions within EMGs at higher contraction forces or the surface EMGs. In Section 2, a general modelling of multichannel systems is revealed and, afterwards, adapted to the EMG signals. Section 3 enlights some of the methods for signal decomposition based on the proposed models. The development is aimed to tackling the EMG decompositions. Simulation results are gethered in Section 4, whereas Section 5 concludes the paper with comparisons and discussion about a foreseen application to the real EMGs.

2 Multichannel Models of Superimposed Signals

Denote the output signal of a multichannel system as the following superimposition:

$$y(n) = \sum_{i=1}^{K} y_i(n - n_i) = \sum_{i=1}^{K} h_i(n) * x_i(n - n_i) \tag{1}$$

where K stands for the number of linear, time-invariant (LTI) channels with unit-sample responses $h_i(n)$, shifted input excitations $x_i(n\text{-}n_i)$, contributing signal components, $y_i(n\text{-}n_i)$, to a single output $y(n)$, and * means convolution. Such a description originates in a multiple-input/single-output (MISO) model depicted in Fig. 1.a.

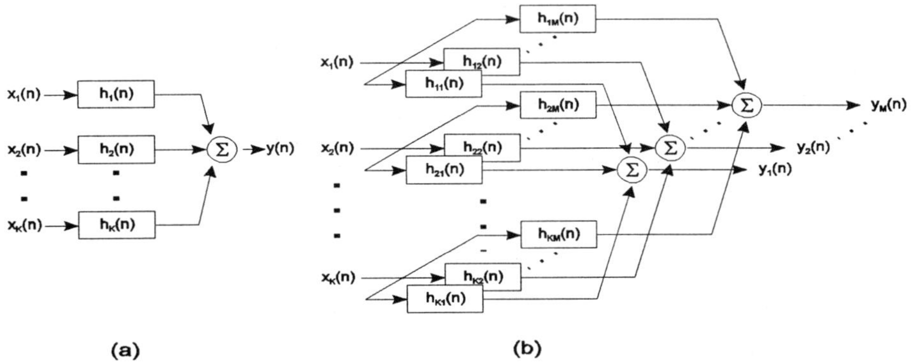

Fig. 1. Multichannel modelling: (a) MISO model, (b) MIMO model.

An extension of the model appears when multiple system outputs are available:

$$\mathbf{y}(n) = \sum_{i=0}^{\infty} \mathbf{H}^T(i)\mathbf{x}(n-i) \tag{2}$$

where

$$\mathbf{y}(n) = [y_1(n), y_2(n), \ldots, y_M(n)]^T$$

a vector of M system output signals,

$$\mathbf{H}(n) = \begin{bmatrix} h_{11}(n), h_{12}(n), \ldots, h_{1M}(n) \\ h_{21}(n), h_{22}(n), \ldots, h_{2M}(n) \\ \vdots \\ h_{K1}(n), h_{K2}(n), \ldots, h_{KM}(n) \end{bmatrix}$$

a matrix of channel unit-sample responses, and

$$\mathbf{x}(n) = [x_1(n-n_1), x_2(n-n_2), \ldots, x_K(n-n_K)]^T$$

a vector of K system input excitations. This structure corresponds to a multiple-input/multiple-output (MIMO) model shown in Fig. 1.b.

Modelling superimposed signals with MISO or MIMO models assumes signal components be equal to the system channel responses, $h_i(n)$ or $\mathbf{H}(n)$, which are excited by pulse trains, i.e.

$$x_i(n) = w_i(n),$$

in such a manner that every pulse marks the time instant of appearance of the corresponding signal component inside the signal under investigation. A MISO model is used when only a single observation is available, e.g. signal measurement with only one pick-up, while a MIMO model suits multiple simultaneous observations/measurements.

Various bioelectric phenomena may be modelled this way. If the measuring electrodes are placed relatively far from the signal sources, even single-input/multiple-output (SIMO) modelling is applicable, e.g. in electrocardiogram (ECG) decomposition (Zazula 1995). Otherwise, MIMO modelling has been implemented in the electroencephalogram (EEG) analysis, whereas both MISO and MIMO models seem to be advantageous in the EMG processing.

2.1 Modelling the EMG Signals

Among a variety of EMG models applied, there is an interesting one taking into account a network of resistors (Gygi 1994). It is fed by the innervation pulses and simulates the travelling discharges through a volume conductor, i.e. muscle fibers. A circuit analysis yields the output potentials, i.e. the measured EMG signals, that may be assumed the lowpass filtered versions of an action potential (AP) taken directly from the surface of a single muscle fiber (Gygi 1994). The fiber characteristics depend on the fiber conduction velocity and the distance between the fiber and the measuring point. Such a presentation may be seen as an array of sources emitting APs through the corresponding lowpass filters being mainly shaped only according to the distances between the sources and the measuring electrodes. Fig. 2 depicts the described structure with a MIMO model similar to that one in Fig. 1.b. Therefore, we can employ Eq. 2:

$$\mathbf{y}(n) = \sum_{i=0}^{Q} \mathbf{F}^T(i)\mathbf{x}(n-i), \tag{3}$$

where $\mathbf{F}(\mathrm{n})$ represents filter matrix with elements f_{ij}; $i = 1, \ldots K$, $j = 1,\ldots,M$, $n=0,\ldots,q_f - 1$, corresponding to a lowpass filter between the i-th source and the j-th pick-up, and finite limit of summation, $Q = max(q_f, q_s)$, is introduced because of a finite duration of APs, fixed to length q_s, that constitute

$$\begin{aligned}\mathbf{x}(n) &= [x_1(n-n_1), x_2(n-n_2), \ldots, x_K(n-n_K)]^T \\ &= [w_1(n) * h_1(n-n_1), w_2(n) * h_2(n-n_2), \ldots, w_K(n) * h_K(n-n_K)]^T\end{aligned}$$

with $w_i(n)$ being the innervation pulse train and $h_i(n\text{-}n_i)$ a shifted unit-sample response with the shape of an AP at the i-th source.

The MIMO model from Fig. 2 may as well be shrinked to a MISO version. On the other hand, it can be understood either as a direct connection between the individual APs, $h_i(n)$, and a measured EMG, $y_i(n)$, or as the muscle motor-unit AP (MUAP) building blocks if observing consecutive columns in matrix $\mathbf{F}(n)$.

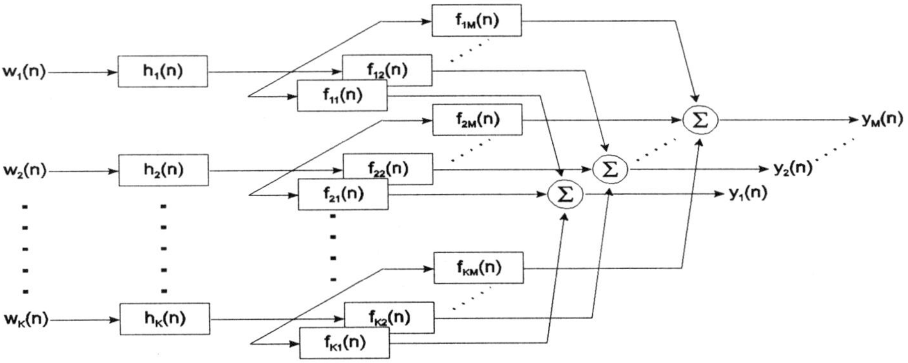

Fig. 2. Multichannel model of the superimposed EMG signal.

3 Identification of multichannel systems

To identify a multichannel system, either SIMO, MISO, or MIMO, it is necessary to determine channel characteristics of the system and, possibly, the input excitation signals. At the start, a single or multiple system output signals, i.e. measurements or observations, are given. Depending on how long the signals are and how "deep" in the model (Fig. 2) we go, deterministic and statistical approaches may be used. The former take fixed signal components $h_i(n)$ as the principal building blocks, while the latter observe the same phenomena as caused by stochastic processes $w_i(n)$. Statistically relevant results may also be obtained only with large enough population for consistency, which, in practice, usually means very long signals to be processed.

3.1 Decomposition of the Superimposed EMGs

There has been a lot of successful approaches to the low-level contraction EMG analysis (Zazula et al. 1995 (1)). Nevertheless, in the case of higher contraction forces or of surface EMG recordings, the superimpositions become too heavy to be decomposed by those approaches.

We decided to evaluate several system identification and signal separation techniques in order to recognize thier feasibility in the superimposed EMG decomposition procedure. Based on the model in Figs. 1 and 2, primarily nonparametric identification methods were used, for in an EMG decomposition the signal components are important, not their parameters. In the sequel, the ideas will briefly be referred to.

3.1.1 Short-Time Cepstral Analysis

The principle of this deterministic method is a running blind homomorphic deconvolution (Zazula et al. 1994 (1)). Starting from the MISO model in Fig. 1.a and Eq. 1, the EMG signal $y(n)$ may be partitioned into subsequent intervals obtained via a sliding rectangular, or other type, window. These intervals are further used in a cepstrum calculation (Oppenheim et al. 1968, Oppenheim et al. 1989). In every interval, some of the signal components $y_i(n)$ are present. We found out that a linear filtering in the cepstral domain can extract only one of these components if

$$A_l^2 > (L-1) \sum_{i=1, i \neq l}^{L} A_i^2,$$

where A_l is the amplitude of the extracted component, A_i the amplitudes of the remaining components, and L the number of all the components in the observed interval (Zazula et al. 1994 (1)). For long intervals of EMG, the condition would seldomly be fulfilled. But if the interval length approximate the length of the longest MUAPs, the number of components, L, might be expected low, thus the possibility of extraction of only one principle component from the observed interval much higher.

At the same time, it has been established that the second cepstral coefficient, either causal or anticausal, observed along the direction of the sliding window changes in a stepwise manner only when a new principal signal component enters the interval under the window. Therefore, this coefficient has been assumed an indication of a new event (MUAP) in the decomposed EMG (Zazula et al. 1994 (1)).

3.1.2 Wavelet Transform

In (Merletti et al. 1992), the wavelet transform with the Hermite-Rodriguez wavelet is mentioned as a stimulated EMG analysis tool giving coefficients that might be taken as features of the analysed waveforms. On the other hand, the obtained transform with its time-frequency representation offers a better insight into the EMG signal composition. Observing the time-frequency picture in cross-sections at different amplitude levels, significant patterns appear in conjunction with different MUAPs. The technique may at least help in localizing the EMG events, similar to the short-time cepstral analysis, although adopting well known peel-off procedure (Zazula et al. 1995 (1)). with pattern recognition in different amplitude cross-sections can benefit as a preprocessing step in the complex decomposition of the superimposed EMGs.

3.1.3 Modelling with Iterative Multimodal Search

Yet another deterministic approach studied supposes filter characteristics $f_{ij}(n)$ and APs $h_i(n)$ in Fig. 2 known. What is unknown, are source locations (depth parameters of filters) and thier delays n_i (Fig. 2 and Eq. 3). Therefore, searching in a two-dimensional parametric plane has to be introduced. Because of the multimodal nature of the problem, a special iterative procedure was tested with the following algorithm:

```
repeat
    synthetize a basic AP;
    for all possible delays do
        compute the error function via a distance
        between the shifted AP and the observed EMG;
    end
    find minimum in the error function and the corresponding delay;
    with this delay do
        for all possible depths do begin
            calculate a lowpass filter for the actual depth;
            use it in filtering the basic AP;
            compute a new error function between
            the filtered AP and the observed EMG;
        end
    find minimum in the new error function and the corresponding depth;
    peel off the observed EMG an AP obtained at the delay and depth found;
until distance between the original EMG and the  model output is higher than
        in the previous step.
```

The basic APs and filter characteristics were generated according to the findings in (Martinez et al. 1995).

3.1.4 Higher-Order Statistics

Finally, we investigated the proposed model in Fig. 2 by higher-order statistics. It means dealing with blind system identification again. The excitation pulse trains $w_i(n)$ were considered Bernoulli, zero-mean white noise, which corresponds to the real EMGs (Gygi 1994).

Signal decomposition was foreseen in the MISO and MIMO models (Zazula et al. 1995 (2)) using the iterative and the multivariate C(q,k) formula, respectively. Recapitulate from (Giannakis et al. 1994). the principles of the MIMO system identification which could be implemented with multielectrode EMG recordings.

In the MIMO case, we deal with the output vector y(n) which is stationary M-variate, non-Gaussian MA(q) process given by

$$\mathbf{y}(n) = \sum_{k=0}^{q} \mathbf{H}(k)\mathbf{w}(n-k) + \mathbf{v}(n), \tag{4}$$

where $\mathbf{w}(n)$ is an input vector of zero-mean and non-Gaussian components $w_m(n)$, $m = 1,...,K$, with the third-order temporal independence. $\mathbf{v}(n)$ is an M-variate, Gaussian, zero-mean process with components $v_m(n)$ and independent of $\mathbf{w}(n)$. $\mathbf{H}(k)$ are $M \times K$ matrices of full rank K ($M \geq K$).

In the identification procedure the third-order output cumulants are used, defined for the stationary M-variant process $\mathbf{y}(n)$ as the $M \times M$ matrices

$$\mathbf{C}_m(\tau_1, \tau_2) = E\{\mathbf{y}(i + \tau_1)\mathbf{y}^T(i)y_m(i + \tau_2)\};\ m = 1, \cdots, M, \tag{5}$$

where $y_m(n)$ denotes the m-th component of the vector process $\mathbf{y}(n)$. Following the derivation (Giannakis et al. 1989), the MA coefficient matrices $\{\mathbf{H}(k)\}_{k=1}^{q}$ are given by the closed-form expression:

$$\mathbf{H}(k) = \mathbf{L}^{(i)T}(q, k)\mathbf{L}^{(i)}(q, 0)[\mathbf{L}^{(i)T}(q, 0)\mathbf{L}^{(i)}(q, 0)]^{-1}, \tag{6}$$

where

$$\mathbf{L}^{(i)}(q, k) = [\mathbf{c}_1^{(i)}(q, k), \cdots, \mathbf{c}_M^{(i)}(q, k)] \tag{7}$$

and $\mathbf{c}_l^{(i)}(q,k)$ denotes the i-th column of the matrix $\mathbf{C}_m^*(q,k)$. Derivation 6 assumes $\mathbf{H}(0)=\mathbf{I}_{MxK}$. This is equivalent to both temporal and spatial third-order independence among components $w_i(n)$. Matrix $\mathbf{C}_m^*(q,k)$ is obtained from $\mathbf{C}_m(q,k)$ in such a way that only first K columns are considered, the last M-K columns having been proven to be zero. When $\mathbf{H}(q)$ is determined, the input cumulant matrix can be obtained as

$$\mathbf{\Gamma}_m = [\mathbf{H}^T(q)\mathbf{H}(q)]^{-1}\mathbf{H}^T(q)\mathbf{C}_m^*(q, 0);\ m = 1, \cdots, K. \tag{8}$$

4 Simulation Results

Some experiments using the methods from the previous section are surveyed here. We concentrated on artificial EMG signals synthetized out of basic AP waveforms $x(n)$ (Martinez et al. 1995):

$$x(n) = -1.8162(6n(1 - un) + u^2n^3)e^{-(un+7)};\ n = 0, \cdots, q_s, \tag{9}$$

where u corresponds to the conduction velocity (in our experiments fixed to u = 3.7 m/s). These APs are then fed into the corresponding filter network with the following characteristics (Gygi 1994, Martinez et al. 1995):

$$f_{ij}(n) = \frac{\frac{1}{4}\pi\sigma}{[d^2 + n^2]^{\frac{1}{2}}};\ n = 0, \cdots, q_f, \tag{10}$$

where d denotes the depth of the i-th source regarding the measurement position j and σ is the conductivity of the surrounding medium.

Substituting Eqs. 9 and 10 into Eq. 3, an EMG simulator following the scheme in Fig. 2 appears. To demonstrate the capabilities of the aforementioned decomposition approaches, we generated two artificial EMGs. The first one has been used in deterministic sense and built as a one-channel output according to Eqs. 3, 9, and 10. The delays and depths of the sources included may be seen from Table 1, the original signal itself, however, is shown in Figs. 3 and 5.

For higher-order statistics, a MIMO(2,3) model from Fig. 1.b has been employed with Bernoulli excitation (noise) (Zazula et al. 1994 (2)) on two inputs and the channels h_{11} ,...,h_{23} as stated in Table 2. The synthetized EMGs were of length of 16384 samples.

Preliminary results are delineated as follows. Short-time cepstral analysis, wavelet transform, and iterative multimodal search have been performed on the first mentioned signal. Outcomes are depicted in Figs. 3, 4, and 5, with left parts of the figures having been obtained on the noise-free signal, while the right parts belong to the analysis of the signal with additive white noise at SNR of 30 dB.

Fig. 3, left part, shows the original signal with the starts of the individual APs marked by short lines above and the sequence of the second cepstral coefficient as a dotted line. It is evident that discontinuities in the dotted line coincide with actual appearances of the APs where the superimpositions are not total. The low-amplitude APs are also skipped because of the overwhelming higher ones.

Additional discontinuities in the sequence of the second cepstral coefficients may be attributed to the points where a principal component vanished out of the observed interval, but the next following component has not become principal yet. The analysis of the noisy signal, however, fails in getting useful information on the components location (Fig. 3- right).

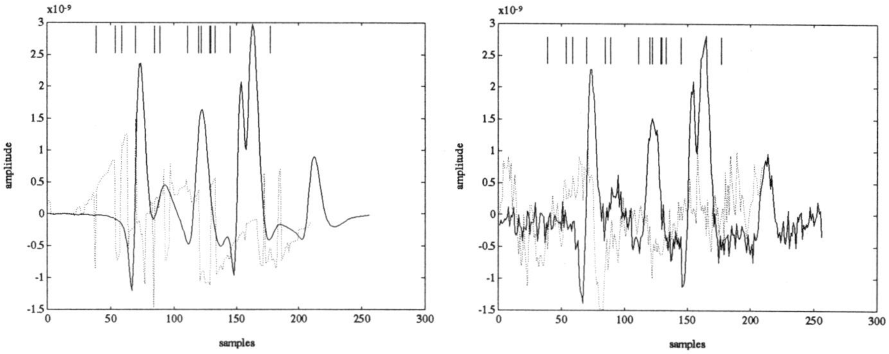

Fig. 3. Short-time cepstral analysis: the original signal (solid line) with markation of the individual APs and the second cepstral coefficients (dotted line); noise-free case left, additive noise at SNR of 30 dB right.

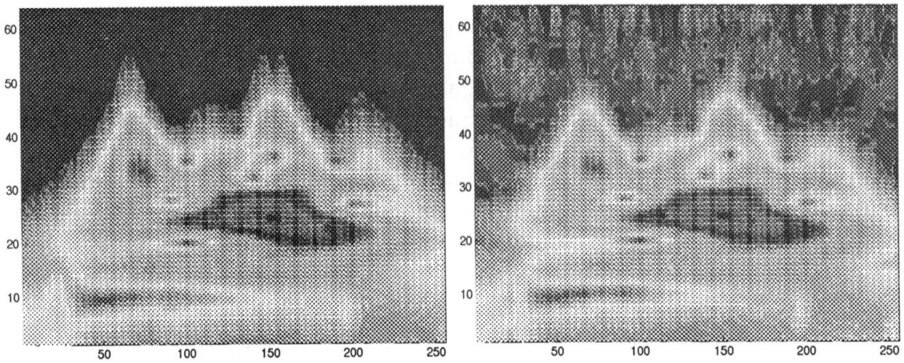

Fig. 4. Time-frequency presentation: noise-free case left, noisy case right.

In Fig. 4, a time-frequency presentation is obtained by the wavelet transform using modulated Gaussian function. The signal analysed was generated with two very similar groups of APs that could possibly be recognized as the same MUAPs at positions 50 and 130 in the original signal. Due to severe overlappings, the pattern from position 50 in Fig. 4 is not recognized at position 130 in the same shape. But apparently additive noise doesn't corrupt the vital part of the time-frequency presentation (Fig. 4- right).

Iterative parametric search produced delays and depths arranged in Table 1 along with the original data for the signal pocessed. Another view of this approach may be seen in Fig. 5, where the original signal is in solid line and the one rebuilt according to the decomposition results in dotted line. As seen, additive noise of -30 dB doesn't disturb the recognition significantly.

The higher-order statistical procedure has been applied to the second type of synthetized EMG described at the beginning of the section. All six channels were identified as in Table 2. The decomposition results are designated by hat (^) signs and accompanied by standard deviation ($\sigma_{\hat{h}_{ij}}$)

Original parameters														
Depth [mm]	1	3	4	2	1	3	4	2	3	2	7	4	8	1
Delay [ms]	1	16	21	51	82	92	107	139	73	47	32	84	95	91
Parameters estimated in noise-free case														
Depth [mm]	1	3	4	2	1	2	4	2	3	3	6	6	-	1
Delay [ms]	1	17	21	49	82	94	107	139	76	49	48	81	-	90
Parameters estimated in the case of SNR of 30 dB														
Depth [mm]	1	3	5	2	1	2	5	2	3	3	-	6	-	1
Delay [ms]	1	17	21	49	82	94	107	139	78	48	-	71	-	90

Table 1: Results of the iterative parametric search.

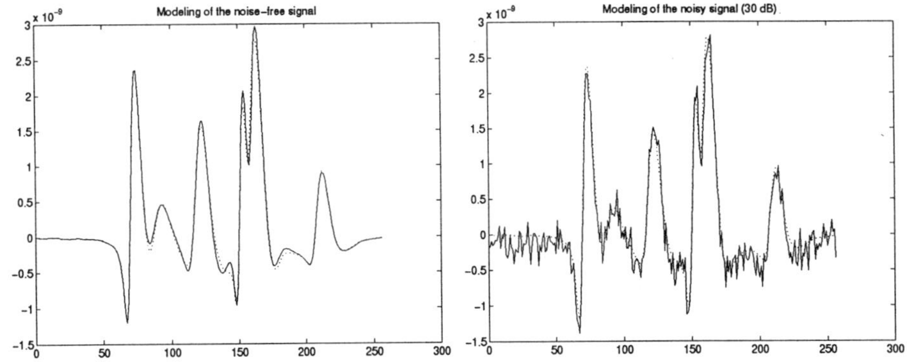

Fig. 5. Comparasion of the original (solid line) and the reconstructed signal after parametric search (dotted line); noise-free case left, noisy case right.

5 Discussion and Conclusions

The simulation results from Section 4 allude a few suggestions for further investigation of the superimposed EMGs.

First, wavelet transform, iterative parametric search, and higher-order statistics, latter by its nature, are sufficiently robust. Short-time cepstral analysis, on the other hand, is very noise sensitive.

Second, the deterministic approaches applied have a reasonable computational complexity of order O(FFT). Decomposition via higher-order statistics demands, however, very long signals and, consequently, extremely long processing times. With high-contraction real EMGs sampled at 5 kHz, the necessary signal length is estimated over 10^6 samples per channel, i.e. per decomposed component, which approximately means 4 minutes of stable and steady multichannel EMG recording.

Third, the iterative parametric search and the higher-order statistics are able to produce a thorough decomposition to the signal primitives, whereas cepstral analysis and wavelet transform may serve more or less only as preprocessing tools extracting preliminary information on shapes and time instants of appearance of the signal components.

Fourth, the iterative parametric search is heavily dependent on a priori knowledge about the shapes of APs and the filtering effects induced by the muscle and measurement characteristics. Nevertheless, this knowledge may be obtained by application of other three methods investigated.

Finally, the decomposition results on the real EMGs would be method-dependent. While higher-order statistics would statistically approximate the repeated waveforms of MUAPs encountered, the iterative parametric search could only rely upon the basic APs, so an additional step in order to combine them into the corresponding MUAPs would be necessary. The decomposition results of the cepstral and wavelet approaches cannot be attributed neither MUAPs nor basic APs without careful further consideration.

	sample values					sample values			
h_{11}	1	-3.3044	2.7310	-0.2787	h_{21}	1	-1.8296	1.0746	-0.2049
$\widehat{h}_{11}$	1	-2.5230	1.9828	-0.1798	$\widehat{h}_{21}$	0.6196	-1.2746	0.7278	-0.7125
$\sigma_{\widehat{h}_{11}}$	0	0.5734	0.5231	0.0689	$\sigma_{\widehat{h}_{21}}$	0.1762	0.6507	0.6310	1.0809
h_{12}	1	-1.6137	0.1673	-0.0039	h_{22}	1	-3.2981	3.0490	-0.5376
$\widehat{h}_{12}$	0.7995	-1.2397	0.1610	-0.0007	$\widehat{h}_{22}$	1	-3.2172	2.8122	0.0475
$\sigma_{\widehat{h}_{12}}$	0.2231	0.3184	0.1496	0.1541	$\sigma_{\widehat{h}_{22}}$	0	1.8286	1.8637	0.5239
h_{13}	1	-4.5592	6.8043	-3.3039	h_{23}	1	-3.9547	5.1403	-2.2009
$\widehat{h}_{13}$	1.4374	-3.9235	5.0570	-2.2191	$\widehat{h}_{23}$	1.0812	-4.3740	6.1798	-2.7986
$\sigma_{\widehat{h}_{13}}$	0.4514	0.3623	1.1084	0.6480	$\sigma_{\widehat{h}_{23}}$	1.1799	1.7657	4.3968	1.9458

Tabelle 2: Identification for Bernoulli noise, output signals were $N = 128*128$ samples long, $h_{ij}(n)$ generated randomly with length of 4 samples.

References

Giannakis, G. B., Inouye, Y., and Mendel, J.M. (1989) Cumulant Based Identification of Multichannel Moving-Average Models. *IEEE Trans. on Automatic Control*, **34:** 783-787.

Gygi, A. (1994) Analyse des Nadel- und Oberflächen-Elektromyogramms mittels Statistiken h"herer Ordnung. PhD Thesis Nr. 10863, ETH Zürich.

Hsueh, A. C. and Mendel, J. M. (1985) Minimum-Variance and Maximum-Likelihood Deconvolution for Noncausal Channel Models. *IEEE Trans. on Geoscience and Remote Sensing*, **GE-23**: 797-808.

Korosec, D., Sostaric, A., and Zazula, D. (1995) A Survey of Methods for Electromyogram Decomposition. In: W. Kropatsch, F. Solina *Proceedings of Visual Modules Workshop*, R. Oldenburg Verlag, Wien-München, pp. 294-303.

Korosec, D., Zazula, D., and Sostaric, A. (1992) Studija dekonvolucije signalov s pomocjo kompleksnega kepstra (in Slovene). In: *IEEE Proc. Electrotechnical and Computer Conf*, Portoroz, Slovenia, pp. B233-236.

Martinez, C., Zazula, D., and Korosec, D. (1995) Surface EMG Forward and Inverse Filter Models. In: *IEEE Proc. Electrotechnical and Computer Conf.*, Portoroz, Slovenia, pp. B385-388.

Mendel, J. M. (1991) Tutorial on Higher-Order Statistics (Spectra) in Signal Processing and System Theory: Theoretical Results and Some Applications. *Proc. of the IEEE*, **79:** 277-305.

Mendel, J. M. (ed.) (1991) A Prelude to Neural Networks: Adaptive and Learning

Systems. PTR Prentice Hall, Englewood Cliffs.

Merletti, R. and Lo Conte, L. R. (1992) Advances in Processing of Surface Myoelectric Signals. In: *Symposium New developments in rehabilitation technology research of the locomotor system*, Enschede, The Netherlands, pp. 2-27.

Oppenheim, A. V., Schafer, R. W., and Stockham T. G. (1968) Nonlinear Filtering of Multiplied and Convolved Signals.l *Proceedings of the IEEE*, **56:** 1264-1291.

Oppenheim, A. V. and Schafer, R. W. (1989) Discrete-Time Signal Processing.Prentice-Hall Inc., Englewood Cliffs.

Rioul, O. and Vetterli, M. (1991) Wavelets in Signal Processing. *IEEE Signal Processing Magazine*, pp. 14-38.

Swami, A., Giannakis, G. B., and Mendel, J. M. (1990) Linear Modelling of Multidimensional Non-Gaussian Processes Using Cumulants. *Multidimensional Systems and Signal Processing*, pp. 11-37.

Wood, J. C. and Barry, D. T. (1994) Radon Transformation of Time-Frequency Distributions for Analysis of Multicomponent Signals. *IEEE Trans. on Signal Processing*, **42:** 3166-3177.

Yau, S. F. and Bresler, Y. (1992) Worst Case Cramér-Rao Bounds for Parametric Estimation of Superimposed Signals with Applications. *IEEE Trans. on Signal Processing*, **40:** 2973-2986.

Yellin, D. and Weinstein, E. (1994) Criteria for Multichannel Signal Separation.*IEEE Trans. on Signal Processing*, **42:** 2158-2168.

Zazula, D., Korze, D., Sostaric, A., and Korosec, D. (1994) Decomposition of the Superimposed Electromyograms at Higher Contraction Forces and Muscular Fatigue, First Technical Report (Associated Contract to RAFT). Faculty of Technical Sciences, Maribor, Slovenia.

Zazula, D. (1995) Cepstral Modelling and Decomposition of the Multilead ECG Signals. In: *Proceedings of System, Modelling, Control*, **2**, Zakopane, Poland, pp. 416-421.

Zazula, D., Korosec, D., and Martinez, C. (1995) Decomposition of the Superimposed Electromyograms at Higher Contraction Forces and Muscular Fatigue, Third Technical Report (Associated Contract to RAFT). Faculty of Electrical Engineering and Computer Science, Maribor, Slovenia.

Zazula, D. and Korze, D. (1995) Higher-Order Cumulants in System Identification and Signal Decomposition. In: W. Kropatsch, F. Solina *Proceedings of Visual Modules Workshop*, R. Oldenburg Verlag, Wien-München, pp. 275-284.

Ziolkowski, A. (1984) Deconvolution. D. Reidel Publishing Company, Dordrecht.

Chapter 6

Spasticity: Pathophysiology, Evaluation, and Treatment

Which Spinal Cord Neurophysiologic Mechanisms are Responsible for Spasticity?

P.J. Delwaide, G. Rapisarda, A. Lozza
University Department of Neurology,
Hôpital de la Citadelle, Liège, Belgium

Abstract - Electrophysiological tests applied non invasively to spastic patients indicate multiple changes: alpha motoneurone excitability is increased, presynaptic, reciprocal and Renshaw (recurrent) inhibitions are reduced. A special attention is paid to non-reciprocal (Ib) inhibition whose reduction is nicely correlated with muscle stiffness felt during passive mobilization but is poorly correlated with tendon jerks briskness.

1 Introduction

From a clinical point of view, spasticity has been defined as a motor disorder encompassing brisk tendon jerks (sometimes clonus) and a velocity-dependent muscle hypertonia during stretch (Lance, 1980) that affects certain muscle groups preferentially. It has long been considered that both components of spasticity are explained only by a facilitated and/or disinhibited direct Ia pathway to motoneurons. This assumption is based on unsatisfactory animal models but can be verified in humans by electrophysiologic techniques (Delwaide et al. 1980). In fact, in the last twenty years, non invasive techniques have been developed which enable to study several well indentified spinal mechanisms controlling excitability of the myotatic reflex arch. Most of these tests lend to quantitative results so that norms, with confidence intervals, may be defined in control subjects. If results of these tests differ significantly in patients suffering from spasticity, it can be inferred that the mechanism under study is modified in that situation. It is thus possible to review five of the neurophysiological mechanisms which could, according to animal physiology (Pierrot-Deseilligny and Mazieres, 1985), explain spasticity. Theoretically, a single one could be enough but they might be combined in variable proportions. These electrophysiological techniques have largely been applied to spastic patients. The results so far obtained allow a better understanding of the spinal mechanisms which contribute to spasticity. A reservation is however necessary: the conclusions are only valid to interpret spasticity at rest. When patients try to contract their muscles voluntarily, many changes in the pathophysiological profile may be anticipated and they depend on the type and the number of lesioned descending motor fibers.

2 Alpha Motoneurone Hyperexcitability

If the motoneurones (MN) were in a chronic state of increased depolarization, for example because of a change in their biophysical properties, they would be nearer to threshold of discharge and respond to weaker afferent stimuli, providing an explanation for brisker reflexes. On the other hand, permanent increase of excitatory inputs, coming from primary afferents or interneurones would increase to excitability level of the final common pathway.

In recent years, attention has been drawn in animal to long-lasting excitability changes in the motoneurones secondary to disappearence of corticospinal influences. These motoneuronal properties are contingent upon innervation by serotonergic or noradrenergic pathways. The monoamines would act by decreasing a K^+ conductance and induce self-sustained firing (Eken et al. 1989; Nielsen and Hultborn, 1993).

In man, these modifications could be reflected by increased amplitude of the F wave (due to backfiring of MNs activated antidromically) and a higher H Max/M Max ratio (which measures the number of MN in the motoneural pool which can be activated by the Ia pathway before occlusion occurs in motor fibers). However, these clinical neurophysiologic techniques do not allow discrimination between alteration of MNs biophysical properties and increased depolarization resulting from changes in synaptic activities influencing cells discharge. The exact contribution of each of these mechanisms should be further defined.

3 Gamma Motoneurone Excitability

An increased gamma motoneurone excitability has long been advocated as responsible for spasticity (Rushworth, 1961). That idea was derived from animal data indicating that the gamma system contributes to decerebrate rigidity and on results of 2 methods applied to spastic patients. However, decerebrate rigidity is not a valid model of human spasticity and the methodology of ancient studies performed in man has been strongly criticized, making their conclusions very disputable.

A less controversial method of evaluating gamma activity is the direct recording in man of single Ia fiber activity (microneurography). Unfortunately, this time-consuming technique has been applied so far to a very limited number of patients. In those who were studied Hagbarth et al. (1973) did not observe any increased discharge which would reflect changes in gamma activity. Further microneurographic studies are necessary before the real role of the gamma system is assessed. However, at present, evidence indicating a consistent change in gamma innervation is lacking.

4 Reduction of Presynaptic Inhibition Acting on Ia Afferents

Presynaptic inhibition acting on Ia afferents results in a reduced release of neurotransmitter onto MN. This presynaptic inhibition, mediated through an interneurone, is influenced both by peripheral and supraspinal afferents and normally attenuates the Ia effects on MNs. Consequently, a reduction of presynaptic inhibition could theoretically make the myotatic arc more excitable because it is desinhibited.

In a normal man, vibratory stimulation of a muscle inhibits its monosynaptic reflex. In agreement with animal experiments (Gilles et al. 1969), it has been shown that this inhibition reflects the mechanism of presynaptic inhibition on Ia fibers (Delwaide, 1971). All research workers who have studied vibratory inhibition in chronic spastic patients have reported a significant reduction (Delwaide, 1971; Burke, Ashby, 1972; Iles, Roberts, 1986; Ashby, Wiens, 1989; Ongeboer de Visser et al. 1989; Koelman et al. 1993). The differences with age-matched normal subjects are clear-cut as they are between both legs in hemispastic patients. However, no good correlation has been found between reduction of vibratory inhibition and intensity of spasticity, as assessed by Ashworth's scale. Correlation is better with tendon jerk intensity. However, the results indicate that presynaptic inhibition is clearly reduced in established spasticity.

Using another technique, Faist et al. (1994) have confirmed a reduction of presynaptic inhibition in paraplegic patients but not in hemiplegics. To explain the difference, they have proposed that vibratory inhibition also depends on postactivation depression following repetitive synaptic transmission.

5 Reduction of Recurrent (Renshaw) Inhibition

This mechanism can be studied by an ingenious technique devised by Pierrot-Deseilligny et al. (1976). Lesions in descending pathways, especially in spinal cord diseases, could reduce activity of Renshaw's cells and explain hyperexcitability of the myotatic arc by removal of a tonic inhibitory mechanism acting on MN.

Recurrent inhibition is not reduced at rest in hemiplegic patients (Katz, Pierrot-Deseilligny, 1982) whereas, in spinal cord injuried patients, reinforcement of recurrent activity has been reported (Shefner et al. 1992). Taken together, the results do not support the view that a reduction in recurrent inhibition - which is theoretically necessary to explain hyperexcitability of the myotatic reflex - is mandatory for spasticity.

6 Reduction of Short-Latency Ia Reciprocal Inhibition

If less active, Ia inhibitory interneurones would deprive MN of a background of postsynaptic inhibition and, hence, explain an enhancement of excitability of the stretch reflex pathway. In addition, selective contractions of antagonistic muscles would be more difficult, a fact which has been clearly documented in spasticity.

In man, functioning of Ia inhibitory interneurones is studied by conditioning monosynaptic reflexes by feeble stimulation of a nerve originating in an antagonist muscle (Tanaka, 1974). Using this technique, it has been shown that short latency reciprocal inhibition from flexors to extensors is reduced in spasticity, both in upper and lower limb (Delwaide, 1985; Nakashima et al. 1989; Artieda et al. 1991; Crone et al. 1994). However, that conclusion is not supported by all the publications (Boorman et al. 1991). As changes in Renshaw inhibition are not prominent - Renshaw cells inhibit normally Ia inhibitory interneurones - it is likely that modification in Ia reciprocal inhibition reflects a lack of facilitatory drive normally exerted by descending spinal pathways.

This reduction, combined with a reduction of presynaptic inhibition is important to interpret co-contractions of antagonist muscles but is also to be taken into account in pathogenesis of spasticity.

7 Reduction of Non-Reciprocal (Ib) Inhibition

Physiologists have originally studied interneurones activated by Ib fibers originating from Golgi Tendon organs and producing inhibition on extensor motor nuclei at the same time as facilitation of flexor ones. However, projections onto these interneurones and their actions on motoneurones has proved to be more complex. Other afferents (Ia, skin, joint...) converge on the same interneurons which , in turn, have variable actions on motoneuron pools. It is now advisable to consider a so-called "non reciprocal inhibition" (Harrison and Jankowska, 1992) rather than to discuss it in terms of Ib afferent action. The role of this non reciprocal inhibition has been reviewed by Jankowska (1992).

There is also a technique to test non reciprocal inhibition in humans. It is based on the assumption that afferents originating in medial gastrocnemius muscle send only Ib projections into the soleus MN pool. If the soleus H reflex is conditioned by prior stimulation at low intensity (in order to activate the largest fibers only) of the gastrocnemius medialis nerve, reduction of H reflex amplitude reflects intensity of non reciprocal inhibition (Pierrot-Deseilligny et al. 1981).

Clear cut differences appear in the results of this test when applied to control and spastic subjects. In hemiplegic patients, the normal inhibition is either reduced or replaced by facilitation on the affected side (Delwaide and Oliver, 1988). Reduction of non reciprocal inhibition is confirmed in paraplegics even if, in a recent paper, differences do not reach a significant level (Downes et al. 1995). In patients presenting a definite upper motoneuron syndrome with brisk reflexes but hypotonia, non-reciprocal inhibition is not reduced but, once stiffness during passive mobilization develops, inhibition in the Ib test disappears to be replaced by facilitation. It can be concluded that non-reciprocal inhibition is markedly reduced in upper motoneuron syndrome provided that stiffness is clinically present. No good correlation exists between departures from normal values and briskness of tendon jerks.

8 Correlation between Pathophysiological Disorders and Clinical Signs

Spasticity is thus associated with several pathophysiological disturbances at the spinal level. It is interesting to investigate whether intensity of hypertonia and tendon jerks correlates in a satisfactory manner with changes in a single test, i.e. a particular pathophysiological mechanism. Before this, it is worth to establish whether the abnormalities are or are not linked and whether they evolved in parallel. This is not the case because no correlation can be found between the results of the various tests as has been demonstrated earlier (Delwaide, 1985).

In a work in progress, we are repeating a battery of 4 electrophysiological tests in a control group and in a series of 50 patients suffering from an upper motoneurone syndrome, some with muscle hypertonia, others with normal tone or even hypotonia. The tests are: H/M ratio, vibratory inhibition, reciprocal Ia inhibition and autogenic Ib inhibition. The results are correlated with brikness of tenson jerks and spasticity intensity assessed by Ashworth's scale.

The best correlation coefficient is found between vibratory inhibition of tendon jerk briskness. If the patients are separated into 2 groups according to presence or absence of hypertonia, a good correlation coefficient (0.7) appears between intensity of stiffness and modifications of the non-reciprocal (Ib) inhibition test. On the other hand, correlation between these latter and tendon jerk briskness is very poor (table 1).

	Vibratory inhibition	**Ib test**
Tendon jerk briskness	Good	Poor
Velocity Dependent stiffness	Poor	Good

Table 1: Correlations between 2 clinical signs and the results of 2 electrophysiological tests

As the best correlation coefficient is between stiffness and non-reciprocal inhibition, it is very likely that reduction in non reciprocal inhibition plays a major role in explaining hypertonia. It has long been shown that exaggerated tendon jerks and tonic stretch reflexes, which reflect stiffness are not well correlated (Dohrman, Nowak, 1974). In addition, the neurophysiological mechanisms of the 2 signs seem distinct, at least quantitatively. It is thus logical to consider separately the 2 signs and to restrict the term spasticity to the velocity-sensitive stiffness felt during passive mobilization.

References

Artieda, J., Quesada, P., Obeso, J. (1991) Reciprocal inhibition between forearm muscles in spastic hemiplegia. *Neurology*, **41**, 286-289

Ashby, P. and Wiens, M. (1989) Reciprocal inhibition following lesions of the spinal cord in man. *J Physiol*, **414**, 145-157

Boorman, G., Hulliger, M., Lee, R. G., Tako, K., and Tanaka, R. (1991) Reciprocal Ia inhibition in patients with spinal spasticity. *Neuroscience Letters*, **127**, pp 57-60.

Burke, D., Ashby, P. (1972) Are spinal "presynaptic" inhibitory mechanisms suppressed in spasticity ? *J Neurol Sci*, **15**, 321-326

Crone, C., Nielsen, J., Petersen, N., Ballegaard, M., and Hultborn, H. (1994) Disynaptic reciprocal inhibition of ankle extensors in spastic patients. *Brain*, **117**, 1161-1168

Delwaide, P. J. (1971) *Etude expérimentale de l'hyperréflexie tendineuse en clinique neurologique*. Editions Arscia, Bruxelles, 324p.

Delwaide, P. J., Martinelli, P., and Crenna, P. (1980) Clinical neurophysiological measurement of spinal reflex activity. In: R.G. Feldman, R.R. Young, W.P. Koella (eds) *Spasticity: disordered motor control.* Year Book Medical Publishers, Chicago, pp 345-371

Delwaide, P. J. (1985) Electrophysiological testing of spastic patients: its potential usefulness and limitations. In: P.J. Delwaide, R.R. Young (eds) *Clinical Neurophysiology in Spasticity*. Elsevier Science Publishers, Amsterdam, pp 185-203

Delwaide, P. J. and Oliver, E. (1988) Short-latency autogenic inhibition (Ib inhibition) in human spasticity. *Journal of Neurology, Neurosurgery and Psychiatry*, **51,** pp 1546-1550

Downes, L., Ashby, P., and Bugaresti, J. (1995) Reflex effects from Golgi tendon organ (Ib) afferents are unchanged after spinal cord lesions in humans. *Neurology*, **45**, pp 1720-1724

Dohrman, G. J. and Nowak, K. W. J. (1974) Relationship between various clinical signs in lesions of the descending motor system (a statistical study). *Dis Nerv Syst*, **35**, pp 375-377.

Eken, T., Hultborn, H., and Kiehn, O. (1989) The plateau potentials and their role in regulating motoneuronal firing. In: J.H.J. Allum, M. Hulliger (eds), *Progress in Brain Research*, vol. 80, Elsevier Science Publishers B.V, Amsterdam, pp. 257-267.

Faist, M. D., Mazevet, D., Dietz, V., and Pierrot-Deseilligny, E. (1994) A quantitative assessment of presynaptic inhibition of Ia afferents in spastics. Differences in hemiplegics and paraplegics. *Brain*, **117**, 1449-1455

Gillies, D., Lance, J. W., Neilson, P. D., and Tassinari, C. A. (1969) Presynaptic inhibition of the monosynaptic reflex by vibration. *J Physiol (Lond)* **205**, 329-339

Hagbarth, K. E., Wallin, G., and Lofstedt, L. (1973) Muscle spindle response to stretch in normal and spastic subjects. *Scan J Rehabil Med*, **5**, 156-159.

Harrison, P. J. and Jankowska, E. (1985) Sources of input to interneurones mediating group I non reciprocal inhibition of motoneurones in the cat. *J Physiol*, **361**, pp 379-401

Iles, J. F. and Roberts, R. C. (1986) Presynaptic inhibition of monosynaptic reflexes in the lower limbs of subjects with uppere motoneurone disease. *J Neurol Neurosurg Psychiat*, **49**, 937-944

Jankowska, E. (1992) Interneuronal relay in spinal pathways from proprioceptors. *Prog Neurobiol*, **38**, 335-378

Katz, R. and Pierrot-Deseilligny, E. (1982) Recurrent inhibition of alpha-motoneurones in patients with upper motor neuron lesions. *Brain*, **105**, 103-124.

Koelman, J. H. T. M., Bour, L. J., Hilgevoord, A. A. J., van Bruggen, G. J., and Ongerboer de Visser, B. W. (1993). The soleus H-reflex and clinical signs of the upper motoneuron syndrome. *J Neurol Neurosurg Psychiatry*, ***56***, 776-781

Lance, J. W. (1980) Symposium Synopsis. In: R.G. Feldman, R.R.Young, W.P. Koella (eds). *Spasticity: disordered motor control.* Year Book Medical Publishers, Chicago, pp 485-494.

Nakashima, K., Rothwell, J. C., Day, B. C., Thompson, P. D., Shannon, K., and Marsden, C. D. (1989) Reciprocal inhibition between forearm muscles in patients with writer's cramp and other occupational cramps, symptomatic hemidystonia and hemiparesis due to stroke. *Brain*, **112**, pp 681-697

Nielsen, J. and Hultborn, H. (1993) Regulated properties of motoneurons and primary afferents: new aspects on possible spinal mechanisms underlying spasticity. In: A.F. Thilmann, D.J. Burke, WZ Rymer (eds), *Spasticity: mechanisms and management.* Springer-Verlag, Berlin, pp 177- 191

Ongeboer de Visser, B. W., Bour, L. J., Koelman, J. H. T. M., and Speelman, J. D. (1989) Cumulative vibratory indices and the H/M ratio of the soleus H-reflex: a quantitative study in control and spastic subjects. *Electroencephalogr Clin Neurophysiol, 73*, 162-166

Pierrot-Deseilligny, E., Bussel, B., Held, J., and Katz, R. (1976) Excitability of human motoneurones after discharge in a conditionning reflex. *Electroencephalogr Clin Neurophysiol* , **40**, 279-287

Pierrot-Deseilligny, E., Morin, C., Bergego, C., and Tankov, N. (1981) Pattern of group I fibres projections from ankle flexor and extensor muscles in man. *Exp Brain Res*, **42**, 337-350

Pierrot-Deseilligny, E. and Mazieres, L. (1985) Spinal mechanisms underlying spasticity. In: P.J. Delwaide, R.R. Young (eds), *Clinical Neurophysiology in Spasticity, Restorative Neurology*, vol. 1, Elsevier, Amsterdam, pp 63-76.

Rushworth, G. (1961) Spasticity and rigidity: an experimental study and review. *J Neurol Neurosurg Psychiatry*, **23:** 99-118.

Shefner, J. M., Berman, S. A., Sarkarati, M., and Young, R. R. (1992) Recurrent inhibition is increased in patients with spinal cord injury. *Neurology*, **42**, 2162-2168.

Tanaka, R. (1974) Reciprocal Ia inhibition during voluntary movements in man. *Exp Brain Res*, **21,** 529-540

Biomechanical and Neurophysiological Implications on Spasticity Assessment

M. Osio[1], M. Ferrarin[2]
[1]First Neurologic Clinic, University of Milan. "L Sacco" Hospital. Milan, Italy
[2]Bioengineering Centre, Don Gnocchi Pro Juventute Foundation IRCCS, Polytechnic of Milan, Milan, Italy

Abstract - Spasticity is a positive sign present in the upper motorneuron syndrome related with hyperexcitability of the stretch reflex, but some neurologists includes flexor spasms from exteroceptive origin in its definition.

From the pathophysiological point of view hyperreflexia is best related with reduction in vibratory inhibition, whereas velocity dependent increased tone with reduction of the Ib non-reciprocal inhibition. It is a common clinical evidence that these are poorly related one each other in different patients. Otherwise, different lesional pattern of the descending pathways acting on the motorneuronal excitability (vestibulo-spinal, reticulo-spinal, rubro-spinal,...) associated with the pyramidal lesion give rise to different motor clinical features.

Thus, a complete neurophysiological assessment must take in account the different pathophysiological mechanisms at the origin of the sign "spasticity" in each patient.

1 Introduction

In clinical neurology, spasticity is defined as a pathological increase of muscle tone during passive movement of limbs and increase of stretch reflexes (Lance 1980).

Spasticity is an accessory disturbance related to the lesion of the pyramidal level of the motor functions. Experimental evidences showed that isolated lesions of the pyramidal tract may produce hypotonia (Tower 1940). Thus the lesion of the pyramidal tract produces weakness and give rise to spasticity only when associated to an unbalanced or interrupted control of the muscles tone exerted by the inhibitory and excitatory centers of the brain stem.

The clinical variability of spasticity and the motor recovery depend on the amount of those descending pathways involvement (Fries et al. 1993) and on the affection of afferent control loops, spinal interneurons and motor units.

Since spasticity take rise from such heterogeneous factors, its diagnosis and assessment was mostly clinical.

Clinicians intent on the repeated evaluation of spasticity by means of various manoeuvres and tests may observe that individual findings vary very widely during the day and in different days in the same subject. In addition the grading of each test is subjective and classification is often coarse. The introduction of analogic assessment scales (Ashworth, Barthel) simplifies evaluation of spasticity but has the disadvantages of subjective repeated assessment and poses difficulties in communication of the results to other examinators.

Therefore, many researchers, interested both in clinic and in pathophysiology, introduced electrophysiological tests, in order to standardize spasticity assessment (Delwaide et al. 1980, Pinelli et al. 1989, Abbruzzese 1990).

2 Neurophysiological and biomechanical assessment

As mentioned before, spasticity derives from a complex interaction of many segmental and supra-segmental components. Only when all the factors that affect muscle tone have been measured, it is possible to extract parameters that correlate better with patients features.

Neurophysiological assessment of spasticity is based upon biomechanical and electromyographic (EMG) recordings during both *kinesiological* and *reflexological* conditions.

2.1 EMG recordings of spinal activities

2.1.1 Direct evaluation of the α-motorneuron excitability

a) F wave evaluation

The features of the F wave from flexors and from extensor muscles is a test of the alpha motorneuron pool (Schiller et al. 1978). In spastic patients F wave amplitude during a repeated stimuli shows an enhanced mean value (Eisen et al. 1979). Nevertheless such parameter is not specific of spasticity, since it was enhanced in parkinsonian patients with plastic hypertonia too (Abbruzzese et al. 1975).

2.1.2 Monosynaptic reflexes

The most classic example of a monosynaptic reflex is the phasic stretch reflex elicited in man by tendon percussion. The mechanical stimuli discreetly stretches the muscle spindles activating their primary endings. Activation of the primary endings generate action potentials that are conveyed to the spinal cord by large diameter afferent nerve fibers, the 1a nerve fibers. In the spinal cord they establish excitatory monosynaptic connections to alpha motorneurons innervating homonymous and synergist muscles and inhibitory connections, through an inhibitory interneuron, to alpha motor neuron of antagonistic muscles.

a) Tendon reflex (T)

In clinical neurophysiology a tendon reflex can be elicited in a standardized way by using electromechanical hammers, attached at the same distance from the tendon and striking from the same angle with the same force. To record the reflex responses may be used both biomechanical and EMG recordings but the last ones are usually preferred. The T response may be related to the amplitude of the maximal motor response elicited by direct electrical stimulation of all the alpha motor neurons innervating the same muscle. The ratio between these two values (Tmax/Mmax) is an indicator of the excitability of the myotatic arc in toto (Pinelli 1975).

b) Hoffmann reflex

Hoffmann reflex (H reflex) is a reflex EMG response obtained stimulating 1a afferent fibers innervating the muscle spindles from the homonymous muscle. During stimulation of a mixed nerve (usually sciatic nerve) with increasing current intensity , 1a fibers are stimulated first and at a critical stimulation values a response is elicited in a muscle innervated from the nerve stimulated (usually soleus) after a latency depending on the length of the reflex arc. When the stimulus intensity raise, the amplitude of the H reflex first increases and then decreases, while the response related to direct stimulation of motor fibers (M response) develops. The ratio of the maximal amplitudes of the H reflex and the M response (H max/ M max) expresses the excitability of that portion of the myotatic arc that lies proximal to the muscle spindles (Delwaide 1971).

Technical factors can change H reflex amplitude. Therefore it is important to standardize stimulation and recording procedures. In order to standardize the test we recorded in 9 normal subject (5 F and 4 M; 24-34 years old) H reflex responses.

Subjects were sitted on a comfortable armchair with head supported and not rotated and arms supported. Hip angle was 90°, knee angle of 120° (60° flexion) and ankle angle was 90°. Recordings were obtained with surface EMG pregelled electrodes fixed on the soleus muscle 4 cm apart. Stimulation was applied to the posterior tibial nerve in the popliteal fossa and held in place by a roll of gauze fixed in the popliteal fossa with velcro bands placed around the knee. Stimulus duration was 1 msec and stimulus intensity varied from 0 mA to the value needed to obtain M max response. Stimulation intensity was increased with steps of 1 mA each. For each value of stimulation intensity were delivered five stimuli with frequency of stimulation of 1 shock per five seconds.

For each subject were measured H max amplitude; Standard Deviation (SD) of the amplitude values obtained from the 5 stimuli at which H max amplitude was obtained; M max amplitude; Hmax/Mmax ratio; Differential threshold (DELTA) at which the first H response and the first M response were recorded.

Results were as follows: Hmax/Mmax ratio was 0.47$\pm$ 0.09, SD was 18.0$\pm$ 8.3% of the H max amplitude and DELTA was 1.4$\pm$0.9mA.

In 4 paraplegic patients we studied, Hmax/Mmax ratio changes proportionally to the level of spasticity clinically expressed and to the amount of antispastic treatment. In patients with complete lesion were recorded SD values lower that 10% whereas in incomplete lesions were recorded normal SD values. DELTA values, even if often higher than 2 mA, were not significantly different from the control group (Ferrarin et al. 1994).

Because of monosynaptic connections with alpha motor neurons the amplitude of H reflex usually reflects the facilitation or inhibition of the alpha motor neurons. This is true only when presynaptic inhibition, which acts upon the terminal arborizations of the 1a fibers, remains constant.

A good method to evaluate the degree of the presynaptic inhibition acting on the 1a afferent fibers is the application of a vibratory stimulus (100 Hz) to the tendon of a muscle, when a monosynaptic H reflex is elicited on the same muscle (vibratory inhibition). During such procedure a marked inhibition of the H reflex is observed in normal subjects.

We measured the vibratory inhibition with the same technique described for H reflex in 11 health subjects both on the H max reflex and on the H reflex with amplitude half times the H max (H/2). Vibratory inhibition decreased the H max amplitude of the 11.7$\pm$9.2%, and the H/2 amplitude of the 26.6$\pm$19.0%. In paraplegic patients there was no or little inhibition, except in one subject with incomplete lesion (Ferrarin et al. 1994).

c) Tonic vibration reflex

Muscle spindles can be stimulated not only by a short phasic stretching, but also in a more prolonged, tonic manner. Vibration of a tendon usually results in a low amplitude continuous reflex EMG activity in the stimulated muscle (tonic vibration reflex or TVR). TVR can be elicited in almost every muscle. The TVR results from the conjunction of monosynaptic activation of the motor neurons and polysynaptic activation through interneurons. Therefore it could be used to explore indirectly the reactivity of certain interneurons (Delwaide et al. 1980).

2.1.3 Polysinaptic reflexes

Various exteroceptive reflexes can be elicited by stimulation of skin, skin nerve or mixed nerve. The intensity of stimulation (delivered as a single shock or as train of stimuli) should evoke a tactile or a painful sensation (Young 1973).

In the cephalic segment the most studied reflex is the blink reflex that explores a bilateral trigemino-facial reflex arc (Kugelberg 1952).

Stimulating the upper extremities, cutaneous reflexes are elicited fairly easily (Campier 1974, Caccia et al. 1990, Caccia et al. 1991, Reis 1961, Shahani 1970). In the lower extremity, several polysynaptic reflexes were described following stimulation of mixed or skin nerves. The EMG studies of the Babinski reflex showed less than normal activity in extensor hallucis brevis muscle; activity in the flexor hallucis brevis even if less than normal and activity of extensor hallucis longus that did not occur in normal subjects (Vangijn 1976).

By stimulating the sural nerve Hugon (Hugon 1973) elicited reflexes first in the short head of biceps femori muscle, then, with a more intense stimulation, in tibialis anterior muscle. Depending on the stimulus intensity, either a short latency response (RA II) is evoked by painless stimulation or a delayed reflex (RA III) is induced by painful stimulation.

We obtained the same results from normal subjects with a stimulation technique similar to that used by Hugon and recording contemporary from biceps femori, quadriceps femori, tibialis anterior and soleus muscles of both legs. Exaggerated flexor reflexes are easily triggered by peripheral inputs in paraplegic patients. Appling the test on paraplegics we observed that the response threshold was lowered and that there was a change in the EMG pattern of the muscles that responded to the stimulus. In fact distal muscles (tibialis anterior) were activated at lower threshold with respect to proximal ones (biceps femori) and in some patients a co-contraction of tibialis anterior and soleus muscles could indicate a loss of reciprocate inhibition mechanisms. When repeated in standing (sustained) position the test did not showed differences in evoked EMG pattern.

EMG reflex activity was never recorded from the lower limb contralateral to the site of stimulation (Ferrarin 1994).

2.2 Supraspinal influences

A great amount of data suggests that spasticity is not confined only to changes in segmental excitability but reflects also changes in descending control pathways (Delwaide et al. 1984, Martinelli et al. 1979).

If this sentence could be easily accepted for patients with cerebral lesions causing spasticity is not obviously acceptable for spinal cord injured patients where the supraspinal control is supposed to be lost. However, also in paraplegic patients, it is important to evaluate how supraspinal influences may modulate reflex activities of the spinal cord below the lesion.

The assessment of the supraspinal descending influences includes:

a) the cortical magnetic or electrical stimulation, which evokes compound muscle action potentials (CMAPs) from the muscles related to the activated motor cortex. Some reports suggest that the threshold values of the CMAPs obtained from magnetic cortical stimulation are strictly related with stretch reflex enhancement (Abbruzzese et al. 1989, Osio et al. 1992).

b) the indirect evaluation of vestibulo-spinal and reticulo-spinal pathways.

The application of caloric vestibular stimulation (water at 44°C) induces in normal subjects a bilateral facilitation of the H reflex evoked from the soleus muscles. During the following nystagmus phase, activated from the labyrinthine stimulation, such facilitation persists (Delwaide 1977).

In some paraplegic patients with incomplete spinal lesion a certain degree of facilitation of the H reflex was recorded during the test (Ferrarin et al. 1994).

The stimulation of the neck muscles with a long train of electrical stimuli (80 Hz frequency, intensity below the motor threshold) modifies the excitability of the soleus muscle H reflex. In normal subjects the stimulation of the neck muscles inhibits the homolateral and facilitates the contralateral soleus muscle H reflex. these H reflex excitability changes last for about 30 minutes after the end of neck muscles stimulation (Osio et al. 1993).

2.3 Changes in EMG activity

2.3.1 Active movements

Obviously it is possible to use these tests only if a certain degree of voluntary movements is maintained.

The simple analysis of the EMG signal recorded during an alternate voluntary movement of a body segment in spastic patients, shows a clear increment in the duration of the EMG burst of both weak and spastic muscles.

In the same way, ballistic spastic arm movements maintain the alternate pattern of EMG activity, but are slower. EMG bursts are longer in duration and higher in amplitude (Angel 1975, Sahrmann et al. 1977).

2.3.2 Passive movements

Using special equipment with motor torque, goniometers, force transducers and EMG recordings of both agonist and antagonist muscles it is possible to measure the initial position of the limb, the amplitude, the velocity and the degree of the displacement, the resistive and the applied forces, and the degree of relaxation and the reflex activities evoked in the muscles during the dynamic or the static phase of the test.

The resistance that is developed during a passive movement depends from:

1) the mass of the moved segment;
2) the biomechanical properties of the muscles and of the soft tissues;
3) the neural activity (including reflexes) occurring in the course of movements

Long muscle stretches (duration >40-50 msec) elicits 2 or 3 peaks of activity in the rectified EMG in some muscles. These peaks are designated M1 (short latency reflex), M2 and M3 (long latency reflexes). M1 corresponds to the phasic stretch reflex elicited by a muscle stretch of short duration, whereas the origin of the long latency reflexes M2 and M3 is uncertain. Most investigators favour the theory that the long latency reflexes is a long loop reflex involving a transcortical route, other authors emphasize that the long latency reflexes may be of polysynaptic spinal origin (Marsden 1983, Marsden 1973, Tatton et al. 1978).

Burke and Coll. (Burke et al. 1970) studied the stretch reflex in the quadriceps muscle of spastic subjects. They affirmed that stretch reflex was determined by three factors:

1) velocity dependent excitation;
2) length dependent inhibition;
3) fatiguability.

On repeated testing stretch reflex fatigued until a baseline level was obtained.

As the velocity of stretch increased, the magnitude of the stretch reflex increased. On cessation of movement, reflex activity died away (the dynamic phase of stretch reflex was not followed by a static phase).

The magnitude of the stretch reflex was shown by both linear and sinusoidal stretching to be inversely proportional to the initial length of the muscle if the velocity of the stretch remained constant.

He concluded that the length dependent inhibition of stretch reflex arises in secondary spindle endings, and that this inhibition underlies the clasp-knife phenomenon.

A simple method to measuring and evaluating spasticity of the thigh muscles by provoking the stretch reflex during the passive swing of a limb is the pendulum test (Wartemberg test).

The pendulum testing of spasticity was found to be especially useful to evaluate anti spastic treatments. The number of total oscillations, the total swing time, relaxation index and other biomechanical parameters are measured. Relaxation index (the ratio between the magnitude of the first drop and the magnitude of the initial angle) was found to be the best index (Bajd et al. 1984).

The association of the EMG recordings from flexor and extensor muscles of the leg permitted to introduce an evaluation of the neural reflex component connected with the passive swing of the leg. In normal subjects EMG activity does not occur, whereas in spastic patient a defined stretch reflex appears (Bajd et al. 1984).

We developed a biomechanical and electromiograpich method to assess thigh muscles spasticity with the Wartemberg test (Ferrarin et al. 1993). This test is now part of the complex battery of tests that we use in the evaluation of spastic patients.

3 Conclusions

This review suggests that only applying a complete neurophysiological and biomechanical assessment it is possible to evaluate quantitatively the features of spasticity in patients with upper motor neuron syndromes. The more significant data collected in the assessment of each patient should be compared in repeated evaluation in order to follow up patient features and eventually to test the effects of treatments.

References

Abbruzzese, G., Vische, M., Ratto, S., Abbruzzese, M., Favale, E. (1985) Assessment of motor neuron excitability in Parkinsonian rigidity by the F wave. *J Neurol*,**232**: 246-249.

Abbruzzese, G., Dell'Agata, D., Morena, M., Primavera, A., Favale, E. (1989) Studio elettrofisiologico delle vie motorie centrali nelle sindromi lacunari. Osservazioni preliminari. Atti Riunione Primaverile Soc Ital EEG Neurofisiol Clin, Roma p13.

Abbruzzese, G. (1990) Spasticità: stato dell'arte della valutazione neurofisiologica. *Europ Med Phys*, **26**:115-119.

Angel R.W. (1975) Electromyography during voluntary movement. The two burst pattern. *EEG Clin Neurophysiol*, **36**:433-438.

Bajd, T., Vodovnik, L. (1984) Pendulum testing of spasticity. *J Biomed Eng*, **6**:9-16.

Burke, D., Gillies, J.D., Lance, J.W. (1970) The quadriceps stretch reflex in human spasticity. *J Neurol Neurosurg Psychiatry*, **33**:216-223.

Caccia, M.R., Osio, M., Tornaghi, R., Viganò, A., Tommasi, P. (1990) Electropysiological observations on the palmomental reflex in normal neonates. *Neurophysiol Clin*, **20**:455-462.

Caccia, M.R., Osio, M., Mangoni, A. (1991) The palmomental reflex from mechanical stimulation in normal humans. *EMG Clin Neurophysiol* **32/1**:151-156.

Campier, J., Dehen, H., Bathien, N. (1974) Upper limb cutaneous polysynaptic reflexes. *J Neurol Sci*, **22**:39-49.

Delwaide, J.P. (1971) Etude experimentale de l'hyperreflexie tendineuse en clinique neurologique. Arsica, Bruxelles.

Delwaide, P.J. (1977) Excitability of the lower myotatic arcs under the influence of caloric labyrinthine stimulation, *J Neurol Neurosurg Psychiatry*, **40**:970-974.

Delwaide, P.J., Martinelli, P., Crenna, P. (1980) Clinical Neurophysiological Measurement of Spinal Reflex Activity. In: R.G. Feldman, R.R. Young, W.P. Koella (eds) *Spasticity: Disordered Motor Control*, Year Book Medical Publisher, Chicago and London, pp.345-371.

Delwaide, J.P., Crenna, P. (1984) Cutaneous nerve stimulation and motorneuronal excitability: II evidence for non-segmental influences. *J Neurol Neurosurg and Psychiatry*, **47**:190-196.

Eisen, A., Odusote, K. (1979) Amplitude of the F wave: a potential means of documenting spasticity. *Neurol*, **29**: 1306- 1309.

Ferrarin, M., Frigo, C., Osio, M., Crenna, P., Pedotti, A., Mangoni, A. (1993) Assessment of spasticity by an integrated system for the analysis of pendular motion and EMG activity. *EEG Clin Neurophysiol*, **2**:S66.

Ferrarin, M., Osio, M., Abello, G., Cardini, R., Crenna, P., Pedotti, A, Mangoni, A. (1994) Batteria di test neurofisiologici e biomeccanici per la valutazione di pazienti paraplegici ai fini dell'ortesizzazione ibrida. *Eur Medicophysica*, **30**(4):193-204.

Fries, W., Danek, A., Sheidtmann, K. and Hamburger, C. (1993) Motor recovery following capsular stroke. Role of the descending pathways from multiple motor areas. *Brain*, **116**:369-382.

Hugon, M. (1973) Exteroceptive reflexes to stimulation of the sural nerve in normal man. In: J.E. Desmedt (ed.) *New Developments in Electromyography and Clinical Neurophysiology*, **3,** S Karger AG, Basel, pp. 713-729.

Kugelberg, E. (1952) Facial reflexes. *Brain*, **75**:385-396.

Lance, J.W. (1980) Pathophysiology of spasticity and clinical experience with baclofen. In: R.G. Feldman, R.R. Young and W.P. Koella (eds.) *Spasticity: Disordered Motor Control*, Year Book Medical Publisher, Chicago and London, pp. 185-203.

Marsden, C.D., Merton, P.A., Morton, H.B. (1973) Is the human stretch reflex xortical rather than spinal? *Lancet*, **1**:759-761.

Marsden, C.D., Rothwell, J.C., Day, B.L. (1983) Long-latency automatic responses to muscle stretch in man: origin and function. In: J.E. Desmedt (ed.) *Motor Control Mechanisms in Health and Disease*, Raven Press, New York, pp. 509-539.

Martinelli, P., Delwaide, P.J., De Pasqua, V. (1979) Reflexes du muscle soleaire evoques par la stimulation du nerf tibial posterieur versus reflex tendineux chez l'homme. *Rev Electroencephalogr Neurophysiol*, **9**:72-76.

Osio, M., Forni, M., Mini, M., Caputo, D., Mangoni, A. (1992) Magnetic Cortical Stimulation in multiple sclerosis patients with prevalent pyramidal signs and with cerebellar-pyramidal signs. 6th Europ Congress of Clin Neurophysiol. Lisbon 19-22 Sept 1992.

Osio, M., Alpini, D., Mangoni, A. (1993) Transcutaneous electric stimulation of the cervical muscles evokes cervico-spinal reflexes in normal adults. *EEG Clin Neurophysiol*, 2:S30.

Pinelli, P. (1975) L'apporto EMG nella valutazione della spasticità: criteri differenziali e quantitativi. *Il Pensiero Scientifico*, **60**:13-25.

Pinelli, P., Di Lorenzo, G. (1989) Electromyographic Assessment of Spasticity. *Ital J Neurol Sci*, **10**:137-144.

Reis, P.J. (1961) The palmomental reflex. *Arch Neurol*, **4**:486-495.

Sahrmann, S.A., Norton, B.J. (1977) The relationship of voluntary movement to spasticity in the upper motor neuron syndrome. *Annals of Neurol*, **2**:460-465.

Schiller, P.H., Stalberg, E. (1978) F responses studied with single fibre EMG in normal subjects and spastic patients. *J Neurol. Neurosurg. Psychiatry*, **41**:45-53.

Shahani, B.T., Burrows, P., Whitty, C.W. (1970) The grasp reflex and preservation. *Brain*, **93**: 181-192.

Tatton, W.G., Bawa, P., Bruce, I.C., Lee, R.G. (1978) Long-loop reflexes in monkeys: an interpretative base for human reflexes. In: J.E. Desmdt (ed.) *Cerebral Motor Control in Man: Long Loop Mechanisms*, Karger, Basel, pp. 229-245.

Tower, S.S. (194) Pyramidal lesion in the monkey. *Brain*, **63**:36.

Vangijn, J. (1976) Equivocal plantar responses: a clinical and electromyographic study. *J Neurol Neurosurg Psychiatry*, **39**:275-282.

Young, R.R. (1973) The clinical significance of exteroceptive reflexes. In: J.E. Desmedt (ed.) *New Developments in Electromyography and Clinical Neurophysiology*. S Karger AG, Basel, **3**:697-712.

A New Biomechanical Approach to Pendulum Test for Spasticity Evaluation

M. Ferrarin[1,2], M. Osio[3], G. Abello[2]
[1]Dipartimento di Bioingegneria, Politecnico di Milano, Milano, I
[2]Centro di Bioingegneria, Fond. Pro Juventute Don Gnocchi, Milano, I
[3]Unità di Riabilitazione Neurologica, Fond. Pro Juventute Don Gnocchi, Milano, I

Abstract - In this paper a new biomechanical approach to implement the pendulum test for spasticity assessment is presented from a methodological point of view. The use of an automatic Motion Analysis System to acquire lower limbs movements allowed to detect kinematic data without interferring with patient movements and minimising the duration of the experimental session. Moreover the implementation of a skeletomuscular model of legs permitted to compute muscle length and lengthening velocity during pendular movements. Surface EMG signals of thigh muscles were acquired simultaneously to kinematic analysis allowing the definition of correlation parameters between neuromuscular events and lengthening muscle state. Examples of results obtained from a group of paraplegic patients with Spinal Cord Injury and from a control group of healthy subject are here presented.

1 Introduction

Several pathologies of Central Nervous System are characterised by "a velocity-dependent increase in tonic stretch reflexes with exaggerated tendon jerks" (Lance, 1980 [27]) a syndrome known as spasticity. Clinically it is expressed by an increase of muscle tone during passive stretch movements.

A need for an objective measurement of spasticity is unquestioned to quantify the effects of any antispastic treatment (pharmacological, kinesiological, electrical stimulation, etc). Several pathological mechanisms can be responsible for spastic phenomena [1,2] and some of them can be present simultaneously. Different methods have been developed to assess the level on patient, each of them, probably, being testing different features of spasticity as shown by the low cross-correlation of the scores [3].

The most common clinical test to quantify spasticity are based on passive manoeuvres (FPM-Fast Passive Movement, tendon jerk, etc.) performed by physical therapist in order to evaluate the muscle resistance to stretch movements and the amount or duration of clonus, but even with the introduction of quantitative scale (Ashworth [4], Pedersen [5]) and their subsequent modifications with additional intermediate grade [15] there are difficulties in data comparison because of subjective assessment and high variability.

Spasticity evaluation can be performed in a more quantitative way with neurophysiological or with biomechanical procedures, the latter being closer to the classical clinical evaluations in their implementation. Our approach to neurophysiological testing of spasticity are described elsewhere in this book [7].

Concerning biomechanical methods, the pendulum test [8], in which the stretch reflex of knee extensor muscles is provoked by a passive swing of the leg, is particularly attractive since it is simple to be performed, completely untroublesome for the patient and meaningful indices can be easily obtained. For these reasons it was used in several studies both for research and for clinical applications. Bajd and Vodovnik [10] and Katz et al. [22] computed pendulum indices in hemiplegic patients after a stroke and in paraplegic patients with spinal cord injury, comparing them with data taken from healthy subjects. Several groups (Andrews et al. [13], Bajd et al. [17,18], Robinson et al. [19,20] and Kawamura et al. [21]) used the pendulum test to quantify the effects of surface electrical stimulation on spasticity level in patients with spinal cord injury. Brown et al. [11,12] reported data acquired with the pendulum test on elderly stroke and Parkinsonian patients and healthy elderly subjects in order to verify the capability of the test to distinguish between spasticity and rigidity.

After a brief historical review about pendulum test methodologies, the main disadvantages of classical implementation will be underlined and then a new method to perform it with an integrated system for the analysis of movements and EMG activity will be described. Results obtained by its application on Spinal Cord Injured patients and five healthy subjects as control will be presented too.

2 Methods

2.1 Review on Pendulum Test development and main parameters

The pendulum test was firstly proposed by Wartenberg in 1951 [8] and it is commonly performed still in its original form hereunder described. The patient was lying on his back with the legs hanging over the edge of a table. The examiner lifted the patient's leg until the full extension of the knee was achieved and then he released it allowing the leg to swing freely. Comparing with healthy subject, spastic patient presented a lower number of swings and a reduced swinging time. In Wartenberg's paper the test was only evaluated qualitatively.

In 1958 Boczko and Mumenthaler [15] quantified the pendulum test by recording on a film of a slowly moving camera the swinging movements of a light fastened to the big toe. An Amplitude Quotient was defined to evaluate the extent of braking during the first pendulous movement.

The use of an electrogoniometer to assess knee joint movements during the pendulum test was introduced by Bajd and Bowman in 1981 [18] and since then it was commonly adopted for its simplicity and low cost [10]. One side of the electrogoniometer was fixed to the calf of the subject and the other to the table, assuming the thigh to be fixed with table surface; special arrangement were used to allow the calibration of device rotation axis with the knee joint rotation centre and to avoid bending stresses on the bars arising because of the movement of joint rotation centre during the swinging of the leg. A tachometer was also used to measure the angular velocity of the joint; alternatively it could be computed by analogue (electronic) or digital (software) derivation. Finally surface EMG of quadriceps muscle were recorded. All data were collected through an A/D converter by a microcomputer where all elaboration and data presentation were performed [16].

Several indices were defined on the basis of data acquired during the pendulum test and most of them refer to knee goniogram (time course of knee joint angular displacement during the pendular movements) and tachogram (time course of knee joint angular velocity), shown in fig.1 for an healthy subject. The main proposed parameters are: Amplitude Quotient, Relaxation Index (RI), first maximum of the goniogram, first maximum and first minimum of the tachogram, first swing angular acceleration, rebound angular acceleration (maximum value during the rebound from the first swing), number of swings, area between goniogram and resting angle and time duration of oscillations. However only for the RI it has been reported a minimal variability in repeated measures, an acceptable correlation with clinical score of spasticity and good correspondence between changes in its value and changes in the spastic condition of the patient [11,22,23,24].

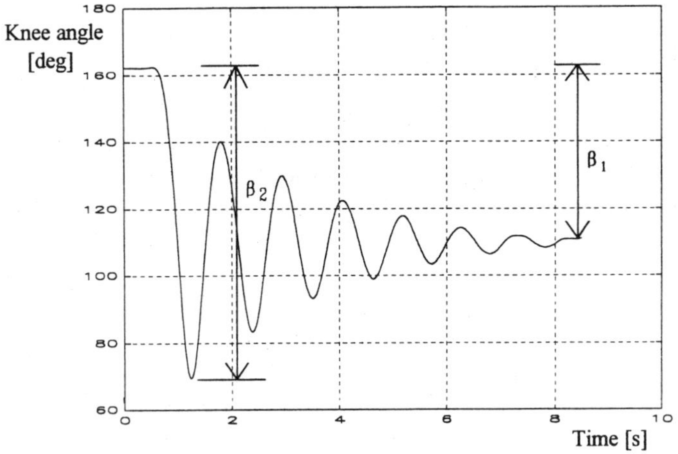

Fig. 1. Knee goniogram of an healthy subject.

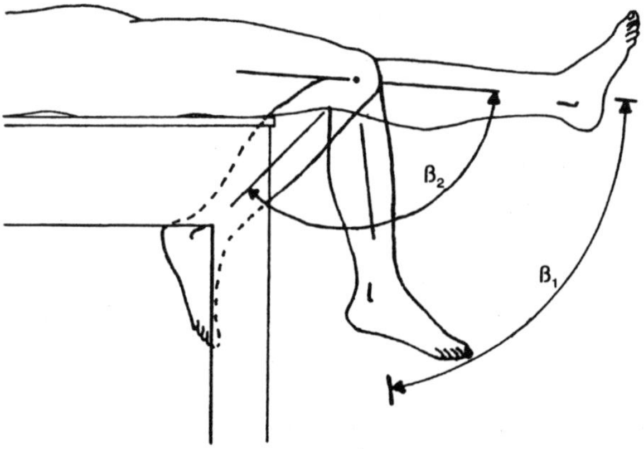

Fig. 2. Angles schematization for the definition of the Relaxation Index.

The Relaxation Index is defined [18] as the ratio between the magnitude of the first swing (starting angle - first minimum) and the magnitude of the starting angle respect the resting angle (starting angle - resting angle), as shown in fig. 1 and 2. That is:

$$RI = \frac{\varphi_0 - \varphi_1}{\varphi_0 - \varphi_f} = \frac{\beta_2}{\beta_1} \tag{1}$$

where:

φ_0 = Starting Angle;
φ_1= First Minimum of goniogram;
φ_f= Resting angle;

The meaning of RI is to quantify the braking effect of extensor muscles on knee joint during the flexion movement in the first swing of the leg: bigger the muscle braking action is, smaller the RI is. In healthy subject the amplitude of RI was found to be 1.6 or more while in spastic patient smaller values are generally found, because of their exaggerated stretch reflexes. For this reason Bajd et al. [18] proposed a Normalised Relaxation Index (NRI) obtained dividing RI by 1.6:

$$NRI = RI / 1.6 \tag{2}$$

Thus NRI > 1 would signify a non-spastic limb whereas NRI < 1 would quantify the spasticity level. On the other hand, the normal value 1.6 depends by the protocol used to perform the test (patient position, number of warming-up swings, etc.), by the measuring system configuration (instrument characteristics, sampling rate, kind of filtering on acquired data, etc.), and by the age of the subjects [11]. For example Brown et al. [11] performed the pendulum test in three different back position (supine, semi-supine and sitting) in two groups of healthy subjects: elderly (mean age 68.5) and young adult (mean age 22). They reported RI mean values between 1.47 and 1.55 in the elderly subjects and between 1.56 and 1.69 in the young adult subject group, depending by the back position but without any clear trend. As a general rule each laboratory is therefore raccomanded to compute its own normative values for different clusters of age.

Concerning the other parameters coming out from the pendulum test, they are not so widely used as the RI because there are big differences in normative values reported by different authors: for instance the first maximum of the tachogram (peak of angular velocity during the first swing) was found in the range between 11 and 17 rad/s by Bajd et al. [10] and in the range between 4.9 and 5.2 rad/s for young adult and between 5.3 and 6.4 rad/s for elderly subject by Brown at al. [11]. The big differences between these studies can not be easily explained, even taking into account some differences in the experimental procedure: in particular the values reported in Bajd's work seems really too high for having any reasonable significance. Moreover all the parameters computed on the basis of angular velocity depend on the derivative procedure adopted, and in particular peak of velocity are very dependent on the filtering procedure performed on acquired data, preventing an easy definition of reference values.

For all these reasons the most widely used parameter is the Relaxation Index and all studies about pendulum test refer to it.

Nevertheless its wide application the classical implementation of the pendulum test presents some disadvantages here summarised:

a) it needs the positioning of an electrogoniometer on the patient leg, with an adequate device calibration,

b) in Bajd's protocol, to which all the subsequent works refer to, the angle measured with the electrogoniometer is the absolute angle between the shank and the horizontal direction, and not the real knee flexion-extension angle, since the thigh is not completely fixed on the table,

c) the analysis of the knee angle gives only an approximation of changes in length of biarticular muscles like Rectus Femoris, since it depends by the hip angle too,

d) RI alone doesn't distinguish between length and lengthening velocity dependence of spastic reflexes.

Attempting to face to these drawbacks we proposed [25] a new implementation of the Pendulum Test together with a modelization of muscles length for the definition of new parameters.

2.2 New Implementation and Elaboration

In order to overcome the acquisition problems (issue a), to guarantee the correctness on angle measurements (issue b) and to provide a simultaneous computation of knee and hip angles (issue c) the use of an automatic Motion

Analysis System to perform data acquisition has been introduced. Kinematic data are collected with an ELITE system (BTS, Italy) and Electromyography with an 8 channel telemetric system (TELEMG, BTS, Italy): the dedicated hardware is able to recognise in the TV field of view the shape of small retroreflective markers (10 mm.) glued on significant landmarks on the subject's body and to compute their 3-Dimensional coordinates with an accuracy of less than 1mm. For Pendulum Test acquisition markers are glued in correspondence with iliac crest, femoral great trochanter (hip), lateral femoral epycondyle (knee), lateral malleolus (ankle) and fifth metatarsal head. A couple of TV cameras, working at a sampling rate of 100Hz, are used for each side of the body in order to alternate the test on each leg without any recalibration. EMG signals are recorded from Rectus Femoris (RF), Vastus Medialis (VM), long head of Biceps Femori (BFCL) and SemiMembranosus (SM) muscles using surface electrodes (bandwidth 10 - 200 Hz). EMG signals are then sampled at 500Hz and sent to a PC were are collected together with kinematic data. In fig.3 a patient during an acquisition trial is shown: markers and electrodes positioning are visible on patient legs together with the TV recording cameras.

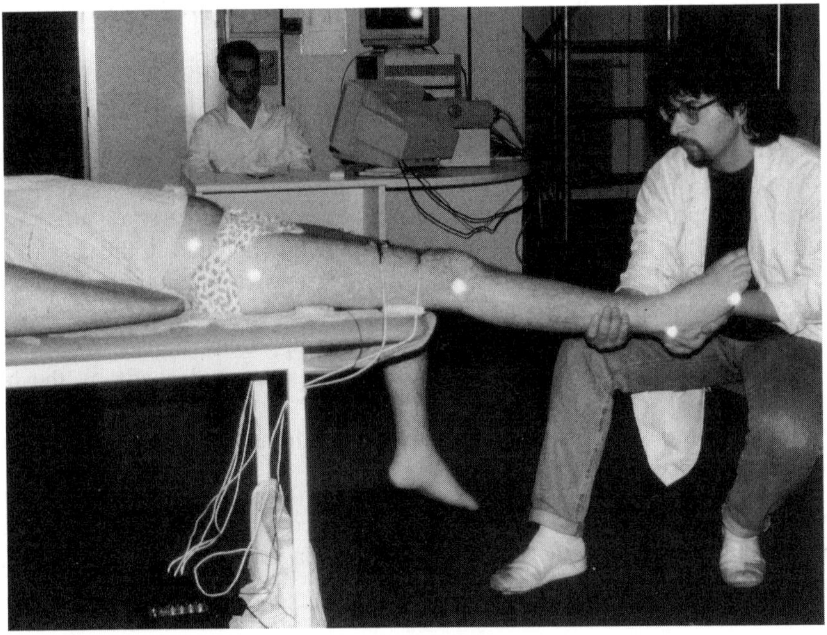

Fig. 3. Photograph of a patient during the Pendulum Test.

Ten warming up swings are firstly performed to bypass any initial irregular phase and then ten swings for each leg alternately are captured, waiting 30 seconds between each swing. Starting from marker trajectories and some anthropometrical parameters of the patient the internal rotation center of ankle, knee and hip joints are then computed. Flexion/extension movements of the three joints are then computed and angular velocities are finally obtained through numerical differentiation.

The geometrical model of the main lower limb muscles proposed by Frigo and Pedotti [26] and shown in fig.4 has been implemented permitting the length and lengthening velocity of each muscle to be estimated from acquired data.

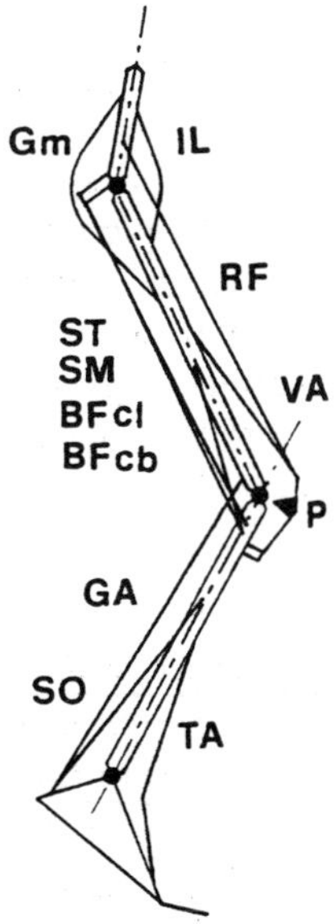

Fig. 4. Muscle modelization used to compute change in length during movement (from Frigo, 1992 [29]).

The parameters extracted by the developed software are the following:

- ARI (Angular Relaxation Index), computed on the basis of the knee goniogram,
- LRI (Length Relaxation Index), defined on the muscle length graphic with the same principle used on the goniogram for the ARI,
- AT (Angle Threshold) and AVT (Angular Velocity Threshold), respectively defined as the knee angle and angular velocity in correspondence with the onset of the EMG burst,
- LT (Length Threshold) and LVT (Lengthening Velocity Threshold), respectively defined as the muscle length and lengthening velocity in correspondence with the onset of the EMG burst.

The last four parameters concern specifically the trigger of the muscle stretch reflex and are computed taking into account the different delay of the arch reflex in each muscle: they are useful to distinguish between length and lengthening velocity dependence of spastic reflexes (issue d). Obviously they can be calculated only on the muscles analysed with EMG recording, while the LRI can be computed on all muscles.

All parameters are computed automatically for each trial of a session and are then presented in trend graph (bar diagram), in order to analyse their consistency.

3 Results

In this section some graphs obtained from spinal cord injured patients will be presented to show a sample of results coming from this methodological approach.

In tab.1 the general characteristics of analysed subjects are reported. All patients are paraplegics (age: 30.7 ± 9.0) with a level lesion ranging between C7 and T9. Two of them are under pharmacological antispastic treatment (Baclofen), able to reduce spasticity at a very low level as shown by Ashworth score (measured on knee joint). A group of healthy subjects were also analysed to obtain reference data.

Table 1 - Subject characteristics

Subject	Sex	Age	Spinal Cord Lesion Level	Antispastic Treatment	Ashworth Score
A	m	43	C7 (*)	no	3
B	m	39	T9 (*)	no	3
C	m	24	T4	yes	1
D	m	20	T8	yes	0
E	m	26	T6	no	1
F	m	32	T9	no	2
Healthy Subjects (n=4)		25.8±3.6			

(*) Denotes an incomplete lesion

Each of the next figures is composed by the following three groups of graphs: (1) EMG activity of the interesting muscles, (2) muscle displacement (both (1) and (2) are characterised by the initials of muscle name) and (3) knee joint displacement (the last graph on the bottom of each figure). In each displacement graph the solid line represent muscle length (in graph (2)) or knee angle (in graph (3)), and the dotted line represent the muscle lengthening velocity or knee angular velocity respectively. Scales on the left refer to linear (mm/s) and angular velocity (deg/s), while on the right to length (mm) and angle (deg). Little circles point out values used to define the Relaxation Indices.

In fig.5 a typical graphic output obtained from an healthy subject is shown: length graph of Rectus Femoris and SemiMembranosus muscles are presented together with EMG signals showing neither voluntary nor reflex activity. The knee goniogram is characterised by 8 swings, a total oscillation time of 9 sec and an Angle Relaxation Index of 1.7: all these values are within the normal range reported in literature. The muscle length graph show a typical phase opposition in the stretching of antagonistic muscle, with a max stretch velocity of 119.2 mm/s for RF and 275.7 mm/s for SM. Both velocities are over the range of minimal velocity (3-113 mm/s) able to produce a stretch reflex as reported by Burke et al. [28]. The Length Relaxation Index is 1.23 for RF and 2.05 for SM.

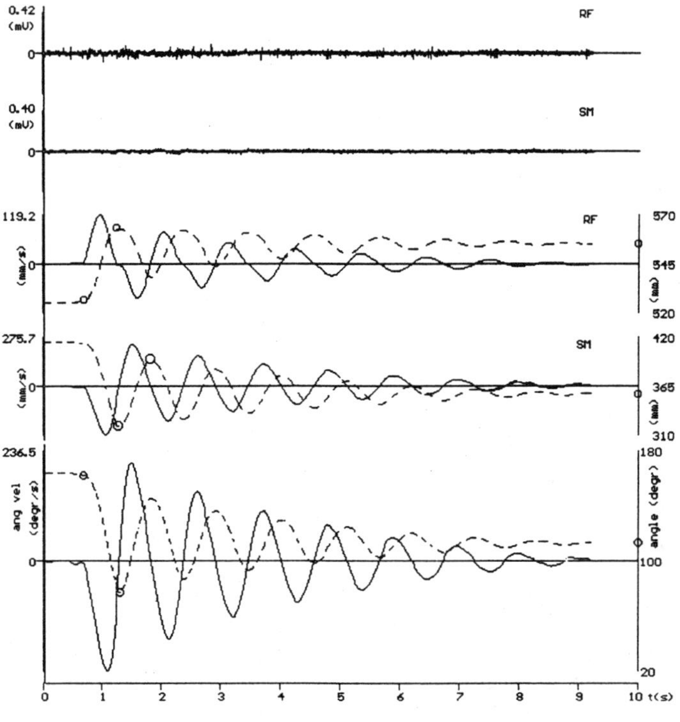

Fig. 5. Results on a healthy subject: EMG signals on RF and SM muscles, length and lengthening velocity of RF and SM, knee angle and angular velocity. No muscle activation is present. Parameters are: ARI=1.7, LRI_RF=1.23, LRI_SM=2.05.

In fig.6 a trial performed on patient E (right leg) with a mild level of spasticity (Ashworth score = 1) is shown. The correspondent ARI is 1.47 while the LRI of RF is 1.08, both lower than normal and in coherence with the knee angular movement that is similar to the normal one but with a higher damping behaviour. This is due to the RF reflex activity arising in correspondence of the maximal stretching velocity (LVT=162.4 mm/s, AVT= -244 deg/s), as shown by the synchronisation vertical line. The LRI of RF is 1.08 The EMG signals of the other muscles show no activation.

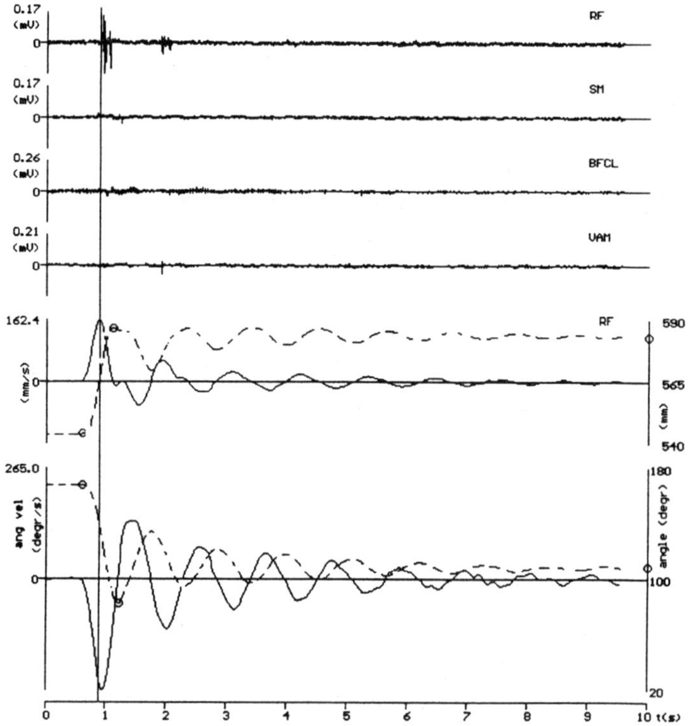

Fig. 6. Patient E, right leg, with a moderate level of spasticity (Ashworth=1). Stretch reflexes are present on RF muscle during the first (AVT=-244deg/s, LVT=162.4mm/s) and second swing, while no activation is present on the other muscles. The other parameters are ARI = 1.47, LRI_RF = 1.08.

In fig.7 the results of left leg on patient A, with a medium level of spasticity are shown. Compared to patient E, it is clear a lower velocity threshold of stretch reflex on RF muscle (LVT=115mm/s, AVT= -153deg/s) and the persistence of EMG activation also for the subsequent 5-6 swings. The more dumped oscillation pattern leads to an ARI of 0.99 and an LRI of 0.98 for RF muscle.

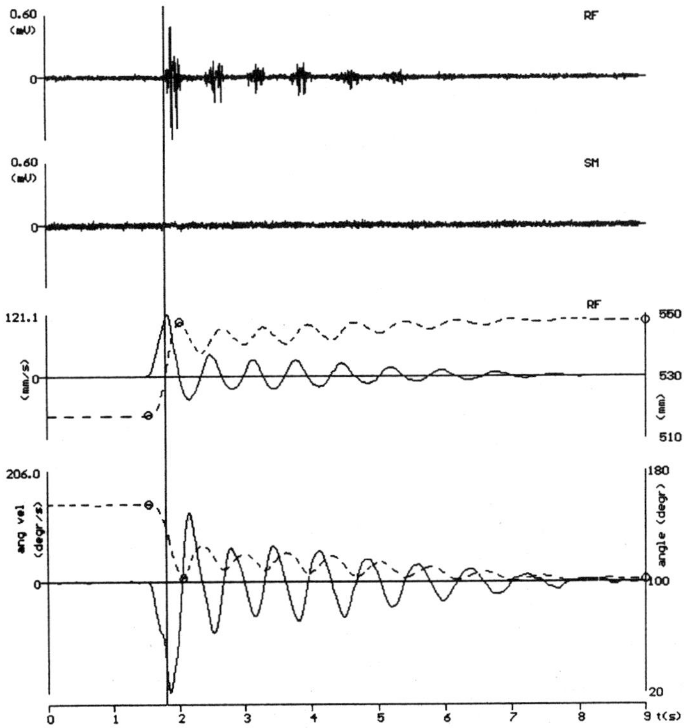

Fig. 7. Patient A, left leg, with a medium level of spasticity. Stretch reflexes are present on the first 6 swings of RF muscle. ARI=0.99, LRI_RF=0.98, AVT_RF= -153deg/s, LVT_RF=115mm/s.

It is interesting to note that the right leg of the same patient presents a different pattern, nevertheless the ARI and the LRI of RF are quite similar in both limbs. As shown in fig.8, in fact, (a) the velocity threshold of RF activity is higher (LVT=121mm/s), (b) it is no more present the multiactivation of RF in the later swings and, on the contrary, (c) there is an activation of SM muscle in correspondence of the maximal stretching velocity (LVT=134mm/s). These different behaviours can be studied only by means the simultaneous analysis of EMG activity and change in muscle length.

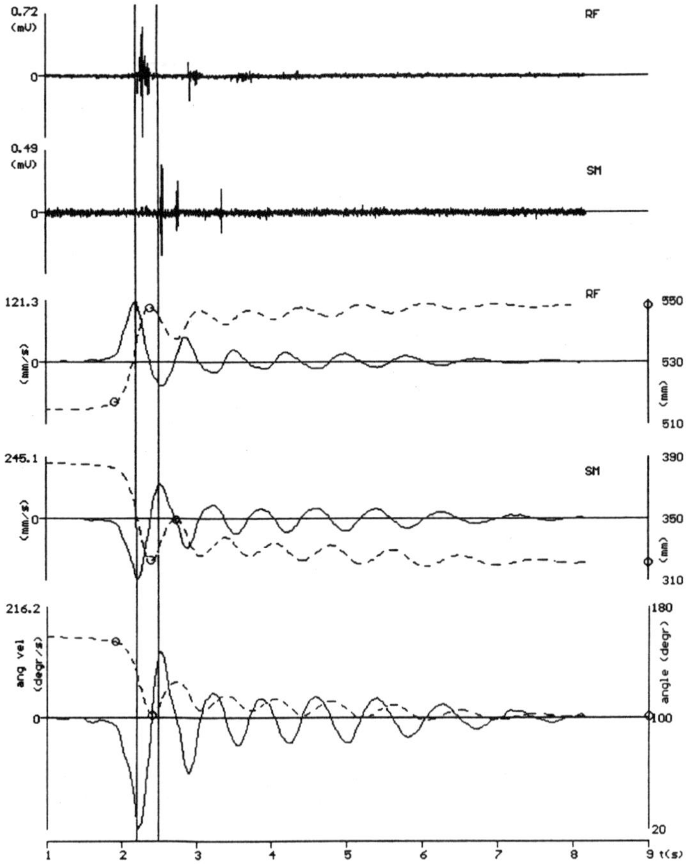

Fig. 8. Patient A, right leg, medium level of spasticity. Reflexes are present on both RF and SM muscles, each of them in correspondence of maximum stretch velocity (LVT is 121mm/s for RF and 134mm/s for SM). ARI=0.98, LRI_RF=0.98.

Fig.9 shows a pattern of severe spasticity (patient B, right limb, Ashworth scale = 3), characterised by a very low threshold in velocity on RF stretch reflex (LVT=91mm/s, AVT= -125deg/s) which produce a high breaking effect on the oscillations. The reflex activation of RF is able to stop the knee joint during the first flexion (at 143 deg) before the achievement of the resting angle (passage from the vertical line) and even to produce 10 deg of extension. Number of swings and time duration of oscillations is highly reduced respect all the previous patients. Note that the spasticity is present selectively only on RF as shown by the absence of EMG signals in the other analysed muscles.

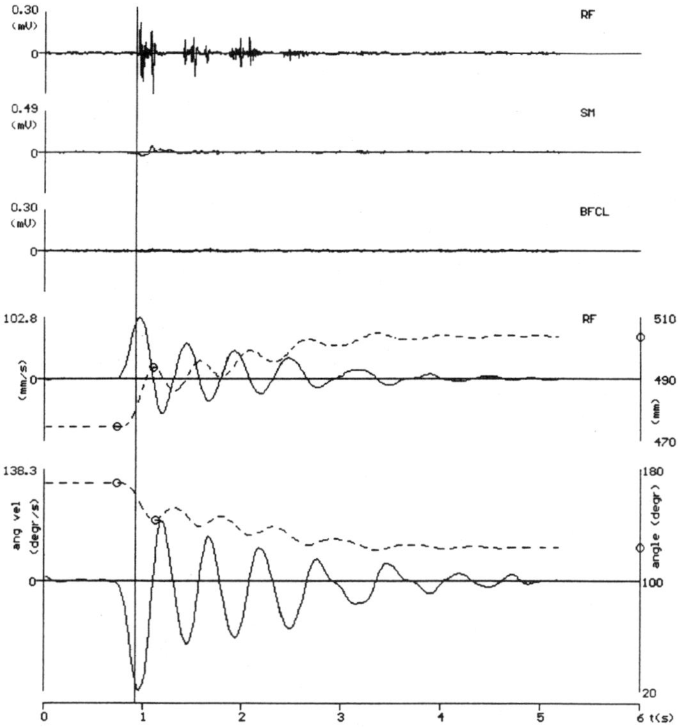

Fig. 9. Patient B, right limb with severe spasticity (Ashworth = 3). AVT= -125deg/s, LVT_RF=91mm/s, ARI=0.59, LRI_LF=0.66.

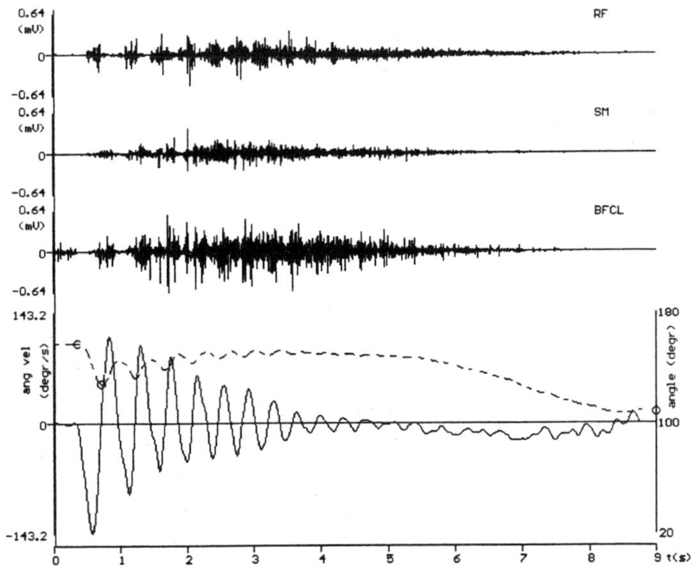

Fig. 10. Pattern with co-contraction of antagonistic muscles followed by slow knee flexion.

In fig.10 a different pattern sometimes found in patient with severe spasticity level is shown. In a first phase (up to 2 sec) it is characterised by a phasic and alternate activation of knee extensor (RF) and flexor (SM, BFCL) muscles, in accordance with the stretching effect of the joint movements on each muscle. Subsequently the oscillation frequency increase and the phasic activation blend in a tonic co-contraction of the antagonistic muscles with a stiffening effect on the knee joint that stops it in extended position. Finally, when the extensors activity decrease, it starts to flex slowly towards the resting position. In few cases a clonus not self exhaustible starts and the acquisition is manually stopped. When these complex patterns are present only by means of a global approach it is possible to characterise the phenomenon, since the classical ARI lose any significance if considered by itself.

In table 2 the ARI, LRI and velocity threshold parameters for Rectus Femoris muscle are shown for all patients and control group. They are computed as the average values on ten trials of an evaluation session.

Table 2 - Mean values of Relaxation Indices and EMG based parameters

Subject	ARI		LRI on RF		AVT on RF [deg/s]		LVT on RF [mm/s]	
	Right	Left	Right	Left	Right	Left	Right	Left
A	0.95	1.00	0.98	0.97	-164.1	-162.2	105.8	108.5
B	0.82	0.93	0.88	0.96	-167.3	-190.3	119.0	130.0
C	1.38	1.53	1.15	1.19	-246.7	-259.2	175.4	179.4
D	1.82	1.81	1.17	1.17	(*)		(*)	
E	1.49	1.49	1.09	1.07	-251.0	-253.1	162.0	155.2
F	1.19	1.22	1.04	1.04	-234.1	-213.2	145.8	127.1
Healthy S. (n=4)	1.73±0.06		1.21±0.02		(*)		(*)	

(*) No activation of stretch reflex

4 Discussion

Table 2 show a good correlation between ARI, LRI and threshold parameters: with few exceptions higher the Relaxation Indices are, higher the velocity threshold of stretch reflex are. Comparing these data with Ashworth score a good correlation with clinical evaluation is also found.

The ARI range found in the group of healthy subjects is similar to what reported in literature [10,23] with a slight increase due to the different way of measuring knee angle (absolute vs. relative) as explained previously (issue b).

Patient D shows complete absence of spasticity (Ashworth = 0, ARI even bigger than normal) with no reflex activities elicited on leg muscles. Patient C and E show a low level of spasticity (Ashworth = 1) with a high velocity threshold. In particular patient C and D were treated with anti spastic drugs whose effects are quite clear: it is possible to hypothesise the use of Pendulum Test to find the best dosage, optimal compromise between desired effects and secondary drawback. Patient F is characterised by a moderate level of spasticity (Ashworth = 2) and an intermediate velocity threshold. The patients A and B present a quite high level of spasticity (Ashworth = 3) with different typology: patient A has the lowest velocity threshold of stretch reflex while patient B is characterised by a higher threshold with a bigger breaking action of RF.

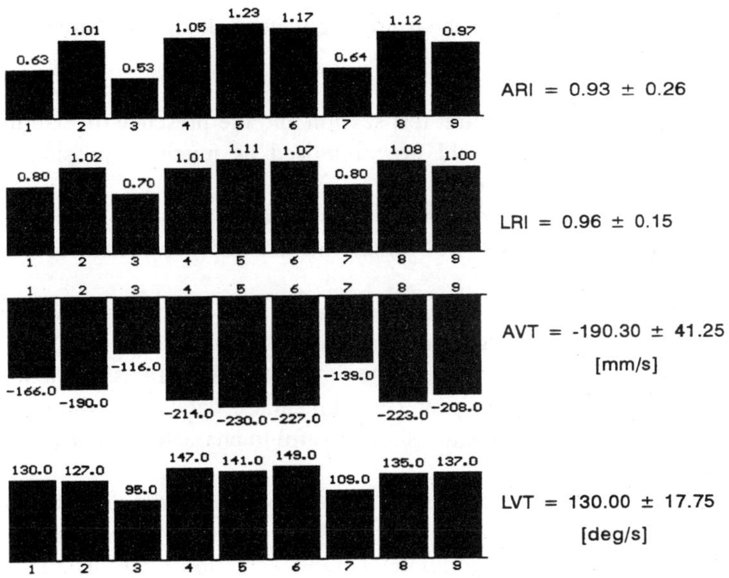

Fig. 11. Trend graph of Relaxation Indices and velocity threshold parameters on Rectus Femoris within one experimental session (patient B).

Some patients show a repetitive pattern of reflex response during a session while others present big differences from one swing to the next one. This is the case, for example, of patient B whose trend graph relative to one acquisition session is presented in fig.11: the diagrams show (from up to down) ARI, LRI, AVT and LVT from the first to the last trial of the same experiment. There is a good inter-parameter coherence with a low data consistency. This variability is very dependent from the actual state of the patient that is highly influenced by hardly controllable variable (his psychological relaxation, tiredness, bowels state, etc.). For this reason the total duration of an experimental session should be as short as possible. Moreover the variability could be partially explained by the presence of biarticular muscles (Rectus Femoris and hamstrings) whose length and lengthening velocity depend also on hip joint position and movement. For example we found that a modification of only 5 degrees in the hip angle during the test provokes a drastic change in the movement pattern. With the present experimental protocol we are able to assess both legs in a short time (around 45 minutes included patient preparation, warming-up and 20 acquired trials) without any device calibration on the patient and with the possibility to look simultaneously also at the hip joint.

5 Conclusions

From the above discussion the following methodological considerations can be derived:

1) time duration of pendulum test session and the presence of external devices mounted on the patient should be minimised as much as possible to reduce uncontrollable influencing factors;

2) the approximation of knee angle with the absolute angle of the shank is not neglectable since the thigh is not fixed with the table: it influences the value of pendulum test parameters;

3) the computation of muscle length permit to analyse the length and lengthening velocity dependence of spasticity;

4) EMG signals are very useful to interpret goniograms particularly when different response patterns appear from kinematic data: they allow to compute new parameters (stretch reflex threshold) useful to characterise spasticity.

Our feeling is that for a good interpretation of pendulum test data and to expand its evaluative potentiality a more global and user friendly assessment set-up than the classical electrogoniometer implementation is needed. Since motion analysis system are more and more widespread in clinical environment for gait analysis, we are suggesting to use them also for this purpose. In this paper our methodology has been presented and some results have been shown to demonstrate its usefulness. In addition to the previous considerations the presented approach has the further advantage of allowing more elaboration to be performed such as the dynamic evaluation of joint moments and powers and the correlation of these variables with the muscles activity.

References

[1] Abbruzzese, G., (1990) Spasticity: the state-of-the-art of neurophysiological evaluation, Europa MedicoPhysica, 26(3): 115-119.

[2] Chapman, C. E. and Wiesendange,r M. (1982) Physiological and anatomical basis of spasticity: review, Physiother. Can., 34: 125-136.

[3] Baxendale, R. H., (1996) A comparison of clinical and biomechanical assessment of spinal spasticity", this volume.
[4] Ashworth, B. (1964) Preliminary trial of carisoprodol in multiple sclerosis, Practitioner, 192: 540-542.
[5] Pedersen, E. (1969) Spasticity: mechanism, measurement and menagement. Springfield: CC Thomas, 36-54.
[7] Osio, M. and Ferrarin, M. (1996) "Biomechanical and Neurophysiological implications on spasticity assessment", this volume.
[8] Wartenberg., R. (1951) Pendulousness of the leg as a diagnostic test, Neurology, 1: 18-24.
[9] Bajd, T. and Bowman B. (1982) Testing and modelling of spasticity, J. Biomed. Eng., 4: 90-96.
[10] Bajd, T. and Vodovnik, L. (1984) Pendulum testing of spasticity, J. Biomed. Eng., 6: 9-16, 1984.
[11] Brown, R. A., Lawson, D. A., Leslie, G. C., and Part, N. J. (1988) Observations on the applicability of the Wartenberg pendulum test to healthy elderly subjects, J. Neurol. Neurosurg. Psychiat., 51: 1171-1177.
[12] Brown, R. A., Lawson, D. A., Leslie, G. C., MacArthur, A., MacLennan, W. J., McMurdo, M. E. T., Mutch, W. J., and Part, N. J. (1988) Does the Wartenberg pendulum test differentiate quantitatively between spasticity and rigidity? A study in elderly stroke and Parkinsonian patients, J. Neurol. Neurosurg. Psychiat., 51: 1178-1186.
[13] Andrews, B. J., Bajd, T., and Baxendal R.H. (1986) Cutaneous electrical stimulation and reductions in spinal spasticity in man, J. Physiol. 367: 86P.
[14] Lin, D. C. and Rymer, W. Z. (1991) A quantitative analysis of pendular motion of the lower leg in spastic human subjects", IEEE-BME, 38(9): 906-918.
[15] Bohannon, R.W. and Smith, M.B. (1987) Interrater reliability on modified Ashworth scale of muscle spasticity, Phys. Ther., 67: 206-207.
[16] Mulvey, N., Quinn J., Andrews B.J., and Bajd T. (1984) "A microcomputer based instrument for pendulum testing of spasticity". In: Jordan M.M., Perkins W.J. (eds.), Computer-aided Biomechanical Imaging and Graphics Physiological Measurement and Control. London: The Biological Engineering Society.
[17] Bajd T., Gregoric M., Vodovnik L., and Benko H. (1985) Electrical stimulation in treating spasticity resulting from spinal cord injury, Arch. Phys. Med. Rehabil., 33: 515-517.
[18] Bowman, B. R., and Bajd, T. (1981) Influence of electrical stimulation on skeletal muscle spasticity, in: Proc. VII Int. Symp. on External Control of Human Extremities, Dubrovnik, Yugoslav Comittee for Electronics and Automation, 567-576.
[19] Robinson, C. J., Kett, N. A., and Bolam, J. M. (1988) Spasticity in spinal cord injured patients: 1. Short-term effects of surface electrical stimulation, Arch. Phys. Med. Rehabil., 69: 598-604.

[20] Robinson, C. J., Kett, N. A., and Bolam, J. M. (1988) Spasticity in spinal cord injured patients: 2. Initial measures and long term effects of surface electrical stimulation", Arch. Phys. Med. Rehabil. 69: 862-868.
[21] Kawamura, J., Ise, M., Matsuya, M., Tagami, M., Ezaki, S., and Nishihara, K. (1987) Clinical use of electrical stimulation for reducing spinal spasticity, in: Proc. IX Int. Symp. on External Control of Human Extremities, Belgrade, Yugoslavia, 353-362.
[22] Katz, R. T., Rovai, G. P., Brait, C., and Rymer, W. Z., (1992) Objective quantification of spastic hypertonia: correlation with clinical findings, Arch. Phys. Med. Rehabil., 73: 339-347.
[23] Baxendal, R.H. (1992) Pendulum testing for spasticity, in: Restoration of walking for paraplegics. Recent advancement and trends. (Eds.) A. Pedotti, M. Ferrarin. Edizioni Pro Juventute, Milano - IOS Press, Amsterdam, 139-142.
[24] Bohannon, R. W. (1987) Variability and reliability of the Pendulum Test for spasticity using Cybex II isokinetic dynamometer, Phys. Ther., 67: 659-661.
[25] Ferrarin, M., Frigo, C., Osio, M., Crenna, P., Pedotti, A., and Mangoni, A. (1993) Assessment of spasticity by an integrated system for the analysis of pendular motion and EMG activity, XIII International Congress of EEG and Clinical Neurophysiology, 30 August-5 September 1993, Vancouver, Canada. Electroenchep. Clin. Neurophysiol., 87(2): S66.
[26] Frigo, C. and Pedotti, A. (1977) Determination of muscle length during locomotion, in: Biomechanics VI-A, (Eds.) Asmussen E., Jorgensen K., University Park Press, Baltimore, 355-360.
[27] Lance, J. W. (1980) Symposium Synopsis, in: Spasticity: Disordered Motor Control. (Eds.) Feldman RG, Young RR, Koella WP. Year Book Publishers, Chicago, 485-494.
[28] Burke, D., Gillies, J. D., and Lance, J. W (1970) The quadriceps stretch reflex in human spasticity, J. Neurol. Neurosurg. Psychiat., 33: 216-223.
[29] Frigo, C. (1992) Methods for gait analysis, in: Restoration of walking for paraplegics. Recent advancement and trends. (Eds.) A. Pedotti, M. Ferrarin. Edizioni Pro Juventute, Milano - IOS Press, Amsterdam, 95-107.

A Comparision of Clinical and Biomechanical Assessments of Spinal Spasticity

R. H. Baxendale
Institute of Physiology, University of Glasgow, Scotland

Abstract - One of the greatest fears concerning the introduction of electrotherapy is that the process may in some way make the condition of the patient worse. The establishment of a new National Spinal Injuries Centre in Glasgow has required us to gain the confidence of a new group of clinicians unfamiliar with functional electrostimulation and to have our activities approved by new safety and research ethics committees. For many years now patients have reported that electrostimulation has beneficial effects in that their spasm is reduced. We sought to quantify the intensity of spasm before and after a period of electrostimulation to prepare muscle for a program of standing and walking with the aim of observing whatever changes might occur in the background spasm. These experiments compared the spasm as detected by several conventional clinical tests and a modified pendulum test. Almost no correlation could be detected between the results of different tests performed on the same patient on the same day. Neither was any detectable trend in the spasm before and after electrostimulation found. There was no evidence that electrostimulation made spasticity worse. It was concluded that each test must detect different features of spasticity and that these can vary independently.

1 Introduction

Unfortunately, spinal injury is an increasingly common condition in western societies, affecting over 100,000 citizens in the European Community. The pattern of incidence is largely due to accidental injury often in road traffic accidents and also reflects the relatively long life expectancy on these patients, which can now approach that of the uninjured members of the community. The spinal injury has many consequences such as loss of voluntary movement and sensation, muscle wasting and urinary problems but the residual involuntary muscle tone and movements known as spasticity is the principal concern of this article. Spastic contractions may be long lasting and lead to skeletal deformity or they may be brief and intense jerks of the limbs which disturb sleep or make other activities like transfers from a bed to a wheel-chair difficult.

Spasticity is a major concern of those interested in rehabilitation of the spinal cord injured man. Particularly, of those interested in reconstructing movements by electrical stimulation strategies since any programmed movement may be destroyed by an unexpected spasm. In addition, there is the fear than stimulation strategies may make spasticity worse. These concerns led us to investigate the changes in spasticity in a group of patients during their preparation for entry in a programme preparing them for FES assisted walking. We attempted to measure how intense their spasm was at weekly intervals to seen if it was affected by the stimulation. Several conventionally employed tests of spasticity were used and these measurements we compared with the patients own views of their condition.

In general patients, physiotherapists, clinicians and researchers thought that the frequency of spasm was if anything reduced by the muscle training associated with the programme, but that the intensity of any spasm might have been greater. The increased force could be due to the same neural activity generating more force from a strengthened muscle. In addition, there were repeated comments by the patients that their spasm was less troublesome, particularly during the night when their sleep was less disturbed. Whilst these statements were supported by patient diaries it was impossible to make any definitive statement about spasm and training. We hoped the repeated testing would answer this question but the results of the tests employed showed very little agreement and we conclude that there is still no single definitive measurement which can define the intensity of muscle spasm.

2 Methods

The experiments were reviewed and approved by the local research ethics committee. Repeated tests were performed on 6 volunteers who had suffered injury to their spinal cords at least 4 years before the experiments began. Their condition was stable and they were not taking any spasmolytic drugs. Their clinical details are summarised in table 1.

Patient	Sex	Age	Lesion Level	Age of Lesion
A	M	19	C4	4 years
B	F	32	L1	12 years
C	M	35	T12	7 years
D	M	35	C4	21 years
E	F	39	T6	8 years
F	F	28	T12	8 years

Table 1. Summary patient details.

The patients attended the laboratory on 5 occasions. On each day conditions were kept as closely standardised as possible. Tests were performed in the same sequence, by the same experimenters, with the same rest intervals to minimise any carry over effects or variation between observers. The following tests were conducted:

1. Patellar and achilles tendon jerks.
2. Ashworth tests of the range of joint motion
3. Fast passive movement of the knee joint. (FPM.)
4. A modified Wartenberg pendulum test.

The patellar tendon jerks and those features of the Ashworth tests related to the range of movement at the knee were compared with tests 3 and 4 to complete the overall picture of quadriceps spasticity. The tendon jerks, Ashworth and FPM performances were rated on a scale where 1 indicated normal, 2 mild spasticity, 3 moderate spasticity and 4 severe spasticity. This provided data of several sorts: the patellar jerk measures the excitability of the segmental monosynaptic reflex pathways by observing the response to very brief, high velocity stretches, the modified pendulum test uses high velocity stretches, but applied for substantially longer, the FPM test is also a quick stretch but slower and more difficult to quantify then the pendulum tests whilst the Ashworth is a slow stretch test. This battery of tests should give information about the responsiveness of the phasic and tonic components of any stretch reflexes in the quadriceps. It also allows comparison of clinically used tests like the tendon jerk and Ashworth with a more biomechanical measure like the pendulum test.

2.1 Modifications to the Pendulum Test

The pendulum test provided quantitative results about the performance of the quadriceps under fast stretch conditions. The patient lay supine with their leg projecting beyond the end of an examination couch. An electrogoniometer recorded knee position and the leg was raised to extend the knee fully before it was released to fall under the influence of gravity. The resulting mechanogram was used to derive the following measures

	Measure	**Definition**
1	Relaxation Index	(max. angle - start angle) / 1.6 x (90° - start angle)
2	Area	area between goniogram and time axis
3	Number of Swings	
4	Maximum Velocity	maximum velocity into flexion
5	Minimum Velocity	maximum velocity into extension
6	Jerk Index	(min angle - max angle) / (start angle - max angle)
7	First Area	between start angle, 90° and time axis
8	Half Period	time from start to 90°
9	Area Ratio	area above time axis / area below time axis.

Table 2. Measures derived from the knee mechanogram during pendulum tests.

The reproducibility of pendulum test measures was evaluated by performing tests on over 50 neurologically normal volunteers and on 15 paraplegic volunteers. The early tests in each case showed distinct trends in the data so that reliable mean values could not be calculated. Specimen data is shown in table 3. This shows that over the first 5 trials there is a distinct increase in relaxation index, maximum velocity and jerk index whilst the half period is progressively reduced.

Test Number	Relaxation Index	Max. Velocity (degrees/sec)	Jerk Index	Half Period (seconds)
1	0.76 ± .11	260 ± 11	0.44 ± .04	0.37 ± .02
2	0.88 ± .03	298 ± 60	0.62 ± .03	0.31 ± .03
3	0.85 ± .03	312 ± 13	0.62 ± .03	0.30 ± .02
4	0.93 ± .03	310 ± 40	0.66 ± .02	0.29 ± .01
5	0.93 ± .03	313 ± 12	0.68 ± .03	0.29 ± .02

Table 3. Summary results of the first 5 pendulum tests showing stabilisation of values by the fifth test.

This led to pendulum tests being modified to allow for a warm up period during which 5 tests were performed but the results discarded. The mean of the next 10 tests was then calculated. With the inclusion of the warm up the results of the test become very consistent in any one session and typically the coefficient of variation was less than 0.1. The large population of normals tested allowed the paraplegic population to be compared with a control population carefully matched for age and sex. Details of this type of comparison are given below in table 4.

Measure	Paraplegic		Normal	
	mean	SD (n=15)	mean	SD (n=15)
Relaxation Index	0.91	.013	1.02	0.03
Area	322	167	345	76.2
Max. Velocity	324	30.8	362	13.6
Min. Velocity	210	51.4	260	25.8
Jerk Index	0.58	0.16	0.69	0.06
Half Period	0.31	0.04	0.28	0.02
Area Ratio	1.90	1.35	1.12	1.12

Table 4. A comparison of mean values for pendulum tests performed in a sample of 15 paraplegic volunteers and an age and sex matched normal control group.

The pendulum tests detected that paraplegic limbs swing more slowly and through a narrower angular range than normal limbs. There was some redundancy in the number of measure taken and attention was concentrated on those most closely related to speed and angle.

2.2 Clinical Ratings

Table 5 shows the spasticity ratings for all six patients as assessed by the three clinical tests before, during and after they participated in a muscle restrengthening programme. In each of the three tests reported in table 5 scoring system is normal = 1, mild spasm = 2, moderate spasm = 3, severe spasm = 4.

	Test	**Left Leg**				**Right leg**		
		Before	**During**	**After**		**Before**	**During**	**After**
a	**FPM**	2	1	2		3	2	4
	Reflex	3	1	2		4	2	2
	Ashworth	2	1	2		2	1	3
b	**FPM**	4	4	4		4	4	4
	Reflex	2	2	2		2	3	3
	Ashworth	2	2	2		3	3	3
c	**FPM**	4	4	4		4	4	4
	Reflex	3	3	3		4	4	1
	Ashworth	3	3	3		4	4	3
d	**FPM**	4	4	4		4	4	4
	Reflex	2	1	3		2	2	1
	Ashworth	2	3	3		3	3	2
e	**FPM**	1	4	4		3	4	2
	Reflex	1	2	1		1	1	1
	Ashworth	1	3	2		1	2	1
f	**FPM**	4	4	4		4	4	4
	Reflex	1	1	4		1	1	1
	Ashworth	1	2	2		1	1	2

Table 5. Summary data from repeated spasticity tests in six patients before during and after a programme of muscle restrengthening. In each test a score of 1 indicates no spasticity and 4 indicates extreme spasm.

The results of these clinical tests were difficult to interpret. In some cases the results of all three tests are very consistent, e.g. subject b. has almost no changes in rating in both legs across all six tests. However, even in this case there is rather less agreement between tests e.g. FPM vs tendon jerks or Ashworth. In other cases, e.g. subject a. left leg, there is good agreement between tests on any one day. In this case the variations between days could be interpreted as changes in the overall intensity of spasm.

In most subjects the results are more mixed and this poses considerable problems of interpretation. The right leg data for subject C in an example of this. The initial measurements agree and indicate severe spasm, but the later measurements diverge sharply with the FPM results continuing to indicate severe spasm whilst the Ashworth scores show a slight improvement but the tendon jerk values are entirely normal. The data emerging here seemed to have little trend and whilst in some cases there was reasonable agreement between the observations this was not generally the true. It is certainly clear that the spasticity in any one patient can be classified very differently even by the same observer on the same day.

Of greatest interest was the very poor correlation between these pendulum tests measures and the clinical measures in the six individuals subjected to repeated testing. Spearman's rank correlation tests were used to look for any association between these data. The results are listed in table 6. Here a value of +1 indicated perfect agreement, 0 indicates no relation and -1 signifies a reverse ordering of data.

Measure	FPM	Tendon Jerk	Ashworth
Relaxation Index	0.144	0.012	0.002
Area	0.093	0.159	0.398
Max. Velocity	0.040	-0.093	0.442
Jerk Index	-0.002	0.219	0.348
Half Period	0.032	0.062	0.479
Area Ratio	-0.160	-0.095	0.446

Table 6. Spearman's correlation between Pendulum test measures of spasticity and the ratings of spasticity made in Fast Passive Movement, Patellar Tendon Jerk and Ashworth tests.

It is clear that there is very poor agreement between the different measures of spasticity. The strongest associations are between the pendulum and Ashworth results. It is very surprising that the relaxation index, which is the most widely used measure from the pendulum test, is not associated with the Ashworth, whilst other pendulum tests features are. Indeed the relaxation index seems almost independent of all the other tests.

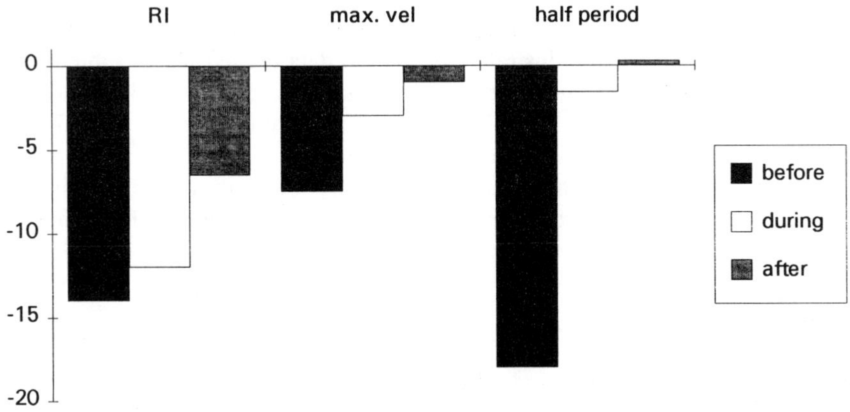

Fig. 1. Pendulum tests results for subject b, left leg before during and after muscle restrengthening. Compare these data with those measured concurrently by clinical tests shown in table 5.

The conclusion to be drawn here must be that either some or all of these tests are relatively insensitive to spasticity or that spasticity is a complex phenomenon and these tests are sensitive to different features which must be largely independent of each other. This is true even within one type of test. Figures 1 and 2 illustrate these points with data derived from a series of pendulum tests. Figure 1 shows illustrative pendulum data the left leg of subject b. The clinical tests

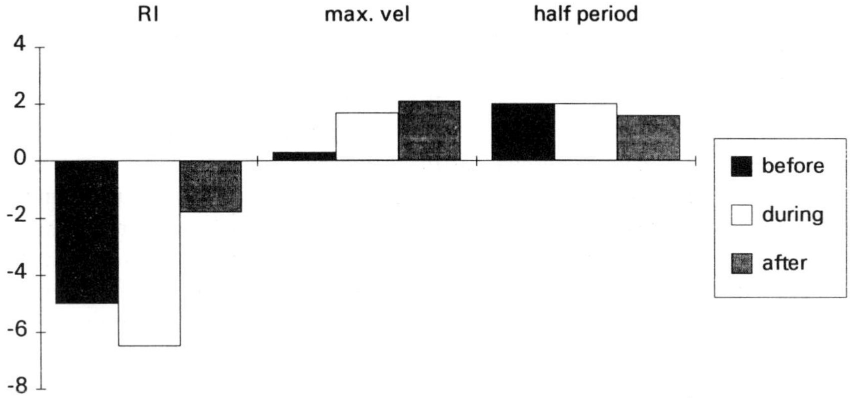

Fig. 2. Pendulum tests results for subject e, left leg before during and after muscle restrengthening. Compare these data with those measured concurrently by clinical tests shown in table 5.

show a pattern of stable moderate to severe spasticity across all three phases of the trial but the pendulum test measures show a substantial progressive reduction in spasm. Figure 2 shows illustrative pendulum data the left leg of subject e. The clinical tests show a pattern of little to no spasm changing to moderate to severe spasm during the trial. The pendulum test measures show little signs of this with a relaxation index which first indicates increased spasm and then returns close to normal by the end of the trial. The velocity of limb movement increases progressively leading one to believe that the knee might almost be hypermobile.

3 Discussion

These data lead one to conclude that some or all of these tests are insensitive to spasticity. Alternatively, spasticity must be complex and these tests are sensitive to different features which must be largely independent of each other. The latter seems the more likely possibility and this presents a substantial problem in assessment of the patient's condition. In some cases all the tests agree in the direction if not the magnitude of the change.

There are several changes in the condition of the skeletomotor system of the paraplegic which might explain this confusing picture. Firstly, there may be changes in the mechanical properties of paraplegics muscle which can masquerade as spasticity. Any increase in fibrous tissue could be mistaken for increased resistance to stretch generated by exaggerated stretch reflexes. Within the nervous system the extra stretch resistance can be generated in response to the velocity or acceleration components of any applied movement or may be generated by sustained length changes as in the tonic stretch reflex. A third neurological explanation could also lie in hyperexcitable motoneurone pool responding in a much less ordered way to any change in physical state. Given the variety of types of damage which the spinal cord may have suffered it is perhaps not surprising that more than one type of reflex response may be observed and that this response pattern may vary trial by trial.

The result of this study was not the one originally sought. Spinal spasticity has proved to be resistant to simple classification. There is no evidence that electrical stimulation for muscle restrengthening or gait restoration has any significant effect on the intensity or frequency of spasm. There is little to be gained by performing a battery of tests since these often generate conflicting data. Our general laboratory practice is to continue with the use of the modified pendulum tests as described here. This is reflects our confidence in the reproducibility of these measurements and the hope of avoiding any observer bias or other error. It certainly does not provide a complete picture of the state of spasm in the subject, merely one can be relatively easily measured.

Parameters Controlling Antispastic Electrical Stimulation: Clinical Application & Theoretical Considerations

G. Vossius, R. Frech
Institute of Biocybernetics and Biomedical Engineering,
University of Karlsruhe, Germany

Abstract - We applied Electrical Stimulation (ES) for therapy of severe spasticity to more than 50 patients, most of them otherwise not more accessible to conventional therapy. A specific therapeutic procedure has been developed along this line. The results proved, that ES is a very good working method for reducing spasticity and the loosening of concomittant contractures. In addition the often high doses of antispastic drugs delivered with its more or less pronounced side effects may be reduced to zero during the stimulation therapy. Patients with temporary paralysis may regain voluntary control in the course of the treatment. The antispastic ES is a refined and elaborate method, resulting from the appropiate adjustment of a multiparametric procedure. It therefore needs special training and experience to handle it. It is interactive with the patient, who normally executes it daily at home. The method adds to the normal procedures of physio- and occupational therapy in the rehabilitation of patients with severe secondary symptoms of paralysis. The theoretical background of the developement of spasticity and its consequences for the therapy are discussed.

1 Introduction

About since 40 years more systematic attempts have been made to treat sypasticity by Electrical Stimulation, ES, (Lee and McGovern, 1950; Levine, 1952). The most elaborate and effective procedure was developed by Hufschmidt (1968; 1969). He treated from cranial to caudal the parts of the motor system afflicted by spasticity with multichannel stimulation at low frequencies timed in specific patterns. But his attempts and the ones of others didn´t get wider recognition, because the method is elaborate and time demanding, and might result in an amplification of the spastic reaction if applied wrongly. He also published and documented his procedure and results rather scarcely. In addition old prejudices of neurologists resulted in the rule, that ES enhances spasticity and should therefore not be used. On the other hand, with the development of the method of Functional Electrical Stimulation, FES, observations compiled, that moderate degrees of spasticity might be favourably influenced by ES. This resulted also in systematic investigations to diminish spasticity via ES, i.e. by Bajd et al. (1985; 1984) or Stefanovska et al. (1989), which proved the usefullness of the method in a number of cases.

In 1986 (Vossius *et al.*, 1989) we started, mainly together with the Rehabilitation Clinic Karlsbad-Langen-steinbach, to look systematically in the possibility to diminish spasticity by ES. These investigations led to the development of a refined multiparametric procedure, which allowed to reduce very severe spastic states, no more accessable to other therapeutic actions, to such a degree, that the musculature was more or less completely relaxed. Concomittant the often high doses of antispastic medication could be reduced to zero. In addition physio- and occupational therapy could be restarted again (Vossius, 1989; Vossius 1990).

In general handicapped and patients with paralysis may benefit in multiple ways from ES besides the special case of FES as indicated by figure 1:

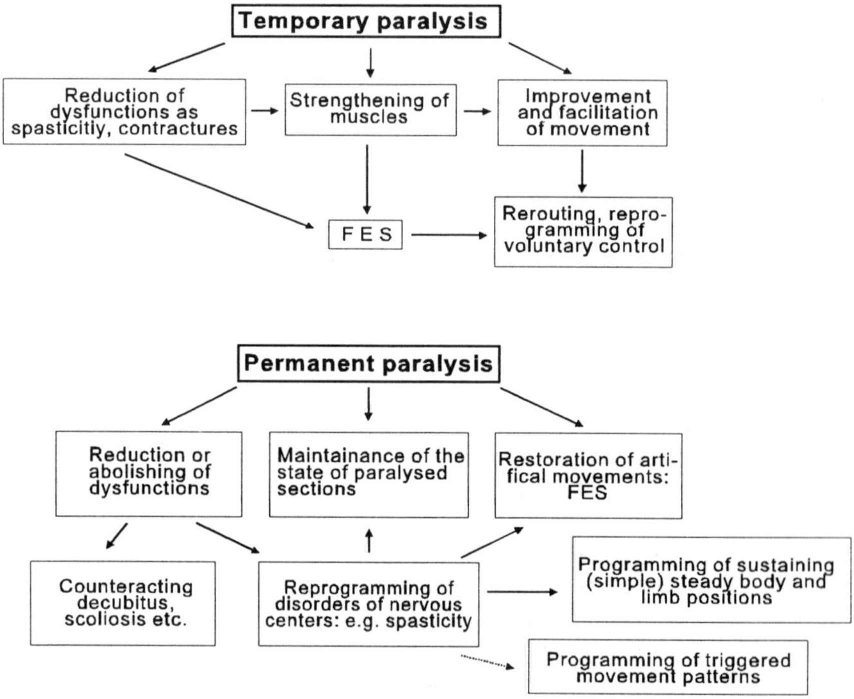

Fig. 1. Use of electrostimulation in case of temporary and permanent paralysis

This paper will concentrate on the treatment of spasticity, the other applications are covered elsewhere (Vossius, 1990; Vossius *et al.*, 1990; Vossius, 1992).

2 Clinical Procedure

Spasticity may be of different significance to the patient:

1. It may bother him not at all or not very much and, as a positive side effect, keep the muscles affected at a certain training state.
2. It may support the execution of some functions, e.g. an extensor spasticity of the lower limb may allow the patient to stand for a shorter time span and to change from one location to an other.
3. It may progressively reduce not only the range of mobility but the total quality of life so far at his command.

The application of ES on spasticity should be limited to point 3.

Before starting with the installation of the antispastic ES routine, a test procedure of the grade of the spasticity has to be established in order to be able to judge the effectiveness of the antispastic ES. In most cases spasticity includes a number of muscles with respective degrees of freedom and may have tonic and phasic components. Therefore the assessment of its severeness, in order to adjust the ES-procedure, may not be achieved by measuring just one parameter as the pendulum test of the lower leg allows (Bajd and Vodovnik, 1984). Therefore for each individual spastic manifestation a special test set has to be established using a graded scale, and allowing this way a judgement of the effectiveness of the ES.

We have found the following parameters to be useful for grading the spastic response to a manual trigger:

- Easiness to trigger off spasticity
- Speed and degree of contractions of phasic spasticity
- Force needed to overcome tonic spasticity
- Duration of the contractions
- Repetition of the contractions
- Spreading to other muscles (groups)
- Subjective feeling of the patient, although often of limited use

In addition the assessment of the duration and the degree of the "carry over" effect at longer time intervals.

The parameters influencing the therapeutic effect of ES on spasticity are the following, as treated more extensively in (Vossius *et al.*, 1989; Vossius, 1989; Vossius, 1990):

- Positioning of the patient in a relaxed mode
- Stimulation site
- Electrode size
- Pulse-duration
- Pulse-frequency
- Pulse-amplitude
- Combination of stimulation sites
- Continuous or intermittent stimulation
- Duration of one stimulation session
- Repetition of sessions

The stimulus has to be set to such an amplitude that the muscles respond only with a slight twitch. The more pronounced the spastic manifestation is, the more the stimulation frequency has to be lowered down to 2 - 0,5 cps. During the installation of the stimulation procedure and the training of the patient and his caretaker in the use of the method, which may take one to three weeks every day for two to three hours, the following has to be observed:

- Every 10 to 20 minutes the spastic response to a trigger is checked. In case of an improvement stimulation is continued until no further improvement can be observed. This time span is used as the basis of every days application, in most cases 45 to 60 minutes.
- It is important to observe the stimulation effects, and if adverse effects effects occur, the stimulation parameters and sites have to be changed.
- In case of fatigue during antispastic stimulation, in advance a preliminary mild training procedure is necessary. Stimulation leading to exhaustion of the muscle should definitely be avoided.
- The testing procedure is repeated with varying electrode combinations until a satisfying result is obtained or the procedure is terminated because any improvement is missing. In the latter case, provided spasticity is not intensified, the procedure may be repeated for a number of days, after which sometimes positive effects may occur. So far we had always positive indications of success during the first session.
- In case of instantaneous relief the duration of the carry over effect is evaluated and the effectiveness of a repetitive stimulation is determined.

As a next step it is investigated whether an intermittent stimulation pattern of 5-10 sec on/off cycles with a slow linear rise and decay of the stimulus is more effective than continuous stimulation.

In the course of the therapy the stimulation frequency may be increased (up to 20 Hz), and consecutively the stimulation amplitude, till a functional state is achieved. Concomitant the antispastic medication may be slowly lowered to zero (see also figure 3).

There are not any universal rules for the selection of the above listed stimulation parameters, i.e.:

- In many cases the stimulation of the dermatom areas associated to antagonistic muscles is successful, sometimes the direct stimulation of the spastic muscles turns out to be more effective, e.g. in case of extensor spasticity of the thigh the stimulation of the m. quadriceps possibly in combination with stimulation of the glutei muscles may be effective whereas stimulation of their antagonists (the hamstrings) fails.
- Extreme low frequencies may be inadequate compared to those of about 0.5 - 2 Hz; higher frequencies may tend to elicit spasticity.
- Stimulation sessions of long duration - longer than 60 minutes - seem to be less effective than shorter ones (30 - 60 minutes).
- The stimulation sites most effective may vary with time.

Following this procedure we treated so far more than 50 patients. The disorders are including spinal cord lesions, brain damage, congenital cerebral palsy, stroke, virus infections of the CNS, multiple sclerosis and other degenerative diseases of the nervous system, spasticity of the vocal cord and stiff sore neck. In most of the cases the spasticity was no more accessable to any other therapy. In all but three cases the spastic state could be decreased to such an extent that it was of no further importance, and functional use of the afflicted muscle groups was achieved. Three handicapped with a pronounced incomplete paralysis experienced a diminution of the spasticity, but no remarkable functional improvement. In all but two cases of multiple sclerosis the antispastic medication

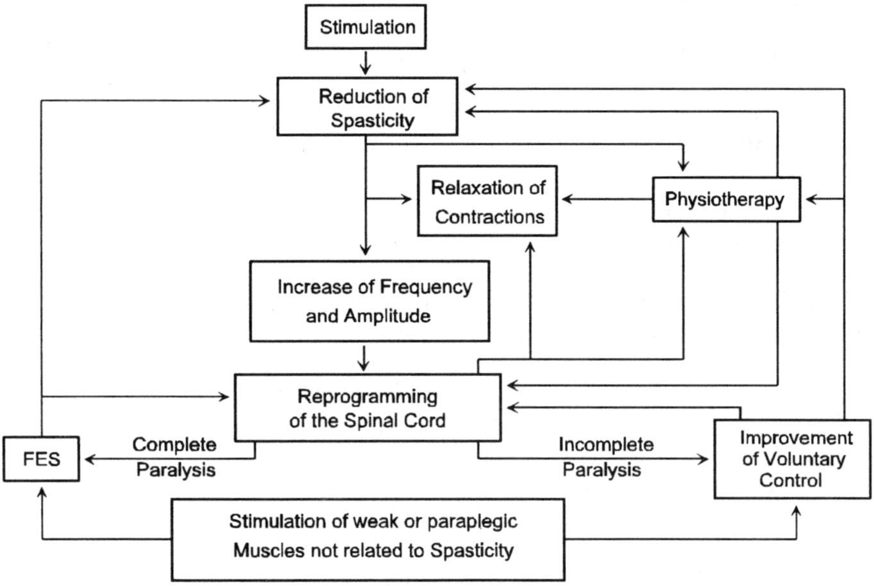

Fig. 2. Therapeutic concept of reducing spasticity by electrical stimulation

could be reduced to zero. The later two could be reduced to very low doses till today during the three years ES is being applied, and their mobility markedly improved.

Our experiences being gained so far may be summed up by figure 2, showing also the interaction of the method of ES with Physio- (and Occupational) therapy (see also figure 3):

3 Theoretical Considerations

A commonly accepted definition of spasticity does not exist. Generalising the observations one may define:

Spasticity is a self eliciting, self sustaining, not voluntarily controllable motor activity, which may also be provoked by unspecific stimuli.

A number of causes based on neurophysiological observations are discussed as origin of the developement of spasticity (Bajd and Vodovnik, 1984; Benecke and Noth, 1986; Vossius, 1990), i.e.:

- Lacking inhibition on the spinal (inter-) neurons
- Changes of excitability of interneurons
- Sprouting of excitative synapses of interneurons
- Receptor hypersensitivity
- Changes of muscle fibres

A number of phenomena observed when treating spasticity are incompatible with these causes, i.e.:

- Direct loosening effect of different therapeutic procedures
- "Vojta"-effect
- "Carry-over" effect following ES
- Long term changes of the state of spasticity by ES

Therefore we summed up the phenoma observed in the course of our therapeutic experiences in a working hypothesis:

Spasticity results from an uncontrolled self-organisation of the neural network of the spinal cord around old primitive reflex-pathways due to lacking or incomplete control by the higher motor centers.

The functional coupling of the higher centers with the spinal level seems to be rather weak and "vulnerable".

If this hypothesis is correct, the diminution of the spastic state of the interneuronal network of the spinal cord results from an interference of the afferent pattern of the muscular sensors elicited by the stimulation. This change of state is enhanced by the daily repetition of the antispastic stimulation and allows in the course of time to increase slowly the stimulation frequency and in doing so the strengthening of the effect. In case of a spinal cord injury the application of FES is finally permitted. In case of a temporary paralysis this may have two effects: one is the change of state of the interneuronal network, the other is the reopening of functionally (not physically!) interrupted motor connections between the spinal cord and the higher motor centers of the brain. These two effects together may result in the complete restoration of voluntary motor control.

This approach allows the classification of the cases treated in at least 4 categories (see figure 3; in this figure the steps of progression of the therapy and the time span each step needs are indicated roughly. The stimulation was executed daily for 45 to 60 min by the patient himself at home.)

In case of a complete lesion of the spinal cord, it might be possible to reprogram the network of the spinal cord in such a way, that it will be converted into an useful activation state. One of our quadroplegic handicapped demonstrated this: He applied FES for executing a grip during years. In the beginning his hand had a pronounced extensor spasticity. This was in the course of time converted into a grip movement, which he could trigger by pressing his shoulder on the backrest of his wheelchair. (Such automated movement patterns may also be observed in centrally paralysed handicapped being very active in sports. With them this mechanism is used involuntarily to stabilise their spine during the execution of fast movements.)

Taking into account the control system aspects diseases and injuries leading to paralysis and afflicting voluntary motor control have not only physio-pathological but, equally important, functional - control aspects. In the course of the healing process the importance of the physio-pathological aspects are decreasing whereas the functional losses of control due to the paralysis are remaining or increasing. These functional losses or restrictions are apparently often more extended than they have to be due to what is physically afflicted. In order to gain a therapeutic access to this diseased functional domain, it is essential to align the treatment according to the laws controlling this domain. Figure 4 gives a general hierarchy of the stages of voluntary motor control in man and the levels at which certain dysfunctional effects might be located (Vossius *et al.*, 1995). This figure represents not yet the state of secured knowledge but rather a guideline along which observed phenomena might be arranged and appropriate therapeutic measures be taken.

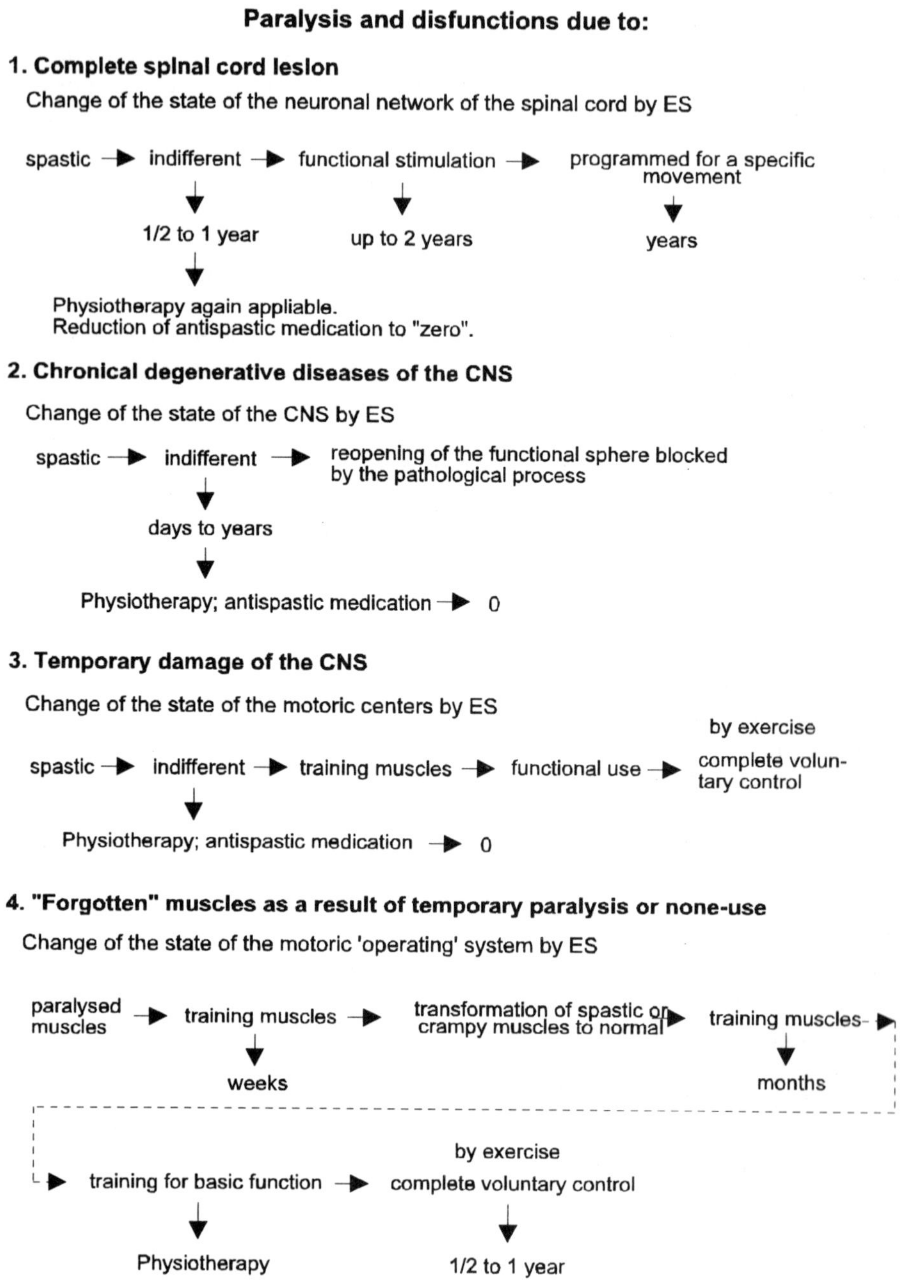

Fig. 3 Paralysis and disfunctions

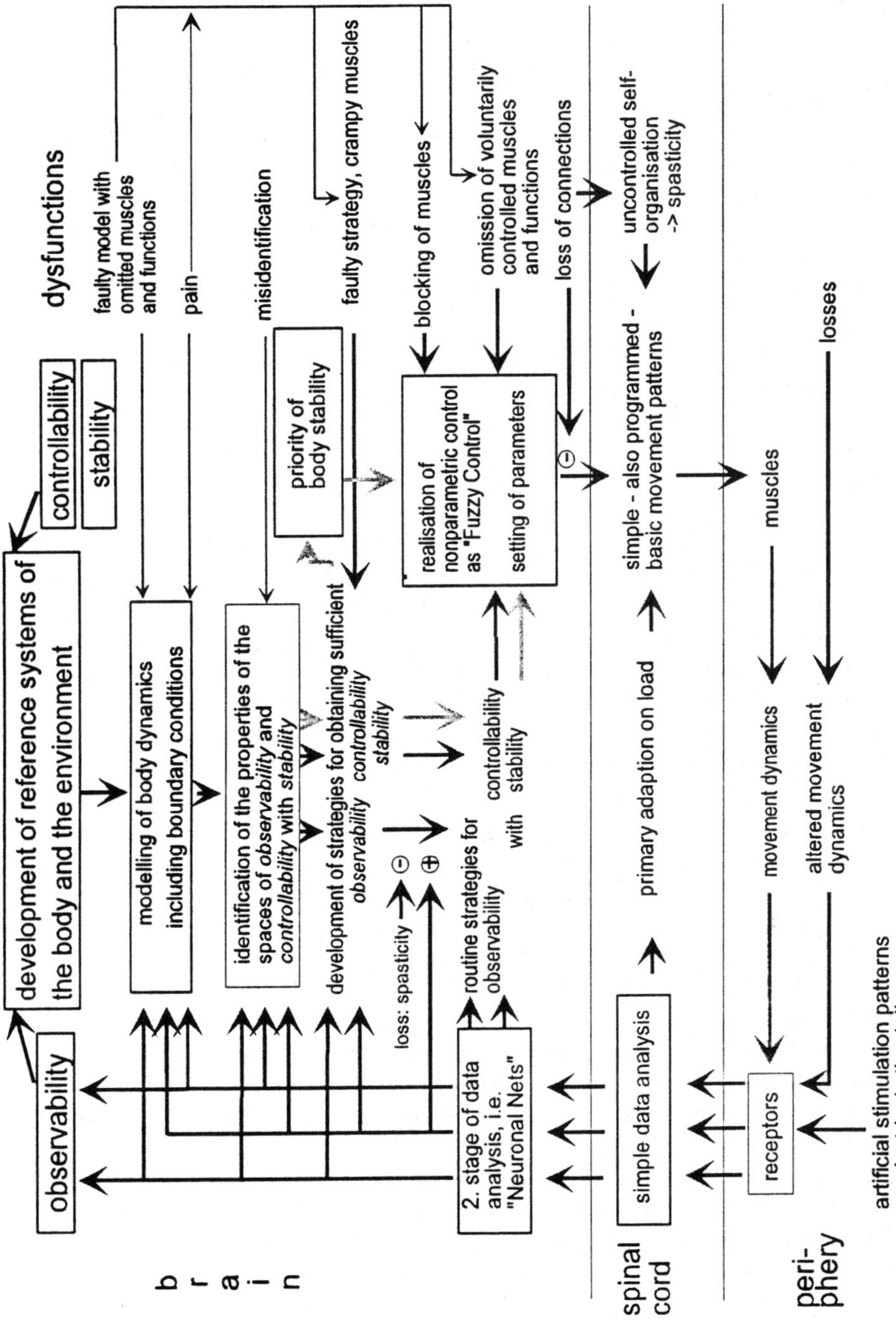

Fig. 4 General hierarchy of the stages of voluntary motor control in man and the levels at which certain dysfunctional effects might be located

References

Bajd, T. and Vodovnik, L. (1984) Pendulum testing of spasticity. Journal of Biomedical Engineering 6, 9-16.

Bajd, T., Gregoric, M., Vodovnik, L., and Benko, H. (1985) Electrical stimulation in treating spasticity resulting from spinal cord injury. Archives of Physical Medicine and Rehabilitation 66, 515-517.

Benecke, R. and Noth, R. (1986) Ursachen und Therapie spastischer Syndrome. Nervenheilkunde 5, 106-114

Hufschmidt, H.-J. (1968) Die Elektrotherapie der Spastik. Medizinische Welt 19, 2613-2616.

Hufschmidt, H.-J. (1969) Elektrotherapie spastischer Bewegungsstörungen. Krankengymnastik 21, 1-9.

Lee, W. J. and McGovern, J. P. (1950) Continuous tetanizing currents for relief of spasm. Archives of Physical Medicine 31, 766-770.

Levine M. G. (1952) Relaxing of spasticity by electrical stimulation of antagonist muscles. Archives of Physical Medicine 33, 668-673.

Stefanovska, A., Vodovnik, L., Gros, N., Rebersek, S., and Acimovic-Janezic, R. (1989) FES and spasticity. IEEE-Transactions on Biomedical Engineering 36, 738-745.

Vossius, G., Nanassy, A., and Frech, R. (1989) Beeinflussung der Spastik durch Elektrostimulation. In: Spinale Spastik. Ed. Grüninger, Überreuter Wissenschaft Berlin, 154-161.

Vossius, G. (1989) Diminishing spasticity by peripheral electrical stimulation. Clinic approach and theoretical considerations. 3rd. Intern. Workshop on Functional Electrostimulation, Vienna, 13-17.

Vossius, G. (1990) Reduction of Spasticity by Electrical Stimulation. A Clinical Approach. Xth International Symposium on External Control of Human Extremities, Dubrovnik, 205-212.

Vossius, G. (1990) Der Einsatz der Funktionellen Elektrostimulation in der klinischen Rehabilitation. Med. Orth. Tech. 110, 244-250.

Vossius, G., Nanassy A, Frech R, and Müller S. (1990) Application of Electrical Stimulation to Clinical Rehabilitation. Xth International Symposium on External Control of Human Extremities, Dubrovnik, 205-212.

Vossius, G. (1992) Significane of the Methodic of FES for the Rehabilitation of Paralysed Patients. 4th Vienna International Workshop on Functional Stimulation, Vienna, Austria, 30-35.

Vossius, G., Frech, R., and Rupp, R. (1995) The consequences of the control structure of voluntary movement on the procedure of therapeutical stimulation 5th Vienna International Workshop on Functional Stimulation, Vienna, Austria, 137-140.

Clinical Considerations on Spasticity and FES

V. Alfieri[1] and A. Alfieri[2]
[1]Dept. of Physical Therapy and Rehabilitation, Ospedale San Gerardo, Monza, I
[2]Villa Gemma Rehabilitation Clinic, Gardone Riviera, I

Abstract - Spasticity manifests in manifold features.

The upper motoneuron disorders, such as hemiplegia, show a typically stereotyped spasticity which frequently involves the flexor muscles of the affected upper limb and the extensors of the lower limb. In these cases therapeutic electrical stimulation (TES) on antagonistic muscles of the spastic ones is generally recommended; the results reported in some papers and presentations strengthen the suggested procedure.

In spinal cord lesions (SCL), spasticity can appear with different peculiarities. Kawamura and co-workers identified 3 types of spasms in the four limbs and two in the trunk and classifies 4 patterns of spasticity in the 4 limbs. We studied 17 SCL patients in relation to their responses to TES. The origin of the lesions were traumatic in 13 patients and viral in 4.

8 patients were cervical, 8 thoracic and 1 lumbar, most of them had neurological signs of complete paralysis. We distinguished 3 kinds of spinal cord spasticity. The first and most frequent type is characterised by clonic contractions in the lower limbs, mostly in extension but often in flexion, usually associated with tonic or clonic spasms in the trunk; this form of spasticity is remarkably reduced when TES is applied on quadriceps ad hamstring muscles in functional sequence. The second type was observed in 1 of the 17 patients and consists of strong tonic extensor spasm of trunk and lower limbs; this type, seen in 2 patients, consists of severe spasms, mostly tonic, 1 prevalently in extension and 1 prevalently in flexion of lower limbs; it is not sensitive at all to TES. The reduction of spasticity is usually of short term, but not always.

1 Introduction

The connection between electrical stimulation (ES) and spasticity should not be regarded as new if only we remember that in 1871 Duchenne (1883) pointed out relaxation of spastic muscles due to ES on their antagonists. In 1952 , Knott and Kabat (1952) published a paper reporting their experience in reducing spasticity using ES on antagonistic muscles, coordinated with therapeutic movements, in stroke patients. The interest in ES and spasticity increased after the classic work of Liberson and coll. (1961) on functional electrotherapy (then called Functional

Electrical Stimulation: FES) for improving gait of hemiplegic patients. In fact, though FES was used by Liberson et al. and by the following users with an orthotic aim, the antispastic FES effect was later remarked (McNeal and Wilemon, 1971; Carnstan and Larson, 1975; Carnstan *et al.*; Alfieri, 1977; Siegfried, 1980).

In 1973 Liberson (1973) and independently Kralj and Grobenik (1973) proposed the use of FES for the recovery of standing and walking in spinal cord injured (SCI) patients. The proposal was put into practice around the end of the seventies and at present a number of SCI patients around the world are standing up and walking assisted by electrically induced muscle contraction, or mostly, by hybrid systems.

Also in this context, a reduction of spastic signs was reported (Bajd and Bowman, 1982; Dimitrijevic, 1983; Kawamura *et al.,* 1987) among other beneficial effects.

Since, according to our knowledge, spasticity appears in different clinical features and probably has different pathophysiological origins in upper motoneuron lesions, and in spite of this, it seems to benefit from ES in any case, we think the subject worthily to be reviewed and supplemented with our personal experience and observations.

From this point, the presentation, ES used with the aim of reducing spasticity will refer to as TES (Therapeutic Electrical Stimulation).

2 Hemiplegia

Hemiplegic spasticity is typical and stereotyped, almost always involving the same muscles: the flexor muscles in the upper limb and the extensors in the lower limb. Nowadays TES is known and accepted in the scientific community as a possible therapy for hemiplegia, multiple sclerosis and some other upper motoneuron affections. Still controversial, however, are two main and crucial topics: i) the muscles to be stimulated and, ii) the duration of relaxation induced by stimulation.

As for the first point, Hufschmidt (1967) maintains the usefulness of direct stimulation of the spastic muscles, while Vodovnik and co-workers (Vodovnik *et al.,* 1984), after the experience of ten patients who applied TES on spastic quadriceps and hamstring muscles, concluded that it is difficult to draw any final conclusion on this topic. Hufschmidt (1967) ascribed his positive results to the excitation of the tendon Golgi organs. But in our opinion it is not conceivable that Ib fibres activation can exceed the facilitation drive exerted by Ia and II group of afferents from spindles as well as that exerted by the alpha and gamma fibres of the same muscle which are stimulated too; this is proven by the prompt, strong and prolonged contraction of the stimulated spastic muscle. Nor can the antispastic TES activity ascribed as Vendensky effect or any other local fatigue effect due to biochemical phenomena; indeed, these effects recede too promptly (seconds for Vedensky effect, minutes for fatigue) to be responsible for an antispastic activity which has longer lasting efficacy.

The majority of Authors suggest that TES should be applied on the antagonistic muscles of the spastic ones.

2.1 Method

Parameters of stimulation: The majority of Authors use trains of impulses modulated in amplitude: duration of single impulses, 0.5-1 msec.; frequency, 30-50 Hz; ramp of modulation, 2 sec.; train duration, 4 sec.; amplitude, sufficient to produce either a slight or a strong contraction (depending on the characteristics of each patient) without allowing the antagonistic spastic muscles to contract; duty cycle, 1/1; length and frequency of sessions. 10-15 min. once a day for 5 days a week, from 20 to 50 and more sessions. In the presence of muscle hypotrophy, the above parameters i.e., amplitude, frequency, duty cycle, must be altered according to the degree of hypotrophy.

Excitable muscles and electrode positioning: The muscles to be stimulated in hemiplegia in order to counteract and reduce spasticity are the paralysed ones, which are hypotonic and tending towards hypotrophy, dominated by central and reciprocal inhibition and antagonist to the spastic muscles. They are usually: deltoid pars media and supraspinatus muscles as antagonists of the pectoralis major; the extensors of the wrist and fingers as antagonistis of flexors; the triceps against the biceps brachili; hamstring versus quadriceps; muscles innervated by the peroneal nerve versus calf muscles.

The positioning of electrodes is described in details elsewhere (Benton *et al.*, 1980; Bajd, 1983; Alfieri, 1992) but here we should like to stress that often the identification and preservation of the best points of stimulation is not easy. This appears to be dependent on two main reasons: the first one is that the muscles are often hypotrophic and in addition, the hypotrophy is often diversified in the different muscles within a muscle group; moreover, neurophysiological signs of peripheral denervation are recorded in a certain percentage of hemiplegics (Stefanic, 1976; Alfieri and Vitale, 1982); the second reason is that the motor points of paralysed non-spastic muscles seem to be very restricted and easily lost. For these reasons great care must be taken in the search of the best points for positioning electrodes.

Evaluation: Spasticity can be evaluated by means of neurophysiological techniques, such as electromyographic recordings of voluntary movements, H reflex, Hmax/Mmax, EMG responses to stretch, F wave, electric and magnetic stimulation of the motor cortex. Unfortunately, these investigation facilities are seldom available in clinical routine practice,i.e., the right environment in which the precise assessing of spasticity is a real necessity.

The pendulum test and the isokinetic procedures are well suited for assessing spasticity, but are not generally practised. Besides, the pendulum test is suitable only for testing spasticity in quadriceps muscle, and isokinetic equipment is not sensitive to small spasticity variations (Knutsson and Alfieri, unpublished experiments).

We are using a new technique, called SRI-test (Stretch Reflex Indicator): the passive hand extension operated by a torque of 1 Nm standardised conditions is measured and data are plotted vs. time by an automatic device. The banal principle on which the evaluation is based is that more the flexor muscles of wrist and fingers are spastic (the prototype device was made for the wrist), the shorter, slower and more jerky the movement will result. The SRI proved to be very sensitive, accurate and repeatable.

2.2 Results

Alfieri (1982) and Alfieri and Vitale (1982) published results regarding a number of hemiplegic patients and showed that TES of antagonistic muscles reduces spasticity in most cases: 90% of 96 cases reported in the first paper, 5 out of 6, compared with 6 cases treated without TES, in the second paper. The first paper refers to the period from March 1973 to February 1977 and the evaluation was only empirical for the most part, while for a minority of cases it was done by means of the Ashworth Scale. In the study reported in the second paper the evaluation was done by means of EMG and the original Ashworth Scale (score from 0 to 4). Both papers reported more or less a reduction of spasticity that lasted at least one month after the end of treatment.

The long lasting effects of TES on hemiplegic patients seems to be confirmed by a study which is actually in progress. The preliminary results of this study have been recently presented by Normell *et al.* (1993).

The same study also confirms which was found by Alfieri (1984), i.e., all the hemiplegic patients treated with TES of extensor muscles of wrist and fingers, independently of the result on spastic restraint, showed a noted reduction or quasi-disappearance of the associated elbow flexion by abnormal irradiation.

2.3 Discussion

Apart from the confirmed effectiveness of TES in reducing hemiplegic spasticity when it is not too hard or not associated with joint stiffness, high muscle stiffness or advanced muscle atrophy, two main features are to be pointed out: i) the remarkable decrease of irradiation and ii) the long duration of the reduction of high reflectivity to stretch of the spastic muscles.

Irradiation is a normal cortical phenomenon, becoming abnormal in intensity and distribution in spastic hemiplegia and other pathological conditions. The fact that it is changed by peripheral ES demonstrates that TES effects are also mediated by the cortex.

This conclusion is important as a starting point for the formulation of a theory on TES and spasticity.

The pathophysiology of spasticity in hemiplegia has not yet been completed clarified. In our opinion, we cannot discriminate between the role played by the cord and the role played by the supra spinal centres and circuits in determining the multiform features and types of spasticity. A lack of supra spinal control, a gammadynamic hyperfacilitation, a reduction of the presynaptic inhibition, a change of activity of the Renshaw interneurons are involved, each one to some unspecified extent; and other unknown mechanisms are likely to interfere. The overall outcome is an excess of facilitating impulses to the "common final path", the alpha-motoneurons. The TES of the antagonistic muscle is certainly able to balance the hyperexcitation of alphamotoneurons through reciprocal inhibition.

But reciprocal inhibition, through the 1a fibres coming from the primary endings of muscle spindles, cannot explain the long lasting antispastic effects of TES (Alfieri, 1992; Alfieri, 1984).

In order to lastingly lessen spasticity it is necessary to repeatedly stimulate physiological mechanisms which are suitable to be influenced, forced, stabilised. One of these mechanisms could be the long loop transcortical reflex mechanism, whose afferent limb is formed by the II group fibres coming from the secondary endings of muscle spindles and whose efferent limb runs along the pyramidal tract (Phillips, 1969; Phillips *et al.,* 1971; Wiesendanger *et al.,* 1975; Wiesendanger, 1978). These afferences are integrated in complex circuits at cortical level among the sensorial, motor and supplementary motor areas and are involved in the fine control and modulation of movements, with great possibilities of restoration and correction. They influence the threshold of pyramidal neurons and are the basis of the transcortical servomechanism which alters the cortical output when the motor programme is suddenly disturbed.

The functions of the different fibres from spindles mentioned are not the only ones; another important function among others, especially pertaining to the II group fibres and secondary endings, is to give perception of the muscle contraction and the length of the muscle at any given moment (the spindle nuclear chain fibres are also called "length measuring fibres").

The fine reflex modulation and control of movement necessarily implies a great amount of inhibitory activity.

If this is true, when we stimulate the spindle afferent fibres of the antagonistic muscles with TES, we possibly trigger a functionally co-ordinated inhibiting activity.

The result depends on what remains and what can be restored of the nervous centres and paths after stroke. Cody *et al.* (1987) shows that in 19 out of 23 patients affected with spasticity in the upper limb from upper motoneuron lesion, the EMG long-latency responses (response M2), ascribed to peripheral stimulation (stretch) of II group fibres are present, though with a more or less reduced amplitude when compared with normal. This means that the related transcortical reflex mechanism of motor control and modulation continues working to a certain extent in the majority of cases, and is available for therapeutical purposes. The Cody *et al.* (1987) experiment associated with the above outlined theory could explain the reasons why a smaller part of spastic patients do not benefit from TES while others benefit from it in different proportions.

3 Spinal Cord Lesions (SCL)

SCL spasticity is not as stereotyped as that of hemiplegia spasticity. It can arise in normal, hyper-or even hypotonic muscles and can appear as tonic, or mostly clonic contractions.

Kawamura *et al.* (1989) studied the spasms of 13 quadriplegic patients. They identified 3 types of spasticity in upper and lower limbs: tonic flexor, tonic extensor, clonic spasms; 2 types in the trunk: clonic and tonic; they also classified 4 patterns of spasticity in the 4 limbs: flexor spasms in upper limbs associated with extensor spasms in lower limbs; extensor spasticity in upper limbs with flexor in lower limbs; extensor in the 4 limbs; flexor in the 4 limbs.

We studied and distinguished different forms of SCL spasticity with relation to their response to electrical stimulation.

3.1 Method

We reviewed the clinical documentation of some SCL patients who have been treated with TES in the last few years. No kind of selection was done except for the based on the completeness of documents evidence.

Thus 17 SCL patients were studied relative to TES effects, 13 of traumatic origin and 4 of viral origin, aged between 21 and 63 with an average age of 37, time elapsed from lesion 3 months to 13 years with an average of about 3 years. The levels of lesions were: 8 cervical, 8 thoracic, 1 lumbar. As for completeness of neurological signs (Frankel Grade), there were: 11 Grade A, 2 Grade B, 3 Grade C, 1 Grade D (see Annex I).

As for spasticity severity, at first we used the categories of the Michigan University Model (MUM) SCI Care System (Table 1), but later, referring to the TES results, we classified our patients with the following grades: spasticity absent, low, medium, high spasticity (Table 2), corresponding to the MUM categories o,1,2, and 3 before TES. The change in terms after electrical treatment is due to the fact that pharmacological administration was no longer the discriminating condition after TES, as TES substituted the drug medication in many cases with positive results, although not always. In any case, the latter was markedly reduced.

level of injury	No.	spasticity severity: 0	spasticity severity: 1	spasticity severity: 2	spasticity severity: 3
C1-C8	8	-	-	5	3
T1-T7	5	1	2	2	-
T8-T12	3	1	-	2	-
L1-S5	1	1	-	-	-
TOTAL	17	3	2	9	3

Table 1. Spasticity severity categories and level of injury of 17 SCL patients.(according to Michigan University Model SCI Care System)

level of lesion	No.	Severity of spasticity: absent or very low	Severity of spasticity: low	Severity of Spasticity: medium	Severity of Spasticity: high
C1-C8	8	-	-	5	3
T1-T7	5	1	1	3	-
T8-T12	3	1	-	2	-
L1-S5	1	1	-	-	-
TOTAL	17	3	1	10	3

Table 2. Severity Grade of Spasticity related to TES before treatment (see text)

All of the 17 patients were treated with TES, 5 for preparation to walking othosis (RGO), the others for strengthening muscles and for the beneficial side effects of electrical training.

The parameters used were: trains of impulses of 600 μsec at 30 Hz lasting 5 sec. with a duty cycle 1/4 for 20 min per muscle group, 2-3 times a day for months at home with a personal stimulator.

The muscle groups stimulated were quadriceps, hamstring muscles and the muscles innervated by the peroneal nerve. Gluteal, abdominal and lumbar muscles were stimulated as well when needed.

Patient n. 8 (see Table 3) was treated with TES on the hamstrings of one side, as antagonist of the tonically spastic quadriceps muscle, and on the peroneal nerve of the other side, in order to evoke the withdrawl a reflex forcing the knee to flex; the stimulation was reciprocated with other side.

The evaluation of spasm intensity was purely empirical, based on the visible force of contraction and on the duration and frequency of spasms directly observed by the medical operators and reported by the patients.

A reduction of about 50% in number and duration of the spastic contractions during the observation period (about 6 hours, from 9 a.m. to 3 p.m., that is the richest spasmogenic stimuli period of the day) was considered a good result.

So the following classes were picked out:

1. spasticity absent or very low;
2. spasticity low=less than 5 spasms;
3. spasticity medium=between 5 and 10 spasms;
4. spasticity high = more than 10 spasms.

We saw that the number of spastic contractions is directly related with the duration and strength of spasticity: less is the number and less are duration and strength of spasms.

No.	age	level and Frankel grade	origin	period from lesion	severity of spasms	results after TES	type of spasticity
1	43	C4 - C	traum.	1y	medium	low	clonic extensor & tonic flexor upper limbs
2	65	C5 - B	traum.	5m	medium	low	clonic extensor lower limbs
3	23	C5 - C	traum.	6y	medium	medium	clonic extens. & flexor
4	33	C5 - A	traum.	4y	high	high	tonic mainly extensor
5	53	C6 - A	viral	5y	high	high	tonic mainly flexor
6	63	C6 - A	traum.	3y 6m	medium	absent	clonic extensor & flexor
7	24	C6 - B	traum.	1y	medium	absent	clonic extensor & flexor
8	21	C7 -C	viral	3y	high	low	tonic extensor lower limbs
9	21	T4 - A	traum.	3y	low	absent	clonic ext. & flex:
10	29	T5 - A	traum.	1y	medium	absent	clonic ext. & flex.
11	39	T5 - A	traum.	13y 6 m	absent	absent	-
12	58	T6 - A	viral	3y 6m	medium	low	clonic exten & flex.
13	46	T7 - A	traum.	6y	medium	low	clonic exten. & flex.
14	40	T8 - A	traum.	1y	medium	low	clonic exten. & flex.
15	30	T9 - A	traum.	1y	medium	low	clonic exten. & flex.
16	35	T10-A	traum.	6m	absent	absent	-
17	45	L2 - D	viral	3m	absent	absent	-

Table 3. Synoptic table of 17 patients with results after TES and kinds of spasms

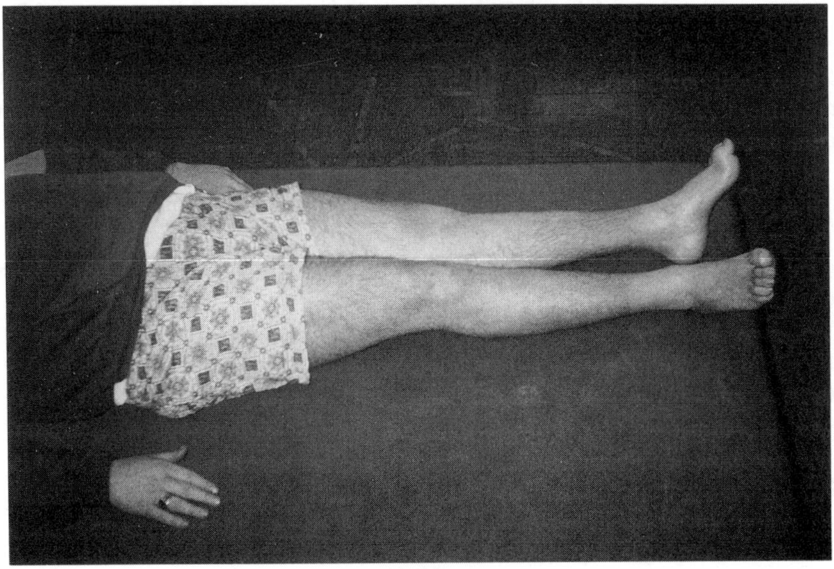

Fig. 1. Patient n.12; quadriceps muscles reflex activity in response to turning posture before TES.

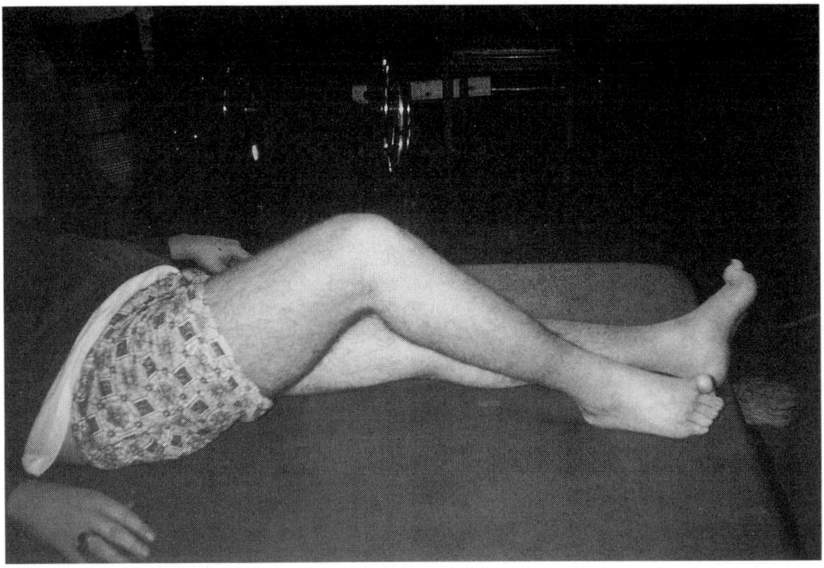

Fig. 2. Same patient of fig.1 and same responses 5 min. after 20 min of TES, reciprocating quadriceps muscle of one side and hamstring muscle of the other side.

The features of spasticity which we identified are included in the general Table 3, where one can note the presence of 3 cases without remarkable spasticity, 11 patients with clonic spasms mostly in the lower limbs, sometimes in extension and sometimes in flexion, 1 with clonic and tonic extensors spasms in the lower limbs and trunk, 1 with tonic extensor spasticity.

We never applied TES simultaneously to agonists and antagonists; this procedure implies a real risk of increasing spasticity. The stimulation must respect a functional sequence.

Some patients were tested by row EMG before and just after TES (figs. 1 and 2).

In this case we administered to the patient two of the most effective stimuli identified by Kawamura in order to provoke spastic contractions: cough and active postural twist.

3.2 Results

The shift of severity categories is illustrated in Table 3. Spasticity did not affect 3 patients, one of them had been paraplegic for 13 years and the lower limb muscles were very atrophic; 10 of the 11 patients with prevailing clonic spasms drew considerable advantages from TES. Only one remained stationary, but we have reason to believe that he did not perform the treatment as prescribed.

Patient n.8 obtained a substantial decrease of his tonic extensor high spasticity, followed by an unmasking of voluntary flexion and extension of the knee (figs. 1 and 2)

Patient n.4 and n.5, affected with high intensity tonic spasticity, showed no improvement from TES.

level of lesion	No.	severity of spasticity			
		absent or very low	low	medium	high
C1-C8	8	2	3	1	2
T1-T7	5	3	2	-	-
T8-T12	3	1	2	-	-
L1-S5	1	1	-	-	-
TOTAL	17	7	7	1	2

Table 4. Severity Grade of Spasticity Related to TES During Treatment

3.3 Discussion

From what has been described above and from our greater experience, we feel that we can characterize 3 kinds of spinal cord spasticity in our SCL patients. This typification is in accordance with Kawamura's.

1. The first kind of SCL spasticity is the most frequently observed and shows mostly clonic contraction in the lower limbs, both in extension and in flexion but with prevalence in extension. This form often includes trunk clonic or tonic contractions; the intensity is usually low or medium, but in some cases it is high. The clonic contractions often begin when the patient is put in a standing position, e.g. when an orthosis is tried on him, or when the patient is sitting down. In this case the contractions are localised particularly in the calf muscles and are likely primed by a "positive support tonic reaction", a primitive tonic reaction pertaining to the first four weeks of human life, emerging again in some pathologic conditions (see Table 4).
2. The first contraction is immediately followed by a fall of tone in the calf muscles causing the fall of the heel; this then provokes a stretch reflex in the calf muscles causing their contraction again, then a fall, and the cycle repeats itself. This form of spasticity is the most sensitive to TES and relaxes easily. TES is usually applied to the quadriceps and hamstring muscles and is often applied to the glutei and peroneal nerve
3. The second kind of spasticity is localised in the antigravitational muscles of the lower limbs and trunk and usually shows a strong tonic contraction in extension; clonic contraction of the calf muscles is sometimes associated when the patient is put into a seated position.
4. This form benefits much from TES, provided that it is applied to the antagonistic muscles, hamstring, and the peroneal nerve, in order to counteract the spasticity of the quadriceps and calf muscles and to provoke flexion of the limb by the withdrawal reaction.
5. The third kind is a severe form of spasticity, showing uncontrollable and untameable spasms of the trunk and legs, often also in the upper limbs in cervical patients, mostly tonic and in flexion in the lower limbs; the spasms can be elicited even by the slightest stimuli. The two patients we observed in these conditions showed no improvement from TES.

Regarding the duration of relaxation in positive cases, Bajd et al. (1984, 1985), Kawamura et al. (1987), Vodovnik et al. (1987) and other authors measured spasticity of SCI patients before and after TES by means of the pendulum test and found a short-term reduction in spasticity not lasting more than 24 hours.
We did not fulfil any measurement regarding this topic, we can however confirm the findings of other authors.

The following cases are exceptions. Patient n. 10, who applied TES for 4 months everyday and then stopped, remained free of spasms for almost 4 weeks; and patient n. 6, who applied TES to the lower limbs for more than one year together with intensive physical exercises, acquired a very good trophism, many new motor abilities and voluntary contraction of quadriceps muscles with force 3. This man, now 65, has not used electrical stimulation nor antispastic medications for about 9 months and he is still free of any kind of spasms.

4 Conclusions

A question arises from the comparison between hemiplegic and spinal cord spasticity.

Why, in the first kind of spinal spasticity can we stimulate agonist and antagonist muscles obtaining relaxation, while in hemiplegic spasticity we must stimulate only the antagonist muscles of the spastic ones?

Another question is: why did patient n. 6 have a kind of spasticity like hemiplegic spasticity, so that we could successfully use the same treatment procedure?

It seems reasonable to postulate that spinal cord spasticity manifests with different features because it has different pathophysiological origins. We think that this will be a challenge for neurophysiologists. Nevertheless, we think that different kinds of spasticity need different electrotherapeutical approaches.

References

Alfieri, V. (1977) La stimolazione elettrica nell'emiplegia. *La Riabil* 10:73-78.

Alfieri, V. and Vitale, A. (1982) EMG and kinesiologic control study on electrical therapy of the hemiplegic hupotonic shoulder. *Proceed 5th ISEK* Cong. Ljubljana, Zdrav Vestn 51: 191-192.

Alfieri, V. (1982) Electrical treatment of spasticity. Reflex tonic activity in hemiplegic patients and selected specific electrostimulation. *Scand J. Rehab Med.* 14: 177-182.

Alfieri, V. (1984) Effects of electrostimulation on stretch reflex and on irradiation of hemiparetic patients*: Proceed 8th Symp on ECHE,* Dubrovnik, pp. 403-407.

Alfieri, V. (1992) La Stimolazione elettrica funzionale. In: *GN Valobra ed: Trattato di Medicina Fisica e Riabilitazione*. Publ. UTET, Torino, Italy.

Benton, L., Baker, L., Bowman, B., and Waters, R. (1980) Functional Electrical Stimulation: A practical clinical guide. Publ. Rancho Los Amigos Rehab Engin Center, Downey, California.

Bajd, T. and Bowman, B. (1982) Influence of Electrical Stimulation on antagonist muscle spasticity. *Proceed 5th Cong ISEK*, Ljubljana, 21-25.6.1982, Zdrav Vestn 51: 153-154.

Bajd, T. (1983) Functional Electrical Stimulation of Extremities. *Publ Stefan Institute*, Ljubljana University, Ljubljana, Slovenia.

Bajd, T. and Vodovnik, L. (1984) Pendulum testing of spasticity. *J. Biomed Eng.* 6: 9-16.

Bajd, T., Gregoric, M., Vodovnik, L., and Benko, H. (1985) Electrical stimulation in treating spasticity resulting from spinal cord injury. *arch Phys Med Rehabil* 66: 515-517.

Carnstan, B. and Larson, L. E. (1975) Electrical Stimulation in a patient with spasticity. EEG and Clin Neurophysiol, *Soc. Proceed* 38: 214.

Carnstan, B., Larson, L. E., and Prevec, T. S.: Improvement of gait following functional electrical stimulation. I. Investigations on changes in voluntary strength and proprioceptive reflexes. *Scand J. Rehab Med* 9: 7-13

Cody, F. W. J., Richardson, H. C., McDermott, N., and Ferguson, I. T. (1987) Stretch and vibration reflexes of wrist flexor muscles in spasticity. *Brain* 110: 433-450.

Dimitrijevic, M. R. (1983) Neurophysiological evaluation and epidural stimulation in chronic spinal cord injury patients. In: *Spinal cord Reconstruction*; eds. CC Cao, RP Bunge and PJ Reier, pp.465-474. Raven Press, New York.

Duchenne, G. B. (1883) Selection from the clinical works. GV. Poore ed, London.

Hufschmidt, H. J. (1967) Electroterapie de la Spasticité, Rev Neurol, Séance Frando-Allemande des 11 et 12 Oct. 1966: 169-170.

Kawamura, J., Ise, M., Matsuya, M., Tagami, M., Ezaki, S., and Nishihara, K. (1987) Clinical use of electrical stimulation for reducing spinal spasticity. In: Popovic D. (ed.): Advances in External Control of Human Extremities IX, Belgrade, Yugoslav Commitee for Electronics and Automation, 353-362.

Kawamura, J., Ise, M., and Tagami, M. (1989) The clinical features of spasms in patients with cervical cord injury. *Paraplegia* 27: 222-226.

Kralj, A. and Grobelnik, S. (1973) Functional electric stimulation a new hope for paraplegic patients. *Bull Prosth Res* 75: 10.

Levine, M. G., Knott, M., and Kabat, H. (1952) Relaxation of spasticity by electrical stimulation of antagonist muscles. *Arch Phys Med Rehabil* 11: 668-673.

Liberson, W. T., Holmquest, H. J., Scot, D., and Dow, M. (1961) Functional electrotherapy:stimulation of the peroneal nerve synchronised with the swing phase of the gait of hemiplegic patient. *ARch Phys Med Rehabil* 42: 101-105.

Liberson, W. T. (1973) Functional electrical stimulation in paraplegics and "reflex walking". *Arch Phys Med Rehabil* 54: 588, 1973 Academy/Congress, abstracts.

McNeal, D. R. and Wilemon, W. K. (1971) Treatment of spasticity through functional Electrical Stimulation. In: *Neuroelectric Research: Electroneuroprosthesis and Non convulsive Electrotherapy*. Eds. DV. Reynolds and AE Sjobert. Publisher Charles C. Thomas, Springfield, Illinois.

Normell, L., Alfieri, V., and Knutsson, E. (1993) Long term effect of therapeutic electrical stimulation (TES) on spastic restraint in patients with hemiparesis. The 50th Cong. of the Swedish Soc. of Medicine, Stockholm.

Phillips, C. G. (1969) Motor apparatus of the baboon's hand. The Ferrier Lecture 1968. *Proceed Royal Soc.* 173: 141-174, London.

Phillips, C. G., Powell, R. P. S., and Wiesendanger, M. (1971) Projection from low-threshold muscle afferents of hand and forearm to area 3a of baboon's cortex. *J. Physiol* 217: 419-446.

Siegfried, J. (1980) Treatment of spasticity by dorsal cord stimulation. *Int Rehab Med* 2: 31-34.

Stefanic, M. (1976) The changes of conduction velocity and excitability of peripheral motor nerves in hemiplegia. *Proceed 5th Intern Symp in Neurol*, Prague.

Vodovnik, L., Bowman, B. R., and Winchester, P. (1984) Effect of elctrical stimulation on spasticity in hemiparetic patients. *Int Rehabil Med* 6: 153-156.

Vodovnik, L., Stefanowska, A., and Bajd, T. (1987) Effects of stimulation parameters on modification of spinal spasticity. *Med Biol Eng & Comput* 25: 439-442.

Wiesendanger, M., Ruegg, D. G., and Lucier, Ge. (1975) Why transcortical reflexes? Le *J Canad des Sc Neurol*, pp. 295-301.

Wiesendanger, M. (1978) Comments on the problem of transcortical reflexes. *J. Physiol* 74: 325-330, Paris.

Pharmacologic Management of Spasticity

S. Sorbi, G. Sorrentino
Department of Neurological and Psychiatric Sciences
University of Florence, Florence, Italy

Abstract - Spasticity is a complex phenomenon expression of an upper motor neuron lesion.Several definitions of spasticity, its complex clinical picture, the lack of quantifiable techniques to monitor therapeutic intervention are factors to be taken into account when we treat spasticity. Current pharmacologic management of spasticity is far from to be satisfactory and generally does not benefit those symptoms that are more disabling for patients with an upper motor neuron syndrome. The focus of this review is on pharmacologic agents that are of practical use for patients with spasticity. *Key Words: spasticity; antispasticy therapy; drugs.*

1 Introduction

Spasticity is a complex phenomenon, often hard to be clinically quantified. In strictly physiologic terms, spasticity is defined as a motor disorder characterized by a velocity-dependent increase in tonic stretch reflexes with exaggerated tendon jerks resulting from hyperexcitability of the stretch reflex (Lance, 1980).

Clinically, the term spasticity is used to refer to a number of unrelated symptoms and signs that occur in patients suffering from an upper motor neuron lesion. It is a complex mixture of so-called negative symptoms, which are due to disconnections of various motor tracts within the central nervous system (CNS), and positive symptoms which are the result of the release of spinal circuits from descending restraints.

From the patient's point of view, negative symptoms, such as weakness, fatigue and loss of dexterity, are the most disabling ones. Moreover, stiffness, flexor spasm and pain, the positive symptoms, can make transfers and sitting impossible or can impair ambulation and self-care.

Nevertheless, spasticity may be useful to the patient improving gait and transfer by masking weakness of the lower limb antigravity muscles.

In managing spasticity the physician must consider all these factors and particularly the relative benefit of therapy versus the disability which originates from spasticity.

Moreover, evaluation of spasticity are based on qualitative or semiquantitative clinical observations (such as pendulum test or the Ashworth scale), but clinical methods suffer from observer bias and all lack of a standard reference point over time, this make more difficult to estimate therapeutic intervention effectiveness.

Finally, since the clinical manifestation of spasticity is related to the locus and to the extent of injury in the central nervous system, and different patho-physiological abnormalities may act in it, several different clinical patterns of spasticity can be encounter, therefore the same therapeutic agents will be not equally effective in all patients (Delwaide, 1985; Delwaide, 1986).

2 Spinal Cord and Neurotransmitters

The pathophysiology of spasticity is not yet well understood, but it appears to include dysfunction of descending pathways that exert control over the motoneurons (e.g. corticospinal, vestibulospinal, reticulospinal).

While synaptic mechanisms and neurotransmitter have been studied in animal models, we have very few data about man, and many of these suggest that some biochemical changes in spinal segments which underline spasticity are peculiar for man (Hultborn and Malmsten, 1983; Naftchi *et al.*, 1979).

Motoneurons, at the anterior horn level, contain high concentrations of choline acetyltransferase, and acetylcholine is their transmitter. Glycine is the neurotransmitter agent responsable for Renshaw inhibition, and it is also the neurotransmitter of the interneurons that mediates reciprocal inhibition during relax action. GABA (gamma-aminobutyric acid) is the neurotransmitter for a more selective form of inhibition, the presynaptic inhibition, but it may also be involved in postsynaptic inhibition at synapses in the spinal cord (Cullheim and Kellerth, 1981). L-glutamate and L-aspartate have been proposed as neurotransmitters with an excitatory function in the spinal cord. There are, moreover, descending cholonergic, adrenergic, and dopaminergic axons which play a less defined role.

Confusion still exists as to which substances are the natural agonists at which synapses, but the logical approach to the pharmacological management of spasticity seems to be the knowledge of which neurotransmitters are involved in it and how we can act to manipulate them.

3 Antispasticity Agents

Several drugs have been proposed to treat spasticity, but only three of them have clearly been demonstrated superior to placebo in the treatment of spasticity: baclofen, diazepam and dantrolene.

We will discuss pharmacologic agents that are of practical use for patients with spasticity.

3.1 Baclofen

Baclofen (para-chlorophenyl gamma-aminobutyric acid) is a powerful neuronal depressant which has been widely used in the clinical practice for control of spasticity since 1967 (Jones *et al.*, 1970). It is probably the best antispasticity drugs for the treatment of spinal causes of spasticity (Pederson *et al.*, 1974).

Baclofen is a GABA-B receptor agonist, and it is believed to work on spinal receptors, presynaptically, reducing the release of excitatory neurotransmitters. However, it also has sites of action more rostrally in the CNS (Yaksh and Reddy, 1981).

Its effect is more evident in segmental reflexes, while intersegmental reflexes (such as flexor spasms) are relatively less sensitive to baclofen.

Moreover, baclofen is believed to have a dose-dependent antinociceptive action, how it has been demonstrated experimentally in intact animals; this has suggested its use in painful syndrome (Henry, 1980).

Baclofen is absorbed rapidly after oral administration. It has a half-life in plasma of about 3 to 4 hours, so it should be administered 3 or 4 times daily to mantain a uniform plasma level.

Dosage varies widely and is difficult to predict for individual patients. Treatment usually begins at 5 mg twice daily and then gradually increased, depending on the response. Maximal dosage is considered 20 mg four times daily, but some times 100 to 150 mg per day may be requested, surprisingly without side effects. Baclofen should be used cautiously in patients with impaired renal function.

Baclofen produces very few long-term side effects which can be prevented, apart from drowsiness, by increasing the dose gradually. In patients with concomitant intellectual impairment higher doses may lead to a confusional state (Smith *et al.*, 1991).

3.2 Intrathecal Baclofen

In order to avoid systemic toxicity and CNS side effects caused by dose levels of orally administered baclofen sometimes required to achieve a therapeutic response, a different route of drugs administration was recently investigated for long-term treatment of severe spasticity (Saltuari *et al.*, 1992).

Surgically implanted pump permitted the delivery of baclofen directly into the subarachnoid space guaranteing high level of drug to diffuse into spinal cord without the side effects of the oral administration.

Several multicenter studies have been published so far, providing clear evidence of the efficacy of intrathecal baclofen in the spasticity of multiple sclerosis and spinal cord lesion (Saltuari *et al.*, 1992; Penn *et al.*, 1989; Coffey *et al.*, 1993). Recently a group from Austria and Italy has shown that intrathecal administration was useful in patients with supraspinal spasticity. The patients of this study were affected by traumatic apallic syndrome, hypoxic apallic syndrome, Little's disease presenting with spastic paraparesis, hereditary spastic paraplegia (Saltuari *et al.,* 1992). This mode of therapy represents a potentially significant advantage over destructive procedures in patients with preserved function or in those unwilling to accept the finality of another surgically induced spinal cord lesion.

3.3 Diazepam

The mechanism of action of diazepam, at the spinal cord level, may be manifested by enhancement of presynaptic inhibition of afferent neuronal terminals in the primary reflex arc. Schmidt et al. (1967) demonstrated, for the first time in 1967, that diazepam increased presynaptic inhibition in cats.

Diazepam, although not having direct GABA-ergic effect, faciliates the post synaptic effects of GABA binding near to the GABA-A receptor and making the receptor more avid for the neurotransmitter.

Many biochemical studies had showen that diazepam, and other BZDs, heighten the affinity of the binding of GABA to GABA-A receptors on CNS membranes (Guidotti *et al.,* 1978; Skerritt and Johnston, 1983).

Diazepam acts in both segmentally and multisegmentally mediated manifestations of spasticity, but some of its well known side effects have limited its use. Some authors recommend to use diazepam together with baclofen when high doses of the latter give not results.

Dosage is started at 2 mg twice a day and then gradually increased until a maximal dosage of 50-60 mg daily.

The most common side effects are drowsiness and ataxia, extensions of pharmacological actions of the drug.

3.4 Dantrolene

Dantrolene acts directly at the level of the muscle fiber. It exerts its action by uncoupling excitation-contraction. It is thought to inhibit the release of calcium ions from the sarcoplasmic reticulum. The block of calcium release is not complete and contraction is never abolished (Ellis and Bryant, 1972). Dantrolene does not affect neuromuscolar transmission but reduces the force of muscle contraction. It may be particularly useful for the treatment of spasticity in patients whose nursing care is made difficult by severe prolonged muscle contraction and who will not be troubled by any concomitant decrease in voluntary power.

Diarrhoea is a frequent side effect of dantrolene, but a more serious one is its potential to cause liver toxicity (Utili *et al.,* 1977). Fatal hepatitis may occur in 0.1 to 0.2 of patients treated with this drug, while a higher percentage, 2%, may experience hepatocellular dysfunction, reversible in many cases.

Usually treatment is started at 25 mg once a day and gradually increased to a maximal dose of 400 mg daily, given in 4 administrations, in increments of 25 mg every 4-7 days.

3.5 Tizanidine

Tizanidine, an oral agent not yet available in all countries, is believed to inhibit spinal polysynaptic pathways, and to reduce the release of interneurons excitatory amino acids (Knutsson *et al.*, 1982). Studies to date suggest that tizanidine is effective at dosage higher than 16-32 mg/day in increasing voluntary strength, reducing spastic restraint, and improving motor performance (Coward, 1981).

Treatment should be startered at 2 mg three times daily and then gradually increased in increments of 2-4 mg every 3-6 days to a maximal dose of 36 mg daily.

The most common side effects are drowsines and dry mouth that usually disappear few days after an increase of dosage(Hutchinson, 1990).

3.6 Other drugs

Other agents which have been studied as antispasticity drugs for different reasons are not of practical interest or, at least, of usual practice.

Some, like the noradrenergic α agonist *clonidine,* reportedly decreased muscular hypertonus, spontaneous spasm and clonus (Maynard, 1986), have not arouse clinician's enthusiasm. Other, like *progabide*, produces many side effects in contrast to an only modest antispasticy effects. The amino acid *L-threonine*, a precursor of glycine, has been used to treat spasticity in familial spastic paraparesis and multiple sclerosis with variable responses (Growdon *et al.*, 1991; Hauser *et al.*, 1992).

More recently, ***botulinum toxin*** has been proposed as an antispasticity agent controlling the troublesome muscle spasm without producing generalized weakness (Barry *et al.*, 1990). It acts presynaptically, inhibiting the release of acetylcholine with an irreversible blockage at the neuromuscular junction level.

However, botulinum toxin appairs potentially more beneficial for patients with isolated troublesome muscle contractions than for patients with generalized spasticity.

4 Conclusions

Spasticity is a complex clinical phenomenon. The pathophysiological mechanisms underlying it are multifactorial and not yet well understood. A number of therapeutic modalities for treatment of spasticity exist, but there are few simple objective methods for evaluating their effects. However, patients with problems attributable to spasticity for which there are potentially effective therapies should be evaluated for these treatments. Studies of the different mechanisms of action of antispasticity drugs has resulted in fundamental new knowledge about the workings of the CNS, these basic discoveries may eventually lead to the development of drugs more useful in countering the effects of upper motor neuron lesions.

References

Barry, J. S., Tsui, J. K. C., Bhatt, M. H., Varelas, M., Hashimoto, S.A., and Calne, D.B. (1990) Treatment of Spasticity with Botulinum Toxin: A Double-Blind Study. Ann Neurol;28(4):512-515

Coffey, R. J., Cahill, D., Steers, W., Park, T.S., Ordia, J., Meythaler, J., Herman, R., Shetter, A.G., Levy, R., Gill, B., Smith, R., Wilberger, J., Loeser, J. D., Chabal, C., Feler, C., Robertson, J. T., Penn, R. D., Clarke, A., Burchiel, K. J., and Leibrock, L. G. (1993) Intrathecal baclofen for intractable spasticity of spinal origin:results of a long-term multicenter study. J Neurosurg; 78: 226-232

Coward, L. (1981) Selective muscle relaxant properties of Tizanidine and an examination of its mode of action. Triangle; 20: 151-158

Cullheim, S. and Kellerth, J. O. (1981) Two kinds of inhibition of cat spinal α-motoneurones as differentiated pharmacologically. J Physiol (Lond), 312:209-224.

Delwaide, P. J. (1986) Electrophysiological testing of spastic patients:its potential usefulness and limitations. In: Clinical Neurophysiology in Spasticity. Eds Delwaide PJ,Amsterdam,Elsevier Science Publishers (BV) Biomedical Division,1986,185-203

Delwaide, P. J. (1985) Electrophysiological analysis of the mode of action of muscle relaxants in spasticity. Ann Neurol. 17:90-95

Ellis, K. O. and Bryant, S. H. (1972) Excitation contraction uncoupling in skeletal muscle by dantrolene codium. Naunyn Schmiedebergs Arch Pharmacol; 274: 107-109

Growdon, J. H., Nader, T. M., Schoenfeld, J., and Wurtman, R.J. (1991) L-threonine in the treatment of spasticity. Clin Neuropharm; 14(5): 403-412

Guidotti, A., Toffano, G., and Costa, E. (1978) An endogenous protein modulates the affinity of GABA and benzodiazepine receptors in rat brain. Nature; 257: 553-555

Hauser, S. L., Doolittle, T. H., Lopez-Bresnahan, M., and Shahani B. (1992) An antispastic effect of threonine in multiple sclerosis. Arch Naurol; 49: 923-926

Henry, J. L. (1980) Pharmacologic studies on baclofen in the spinal cord of the cat. In:Feldman RG, Young RR, Koella WP, eds. Spasticity:disordered motor control. Chicago:Year Book: 437-452.

Hultborn, H. and Malmsten, J. (1983) Changes in segmental reflexes following chronic spinal cord hemisection in the cat. Acta Physiol Scand, 119:423-433.

Hutchinson, R. (1990) A multinational study in general practice to evaluate the effectiveness and tolerability of tizanidine in the treatment of painful muscle spasm. British Jour of Clin Research; 1: 39-48

Jones, R. F., Burke, D., Marosszeky, J. E., and Gillies J. D. (1970) A new agent for the control of spasticity. J Neurol Neurosurg Psychiat; 33: 464-468

Knutsson, E., Martensson, A., and Gransberg, L. (1982) Antiparetic and antispastic effects induced by tizanidine in patients with spastic paresis. J Neurol Sci; 53: 187-204

Lance, J. W. (1980) Symposium synopsis. In: Feldman RG, Young RR, Koella WP eds. Spasticity disordered motor control. Chicago: Year Book Medical Publishers, 485-94.

Maynard, F. M. (1986) Early clinical experience with clonidine in spinal spasticity. Paraplegia; 24: 175-192

Naftchi, R. E., Schlosser, W., and Horst, W. D. (1979) Correlation of changes in the GABA-ergic system with the development of spasticity in paraplegic cats. In Mandel P, DeFeudis FV (eds): GABA: Biochemistry and CNS Function. New York, Plenum, pp 431-450.

Pedersen, E., Arlien-Søborg, P., and Mai, J. (1974) The mode of action of the GABA derivative baclofen in human spasticity. Acta Neurol Scand;50: 665-80

Penn, R. D., Savoy, S. M., Corcos, D., Latash, M., Gottlieb, G., Parke, B., and Kroin, J. S. (1989) Intrathecal baclofen for severe spinal spasticity. NEJM; 320: 1517-1521.

Saltuari, L., Kronenberg, M., Marosi, M. J., Kofler, M., Russegger, L., Rifici, C., Bramanti, P., and Gerstenbrand, F (1992). Long-term intrathecal baclofen treatment in supraspinal spasticity. Acta Neurol Napoli; 14(3): 195-207

Schmidt, R. F., Vogel, M. E., and Zimmermann, M. (1967) Die Wirkung von Diazepam auf die prasynaptische Hemmung und andere Ruckenmarksreflexe. Naunyn Schmiedebergs Arch Pharmacol; 258: 69-82.

Skerritt, J. H. and Johnston, G. A. R. (1983) Enhancement of GABA binding by benzodiazepine and related anxiolytics. Eur J Pharmacol; 89: 193-198

Smith, C. R., LaRocca, N. G., Giesser, B. G., and Scheinberg, L. C. (1991) High dose oral baclofen: experience in patients with multiple sclerosis. Neurology; 42: 1829-1831.

Utili, R., Boitnott, J. K., and Zimmermann, H. J. (1977) Dantrolene-associated hapatic toxicity. Gastroenterology; 72: 610-616

Yaksh, T. L. and Reddy, S. V. R. (1981) Studies in the primate on the analgetic effects associated with intrathecal actions of opiates, α-adrenergic agonists and baclofen. Anesthesiology, 54: 451-467

Management of Spasticity - Southport Experience

B. M. Soni
Spinal Injuries Centre, District General Hospital, Southport, United Kingdom

Abstract - The aim of this study is to review management of spasticity in spinal cord injured patients in the Spinal Injuries Centre at Southport. Evolutionary changes in the management of spasticity are briefly discussed. The use of intrathecal Baclofen using an implanted programmable drug delivery Medtronic SynchroMed system seems a very useful mode of therapy in patients in whom oral agents are either not effective enough or produce intolerable side effects. Sixteen patients have received such implants over the last 3 years in this Centre. Aggregate follow up of 374 months revealed no complication pertaining to system malfunction. There were no medical, surgical or mechanical complications observed in this series. The outcome, especially with regards to intrathecal Baclofen drug delivery systems, is compared with previously published results. It seems that the majority of system related problems can be resolved with uniformity in implanting surgical technique and subsequent meticulous system management. From this observation so far it has been assessed that approximately 5-10% of spinal cord injured patients will require intrathecal drug delivery systems.

1 Introduction

Spasticity is a motor disorder characterised by velocity-dependent increase in the tonic stretch reflex (muscle tone) with exaggerated tendon jerks resulting from hyperexcitability of the stretch reflexes, as one component of the upper motor neuron syndrome (Lance JW). Troublesome spasticity is a common consequence of central nervous system injury, in particular after spinal cord damage, once the spinal shock has resolved. In neurological terms, spasticity is the result of a decreased threshold of responsiveness of motor neurons to proprioceptive input. There are several possible sites of action within the stretch reflex arc which can cause exaggerated stretch reflex activity and produce muscle hypertonia in spastic conditions. These sites include (1) muscle spindle hyperactivity due to increased gamma motor neuron activity; (2)decreased pre-synaptic inhibition, due to impaired descending influence or segmental input, or structural reorganisation of the propriospinal input; (3) alteration in the segmental reflex mechanisms with resulting increased responsiveness of alpha and gamma motor neurons to the input from muscle afferents; (4) impaired suprasegmental influence on alpha motor cells and consequent hyperactivity of alpha motor cells (Milan R, Dimitrijevic).

In the case of a sustained, functionally complete spinal cord injury characteristic neurological findings are muscle hypertonia predominantly of the flexor group muscles, moderate to markedly enhanced deep tendon jerks and sometimes short lasting patellar and ankle clonus. Such findings are regularly observed in spinal cord injured patients. Moderate spasticity has its advantages. Regular muscle contractions produces physical stretch on the periosteum retarding osteoporosis; moderate skeletal muscle spasms helps venous circulation and return, thus, helping to reduce incidence of deep venous thrombosis; spastic lower limb muscles help improve balance for transfers and ambulation. It is the troublesome, excessive, persistant spasticity that requires attention and therapeutic measures. A pyramidal approach practised in this Centre is presented to address spasticity management. (Figure 1).

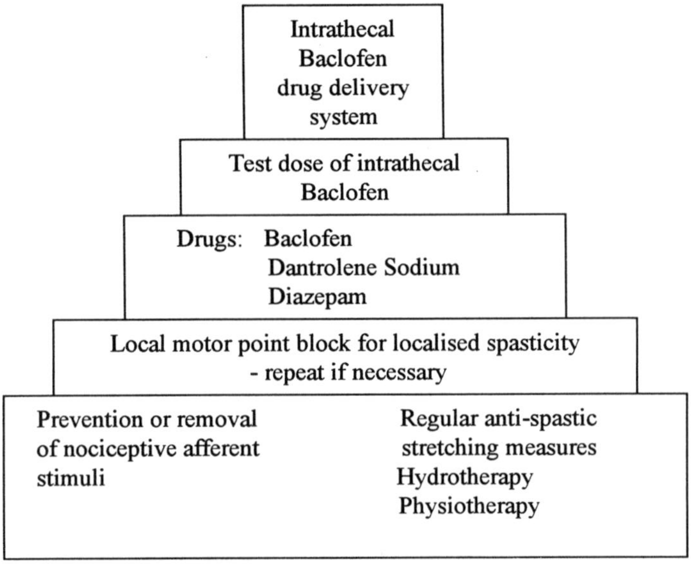

Fig. 1. Pyramidal Approach to Spasticity

Skin ulceration in the form of pressure sore, chronic constipation and voiding disorders in the form of detrusor-sphincter dyssynergy can precipitate or exacerbate spasticity. A vigilant check and examination should be carried out to exclude such disorders prior to increasing antispastic medications. Sudden exacerbation of spasms in a well settled patient requires thorough investigation and treatment of precipitating disorders.

Persistent excessive spasticity produces skin ulceration, chronic constipation and detrusor-sphincter dyssynergy. Thus, a vicious circle is established.

In clinical settings troublesome spasticity produces varied complications in spinal cord injured patients such as:

1. Musculoskeletal system disorders in the form of bad posture, vertebral column deformity, joint contractures and joint dislocations.
2. Chronic constipation which in turn precipitates further spasticity.
3. Spasticity also causes incomplete emptying of the urinary bladder. Such pronounced detrusor-sphincter dyssynergy leads to incomplete emptying of the bladder. Resultant urinary tract disorders further precipitate spasticity/exacerbates spasticity.
4. Spasticity severely restricts rehabilitation, reduces independence and wheelchair mobility. It also produces disturbed sleep, persistant physical discomfort. All such impaired functions leading to significant compromise in activities of daily living and reduced quality of life.

Spasticity may not always be detrimental in that mild to moderate forms may act as a compensatory stabiliser for motor deficit but severe spasticity is invariably detrimental. To achieve comprehensive rehabilitation goals of a disabled person, excessive spasticity needs treatment. The treatment employed in the Spinal Injuries Centre at Southport is reviewed and presented here.

2 Review

This Centre has been providing life long global care for spinal cord injured patients from the north west of England since 1945. It has a catchment population of 5.2 million. In addition, this Centre has an unique national expertise in providing total care for ventilatory dependent tetraplegic patients. Assessment of spasticity is performed on the Ashworth scale and spasms score (Ashworth B). (Table 1).

The treatment of spasticity prior to 1972 included physical antispastic therapy measures in the Unit and in the community. Surgical measures employed then consisted of posterior and anterior rhizotomy, tenotomy and neurectomy and midline myelotomy. The results with the above described surgical measures were either disappointingly short lived or produced further permanent unacceptable neurological loss. Local motor point blockade had also shown short lived results, if any, in treating spasticity.

Intrathecal Phenol injection carried out in a few spinal cord injury patients was found to be imprecise in the effect with loss of reflex activity of bowels, urinary bladder and loss of reflex penile erections. Here again the benefits in controlling spasticity were found to be short lived. Overall these measures were not found beneficial in the treatment of spasticity and are not practised further. Additionally, it would not be justifiable to perform such irreversible destructive procedures in young spinal cord injured patients.

Ashworth Scale:	**GRADE**	**DEGREE OF MUSCLE TONE**
	1	No increase in tone
	2	Slight increase in tone, giving a "catch", where affected part is moved in flexion or extension
	3	More marked increase in tone, but affected part easily flexed
	4	Considerable increase in tone Passive movements difficult
	5	Affected part rigid in flexion or extension
Spasm Score	**GRADE**	**FREQUENCY**
	0	No spasm
	1	Mild spasms induced by stimulation
	2	Infrequent spasms occurring more than once per hour
	3	Spasms occurring more than once per hour
	4	Spasms occurring more than 10 times per hour

Table 1. Clinical Assessment Scales for Spasticity

A brief pharmacokinetic review is discussed regarding commonly used medications presently to treat spasticity in newly injured and old spinal cord injury patients of this Centre.

In light of available knowledge of neurophysiology and neurotransmitter substances, a better understanding of spasticity and drug pharmacokinetics has emerged. Baclofen was introduced in the United Kingdom in 1972.

Dantrolene sodium and Benzodiazipine group of medications were also found successful in the treament of spasticity of spinal and supraspinal origin. Clonidine has shown rather unacceptable medical side effects and has not proven to be of substantial benefit on a long term basis in the treatment of spasticity. Tinazidine trial results are long awaited. Presently Baclofen, Dantrolene and Diazepam form the first line of drug therapy for treatment of spasticity in this Centre.

In 1965 studies of spinal cord pharmacology offered a new approach to the problem of spasticity. The attention was focused on gamma amino butyric acid (GABA) a compound found to inhibit mono and polysynaptic activity in experimental animals (Curtis DR, Watkins JC).

2.1 Baclofen

Gamma amino butyric acitd is a neurotransmitter substance known to inhibit mono and polysynaptic activity in experimental animals (Curtis DR). It is shown to inhibit transmission at GABA-B receptor in humans. Baclofen is an analogue of this GABA central neurotransmitter. The therapeutic effectiveness of Baclofen was, however, limited due to its hydrophilic properties which hindered absorption across the blood-brain barrier and other lipid membranes in the central nervous system. Substitution of a Pchlorophenyl group at the β carbon atom of GABA produced a derivative called Baclofen with enhanced lipophilic properties. This compound was found to cross the blood-brain barrier. The concentration ratio between cerebrospinal fluid and plasma was found to be very low. Baclofen proved effective in the treatment of spasticity of cerebral as well as spinal cord origin. In several double blind trials using Baclofen and Diazepam, Baclofen was found to be more effective and better tolerated and with less long term side effects.

Long term safety data of Baclofen suggested fewer side effects. Oral Baclofen forms the first line of drug treatment for spasticity in this Centre which ranges between 10-120 mgm per day. Baclofen has been found safe to combine with other antispastic medications. The doseage adjustment should be made according to beneficial response and regular assessment.

Dantrolene sodium is also used in this Centre for the treatment of spasticity. Dantrolene acts peripherally at a site beyond the myoneural junction. It produces a dissociation of excitation contraction coupling, probably interfering with the release of calcium from the sarcoplasmic reticulum. This muscle relaxant effect is seen in both fast and slow fibres but is more pronounced in the former. The dosage is increased in 25 mgm increments every week until a satisfactory clinical reponse is established in suppressing spasticity. Liver function tests were carried out prior to and after commencing Dantrolene therapy at regular intervals. Dantrolene is discontinued if at any stage deterioration in liver function test is observed. Dantrolene is used alone or in conjunction with other antispastic medications. Concomitant use of alcohol with Dantrolene is actively discouraged. Dantrolene frequently produces intolerable side effects especially affecting the central nervous system, cardiovascular system and hepatic dysfunctions. In our observation Dantrolene is less well tolerated.

2.2 Diazepam

Diazepam has centrally acting muscle relaxant properties and it facilitates GABA-A receptors post-synaptically. Due to its numerous central nervous system and central respiratory depression side effects, Diazepam is used less frequently in this Centre. Diazepam is used as a third line of medication in the treatment of spasticity.

A regular programme of antispastic stretch measure is implemented during the rehabilitation stage. All these patients are encouraged to continue such measures regularly in their own home. Hydrotherapy and regular passive skeletal muscle stretch measures are actively pursued in this Centre and in the community. Patients are encouraged to contact the Centre in case of exacerabtion of their spasticity.

2.3 Intrathecal Baclofen

It is expected that 5-10% of spinal cord injured patients would require intrathecal drug delivery systems to treat their excessive spasticity. This percentage figure is derived from the experience collated in treating a large number of spinal cord injured patients through this Centre. This percentage of patients with excessive spasticity experience unacceptable side effects of medications or fail to gain any meaningful benefits from conventional oral medication therapy.

Such patients should be offered intrathecal Baclofen drug therapy preferably with programmable drug delivery system. Obviously a successful trial test dose in relieving spasticity is a pre-requiste to such therapy.

Intrathecal use of Baclofen for severe spasticity was first reported by Penn and Kroin in 1984 (Penn RD, Kroin JS). Since then several studies supporting this result have been published. Intrathecal Baclofen has been found to improve supraspinal spasticity, although experience of this aspect is presently limited in this Centre. Intrathecal Baclofen has been found beneficial in the treament of hereditary spastic paraplegia in one of our patients who recieves complex continuous intrathecal Baclofen infusion through a Medtronic SynchroMed programmable pump. Intrathecal Baclofen has been found beneficial in treatment of spinal spasticity as shown by our results.

Baclofen, a GABA analogue, binds to the GABA-B receptor resulting in the inhibition of caclium influx in presynaptic terminals and, thus, suppressing the release of excitatory neurotransmitters. These GABA receptor sites occur widely throughout the central nervous sytem (Price GW). This finding is consistent with observations of profound suppression of both mono and polysynaptic reflexes with intrathecal Baclofen in animal models (Curtis DR, Malik R); although it is argued that intrathecal Baclofen selectively suppressed segmental monosynaptic reflexes, such as the tendon jerks, muscle stretch reflex and the H-reflex.

There is an abundance of GABA-B receptors in the superficial layers of the spinal cord (Curtis DR, Malik R) and this means that intrathecal administration of Baclofen results in a greater than four fold increase in cerebrospinal fluid level with 1% of the oral dose (Penn et al). Measurement of cerebrospinal fluid Baclofen concentration shows lumbar to cervical ratio of 4:1, thus avoiding untoward cerebral effects of the intrathecally administered Baclofen.

A programmable pump allows a desired mode of infusion without changing the solution in the implant chamber. It allows precise adjustment of the drug dosage and variation of the dosage schedule accommodating circardian rhythm used to control spasms at required times. A high incidence rate of complications has been reported with cardis secor, fixed volume pumps in literature (Teddy et al and Gardner et al).

All our 16 patients had a Medtronic SynchroMed programmable pump model 8615. This model has an easy access port which allows withdrawal of cerebrospinal fluid and checking of the tube patency using radiological contrast material, if required. To maintain uniformity and avoid complications, one surgeon performs the pump implantation procedure and maintains meticulous follow up of all the implanted patients (author).

2.4 Test Dose

The policy of the Centre for this procedure is to admit the patient and perform assessment of the spasticity according to Ashworth and spasm scores. A lumbar puncture at L3/4 interspace is performed and 40 μgm of intrathecal Baclofen is administered. Improvement in overall assessment score is concluded as a positive response. The maximum intrathecal Baclofen dose used is 100 μgm.

The patient is mobilised in their wheelchair after the test dose and a subsequent Ashworth and spasm score assessment is made every hour for the following 4 hours. All patients have responded favourabley to the test dose in our practice. Improvement in the assessment score justifies recommendation of implantation procedure with a programmable pump for the treatment of spasticity. The patient is allowed home after 24 hours. As intrathecal Baclofen may suppress reflex detrusor activity close observation is advised. In our practice 2 patients developed urinary retention.

2.5 Implant Procedure

Implantation procedure is performed according to the manufacturer's operating instructions with the following modifications specific to the technique.

1. Subarachnoid access at L3/4 interspace with size 16 Touhey needle is performed not through the midline but through a paramedian approach.
2. Subarachnoid catheter (SynchroMed InDura pack) is advanced up to T10 level without any kink and this finding is confirmed by x-ray screening during surgery.
3. Prior to withdrawal of the Touhey needle a small circular paraspinal muscle fascia flap is raised to tunnel the catheter underneath.
4. Catheter is stabilized in the majority of cases using butterfly connector. This is further stabilized by suturing the connector deep in the paraspinal muscle. The fascial semicircular flap is closed over and several sutures are applied. This procedure not only avoids the catheter from kinking but also secures the catheter firmly.
5. The pump is always implanted under external oblique muscle. I have found this method cosmetically better for the patients. The right iliac fossa remains a place of choice for the pump implantation unless indicated otherwise. The patient is given 3 days of parenteral antibiotic therapy.

The rest of the system management is carried out according to the manufacturer's manual.

Spasticity evaluation is carried out on a regular basis and the dosage adjusted accordingly. Refill procedures are performed aseptically and no atmospheric air is allowed to ingress into the pump chamber. This is achieved using a 0.2 micron particulate, bacterial and air filter during refilling procedure. All oral antispastic medication is gradually withdrawn.

Patients are encouraged to telephone the Centre without hesitation in case of any problem. Normally refill procedures are repeated at 4-6 month intervals. This is achieved by using nit or diluted 3000 μgm/ml Baclofen solution manufactured at the Pharmacy Department of Countess of Chester Hospital, Chester, England. Emergency procedure sheets are given to patients to keep with their implant registration card. Baclofen overdosage signs, along with emergency treatment protocol sheets, are displayed for the Centre staff in treatment areas.

3 Results

Sixteen Medtronic SynchroMed 8615 model pumps along with InDura 8703W (Medtronic) catheter system were implanted over the last 3 years for the treatment of excessive spasticity of spinal origin. The intrathecal Baclofen dose ranges from 40 μgm to 760 μgm per day. The majority of patients have simple continuous infusions, while 3 patients are on complex continuous infusion to accommodate their required diurnal increased Baclofen doseage.

Results have objectively shown significant improvement in Ashworth and spasm scores, improvement in mobility and freedom of movement of all patients. A significant increase in patient's activities of daily living has transpired following intrathecal Baclofen therapy. The results are tabulated in Table 2. They compare favourably when compared with other published series. (Table 3).

This invaluable treatment for patients with excessive troublesome spasticity should not be used by the occasional operator. A well co-ordinated team approach is essential. This opinion expressed by Teddy et al and Gardner et al cannot be overemphasised.

4 Conclusion

Literature reviewed so far suggests satisfactory outcome using intrathecal Baclofen in the management of severe spasticity. The Medtronic SynchroMed programmable drug delivery system has performed well in the 16 patients treated so far. It is a reversible therapy and, with radiotelemetry dosage adjustment, it makes this therapy very versatile and comparatively less risky. So far complications have not been observed with this system. Reviewed literature supports our observation that Medtronic SynchroMed programmable drug delivery system performs far better compared to other available pumps (Gardener B, Teddy P). Complications with SynchroMed Medtronic programmable implantable Baclofen intrathecal drug delivery system have been recorded. Uniformity in modified implanting technique and meticulous follow up technique by one person/team is recommended to minimise or avoid complications with this system as demonstrated by our experience.

Name/ Age	Date of injury	Dia-gnosis	Ashworth /spasm score	Date of implant	Durat-ion of implant	Post-implant Ashworth /spasm score	Post-op infect.	OP episode	Surgical complic	Mech. complic.	Pump/ tube malfunc	Morbid. related to therapy
PS 57	23.3.78	T8 para	5 - 4	1.6.89	78 mth	1 - 0	none	2*	none	none	none	none
BW 69	24.5.91	C6 tetra	4 - 3	3.11.92	36 mth	1 - 0	none	1	none	none	none	none
JH 50	3.9.91	C6 tetra	5 - 4	3.11.92	36 mth	1 - 0	none	1	none	none	none	none
JW 47	24.1.92	C4 tetra	4 - 4	22.1.93	33 mth	1 - 0	none	1	none	none	none	none
BW 29	26.11.89	C6 tetra	5 - 3	23.4.93	30 mth	1 - 0	none	1	none	none	none	none
KM 68	23.3.78	C3 tetra	4 - 4	30.7.93	15 mth	1 - 0	none	1	none	none	none	none
RS 67	9.2.93	C6 tetra	4 - 4	12.11.93	24 mth	1 - 0	none	1	none	none	none	none
JC 58	14.6.93	C4 tetra	4 - 4	30.11.93	24 mth	2 - 1	none	1	none	none	none	none
BS 42	16.2.90	Spas.para	5 - 3	14.1.94	21 mth	2 - 1	none	1	none	none	none	none
BB 68	20.10.93	C7/8 tetra	4 - 4	1.2.94	20 mth	1 - 1	none	1	none	none	none	none
RA 58	1983	T6 para	5 - 3	15.4.94	18 mth	1 - 0	none	1	none	none	none	none
KO 29	6.5.85	C6 tetra	4 - 4	13.5.94	17 mth	1 - 1	none	1	none	none	none	none
WJ 26	10.12.93	C6 tetra	5 - 2	1.7.94	16 mth	1 - 0	none	1	none	none	none	none
JH 23	3.5.93	T5 para	5 - 4	7.7.95	3 mth	1 - 0	none	1	none	none	none	none
AG 28	19.7.84	C5 tetra	4 - 4	8.9.95	2 mth	1 - 0	none	1	none	none	none	none
AS 36	4.9.95	T7 para	5 - 4	26.9.95	1 mth	1 - 0	none	1	none	none	none	none

23.5 months average follow up; 374 months aggregate follow up; * battery exhausted - new pump implanted

Table 2. Results of intrathecal Baclofen therapy - Southport experience

	Teddy et al 1992	McLean (1993)	Gardner et al (1995)	Soni Southport (1995)
No. of patients	46	168	17	16
No. of pump implanted	56	n/a	19	17
Pump removal	n/a	n/a	2	none
Reimplants required	n/a	n/a	2	1*
Re-operation	48	n/a	10	1*
Tube dislodgement	7	12	4	none
Tube disconnection	8	n/a	5	none
Tube kinking, blockage	5	5	6	none
Tube breakage	1	1	1	none
Pump malfunction	3	8	2	none
Significant CSF leak	2	n/a	1	none
Wound haematoma	3	5	1	none
Skin necrosis, breakdown	3	5	none	none
Infection	5	10	none	none
Mild drug overdose	3	6	none	none
Serious drug overdose	2		2	none
Inability to use pump	2	none	none	none
Sacral root trauma	n/a	1	n/a	none
Meningitis	none	5	none	none
Reluctance to use the pump; psychological reason	2	n/a	1	none
Total implant times in months	1165	n/a	567	374
Number of complications	46	58	23	none

n/a = not available   * = battery exhausted

Table 3. Complications - Results Comparison

As complications are related to operator inexperience, it is recommended that specific centre or personnel should only perform this procedure. Standardised operation and follow up protocols can evaluate results and avoid complications and risks. All 16 patients in this Centre, so far, have shown favourable outcome without any complications. Patients have achieved better mobility and quality of life. In our Centre this mode of therapy has replaced irreversible orthopaedic and neurosurgical intervention in cases suffering with severe spasticity.

Troublesome spasticity in spinal cord injured patients could prove detrimental and disabling. Further research in the management of spasticity is called for. Should such research be in the field of neural regeneration, neural transplantation or in the field of local or central electrical stimulation? On the other hand have we found the answer now with intrathecal Baclofen drug therapy?

References

Ashworth, B. (1964) *Practitioner*, **192**, 540

Curtis, D. R. and Malik, R. (1985) The differential effects of Baclofen on segmental and descenting excitation of spinal interneurons in the cat. *Exp-Brain Res* **58**: 333-337

Curtis, D. R. and Watkins, J. C. (1965) *Pharmacology Review*, **17**, 347

Gardner, B. and Jamous, A. (1995) et al. Intrathecal Baclofen - a multicentre clinical comparison of the Medtronic programmable, cordis secor and constant infusion infusaid drug delivery system. *Paraplegia* **33**:551-554

Lance, J. W. (1980) Symposium Synopsis. Feldman RG, Young RR, Koella WP, eds. Spasticity - disordered motor control. *Year Book Medical Publishers, Chicago*: 485

McLean, B. N. (1993) Intrathecal Baclofen in severe spasticity: Review. *British Journal of Hospital Medicine* **49**: 4

Milan, R. and Dimitrijevic. Spasticity. *Scientific basis of clinical neurology*. 108-115

Penn, R. D. and Kroin, J. C. (1965). *Pharmacology Review*, **17**, 347

Pen et al. (1989) *New England Journal of Medicine* **320**: 1517-1521

Price, G. W. and Wilkin, G. P. et al. (1984) Are Baclofen sensitive GABA-B receptors present on primary afferent terminals of the spinal cord? *Nature* **307**: 71-74

Teddy, P. and Jamous, A. et al. (1992) Complications of intrathecal Baclofen delivery. *British Journal of Neurosurgery* **6**: 115-118

Chapter 7

Orthotics and Hybrid Systems

Powered Hip Orthosis

J. Edwards, S. V. S. Rithalia
Orthopaedic Mechanics Research Institute,
University College Salford, Salford, United Kingdom

Abstract - The purpose of this study was to investigate the feasibility of adding externally powered drive units to a reciprocating orthosis in order to extend the walking capability of paraplegics. This included patients with progressive neuromuscular diseases and damaged secondary motor neurones who are unable to benefit from functional electrical stimulation. A design was adopted in which only the hip joints were driven by external power units which worked in conjunction with the patient's own upper body musculature.

Drive was provided by an electronically commutated DC motor powered by a one kilogram weight pack of nickel/cadmium batteries. By connecting this motor directly to the hip joint actuator through a ball screw of 87.5% mechanical efficiency, the use of cumbersome and heavy gear boxes was avoided. The user was able to release both the hip and knee joints for sitting. Furthermore, location of the drive units in space behind and slightly above the hip joints made sitting feasible in most chairs. Use of a new Salford design of unlockable knee joint would enable the subject to walk with knee bending during the swing phase. This was achieved by causing the powered drive to accelerate hip joint flexion during the initial phase of swing. The result was a prototype powered reciprocating orthosis which should enable a more normal pattern of paraplegic walking at faster speeds of progression, greatly reduced patient energy expenditure and whose size and weight make it eminently suitable for use in the community.

1 Introduction

The use of reciprocating or hip guidance orthoses (Yngve *et al.*, 1984; McCall and Schmidt, 1986; Rose *et al.*, 1981) for upright mobility in children has proved to be very successful. However, the clinical experience of prescribing these devices to over 60 adult paraplegics at our Orthotic Clinic in Salford has been that, following an initial flush of enthusiasm, 80% lost interest in continuing regular upright exercise after approximately three years. Even on hard and level ground, adults found that the speed of walking in a reciprocating orthosis was too slow to satisfy the demands of daily living, doffing and donning the device was time consuming and many became excessively fatigued after walking only a few hundred metres.

Functional electrical stimulation (FES) with electrodes implanted around the nerves, or directly onto muscles, offers the potential of overcoming some of these problems (Marsolais and Kobetic, 1987). However, paraplegics with partial lesions who still have sensation in their lower limbs may find this procedure too painful. Furthermore, FES is not effective on muscles with damaged secondary motor neurones, or in many patients with progressive neuromuscular diseases. As an alternative to FES in these cases, we have conducted a feasibility and design study to investigate the benefits of adding external power to drive the hip joints of reciprocating orthoses of the reciprocating gait orthosis (RGO), advanced reciprocating gait orthosis (ARGO) or hip guidance orthosis (HGO) variety (Douglas *et al.,* 1983; Hugh Steeper Ltd., 1991; Watkins *et al.*, 1987). In the first instance, we concentrated on design changes to the Louisiana State University RGO, since this device was being used by the majority of our paraplegics. The present paper dealt with mechanical aspects of that design whilst a paper by Gray *et al.* (1993) described the electronic and control part of the study.

2 General Considerations

Previous publications reporting attempts to power lower limb orthoses have been few in number (Hill, 1977; Miyamoto *et al.,* 1985; Ferrara *et al.,* 1983), and the hardware they describe has tended to be heavy and cumbersome. As a result, they proved impractical for daily use in the community. With a view to producing a more practical solution, it seemed expedient that any use of external power should aim to assist the patient's own residual upper body abilities, rather than taking over the walking process completely. By adopting this approach, it was possible to minimise the size and weight of the orthotic power drive units so that their total mass was acceptable in comparison with that of the lower limbs.

3 Overall Project Plan

Several project sub-divisions were identified with common engineering features that would allow us to develop the study in stages. These started with power to one joint only and then moved on to orthoses capable of greater versatility by powering several joints and adding several passive refinements as follows:

Stage 1 Hip Walker (single drive) - For the initial clinical trials, a single power unit would drive the hip joint on one side of an RGO or ARGO orthosis, with powered movement transmitted to the other hip joint through the existing cables.

Stage 2 Hip Walker (two drives) - After disconnecting the reciprocating orthosis cables, a second drive unit can be added so that the left and right hips can be controlled independently. This would allow the angular velocity of hip movement on the swing side to be independent of that on the stance side (as occurs in normal walking). As a result, a more natural, energy efficient pattern of walking is possible.

Stage 3 Knee Walker - A third stage involving the addition of external power to drive the knee joints as well as, or instead of, the hip would a) enable powered bending of the knee during the swing phase of walking, and, b) provide power to shorten and extend the legs at the knees for sitting and standing, going up and down stairs, or negotiating ramps.

Stage 4 Passive Refinements - Several other design refinements were studied in parallel with the powered approach which involved improvements to the passive mechanisms of present-day reciprocating orthosis designs. This included the development of orthotic knee joints which lock or unlock at appropriate times during the cycle of movement. By this means, paraplegics were able to reduce energy expenditure and improvements of gait pattern by knee bending during the swing phase of walking.

This paper concentrated on the design study involved in stages 1, 2 and 4.

4 Mechanical Design of Powered Hip Walking Orthosis

The purpose of this design was to extend the walking capability of paraplegics beyond that presently provided through the use of reciprocating orthoses. By adding external power drives to an RGO orthosis, our aim was to allow larger numbers of paraplegics to achieve reciprocal walking at near normal speeds and with significantly less fatigue.

Acting in conjunction with a rollator frame or crutches, the arms will assist in overall body balance. Furthermore, by pushing down on the handlebars of these devices, the arms will be required to lift the body during standing up, and to lift the hip of the swinging leg so that the foot clears the ground at the mid-point of the swing phase of walking.

To achieve anything like a normal pattern of gait, the powered orthosis should satisfy the requirements listed in table 1. The data in this table is derived from average values quoted for normal walking (Edwards, 1964; Paul, 1975). The velocity requirement number IV is for the hip of the limb undergoing movement in the stance phase. When the cables are connected this will equal that on the swing side. However, with the cables disconnected in a double drive configuration, it would be beneficial if the maximum velocity achieved on the swing side was 50% greater than that on the stance side.

In order to minimise the weight and size of the drive units, it was inevitable that some design comprises would have to be made which meant that not all of the requirements in table 1 could be satisfied to the full. In making these compromises, it was clear that the angular displacement requirement numbers I, II and III must be satisfied. However, the achievement of sufficient velocity (No. IV) was considered more important than satisfying the torque or acceleration requirements. Acceleration depends on the torque and 50% of the torque is capable of being supplied by the action of the patient's upper body musculature. On the other hand, it is imperative that the external power units should be able to drive the hip joints at speeds which are fast enough to keep up with the patient's own efforts. Otherwise, it will act against forces produced by the patient and cause unnecessary expenditure of muscular energy.

Requirement number	Requirement at each hip joint	Numerical value & units
I	Maximum angular movement in extension	15°
II	Maximum angular movement in flexion	20°
III	Overall maximum angular movement	35°
IV	Maximum angular velocity	1.3 to 1.8
V	(during stance phase)	rad/sec
VI	Angular acceleration for knee flexion in swing phase	40 to 85 NM
VII	Angular deceleration to bring knee into full extension	25 rad/sec^2

Table 1. Numerical design requirements for a powered hip walker orthosis

5 Choice of Power Supply

A feasibility study aimed at selecting a suitable power supply was carried out by Riding (Riding *et al.,* 1991), one of our research team. Pneumatic, hydraulic and electrical power alternatives were considered. The possibility of oil leakage in equipment worn next to clothes suggested that hydraulics was inappropriate. It was also decided not to use pneumatics due to the likelihood of actuator bounce and feedback control problems arising from gas system compressibility. Furthermore, users are likely to experience difficulties of power source replacement when they live some distance from the supplier. Therefore, electrical power became the favoured choice. Several options of supplying electrical power to the orthosis were examined.

The first option was to use a fixed power supply connected to the orthosis with umbilical cables. This technique has been used by previous investigators of powered lower limb orthoses (Ferrara *et al.,* 1983) and involved trailing cables from the patient to large fixed laboratory based power supplies. Although this approach could provide all the power that might be needed for indefinite periods of time, practical problems of umbilical management would restrict the use of such an orthosis to the home. Inside the home, we conceived the possibility of power being supplied through a coiled wire from a small box which follows the patient around the house on an overhead ceiling-mounted strip power supply, rather like the electrified railways. However, trailing cables of any form would be a major barrier against outdoor use.

A second option was to carry a wheelchair size battery power supply on a wheeled mobile vehicle which follows behind the patient when walking out of doors. A short length of coiled cable would link the orthosis to the battery on the vehicle. The vehicle itself could even form part of a wheelchair and could detach itself from the chair, ready to go with the subject as he or she rises into the upright position. However, the problems of designing such a vehicle are several orders of magnitude greater than those of the orthosis, and mobility would still be hindered by umbilical management factors.

It was felt that a more appropriate option for use indoors, as well as for short range trips outside the home, would be to use small, rechargeable battery packs carried on a waist belt, or on a walking frame. This obviates completely the need for trailing wires. Although use of these small batteries would limit the distance that could be walked, the benefits of versatility and independence for the majority of short distance trips would outweigh, in most cases, the penalties of not being able to make the occasional longer journey. In any case, longer journeys are best done in a wheelchair.

Alternatively, if it is necessary to walk further, additional battery packs could be carried over the shoulders in a rucksack. Recharging from a wheelchair mounted power source is also a possibility.

Estimates carried out by Riding (Riding *et al.*, 1991) of the battery power required by adults to drive the hips during walking at slightly reduced walking speeds were of the order of 50 to 100 watts. The energy storage capacity of latest generation nickel/cadmium (NiCad) batteries weighing 1kg is 40 watt hours. The conversion efficiency from battery electrical energy to a mechanical actuator on the brace is likely to be no better than 70%, giving 28 watt hours from a 1kg battery pack. With the paraplegic user providing additional power from the upper body musculature, this should be sufficient to allow walkling for moderate distances up to 1 to 2km before a recharge is needed. On the basis of these estimations, it was considered worthwhile designing and building a prototype orthotic device to be driven by an electric motor powered from a NiCad battery pack.

6 The Motor and Actuator

Practical circumstances require that the motor should be of minimal weight and exhibit a maximal ratio of power output to power input. The motor selected for our prototype design was an electronically commutated, high quality DC motor of appropriate size and weight from Maxon (Interelectric AG, 1993). Using neodymium (NdFe) magnets, this motor gave 100 watts output with variable speeds up to 4450 rpm. The benefits of this motor are that it has high efficiency, good heat dissipation and a life expectancy limited only by ball bearing life.

To generate the required maximum speed of 1.8 rad/sec (or 16 rpm) at the hip joint (see table 1), the mechanical ratio (MR) between the motor and hip joint should be of the order MR = 4450/16 or 278 to 1. To achieve such a large mechanical ratio in one gear box would involve several stages of gearing so that the resulting size and weight of a gear box would be excessive. In addition, mechanical energy losses would be unacceptable. However, theoretical calculations showed that the required mechanical ratio, torque and hip speed can be achieved in one step by adopting a direct drive system through a BALL SCREW. The use of a ball screw system entails minimal weight and size penalties, an 87.5% mechanical efficiency and commercial availability.

7 The Mechanical Design

The location of the externally powered drive units on a reciprocating gait orthosis is shown in fig 1. Each unit is supported by brackets mounted onto the orthosis sacral band, above and behind each hip joint.

The drive motor (D) is mounted on the inside surface of a boss (G) which also houses a deep groove ball bearing for location of the ball screw (P). Motor (D) is connected to the end shaft of the ball screw (P) by a rigid coupling (F). With this arrangement, the weight and length of the drive unit is minimised by using just one ball bearing (J) because any bending moments developed in the screw (D) will also be supported by two internal ball bearings which carry the motor shaft. The magnitude of any such moments are also kept small by mounting the whole drive unit on trunnion shafts (H) having an axis which passes through the centre of the bearing (J). Rotation of screw (P) moves the ball nut (K) linearly away from the motor to flex the hip, or towards the motor to extend the hip. Under normal circumstances, the stroke of the nut would be electronically controlled so that it never impinges against the mechanical end stops of the screw. However, in the event of a control fault, if the nut pushes against the end stop collar (M) or the front face of the boss (G), a rise in electrical current within the motor will cause the motor to be switched off.

The motor is housed within a cylindrical cover so that the assembly can be cooled by air flow from an electric fan (B). The air is drawn in through a slot in the rear aspect of the enclosure and expelled through another slot near the boss. A digital encoder (C) is mounted over the rear shaft of the motor for speed control purposes.

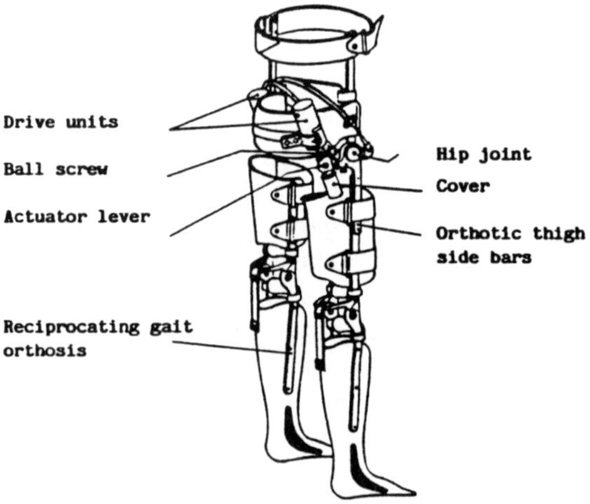

Fig. 1. General arrangement showing location of two electrically powered drive units on an LSU Reciprocating Gait Orthosis. The general construction of each drive unit is shown in fig 2.

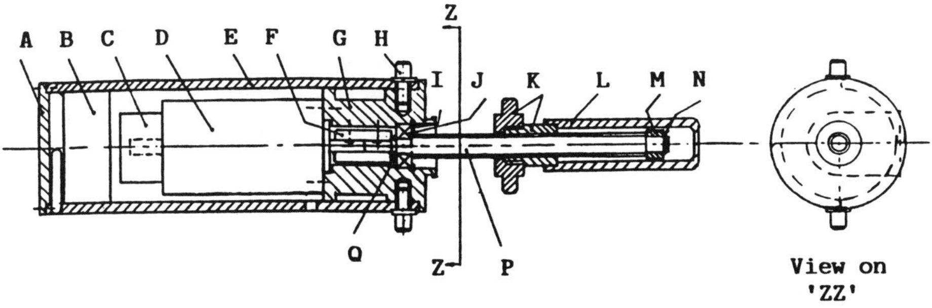

Fig. 2. General construction of electrically powered drive unit.

The general assembly of the system is illustrated in fig 1 and the photograph of fig 3. The nut of the ball screw arrangement is connected via trunnion bearings to the end of a lever which is attached to the existing coupling plate of the RGO hip joint (Durr-Fillauer, 1983). When the hip joint latch plunger is set in its locked position, rotation of the motor will cause the thigh side bars of the orthosis to flex or extend the hip joint, thereby assisting walking. However, disengagement of this plunger allows the hip to rotate freely so that the user can sit down whilst still wearing the orthosis.

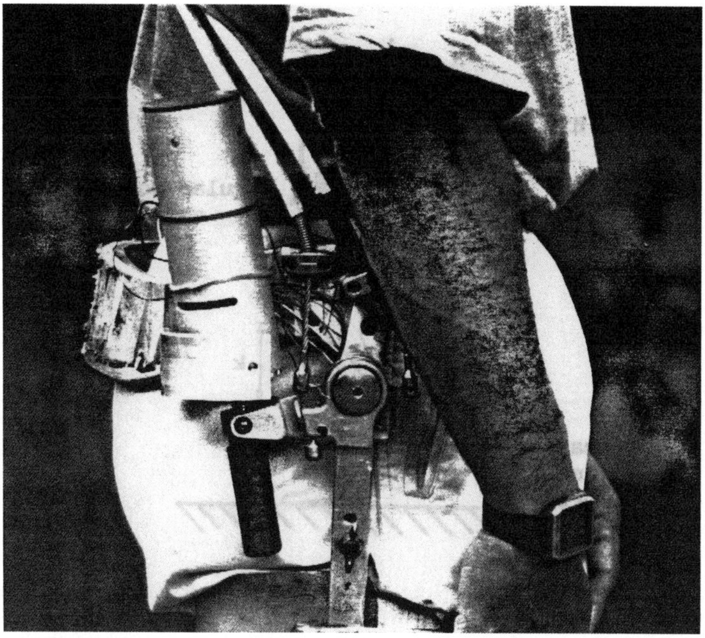

Fig. 3. Photograph of powered orthosis prototype.

In use, the motor will drive the hip of one leg into flexion during the swing phase of walking. This continues until angular displacement transducers mounted on each orthotic hip joint indicate that the end of swing has been attained. The control system electronics will then stop and reverse the motor to cause extension of the hip during the stance phase. This cycle of events is then repeated from the start of the next swing phase.

8 Unlockable Knee Joints

As well as walking with knees fixed in the extended position, as is the convention with existing orthotic designs, the clinical trials of this powered prototype orthosis will also investigate the benefits of using a recent Salford design of lockable/unlockable knee joint (Edwards and Gray, 1993). It operates by releasing the knee joint so that it is free to flex when weight is removed from the limb at the beginning of the swing phase. By causing the powered drive unit to accelerate, the thigh of the swing leg forwards, during the initial part of the swing phase, a rearward acting inertia force will be developed which acts through the centre of mass of the lower leg as illustrated in fig 4. This inertia force creates a bending moment about the knee joint axis which shortens the limb by flexing the knee. This in turn raises the foot to avoid stubbing the toe on the ground at the midswing position. The amount of knee bending can be controlled by changes in angular acceleration of the hip joint, and this can be adjusted by the user. As a result, less effort will be expended in lifting the hip on the swing side.

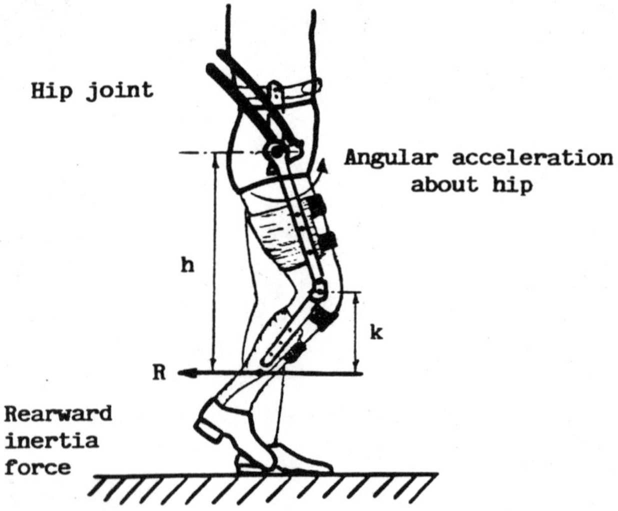

Fig. 4. Diagrammatic illustration of rearward inertia force R acting in response to angular acceleration of the hip joint in flexion during the first half of the swing phase of walking. Shown at the mid swing position, the moment acting to bend the knee is equal to R x k.

During the latter part of the swing phase, the drive unit will be called upon to decelerate the thigh so that the knee becomes fully extended in preparation for the orthotic knee joint to lock again when weight is placed back onto the limb at heel strike.

9 Discussion

The batteries, electronics and control hardware for the powered system were mounted behind the patient on the rear surface of the sacral band of the orthosis. A description of the electrical and control part of the investigation is the subject of an accompanying paper by Gray *et al.* (1993). This paper has been concerned with mechanical aspects of the study.

The weight of each drive unit was 1kg and this was found to be eminently acceptable in comparison to the much greater mass of the abdomen and pelvis, next to which it was mounted. With a maximum outside diameter of 58mm, these units were located comfortably behind and superior to the hip joint, so that they did not interfere with swinging movements of the arms. Yet, because the drive unit body remained in front of the rearmost part of the sacral band as viewed in the sagittal plane (fig 3), the user was able to sit resting against the back support of a chair. The width of the orthosis in the region of the hips as viewed from the front was only 5cm greater than the standard RGO. This still allowed the user to sit between the armrests of their wheelchair and most other seats.

Another benefit gained by fixing the drive units onto the upper portion of the orthosis close to the hip joint centre is that, in this position, linear movements and accelerations are minimised. Therefore, minimal energy is wasted in overcoming the inertia of the added units.

The chosen design for this prototype provides a means of conducting trials to compare the relative performance of different orthotic design configurations. In the first case, only one unit will be used with the drive to one hip joint transmitted to the other hip via the Bowden cables. In a second configuration, the left and right limbs will also be linked together by the cables, but in this case left and right motors will work together in reciprocating unison. In the final case, the cables will be removed so that the left and right legs of the paraplegic can be driven independently, at different speeds and accelerations. The latter arrangement will make significant demands on the control system and may reduce the users capability to assist the drive units in moving the limbs. However, it is likely to produce the most normal pattern of gait.

To date, bench tests have been conducted in the laboratory with the orthosis suspended from its sacral band in a vertical position, and with the leg members free to move under the action of the powered drive units. Plaster casts of similar weight and shape to human lower limbs were strapped into the orthotic legs. The preliminary results of these tests were most promising. Angular rates of movement corresponding to cadences of greater than 60 steps per minute were achieved. Also, a 1kg weight Nicad battery pack driving both limbs continuously via one drive unit and two Bowden cables lasted one hour.

More detailed results from these laboratory tests, as well as from field trials on paraplegic patients, will be the subject of future publications.

References

Douglas, R., Larson, P. F., D'Ambrosia, R. and McCall, R. E. (1983) The LSU reciprocation-gait orthosis. Orthopedics; 6: 834-839.

Durr-Fillauer (1983) LSU Reciprocating gait orthosis - description and application manual. Durr-Fillauer Medical Inc, Chattanooga, Tennessee, USA, 47-49.

Edwards, J. (1964) The mechanics of the joints in the lower limb. MSc(Eng) thesis, University of London, London, p. 429.

Edwards, J. and Gray, J. O. (1993) Powered Hip Orthosis. UK Patent Application No. 9314825, June 1993.

Ferrara, G., Richtshoffer, M., Cabral, J. O., and Marshall, L. (1983) More freedom for the disabled. International Health Magazine, No. 2, Feb 1983, 6-16.

Gray, J. O., Hill, S., and Downes, C. (1993) Powered Orthotics - Part II Electronics and control. Paper presented to Commission of European Communities RAFT Topical Workshop on Muscular Components in Functional Electrical Stimulation, Salford, England, June, 1993.

Hill, J. W. (1977) Hydraulically powered lower limb orthosis. Second CISM/IFT OMM International Symposium on the theory and practice of robots and manipulators. Elsevier, Sept 1977, 182-192.

Hugh Steeper Ltd. (1991) The Steeper advanced reciprocating gait orthosis. Company literature No. L18805, issue 1. Hugh Steeper Ltd., Queen Mary's University Hospital, Roehampton Disability Centre, London, U.K.

Interelectric AG (1993) Maxon motor catalogue Edition 92/93. Interelectric AG, Bruningstrasse 220, CH-6072 Sachsein, Switzerland, 53-60.

Marsolais, E. B and Kobetic, R. (1987) Functional electrical stimulation for walking in paraplegia. J. Bone Joint Surg; 69A: 728-733.

McCall, R. E. and Schmidt, W. T. (1986) Clinical experience with the Reciprocal Gait Orthosis in myelodysplasia. J. Pediatric Orthopedics; 6: 157-161.

Miyamoto, H., Israel, I., Miyamoto, H., Mori, S., Sano, A., and Sakurai, Y. (1985) Approach to a powered orthosis for paralysed lower limbs. Proc. of 1985 International Conference on Advanced Robotics, Tokyo, Japan, 451-458.

Paul, J. P. (1975) Instruments for force measurement. In Techniques for the analysis of human movement. (eds) Grieve J.W., Miller D, Mitchelson, Paul J.P. and Smith A.J; Lepus Books, London.

Riding, D., Edwards, J., and Gray J.O. (1991) First annual report of project on improved and power-assisted ambulation aids for paraplegics. University of Salford, Departments of Electronic and Electrical Engineering and Orthopaedic Mechanics, 1-51.

Rose G. K., Stallard, J., and Sankarankutty, M. (1981) Clinical evaluation of spina bifida patients using Hip Guidance Orthosis. Develop. Med. Child Neurol; 23: 30-40.

Watkins, E. M., Edwards, D. E., and Patrick, J. H. (1987) ParaWalker paraplegic walking. Physiotherapy; 73: 99-100.

Yngve, D. A., Douglas, R., and Roberts, J. M. (1984) The reciprocating gait orthosis in Myelomeningocele. J. Pediatric Orthopedics; 4: 304-310.

On the Improvement Provided by Hip Transversal Rotation on Paraplegic Gait Walking with Reciprocating Orthosis

M. Ferrarin, M. Rabuffetti
Bioengineering Centre, Don Gnocchi Pro Juventute Foundation IRCCS, Polytechnic of Milan, Milan, Italy

Abstract - In this paper the importance of hip transversal rotation during human walking is studied with the goal to improve the effectiveness of paraplegic gait assisted by reciprocating orthoses. Starting from the theoretical influences of this rotation on walking pattern, its real effectiveness is analysed on a paraplegic patient walking with a Reciprocating Gait Orthosis (RGO). Quantitative analysis of gait has been performed during walking both with the classical RGO and with a modified version in which hip transversal rotation is allowed by means of a new prototypal hip joint (R^2GO). Results show improvements on pelvis horizontal rotation and on the vertical displacement of the Body Centre of Mass. The possibility further to improve the prototype are also underlined.

1 Introduction

Several mechanical devices have been recently developed to restore locomotion in paraplegic patients with spinal cord lesion at thoracic level. But only few of them have obtained reasonable results in clinical application, particularly on adult patients, where high cost of locomotion and big efforts on upper limbs remain the main problems to solve. The most innovative systems are mechanical orthosis specifically developed to provide a reciprocating gait pattern, like the Reciprocating Gait Orthosis or RGO (Douglas 1983, Solomonow 1989), developed at the Louisiana State University, New Orleans, the ParaWalker or Hip Guidance Orthosis (Rose 1979) developed at the ORLAU of The Robert Jones & Agnes Hunt Orthopaedic Hospital of Oswestry, England and the Advanced Reciprocating Gait Orthosis or ARGO (Lissene 1990), developed in London by Steeper. All of them, during walking, are characterised by locked knee and ankle joints, while the hip joints are free to rotate only in the sagittal plane, where flexion-extension movements are performed in order to put forward alternatively each leg. The resulting gait pattern can be schematised as in fig.1, where a stiff leg model walking without pelvis rotation is reported. In this case the trajectory of the Body Centre of Mass is characterised by a series of intersecting arcs where the radius is equal to the length of the limbs.

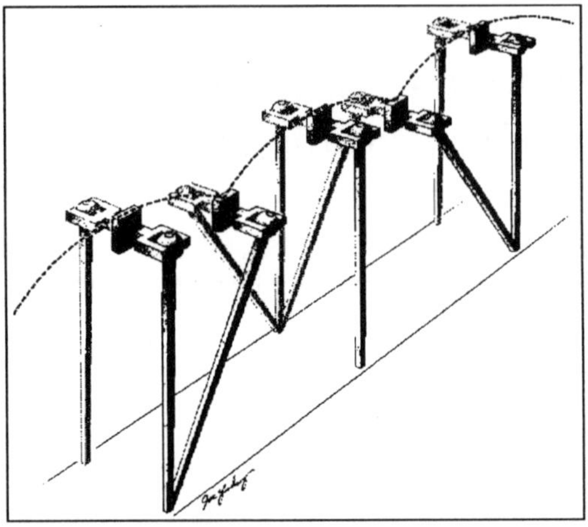

Fig.1. Reciprocating orthosis gait pattern schematisation: bipedal locomotion with stiff legs and without pelvis rotation (from Saunders et al. 1953).

Normal walking, on the other hand, is characterised at each step by an horizontal pelvis rotation around a vertical axis (Saunders et al. 1953), permitted by the anatomical properties of the hip joint that is comparable to a three degrees of freedom spherical joint. In particular, as shown in fig.2, when hip is extending, during the stance phase, it is also internally rotating around the longitudinal axis of the femur, to allow the internal rotation of the pelvis on the horizontal plane. On the contrary, during the swing phase, the hip is flexing and externally rotating to maintain the swinging leg and foot parallel to the progression plane.

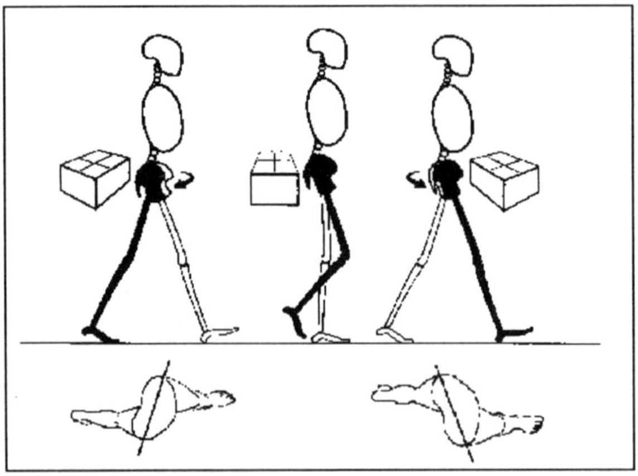

Fig.2. Pelvis rotation during normal walking (modified from Perry 1992).

The advantages of such a pelvic rotation are (Saunders et al. 1953):

1) to reduce the range of hip flexion/extension movements to obtain the same step length;
2) to flatten the arc trajectory of the body Centre of Mass, reducing in this way its vertical displacement.

As a consequence the forces required to change the direction of movement of the Centre of Mass in the succeeding arc of the translation are less when compared to the compass gait and the energetic of walking is therefore optimised.

Purpose of this study was to assess quantitatively the improvements provided by hip transversal rotation in paraplegic gait assisted by reciprocating orthosis.
In order to obtain this goal a kinematic analysis of gait was performed both on a young healthy subject, to have control data on normal walking, and on a paraplegic patient with a complete traumatic Spinal Cord Lesion at T5 level (Ferrarin et al. 1995). He had satisfactorily completed the standard training regime and was a skilled user of a Reciprocating Gait Orthosis since two years. His gait pattern was analysed during walking in two different situations:

- with his own RGO in the classical configuration (without hip transversal rotation)
- and with a new prototype of hip joint fitted in the same orthosis that will be called R^2GO, since it allows both sagittal and transversal rotation of the hip.

2 Materials and Methods

2.1 Hip joint description

In this paragraph the two joint will be described concerning both their technical and kinematic characteristics, in terms of number of allowed degrees-of-freedom (dof). In the classical RGO orthosis (see fig.3) each hip joint is a 1 dof hinge that is free to rotate only in the sagittal plane; it means that the orthosis has two dof in total. As shown in the photograph, a reciprocating mechanism constituted by two steel cables guided inside a conduit is present. The cables are connecting each other joint to induce flexion in one joint when the controlateral is extended and viceversa. In standing posture this double cables system prevents the contemporary flexion of both hips in order to lock the trunk and pelvis and to permit stand with free hands, while during walking it helps the flexion movements of the leg during the swing phase. The presence of this reciprocating mechanism reduces the total number of dof of the system from two to one, because there is a rigid correspondence between right and left hip movements.

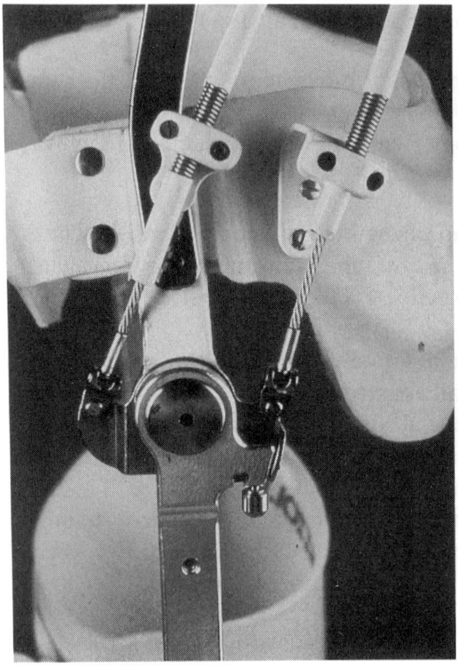

Fig. 3. Hip joint of classical RGO.

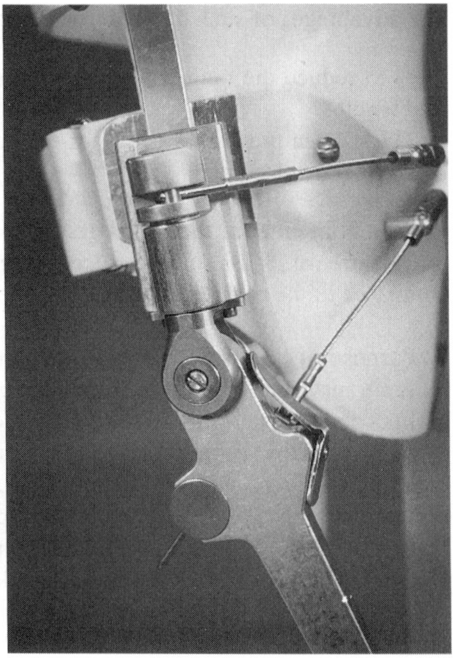

Fig. 4. New hip joint of R^2GO.

In the new joint, developed at the Rizzoli Orthopaedic Workshop of Bologna (Lusvardi et al. 1995) the upper part can rotate around its vertical axis, allowing transversal rotation of the hip, while the lower part can rotate around the horizontal axis thus permitting flexion and extension. These two movements are reciprocally constrained by means of a conic gear-wheel, in which the rotation ratio is 1.5. It means that 10 degrees of transversal rotation correspond to 15 degrees of sagittal rotation; this ratio was chosen as a first compromise between mechanical strength and device dimension. As in normal walking flexion is correlated with external rotation and extension with internal rotation. The two cable reciprocator mechanism is still used to maintain a complete control of hip and pelvis movements.

The number of dof of the orthosis is 4 in principle (2 for each joint) but it is reduced firstly to 2 because of the conic gear and secondly to one because of the reciprocating mechanism: therefore also the R^2GO has only one dof in total. To unlock the mechanism for sitting the subject can push downwards a small lever. As with the classical RGO orthosis static equilibrium is guaranteed with free hands and walking is performed with the support of crutches or walking frame. The gait pattern is different from the pattern associated to the classical RGO only as regard the pelvis horizontal rotation performed at each step.

2.2 Data acquisition

To collect kinematic data an ELITE system (BTS, Milano) was used. It is able to compute the position of small passive markers glued on the patient, by means of a shape recognition performed in real time on TV images acquired with a sampling frequency of 50 Hz (Ferrigno et al. 1985).

Marker displacement on the patient and orthotic structure was the same as in a previous work (Ferrarin et al. 1993): they were attached respectively to the posterior part of the head, shoulders, elbows, wrists, anterior and posterior part of the walking frame, upper part of the body brace, sacral band, ankles and anterior part of the feet. A couple of TV cameras was used for each side to allow a three dimensional analysis of the total body, with an accuracy of less than 1 mm.

In fig.5 the patient during an experimental session is shown together with the stick model derived from marker position. Starting from 3D co-ordinate of each marker a reference system was defined for the pelvis and each leg, then hip joint centres was computed during walking on the basis of a calibration procedure with technical markers. Finally pelvis horizontal orientation respect the laboratory reference system and both sagittal and transversal rotation of hip joint were computed by using Eulerian angles definition (Grood et al. 1983).

One calibration acquisition and ten walking trials were performed at the preferred speed in each experimental session, in order to assess data consistency. For each computed angle, time normalisation on a stride (from one heel strike to the next one) and average values were computed together with the range of standard deviation.

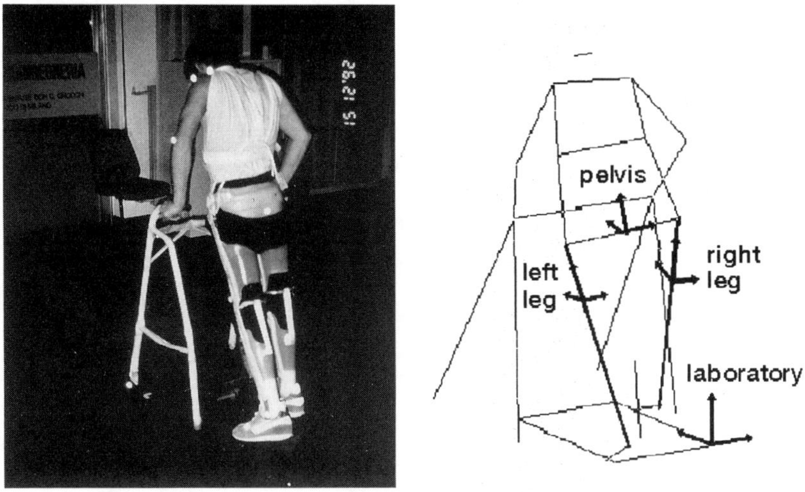

Fig.5. Patient during data acquisition in the gait laboratory (Left).
Stick diagram with co-ordinate reference system of pelvis and legs (Right).

3 Results

Speed of normal subject was around 1.4 m/s while the patient was walking at 0.3 m/s with both orthoses. No large differences on general gait parameters were found comparing RGO and R^2GO, on the contrary we found specific differences in horizontal angle pattern, as it could be expected. In this paragraph the time course of hip angles (both in the sagittal and in the transversal plane) and the pelvis horizontal rotation are presented. Having in mind the particular gear adopted in the R^2GO orthosis, the angle-angle diagram of hip sagittal and transversal rotation are reported too, in order to underline the correlation between the two components of hip movement. In the temporal diagrams time is expressed as percentage of gait cycle from one heel strike to the next one and a stick identifies toe off. All these results will be presented for normal walking, RGO and R^2GO assisted walking.

3.1 Normal subject

Fig.6 shows the results for the healthy subject: time course of hip joint angles on the sagittal (A) and transversal (B) plane, horizontal pelvis rotation (C) and hip angle-angle diagram (D) are reported.

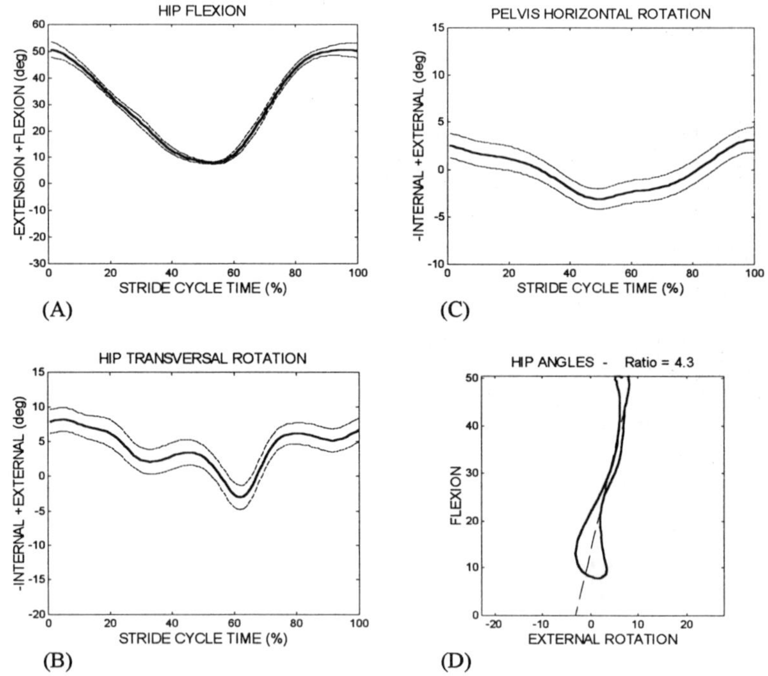

Fig.6. Healthy subject pattern: (A) hip sagittal angle, (B) hip transversal angle, (C) pelvis horizontal rotation, (D) hip angle-angle diagram.

As described in the Introduction, during normal walking hip extension, occurring during the stance phase, is associated with internal rotation, in order to allow the horizontal rotation of the pelvis. During the swing phase, when hip is flexing, the rotation is externally oriented, to maintain the swinging leg and foot parallel to the progression plane. In the second half of the cycle, the pelvis rotates in the other direction, pivoting on the other supporting limb.

Concerning the hip angle-angle diagram, a good correlation between the two rotational components are evident: in this case the angular coefficient of the best regression line provides a sort of ratio between these components. For this subject the ratio is 4.3 meaning that, in average, every 4.3 degrees of flexion/extension correspond 1 degree of external/internal hip rotation.

3.2 RGO walking

In fig.7 the results concerning the paraplegic patient walking with the classical RGO orthosis are shown. While the total flexion/extension range is quite the same as in normal (around 40 degrees), the pattern is very different, characterised by period with constant angle, corresponding to the double support phases during which the cables prevent any hip movement and the patient moves ahead the

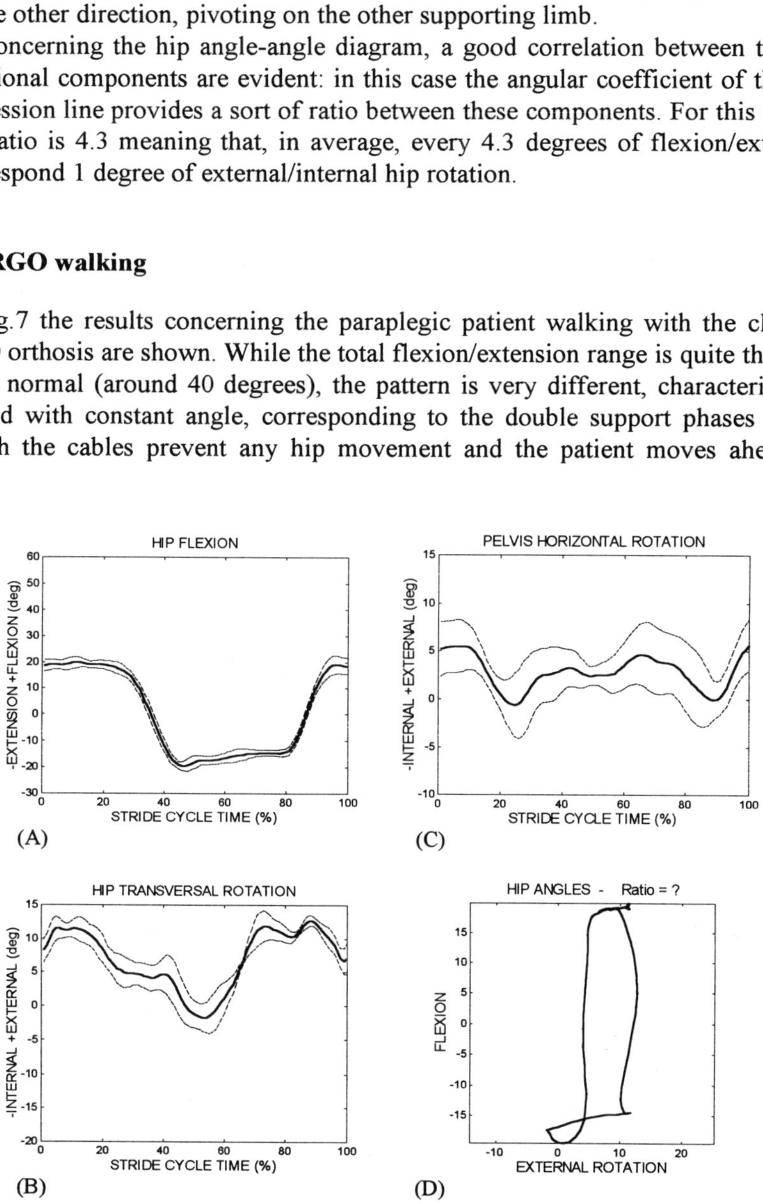

Fig.7. Angular pattern of paraplegic gait assisted by RGO orthosis.

walking frame. These phases are interrupted by extension phase during stance and flexion during swing. Transversal rotation of the hip (B), that is not allowed by the joint, is achieved against the resistance of the orthosis structure.

For this reason the pelvis orientation doesn't follow a good pattern, and during leg swing even goes in counter phase, probably because of the elastic deformations of the caliper section of the orthosis on the supporting limb under patient load.

As a result the hip angle-angle diagram is a loop without any correlation between sagittal and transversal rotation.

3.3 R^{2}GO walking

Finally in fig.8 the results obtained with the patient walking with R^{2}GO are reported. The hip sagittal angle is very similar to the classical RGO, both in range and in shape.

On the contrary the transversal rotation shows a clear cyclic pattern, well correlated with the sagittal movements. The results is an efficient pattern of pelvis horizontal rotation, with an internal rotation on the supporting limb present at each step, even larger than in the normal pattern.

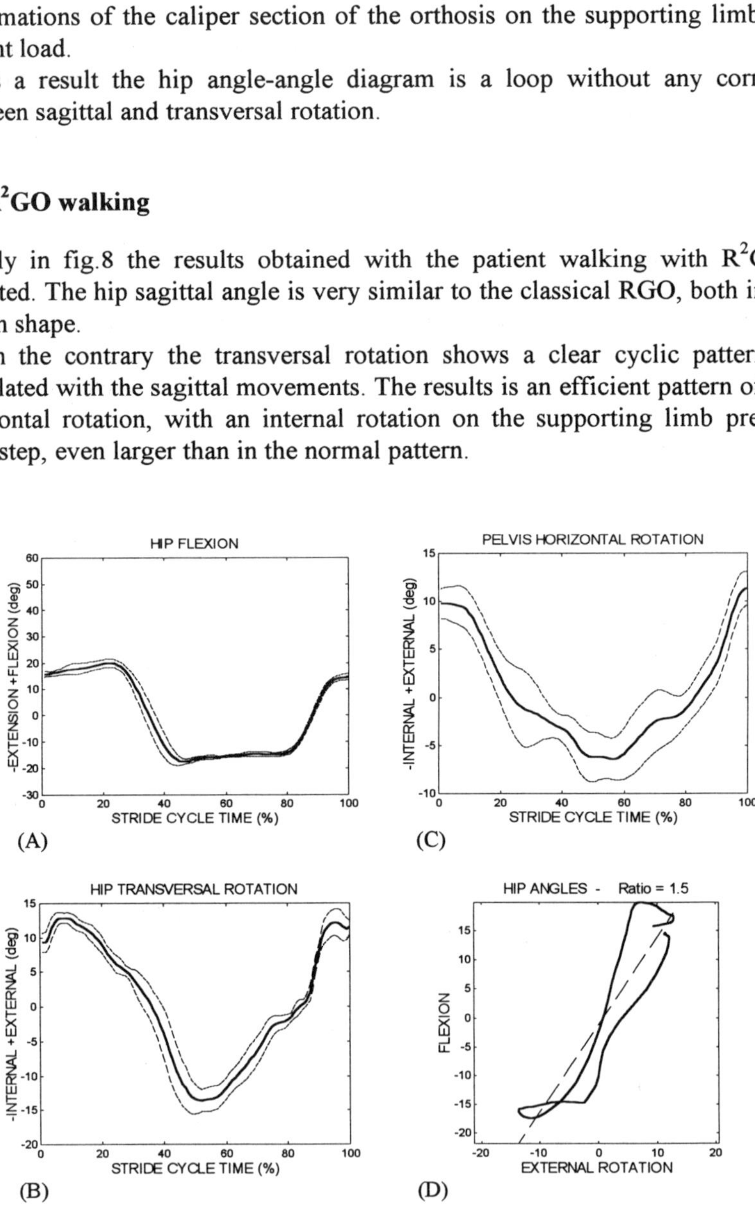

Fig.8. Angular pattern of paraplegic gait assisted by R^{2}GO orthosis.

As a consequence, the hip angle-angle diagram shows a clear linear correlation between the two angular components. The angular coefficient of the best regression line is 1.5, equal to the rotation ratio of the gear, as it was expected.

4 Discussion and Conclusion

In table 1 the comparison of the main found parameters are reported for both orthoses, together with normal values as control. The following conclusions can be observed:

- passing from the classical RGO to the R^2GO orthosis the hip sagittal range of movement is lightly reduced while the transversal one is quite doubled;
- in the R^2GO orthosis the pelvis horizontal rotation range is very increased respect the classical orthosis;
- the ratio between hip sagittal and transversal rotation, not present in the RGO, is 1.5 in the R^2GO orthosis, and it should be increased close to a more physiological value, in order to avoid exaggerated pelvis rotation and dangerous stress to patient hip joint.

Table 1. RGO - R^2GO - Normal gait: result comparison

	Hip sagittal range	**Hip transversal range**	**Pelvis horizontal range**	**Hip rotation ratio**	**CoM vertical displacement [mm]**
RGO	42°	12°	5°	absent	39
R^2GO	37°	25°	18°	1.5	31
Normal	40°	10°	6°	4.3	20

In the last column the vertical range of movement of the body Center of Mass is reported. As it was expected, it is reduced from 39 mm to 31 mm, closer to the physiological one typical of normal walking. This last point should provide an increase in the total efficiency of the gait from an energetic point of view, that it could be verify with direct measurements of energy consumption during walking and/or with the assessment of Ground Reaction Force on feet and arm aids through a dinamometric platform.

From the above considerations the importance of a biomechanical evaluation to paraplegic gait assisted by orthotic system as well as, more in general, to gait assisted by external devices (prosthesis, orthosis, Functional Electrical Stimulation, etc) is evident particularly when design definition and optimal adaptation of the system are investigated.

References

Douglas, R., Larson, P.F., D'Ambrosia, R., Mc Call, R.E. (1983) The LSU reciprocating gait orthoses. *Orthopedics*, 6: 834-839.

Ferrarin, M., Rabuffetti, M., Pedotti, A., Lusvardi, M., (1993) Gait analysis in paraplegics walking with RGO orthosis In: *Book of abstract of Biomechanics XIV ISB Congress*, 4-8 july, 1993, Paris, France, pp.402-403.

Ferrarin, M., Rabuffetti M., Lusvardi M., Pedotti A. (1995) A pilot study on the improvement provided by hip horizontal rotation on reciprocating orthosis for paraplegics. In: *Book of abstract of the XV International Congress on Biomechanics*, 2-6 july 1995, Jyvaskyla, Finland, pp.266-267.

Ferrigno, G.C., Pedotti, A. (1985) ELITE: a digital dedicated hardware system for movement analysis via real-time signal processing. *IEEE Transaction on Biomedical Engineering*, 32(11):943-950.

Grood, E.S., Suntay, W.J.(1983) A joint co-ordinate system for the clinical description of three-dimensional motions: application to the knee. *J Biomech Eng*, 105:136-144.

Lissene, M.A., Peeraer, L., Goditiabolis, F., Lysens, R. (1990) Advanced reciprocating gait orthosis in paraplegic patients. In: J.K. Zupko et al. (eds) *Proc. of the 7th World Congress of the International Society for Prosthetics and Orthotics*, Chicago, p.31.

Lusvardi, M., Varroni, P., Ferrari, A. (1995) The R^2GO: a reciprocating orthosis with 2 degrees of freedom hip joint. In: *Proc. of 8th World Congress of the International Society for Prosthetics and Orthotics*, Melbourne, april 2-7.

Perry, J., (1992) Basic functions. In: *Gait Analysis*, Slack, Thorofare, pp.20-47.

Saunders, J.B.deC.M., Inman, V.T., Eberhart, H.D. (1953) The major determinants in normal and pathological gait. *J Bone Joint Surg*, **35A**(3): 543-557.

Solomonow, M., Baratta, R., Hirokawa, S., Rightor, N., Walker, W., Beaudette, P., Shoji, H., D'Ambrosia, R. (1989) The RGO generation II: muscle stimulation powered orthosis as a practical walking system for thoracic paraplegics. *Orthopedics*, **12**(10): 1309-1315.

Mechanical Orthoses and FES for Patients with Complete Thoracic Lesions

J. Stallard
Orthotic Research & Locomotor Assessment Unit,
RJ & AH Hospital, Oswestry, Shropshire, U.K.

1 Introduction

There are currently three approaches to providing walking for patients with complete thoracic lesions. Reciprocal walking with mechanical orthoses was first described by Rose (1979) and a variety of such devices are now routinely available (Butler and Major, 1987; Douglas et al., 1983; Lissons, 1992). More recently a considerable amount of work has been done in attempting to provide reciprocal walking with pure FES systems (Kralj, 1989; Marsolais, 1987). Since neither of these systems has proven to be entirely satisfactory for every patient other experimental work has been carried out on hybrid systems which combine elements of the other two. Most commonly these have incorporated a standard mechanical orthosis such as the ORLAU ParaWalker or the LSU RGO. In such cases the electrical stimulation of the lower limbs has supplemented the mechanical stability and control provided by the orthosis. All of these three approaches have provided insight to the problems which have to be resolved in order to provide effective walking for thoracic lesion patients. A careful study of the experiences of researchers in those three areas suggest that further improvements can be made provided that proper attention is given to the important parameters of swing leg clearance, overall stability and control.

2 Requirements for Walking

Any type of reciprocal walking, whether it be for normal or handicapped persons, requires the following elements:

1. Swing leg to clear the ground.
2. Cleared leg to swing from extension to flexion.
3. Trunk to translate up and over the stance leg.

The key requirement is that of swing leg clearance. For patients with complete thoracic lesions this is particularly difficult to achieve. However, lack of clearance prevents swing phase, making reciprocal walking impossible. In pure mechanical orthotic systems swing leg clearance is achieved through the use of a hip, knee, ankle, foot orthosis. By crossing the hip such an orthosis will limit adduction when the swing leg is cleared from the ground. The lateral rigidity of the orthosis will influence the walking efficiency because the greater the stiffness the easier it will be to get the swing leg to clear the ground.

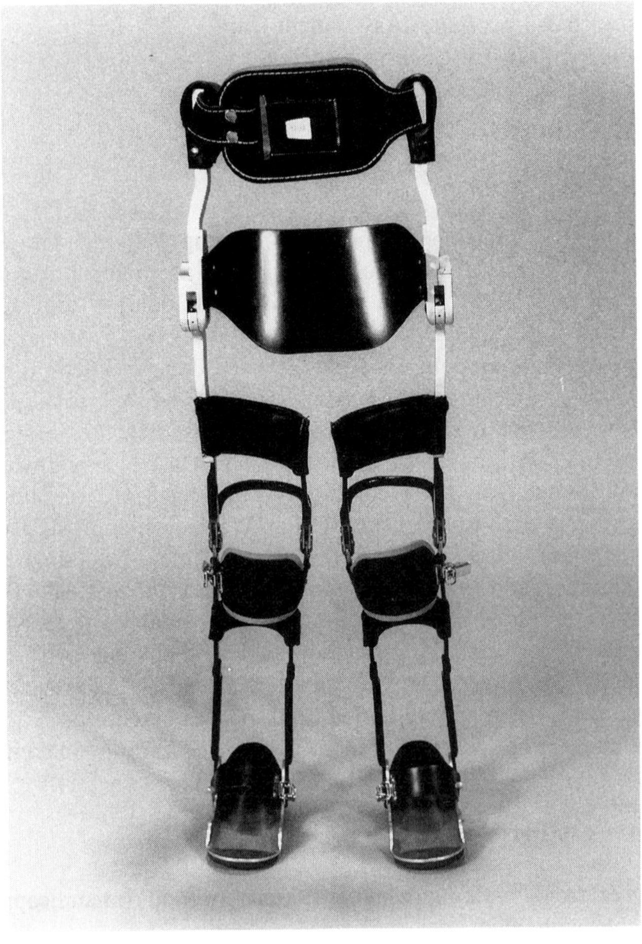

Fig. 1. The ORLAU ParaWalker.

The ORLAU ParaWalker has a structure designed to provide maximum lateral rigidity (Fig. 1). It has the greatest structural rigidity of any of the commonly available reciprocal walking orthoses currently supplied. A number of studies have shown the ParaWalker to have the highest efficiency of walking for mechanical orthoses (Banta, et al., 1991; Bowker et al., 1992; Bernardi et al., 1995). These are summarised in Fig. 2. In each case the energy cost of the ParaWalker is between 70% and 80% of other reciprocating gait orthoses.

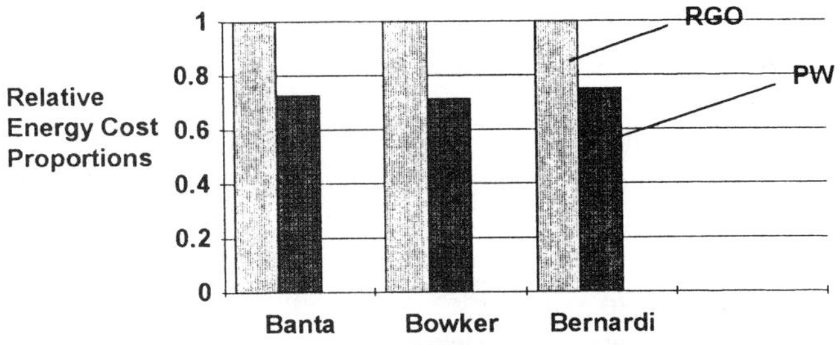

Banta et al (1991). Parawalker: energy cost - . Eur. J. Pediat. Surg. Suppl.1:7-10
Bowker et al (1992).The energetics of paraplegic walking. .Biom. Eng.14:344-350
Bernardi et al (1995).The eff. of walking - using a RGO.Paraplegia, 33: 407-415

Fig. 2. Energy comparisons of walking in RGO and ParaWalker.

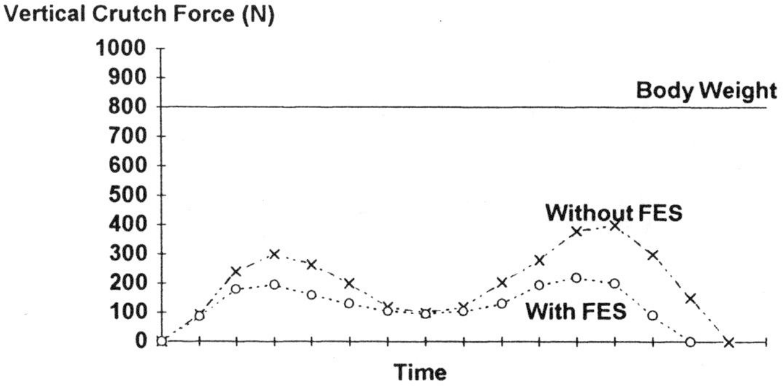

McClelland M R et al (1987). Augmentation of the Oswestry ParaWalker by means of surface electrical stimulation: gait analysis of 3 patients. Paraplegia, 25: 32-38

Fig. 3. Relative crutch impulse with and without FES in a ParaWalker

With pure FES reciprocal walking systems swing leg clearance requires stimulation of the gluteal muscles to ensure that abduction occurs on the stance side so as to permit swing leg clearance. In the main, such systems use walking frames to increase the stability, particularly in the lateral plane, and gluteal stimulation is then sufficient to provide the necessary clearance.

Hybrid systems which combine both mechanical orthoses and FES utilise a combination of gluteal stimulation and mechanical hip bracing. By supplementing mechanical rigidity of the orthosis with gluteal stimulation these systems seek to further improve the efficiency of walking. Several different studies have confirmed that supplementing mechanical orthoses with FES applied to the gluteal muscles canachieve this objective. McClelland et al. (1987) showed that the upper limb effort required to produce effective propulson could be considerably reduced using this technique. They studied vertical ground reaction forces from the crutches during walking and showed that the impulse (force/time integral) required to be generated by the upper limb could be significantly reduced. A typical result is shown in Fig. 3, where an overall reduction of impulse of the order of 35% was achieved. Since many patients complain about fatigue in the upper limbs when walking reciprocally, this is potentially a very advantageous result. Nene and Andrews (1986) reported on 6 patients who had been provided with a standard ParaWalker to which FES of the gluteal muscles had also been added. Fig. 4 shows that in every case except one (patient D), the impulse was reduced with the use of FES. An average reduction in impulse of 19.5% was achieved for those 6 patients.

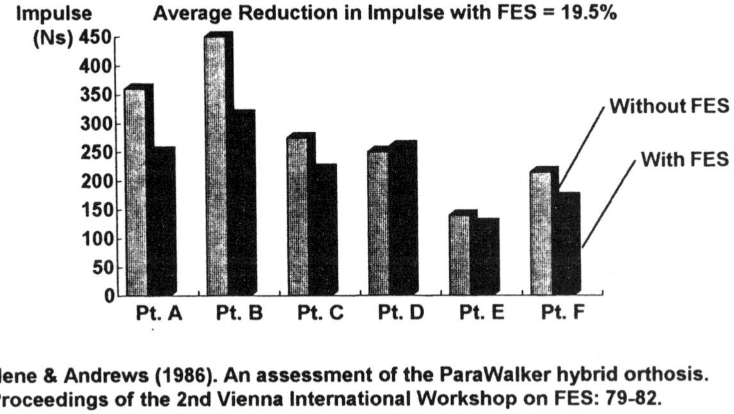

Fig. 4. The influence of gluteal stimulation on upper limb impulse when walking in FES/orthosis hybrid systems

Whilst the reduction in upper limb fatigue, as indicated by a reduction in impulse, is of value, the degree of reduction is not a measure of the overall saving in energy cost. Some of the energy from the upper limbs is transferred to the gluteal muscles by the electrical stimulation. However, the increase in lateral rigidity of the combined system has the potential to bring about overall energy savings. Nene and Patrick (1989) showed that in five patients who had used a hybrid system and a standard ParaWalker, four of them had reductions of between 6% and 9% in energy cost, as measured by oxygen uptake techniques (Fig. 5). The fifth patient recorded no change and, not surprisingly, this was the patient who recorded no significant change in impulse when FES was added.

Similar studies with an RGO device also produced reductions in overall energy cost when FES to the gluteal muscles was used to supplement the standard orthosis. Bernardi et al (1995) reports that average energy cost of walking in the standard RGO is 20 J/kg/metre and that this can be reduced to approximately 18

J/kg/metre with FES and that the average energy cost of the standard ORLAU ParaWalker could be reduced from 16 to 14.5 J/kg/metre with the addition of FES (Fig. 6).

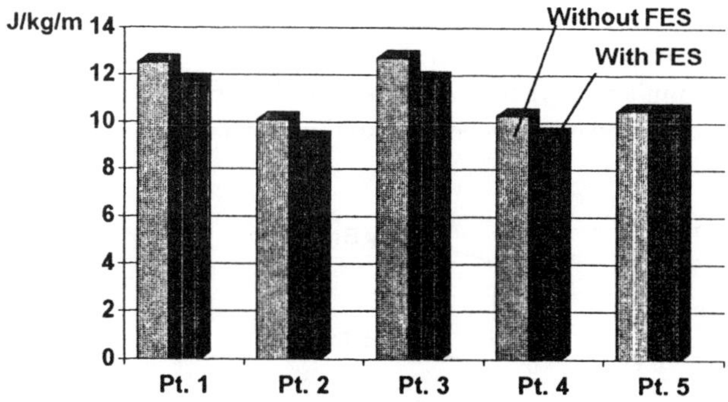

Average Reduction in Energy Cost = 5.88%

Nene & Patrick (1990). Energy cost of locomotion using the Parawalker - electrical stimulation 'hybrid' orthosis. Arch. Phys. Med. & Rehab., 71: 116-120

Fig. 5. Comparisons of relative energy cost of walking with and without FES in the ParaWalker

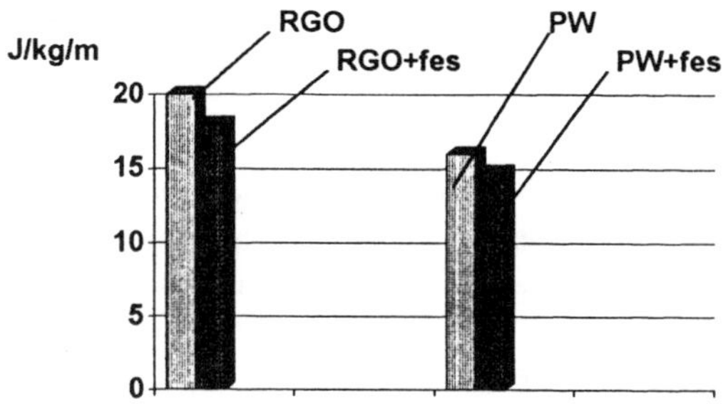

Bernardi,M et al (1995). The effiency of walking of paraplegic patients using a reciprocating gait orthosis. Paraplegia,33:409-415

Fig. 6. Comparison of energy cost changes in RGO and ParaWalker hybrid system.

Despite the reported reductions in energy cost which FES can achieve in hybrid systems, they have not been commonly taken up for routine supply. There are a number of problems which have inhibited their widespread clinical usage:

1. The difficulty of locating the gluteal electrodes accurately.
2. Poor electrode adhesion.
3. The need for careful skin preparation.
4. The inconvenience of signal cables from switches on the crutch or walking frame to the body mounted controller.
5. Cutaneous signal tracking from surface electrodes causing contractions of the abdominal wall muscles.
6. The additional don and doff time required for the FES system.
7. The large additional costs associated with the FES components.

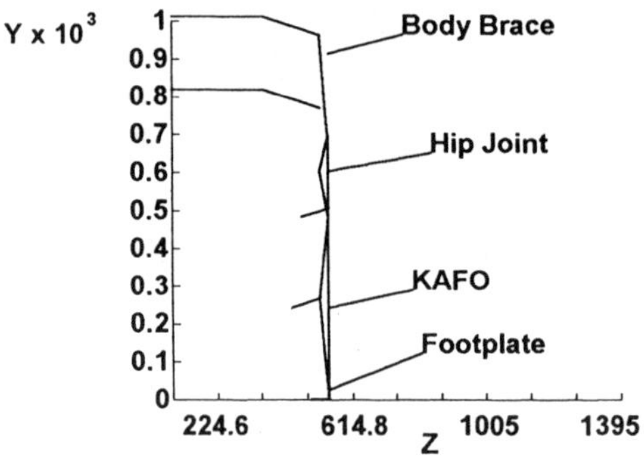

Ferrarin M et al (1993). Estimation of deformation in a walking orthosis for paraplegic patients. Clinical Biomechanics, 8: 255-261.

Fig. 7. The deformation of the ParaWalker during walking by paraplegic patients.

The disappointing clinical uptake of hybrid systems has prompted a re-examination of the principles by which reciprocal walking is provided to paraplegic patients to see whether the improvements can be achieved in other, more simple ways. Ferrarin et al (1993), in a study of three paraplegic patients using three dimensional movement analysis techniques, identified the areas of deformation in pure mechanical devices. Fig. 7 is the direct output from the kinematic analysis and shows that deformations occur both at the hip joint and within the KAFO section of the ParaWalker orthosis. As a result of this study a redesign of the ParaWalker hip joint was undertaken. A four-point bend test in abduction (Fig. 8) showed that stiffness was increased by 70% and that considerable improvements in strength were also achieved. When the new hip joint was mounted within the standard ParaWalker orthosis an overall increase in stiffness of the order of 10% was achieved. As a result the joint was therefore introduced into routine clinical service. A study of the effect of this increased stiffness on relative energy expenditure of walking was undertaken by measuring changes in physiological cost index (PCI). Three adult patients with several years' experience in the original ParaWalker design had their PCI monitored using a standard technique (Nene and Jennings, 1992) immediately prior to routine re-supply. Each was then provided with the new ParaWalker '89 design incorporating an increase in lateral stiffness of 10%. After becoming familiar with their new orthosis relative energy cost measurements were repeated and each patient recorded a significant decrease in PCI (Fig. 9) changing the average result from 1.4 bts/m to 0.98 bts/m. This result is a clear demonstration that more sophisticated mechanical engineering which provides increased lateral rigidity can bring about similar improvements in efficiency to that achieved with FES of the gluteal muscles on orthoses with lower lateral rigidity.

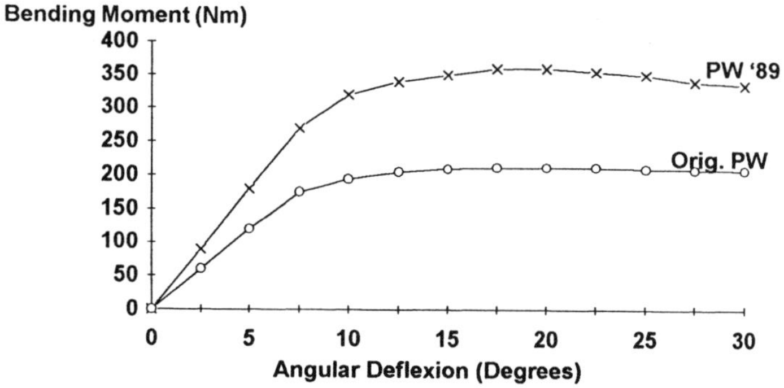

Stallard J, Major R E (1993). The case for lateral stiffness in walking orthoses for paraplegic patients. Journal of Engineering in Medicine, 207: 1-6.

Fig. 8. Mechanical performance of the original and '89 ParaWalker hip joints (4 point bend test in abduction).

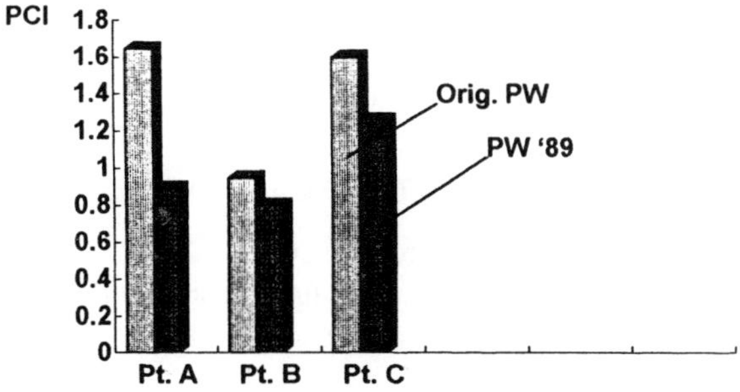

PW '89 is 10% Stiffer than Orig. PW
Average Reduction in PCI for PW '89 = .413

Nene & Patrick (1990). Energy cost of locomotion using the ParaWalker - electrical stimulation "Hybrid" orthosis. Arch. Phys. Med & Rehab., 71: 116-120

Fig. 9. The influence of orthosis stiffness on walking efficiency.

Reported experience with the three types of walking system: conventional mechanical orthoses; pure FES; mechanical orthosis/FES hybrids, suggests that some alternative strategies might now be adopted to make further overall improvements in patient performance. Amongst those worthy of further examination are:

1. Use of stiffer orthoses to effect a swing leg clearance.
2. Use of FES to achieve knee flexion during swing phase.
3. Incorporation of hip joint interlinking to drive reciprocation within a stiffer orthosis.
4. The adoption of implantable technology to reduce the inconvenience of surface electrodes.
5. Acceptance of considerably higher costs (and possibly lower reliability) in order to improve walking effectiveness.

3 Conclusions

Each of the existing approaches to providing walking for paraplegic patients has its own advantages and disadvantages.

Pure FES systems have the following:

Advantages	Maximum convenience Good cosmesis Maximum therapeutic effect.
Disadvantages	High cost Requirement for surgical procedures. Limited fail-safe features Limited walking performance.

FES/mechanical orthosis hybrid systems have the following:

Advantages	Good walking performance Commonly need only crutches for ambulation. Therapeutic effect on muscles.
Disadvantages	Maximum inconvenience Moderate/high cost

Pure mechanical orthosis systems have the following:

Advantages	Good walking performance Ease of supply Fail-safe features Reliability With some systems, use of crutches Proven therapeutic effect relative to bowel function and skin condition
Disadvantages	Poor cosmesis No FES therapeutic effect

In examining the implications of all of the work which is being undertaken in providing walking for paraplegic patients some pointers for the future can be discerned. It is apparent that to achieve continuing progress the following require further examination:

1. Greater synthesis of current approaches.
2. More sophisticated mechanical engineering of orthoses.
3. More miniaturised electronic control systems for implantation (e.g. EC UREKA CALIES Project).
4. Better integration of electronic and mechanical controls.

Following these through will lead to a better understanding of the requirements for pure FES systems and enable real and effective progress to be made.

The benefits of walking for paraplegic patients are now well established (Mazur et al., 1989). It is known that patients can gain therapeutic benefit and maintain acceptable levels of compliance (Moore and Stallard, 1991) provided that treatment systems are effectively delivered. A further improvement in the technology is now required to permit greater numbers of patients to take advantage of the therapeutic and functional benefits of walking. It is still questionable whether this will be achieved mechanically, by FES, or as a hybrid of the two. However, only by taking relevant experience from research conducted on each of these systems can real progress be made in the future.

References

Banta, J. V., Bell, K. J., Muik, E. A., and Fezio, J. (1991) ParaWalker: Energy cost of walking. *Eur. J. Pediatric Surgery,* **1**. Suppl. 1, 7-10.

Bernardi, M., Canale, I., Castellano, V., Di Filippo, L., Felici, F., Marchetti, M. (1995) The efficiency of walking of paraplegic patients using a reciprocating gait orthosis. *Paraplegia,* **33**: 409-415.

Bowker, P., Messenger, N., Ogilvie, C., and Rowley, D. (1992) The Energetics of Paraplegic Walking. *Journal of Biomedical Engineering*, **14(8)**: 344-350.

Butler, P. B. and Major, R. E. (1987) The ParaWalker - a rational approach to the provision of reciprocal ambulation for paraplegic patients. *Physiotherapy*, **73**: 393-397.

Douglas, R., Larson, P., D'Ambrosia, R., and McCall, R. E. (1983) The LSU Reciprocating Gait Orthosis. *Orthopaedics*, **6(7)**: 834-839.

Ferrarin, M., Stallard, J., Palmieri, R., and Pedotti, A. (1993) Estimation of deformation in a walking orthosis for paraplegic patients. *Clin Biomech*; 8: 255-261.

Kralj, A. and Badj, T. (1989) *Functional electrical stimulation: standing and walking after spinal cord injury*. CRC Press, Boca Raton, p. 189.

Lissons, M. A. (1992) Advanced Reciprocating Gait Orthosis in paraplegic patients. *Proceedings of ISPO World Congress*, Chicago, 28 June - 3rd July.

McClelland, M. R., Andrews, B. J., Patrick, J. H., Freeman, P. A., and El Masri, W. S. (1987) Augmentation of the Oswestry ParaWalker by means of surface electrical stimulation: gait analysis of three patients. *Paraplegia* **25**: 32-38.

Marsolais, E. B. and Kobetic, R. (1987) Functional electrical stimulation for walking in paraplegia. *JBJS*, **69:** 728-733.

Mazur, J. M., Shurtleff, D., Menelaus, M., and Colliver, J. (1989) Orthopaedic management of high-level spina bifida. *JBJS*, **71A**: 56-61.

Moore, P. and Stallard, J. (1991) A clinical review of adult paraplegic patients with complete lesions using the ORLAU Parawalker. *Paraplegia,* **29:** 191-96.

Nene, A. and Andrews, B. J. (1986) An assessment of the Parawalker hybrid orthosis. *Proceedings of the 2nd Vienna International Workshop on Functional Electrostimulation*, 79-82.

Nene, A. V. and Jennings, S. J. (1992) Physiological Cost Index of paraplegic locomotion using the ORLAU ParaWalker. *Paraplegia,* **30**: 246-252.

Nene, A. V. and Patrick, J.H. (1989) Energy cost of paraplegic locomotion with the ORLAU ParaWalker. *Paraplegia*, **27**: 125-132.

Rose, G. K. (1979) The principles and practice of hip guidance articulations. *Prosthetics & Orthotics International*, **3**: 37-43.

Stallard, J. and Major, R.E. (1993) The case for lateral stiffness in walking orthoses for paraplegic patients. *Part H: Journal of Engineering in Medicine. Proc Instn Mech Engrs*, **207**: 1-6.

Hybrid FES/Reciprocating Gait Orthosis Design

L. Yang[1], M.H. Granat[1], D.J. Maxwell[1], J.P. Paul[1], D.N. Condie[2], D.I. Rowley[3]
[1]Bioengineering Unit University of Strathclyde, Glasgow, Scotland
[2]Tayside Rehabilitation Engineering Services, Broughty Ferry, Scotland
[3]Department of Orthopaedic Surgery, University of Dundee, Scotland

Abstract - A hybrid orthosis has been developed incorporating a linked hip design which promotes the 2:1 flexion-extension ratio found in normal walking. The FES component of the orthosis acts to aid hip flexion during swing phase. The process by which the optimal brace configuration was determined is described and the results presented. Initial results on speed, stride length, efficiency and crutch loading are presented for paraplegic subjects. The control of FES induced movements was implemented using finite state methods based on EMG data. Artificial intelligence methods are being used to identify an optimal sensor set for the detection of gait states and initiation of state transitions.

1 Introduction

Research and development in the field of electrical stimulation continues to face problems which were present when the concept was first introduced. Obviously until a successful scheme of FES can be guaranteed to a patient receiving it, it is unreasonable for this to involve other than surface stimulation. Consequently, there is difficulty in stimulating only the desired muscles and in producing a muscular response corresponding to the external loading conditions and the physiological parameters relating to muscle contraction such as length/tension relationship and force velocity relationship. Using surface electrodes, high values of stimulation parameters are generally used and the consequent contractions, approaching tetanic states, leads to rapid fatigue. Where reflexes are elicited, habituation is a corresponding problem. These biomechanical features of paraplegic walking are generally understood, but are not universally considered.

Reciprocal gait has been restored in spinal cord injured individuals by both mechanical bracing and functional electrical stimulation (FES). Mechanical bracing is extremely safe and it eliminates the energy demands of maintaining posture however the gait achieved is very slow and has a high energy cost (Bowker et al, 1992). Hybrid FES orthotic systems combine the supportive functions of mechanical bracing with electrical stimulation of the paralysed muscles (Andrews et al, 1989). The hybrid orthosis has low energy demands during stance and uses the preserved muscle mass of the lower limbs to assist in joint flexion resulting in improved ambulatory efficiency.

In this article studies on the two aspects of the development of hybrid FES orthoses are presented: the performance comparison of the different orthotic joint constraints and the corresponding control strategies of muscle stimulation.

2 Analysis

In straight line surface walking of normal humans, there are periodic energy changes between forwards kinetic energy (KE) and potential energy (PE) corresponding to the height of the centre of mass from the ground. Newton's first law indicates that the body remains in its state of rest or of movement in a straight line at uniform velocity unless acted on by an external force. The converse of this is that a person walking at uniform speed requires no propulsive force provided that no aerodynamic effects need to be taken into account. In fact, during walking, the forward velocity (V) frequently is found to vary by approximately +/- 15% corresponding to the successive transitions between double support and single support, first on one leg and then on another, and the fact that the ground to foot force vector is generally not vertical. If a walking speed of 1 m/s is considered:

$$\begin{aligned} \text{change in KE} &= 0.5M(V_{max}^2 - V_{min}^2) \\ &= MV_{mean}\,\text{velocity change} \\ &= M \times 0.3\,kgm^2s^{-2} \end{aligned}$$

where M is the total mass of the body.

The change in potential energy PE during the walking cycle corresponds approximately to a change in the height of the centre of mass of 5cm, thus the change in PE is:

$$\text{change in PE} = Mg\;0.05 = \text{approximately } 0.5M\,kgm^2s^{-2}$$

Thus at 1m/s walking speed, the kinetic and potential energies do not exactly balance. However, if the walking speed is increased to 1.3m/s the balance is exact, and this may well correspond to the self-selected walking speed. Equally, however, if the walking speed is diminished, the imbalance between the two types of energy becomes great. This corresponds to the problem of locomotion of the spinal cord injured (SCI) patient, where the normal flexion and extension of the joints of the leg cannot be used to produce the required changes in height of the centre of mass necessary to allow swinging of the unsupported leg in the swing phase without ground contact. Thus, these patients require to use arm and shoulder muscles to implement the cycle of changes in vertical position of the centre of mass and this results in a correspondingly enhanced rate of fatigue.

Other mechanical problems of the SCI patient include difficulty in initiating the swing phase of locomotion and difficulty in controlling the flexion in the swinging limb leading to instability. Some of the difficulties of paraplegic locomotion may be avoided by the use of a reciprocal gait orthosis (Douglas et al, 1983). The problem with this orthosis, however, relates to the features of normal walking in which the angle of flexion of the thigh in the swing phase leg is within the range 12° extension to 30° flexion, and the reciprocating gait orthosis constrains the angles of flexion and extension to match those of the contralateral leg resulting in a reduced range of flexion/extension and a shorter overall stride length and consequent lower walking speed (Whittle and Cochrane, 1989; Yang et al, 1994). Figure 1(a) illustrates this phenomenon. Yang and coworkers correspondingly devised a mechanism giving a ratio of extension and flexion which could be set at a desired amount and values of 1.5 and 2.0 were chosen. Using these ratios, Figure 1(b) has been constructed to show the diagram corresponding to Figure 1(a) using two different values of this flexion/extension ratio. This is a theoretical graph since the orthosis is attached to soft tissue of the patient and the bony skeleton therefore does not perform the angulation indicated by the theoretical analysis. When comparing the results of this device with those of Jefferson and Whittle (1990) it should be noted that their data correspond to angles measured on the orthosis and the angles in the skeleton of the patient will therefore be different.

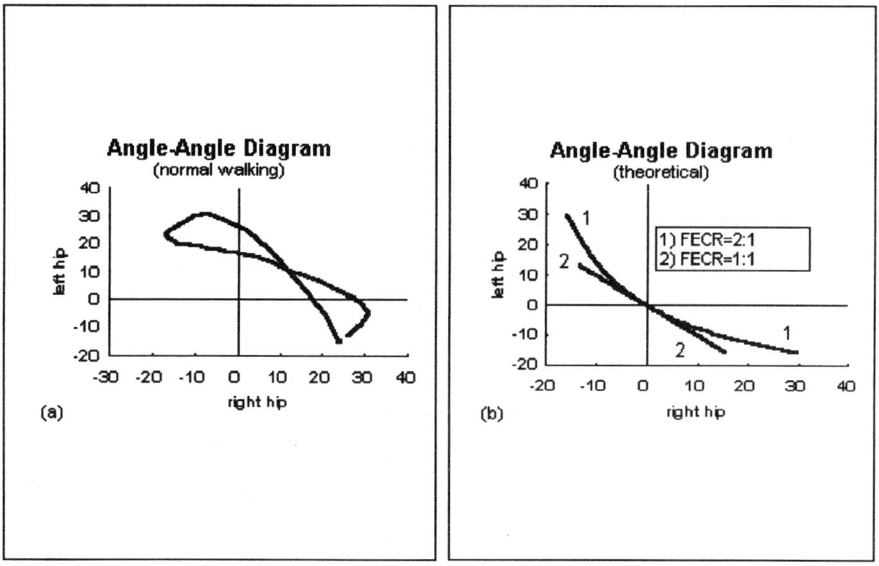

Fig. 1. (a)Relationship between flexion and extension angles of left and right thighs in normal walking. (b)Theoretical relationship between flexion and extension angles of left and right legs in a reciprocating gait orthosis with variable angle relationship. (Adapted from Yang et al, 1994).

3 Investigation

A project was conceived to implement a system using the modified reciprocal gait orthosis in association with functional electrical stimulation applied to selected muscle groups, in an endeavour to reduce the energy cost to the patient in locomotion by making it possible to achieve more rapid walking speeds. The literature contains data on the phasic activity of the muscles of the leg of normal humans in locomotion (Eberhart et al, 1953). However, the proposal envisaged a reciprocating gait orthosis with the possibility of a partially or completely fixing joints at a particular level or leaving them free and no publications were found which could give definitive information on the phasic activity of leg muscles using orthoses of this description. Three young active male volunteers were recruited and fitted with a reciprocating gait orthosis which incorporated the variable ratio mechanism joining the thigh portions at the hip. The knee joints which were provided could be fixed in extension or were free. At the ankle the joints could be fixed at 90° against dorsiflexion, fixed at 90° in dorsiflexion, but free in plantar flexion or completely free.

Gait analysis tools (Vicon, Kistler forceplates, EMG and heart rate measurement systems) were used to collect data from these normal test subjects as they walked in the orthosis at their self-selected speed with combinations of configurations at the knee and ankle as shown in Table 1. From the collected data the Physiological Cost Index (PCI) (MacGregor 1979), walking speed, joint angles, joint moments and ensembled linear EMG envelopes were calculated.

Table 1. Orthosis combinations tested (PF = Plantar Flexion) adapted from Yang et al (1995)

Hip Coupling Ratio	Knee Setting	Ankle Setting	Designation
1:1	Locked	Locked	1HLKLA
1:1	Free	Locked	1HFKLA
1:1	Locked	PF Free	1HLKPA
1:1	Free	PF Free	1HFKPA
2:1	Locked	Locked	2HLKLA
2:1	Free	Locked	2HFKLA
2:1	Locked	PF Free	2HLKPA
2:1	Free	PF Free	2HFKPA
Free	Locked	Locked	FHLKLA
Free	Free	Locked	FHFKLA
Free	Locked	PF Free	FHLKPA
Free	Free	PF Free	FHFKPA

Prior to the tests each subject underwent a training programme for four-point gait using elbow crutches. During the actual tests sufficient time was allocated for the subject to become accustomed to the new joint constraints before any data was collected.

Studies of the performance of four paraplegic subjects walking in the assessment orthosis have also been undertaken. For one paraplegic subject two series of tests have been conducted to compare (1) 2:1 and 1:1 hip ratios using fixed knee and ankle and without FES; (2) with and without FES assisted hip flexion using 2:1 hip ratio and fixed knee and ankle.

Using the hybrid orthosis configuration, hip flexion can be augmented by two means. Stimulation of rectus femoris will contribute both a hip flexing and a knee extending moment. The knee extending moment is not a hindrance as the configuration of the orthosis does not allow knee flexion during swing. Hip flexion can also be achieved using the flexion withdrawal reflex recruited via afferent stimulation of the peroneal nerve. The fact that the knee extensors are not required for stance phase support, due to the mechanical bracing of the orthosis, allows two independent strategies of FES induced hip flexion to be employed.

The endurance of these two independent strategies of hip flexion are determined by separate physiological mechanisms. In the case of efferent stimulation of rectus femoris muscle fatigue due to non-physiological recruitment occurs rapidly. The flexion reflex tends to habituate; its magnitude declining with time and the number of stimuli applied.

In the paraplegic subject for whom preliminary results are presented peroneal nerve stimulation only was applied. For these laboratory tests the subject was connected by an umbilical cable to an IBM personal computer which was programmed with the control algorithms. A finite state controller was implemented in the software with state transitions controlled by the subject via hand-switches mounted on the crutch handles. The subject initiated swing phase of the leg by depressing the switch mounted on the contralateral crutch. Release of the switch stopped stimulation and initiated the stance condition.

4 Results

4.1 Normal Subjects

Although a limited amount of free play was found in the system the performance of the hip coupling mechanism met the design specification. During normal subject trials the subjects walked against the joint motion constraints and applied loads on the coupling system resulting in the deviation of hip angle-angle diagram from its theoretical trajectory (Figure 2). For the coupled hip configuration (1:1 or 2:1) the hip flexion-extension ratio tended to converge to 1:5.

To eliminate the effects of inter-subject variability, the PCI and speed data were normalised as percentages of the overall mean PCI and speed of each subject. The normalized data were then pooled according to the brace configurations and subjected to one-way Analysis of Variance (ANOVA).

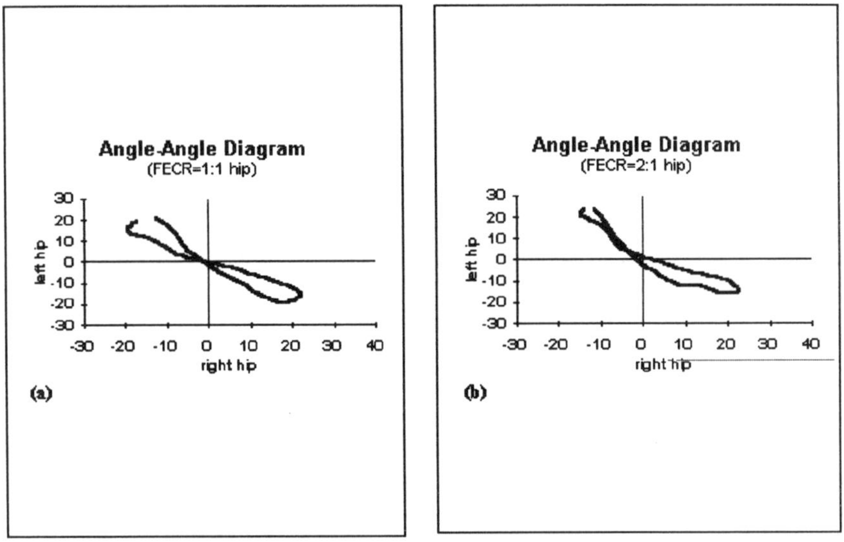

Fig. 2. Angle-angle diagrams for normal subjects walking in a RGO with a fixed hip angle ratio: a) with 1:1 ratio (b) with 2:1 ratio. (Yang et al, 1994)

Table 2. Results from normal subjects (Mean & SE)

Orthosis Configuration	PCI (%)	speed (%)	stride length (m)
free hip	92(±16)	106(±11)	1.031(±0.155)
1:1 hip	115(±34)	95(±15)	1.101(±0.072)
2:1 hip	92(±24)	100(±11)	1.170(±0.075)
LKLA	123(±28)	88(±12)	1.036(±0.142)
FKLA	99(±24)	99(±10)	1.093(±0.099)
LKPA	89(±22)	102(±7)	1.118(±0.126)
FKPA	85(±16)	112(±9)	1.157(±0.080)

Note: Normalised PCI and speed are defined as percentage of the overall means.

For the normal subjects tested the 2:1 hip ratio was associated with a significantly lower PCI ($p<0.01$), higher speed and longer stride length than the 1:1 hip ratio (Table 2). Theoretically the increased step length as a result of the 2:1 configuration would result in more energy being required to move the centre of gravity upwards and forwards over the stance. This was not substantiated by the experimental results.

The LKLA configuration was related to the highest PCI in all knee and ankle configurations. Thus free knee or/and plantarflexion free ankle are desirable in reducing energy cost. During swing phase, knee flexion shortens the leg and ensures the ground clearance of the foot. Alternative ways of ground clearance are either the circumduction of the leg which is awkward or vaulting which results in large excursions of the centre of gravity and a less energy efficient gait. Ankle plantar flexion occurs in early stance phase to achieve a controlled foot flat and in late stance phase which corresponds to a considerable mechanical power generation at the ankle joint. Many existing systems for paraplegic walking use FES to control the free knee joints. Bajd (1993) tested FES assisted ankle plantarflexing at terminal stance phase in paraplegic walking and found that for incomplete paraplegics FES ankle plantar flexion brought about a significant improvement in push-off and roll-off of the stance leg.

Figure 3 shows the integrated EMG patterns for eight muscles in the normal test subjects obtained using surface electrodes. These diagrams represent a pooling of all of the data relating to the different orthosis configurations. It was not found possible to identify specific patterns of muscular activity which differed materially from one orthosis configuration to another. These patterns of muscular activity were used as a guide to programming the multi-channel stimulator so that paraplegic patients could be enabled to use the new reciprocating gait orthosis to explore the optimum configurations in respect of constrained or non-constrained joints.

4.2 Paraplegic Subjects

The hip coupling mechanism worked well with the ratios being 1.9 and 1.05 for theoretical ratios of 2:1 and 1:1 respectively.

The average heart rates and PCIs with a 2:1 hip were consistently lower than those with a 1:1 hip although the hip configurations had different effects on the average walking speed on different days.

The stimulation of the peroneal nerve significantly ($p<0.05$) reduced upper limb effort to 17% from 28% of body weight as indicated by the axial crutch force impulses. The stimulation also tended to reduce physiological cost.

Using the kinetic and kinematic data obtained with the normal subjects and expert paraplegic users, artificial sensor sets for the control of reciprocal gate have been simulated (goniometers, foot switches, accelerometers, crutch load sensors, floor contact switches and upper-body postural indicators). A software programme (MIMIC) generates the virtual sensor outputs from the raw data. This allow critical evaluation of sensor sets before hardware implementation or even development.

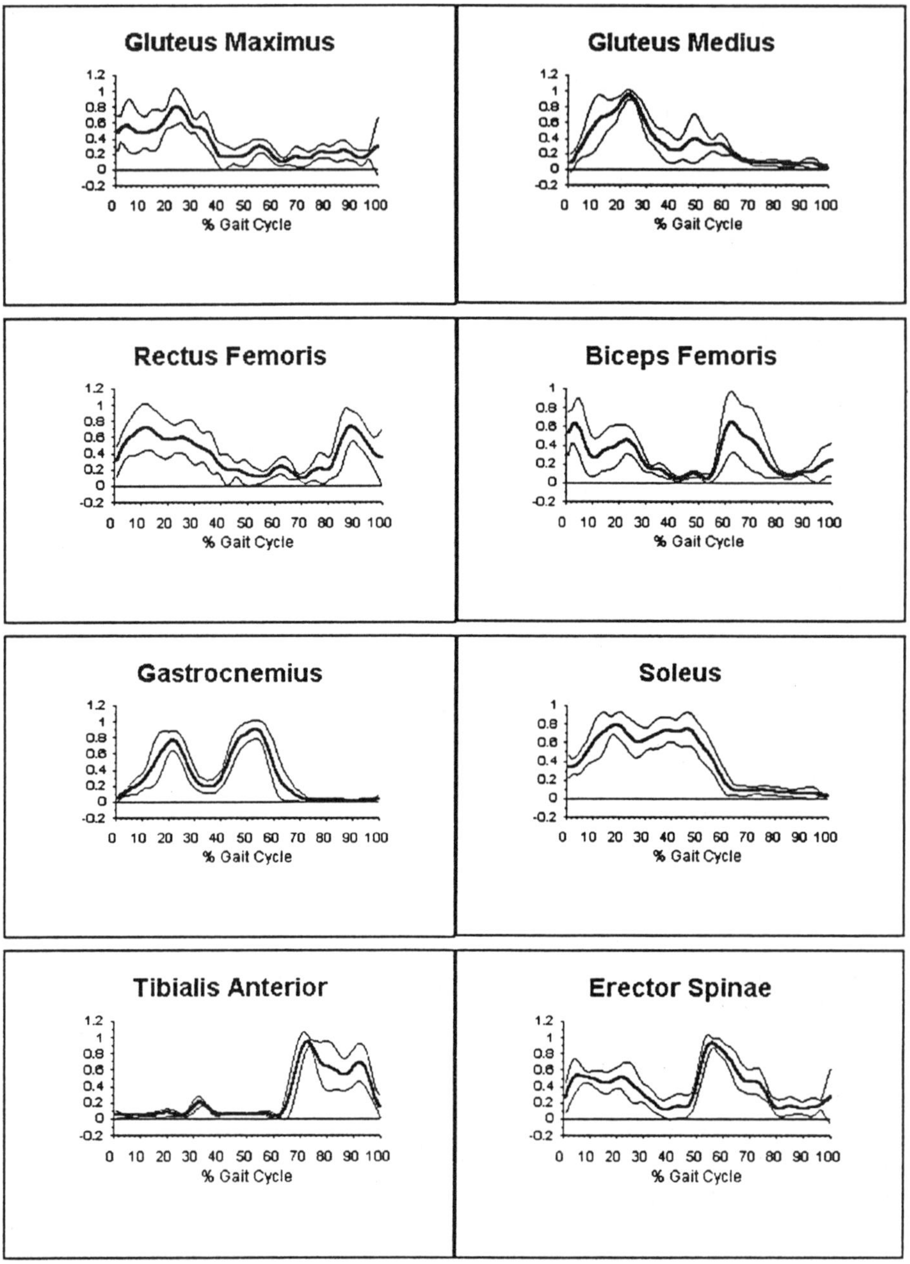

Fig.3. Integrated EMG variation in arbitrary units during a gait cycle commencing at heel strike, averaged over 5 cycles for each of the orthosis configurations in Table 1. Solid line is mean, light lines indicate ± 1SD. (From Yang et al, 1996 with the permission of Journal of Biomechanics).

The activation of muscles during gait is taken from the EMG recordings and hence the transition between different gait states can be defined by EMG signal thresholds. These thresholds are used to define gait state transitions in the training and testing data sets.

The finite state predictions and FES control rules (decision trees) are produced by an artificial intelligence algorithm. This program is a development of *EMPIRIC* (Heller et al, 1993), a symbolic inductive learning program. *EMPIRIC* can employ 'fuzzy' weighting techniques to cope with uncertainty in the training data.

In this way a sensor set and associated decision tree can be identified which is optimal for state transition detection and also robust (indicated by a low rate of false detection). This allows sensors to be evaluated without requiring a large number of laboratory subject tests. However the final selection of sensor set will be the result of laboratory comparisons of implementations of the most successful virtual sensor sets.

Table 3. Results from the paraplegic subjects (Mean & SE)

		Session 1		Session 2	
	FECR	1:1	2:1	1:1	2:1
	FES	none	none	none	none
Test Series 1	PCI(beat/m)	2.7(0.2)	2.2(0.1)	1.8(0.1)	1.6(0.1)
	Speed (m/s)	0.29(0.01)	0.32(0.01)	0.42(0.01)	0.40(0.01)
	Stride Length (m)	1.04(0.02)	1.08(0.02)	1.14(0.02)	1.12(0.02)
	Actual FECR	1.05(0.03)	2.10(0.07)	n/a	n/a
	Crutch impulse (Ns)	n/a	n/a	361(12)	364(9)
	FECR	2:1	2:1	2:1	2:1
	FES	No	HFS	No	HFS
Test Series 2	PCI(beat/m)	4.2(0.2)	2.8(0.2)	3.7(0.2)	3.3(0.1)
	Speed (m/s)	0.31(0.01)	0.34(0.02)	0.31(0.02)	0.36(0.02)
	Stride Length (m)	0.98(0.04)	0.96(0.02)	0.94(0.06)	1.12(0.02)
	Actual FECR	n/a	n/a	1.84(0.09)	2.12(0.07)
	Crutch impulse (Ns)	420(7)	327(6)	431(9)	367(9)

Note: The pairs of data underlined are significantly different at $p<0.05$.

5 Conclusions

The novel hip joint coupling mechanism allowing a more normal flexion-extension ratio proved successful. The addition of FES assisted hip flexion to the orthosis proved the most effective combination.

6 Acknowledgments

This project was supported by "Action Research". The assistance of Dr B J Andrews, Dr R H Baxendale, Mr J Linskell and Mr R Baker is gratefully acknowledged.

References

Andrews, B. J., Barnett, R. W., Phillips, G. F., Kirkwood, C. A., Donaldson, N., Rushton, D. N., and Perkins, T. A. (1989) Rule-based control of a hybrid FES orthosis for assisting locomotion. *Automedica,* 11:175-199.

Bowker P., Messenger N., Ogilvie C., and Rowley, D. I. (1992) Energetics of paraplegic walking. *J. Biomed. Eng.,* 14:344-350.

Bajd, T., Kralj, A., Karcnik, T., Savrin, R., and Obreza, P, (1993) Importance of FES assisted terminal stance phase. *Proc. Ljubljana FES Conf., Slovenian Society of Medical and Biological Engineering, Ljubljana,* 57-60.

Douglas, R., Larson, P.F., D'Ambrosia R, and McCall, R.E. (1983) The LSU reciprocating gait orthosis. *Orthopaedics,* **6:** 834-838.

Eberhart, H.D., (ed) (1953) The pattern of muscular activity in the lower extremity during walking. *Prosthetic Devices Research Report, Series II,* ***Issue 25.*** University of California, Berkeley, USA.

Heller, B. W., Veltink, P. H., Rijkhoff, N. J. M., Rutten, W. L. C., and Andrews, B. J. (1993) Reconstructing muscle activation during normal walking: a comparison of symbolic and connectionist machine learing techniques. *Biol. Cybern.* **69**, 327-335.

Jefferson, R. L. and Whittle, M. W. (1990) Performance of three walking orthoses for the paralysed: a case study using gait analysis. *Prosthet. Orthot. Int.* **14**, 103-110.

MacGregor, J. (1979) The objective measurement of physical performance with long-term ambulatory surveillance equipment. *Proc. 3rd Int. Symposium on Ambulatory monitoring (Academic Press, London),* 29-39.

Nene, A. V. and Patrick, J. H. (1990) Energy cost of paraplegic locomotion using the ParaWalker - electrical stimulation "hybrid" orthosis. *Arch. Phys. Med. Rehabil.,* 71:116-120.

Rose, G. K. (1979) The principles and practice of hip guidance articulations. *Prosth. Orthot. Int.,* 3:37-43.

Whittle, M. W. and Cochrane, G. M. (1989) A comparative elavuation of the Hip Guidance Orthosis (HGO) and the Reciprocating Gait Orthosis (RGO). *Health Equipment Information* **192**, NHS Procurement Directorate, London.

Yang, L., Granat, M.H., Paul, J.P., Condie, D., and Rowley, D.I. (1994) Effects of joint motion constraints on the gait of healthy subjects. *Proc. Conf. 12th Triennial Conf. Int'l Ergonomics Assoc'n, Vol. 3: Rehabil. Ergonomics,* 43-45, Toronto, Canada,

Yang, L., Granat, M.H., Paul, J.P., Condie, D., and Rowley, D.I. (1996) Effects of joint motion constraints on the gait of normal subjects and their implications on the further development of hybrid FES orthosis for paraplegic persons. *J. Biomech.* (in press).

Hybrid System for Upright Mobility with Unlockable Orthotic Knee for Knee Bending during Swing Phase

J. Edwards, A. O. P. Bataweel
University of Salford, Salford, UK
and Spinal Injuries Centre, District General Hospital, Southport, UK

Abstract - An orthotic knee joint was developed which unlocked and allowed the knee to flex when the weight of the body was removed from the leg at the beginning of the swing phase of walking with a reciprocating gait orthosis (RGO). Knee flexion during the ensuing swing phase was achieved by functional electrical stimulation of the flexion withdrawal response, followed by quadricepts muscle stimulation to extend the leg prior to heel strike. A single case study trial of the system was carried out by a man with a complete T6 level paraplegia who has used an RGO for over seven years. Compared with conventional RGO walking, when he used the Unlockable/Lockable (LUK) joint to walk between parallel bars his energy expenditure was reduced by 56%. When the patient walked with a rollator after a further twelve sessions of training with the LUK system, the comparative reduction in his energy expenditure was 36%. However, the forces exerted by his arms on the rollator were reduced by 50%.

1 Introduction

Rehabilitation centres thoughout the world have accumulated considerable experience in the provision of reciprocating orthoses for upright mobility and exercise of spinal cord injured patients (Douglas *et al.,* 1983; Whittle and Cochrane, 1988).

A recent survey on the long term usage of patterns of reciprocating gait orthoses (RGO) among these patients has yielded some disappointing results (Sykes *et al.,* 1995). It was found that 57% gave up using the othosis after an average period of between 24 to 27 months. Furthermore, usage was mainly limited to the home and the distance walked by adult subjects rarely exceeded 50 metres. Such distances are clearly not sufficient to be considered functional.

When asked what limited them from making greater use of the orthosis, both adult and child patients complained that too much physical effort was required. Therefore it was clear that reducing the energy consumption involved in using these devices is a major requirement. The results of gait studies on sujects with paraplegia walking with an RGO in our laboratory suggested that lack of knee bending during the swing phase of walking was a key factor in causing this high level of fatigue. The purpose of the present study was to investigate the effect on energy expenditure of allowing the RGO orthotic knee to bend during the swing phase.

2 Methods of Reducing Energy Consumption

Several authors have reported that use of a hybrid system in which functional electrical stimulation (FES), by skin surface electrodes, in combination with an RGO can reduce the energy expenditure of walking by 30% to 40%. In our clinical work we have adopted a hybrid system developed by Louisiana State University Medical Centre, USA (Solomonow *et al.*, 1989). This system involved stimulation of the quadriceps muscle to assist the forward swing of one leg whilst, at the same time, stimulating the hamstrings of the stance leg to propel the body forwards. In a clinical trial on four paralysed adult subjects, with injury levels ranging from T4 to C1, we measured energy expenditure by a comparative method developed by MacGregor (1979; 1981), called the Performance Cost Index (PCI). This method involved calculating the PCI from the heart rate at steady state walking minus the heart rate at rest, divided by the walking speed. The resulting measure was in units of beats/metre. Isakov *et al.* (1992) used PCI to compare ambulation using a reciprocating gait orthosis (RGO) on its own with that for a combined FES and RGO system. The study reported a reduction of PCI from 2.55 beats/metre with the RGO only, to 1.54 beats/metre with the hybrid system. That represented an energy reduction of nearly 40%.

In our own clinical trial, we found that the reduction in PCI due to the additional use of FES was often considerably less than 20%. Furthermore, with the most proficient RGO users, the faster they were able to walk, the smaller was the benefit of using electrical stimulation. In fact, the patients complained that it held them back.

Equipment Used	RGO	RGO & FES
PCI (bts/m)	2.47	2.44

Table 1. Results of PCI measurement for a patient (A) with a complete T6 level lesion, walking to 0.3 metres/second in a reciprocating gait orthosis, with and without functional electrical stimulation of the quadricepts and hamstring muscles. Units are in beats per metre.

Table 1 is a typical result of PCI measured for a 28 year old man, with a complete T6 level paraplegia, walking in an RGO with and without FES. From a value of 2.47 beats/metre with the RGO alone, the PCI dropped by only 1.2% to a value of 2.44 beats/metre with the hybrid system. The change was not significant.

The most likely explanation for the small change in Table 1 is that these measurements were for a patient (A) who habitually walked at a significantly higher speed than most RGO users. A study by Hirokawa et al (1990) demonstrated that at speeds below 0.32 m/s the RGO and FES were more energy efficient than the RGO on its own. However, when the speed exceeded 0.38 m/s there was no significant difference between use of these two systems. In this case, the walking speed of our patient was just below the threshold at 0.3 m/s. Kinematic studies on this same patient (A) revealed that he had to lift his hip through a vertical displacement of 150 mm at the mid-swing position in order to clear the foot of his extended leg from the ground. This compared with an average lift of only 43 mm in normal subjects of similar age and height. The effect of this excessive lift on the gait pattern of patient A is illustrated in fig. 1. The darker line represents the right leg during the swing phase of walking with an RGO.

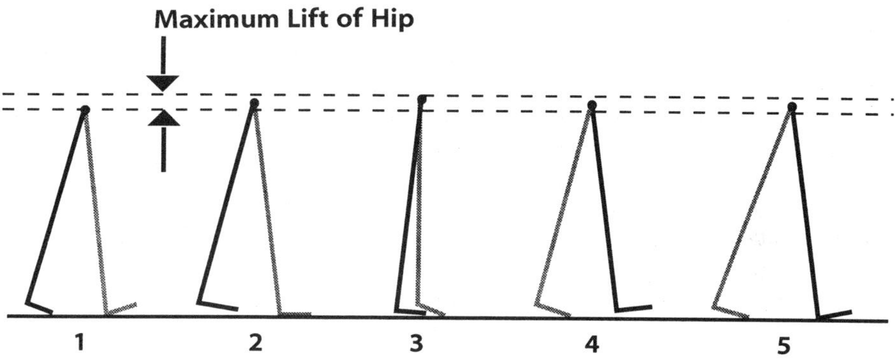

Fig.1. Illustration of consecutive positions of legs during walking with a conventional reciprocating gait orthosis. The knees of both legs are locked in an extended position. The darker line represents the right leg during the swing phase.

Position 1 is at toe off, position 3 at mid-swing and position 5 at heel strike. We see that during the early part of the swing phase, the patient starts to lift his right hip by pushing down on the handle bars of his rollator frame. Maximum lift is achieved at position 3. Due to the transverse stiffness of the RGO sacral band, the patient was restricted from tilting his pelvis in the coronal plane. Therefore, the stance leg (shown by lighter line) was also lifted, causing the left heel to leave the ground. In fact, when patient (A) walked at speeds over 0.3 m/s, the whole of the stance foot, including the toe, would frequently lift completely away from the floor. When this happened the full weight of the body was carried by the arms. Performing such a push up with every step was a very energy consuming activity.

3 Effect of Locking Knees in Extension

Further evidence to support our concept that walking with fixed knees is a key factor causing high energy consumption comes from studies on the ambulation of normal subjects. Ralston (1965) measured oxygen levels in expired gases to demonstrate the effect of restricting knee movement in normal people during walking. When one knee was fixed in the extended position with a brace, the energy expenditure increased by 18%. During similar studies in our own laboratory, we found that when both knees of normal subjects were restricted with light weight braces, the energy consumption increased by an average of 45%.

From the evidence of the foregoing studies, we reasoned that if each leg of an RGO clad subject could be made to bend during the swing phase of walking, then the height through which the patient would have to lift the body centre of gravity at each step would be reduced. This in turn would reduce both the load on the arms and the energy expenditure.

4 Orthotic Knee Joint Design

In order to prove the foregoing hypothesis, we are investigating a variety of design approaches that will allow the orthotic knee joint to unlock and bend at the start of the swing phase, then lock again during the stance phase. This has included user operated designs such as mechanical latches and dog clutches, as well as mechanisms which can be unlocked under computer control such as wrapped spring, electro-magnetic, magnetic particle, friction brake and spragg clutches. To date, our progress has been most rapid with a patented (Edwards and Bataweel, 1993), weight operated design called the Lockable/Unlockable Knee (LUK) joint, as illustrated in fig.2.

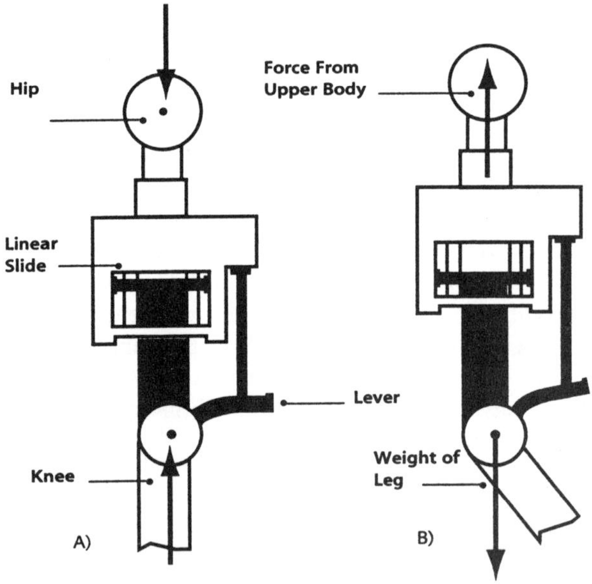

Fig.2. Schematic diagram of Lockable/Unlockable Orthotic Knee (LUK) joint. (A) Under axial compression from body weight the joint is locked. (B) When the upper body is lifted, the joint unlocks, allowing the knee to bend.

The side member of the thigh portion of the RGO was cut above the knee. Across the resulting gap a linear mechanical slide was introduced with a rod or wire connecting the upper side member to a specially hardened, latching lever in the orthotic knee joint. When the assembly was axially compressed by body weight during the stance phase, as in fig. 2(A), the lever was pushed down to lock the joint. However, when the hip was lifted at the start of the swing phase, as in fig. 2(B), distension of the slide operated the lever and unlocked the joint, thus allowing the knee to bend.

Our first prototype slide mechanism was positioned in the orthotic side member just above the joint and below the thigh cuff. This unlocked the joint as required but proved unreliable for several reasons. It used linear ball bearings to minimise sliding friction. However, due to their small size these proved incapable of carrying the high bending moments developed in the stance phase, even when used in pairs. The device was too bulky to be used in the medial side member. Furthermore, it was found that the main axial load to operate the device came from the upper sacral portion of the RGO above the hip joint. Hence the plastic thigh cuff interfered with the axial load transmission.

A MKII prototype design now uses a stronger linear ball slide positioned in the orthotic side bar above the thigh cuff and below the hip joint (fig. 3). This functioned satisfactorily when subjected to the full range of bending moments experienced in practice. Also, it allowed a free joint to be incorporated on the medial side of each knee which gave greater axial torque carrying capacity.

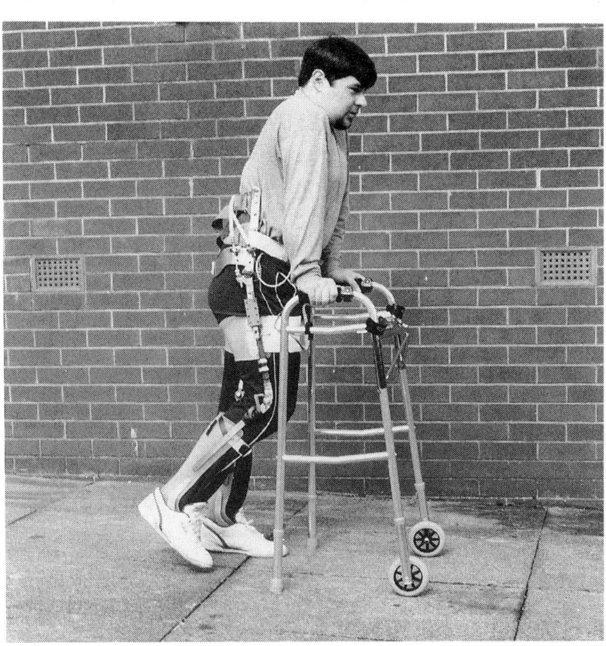

Fig.3. Photograph showing the MKII prototype of the LUK-RGO orthosis with linear slide in orthotic side member above the thigh cuff.

5 Combined FES/LUK-RGO

In conjunction with the Lockable/Unlockable Knee (LUK) RGO we used a six channel FES stimulator system attached to a belt at the patient's waist. This was operated by two push switches, one on each of the rollator handle bars.

At toe off, as the right orthotic knee joint was unlocked, the patient pushed a switch on the right handle bar to stimulate the right peroneal nerve and cause flexion of the right knee. This was followed by stimulation of the right quadricepts muscle after a delay of about 0.5 second, in order to extend the leg in preparation for heel strike. Quadricepts stimulation was maintained into the early part of the stance phase to ensure that the orthotic knee joint was firmly locked after experiencing the impact of heel strike.

6 Results

A single case study was carried out in which this LUK-RGO was used by a man with a complete T6 level paraplegia (Patient 'A'). He was first trained between parallel bars to gain confidence of walking with a knee bending swing phase. Initially, the knee joint of just one leg was allowed to bend. Then after a few weeks, he began to walk with both the left and right LUK joints operating. Once the patient was confident between parallel bars, he was allowed to progress onto walking with a rollator. Objective assessments were carried out at three or four week intervals. These included menasurement of the forces exerted by the upper and lower limbs using a strain guage instrumented rollator and Kistler force plates. Energy expenditure was also measured by the Performance Cost Index (PCI) method (MacGregor, 1981).

Compared to conventional RGO walking, the peak vertical forces exerted by the arms in order to clear the feet from the ground were reduced by 30% when using a LUK-RGO without FES, and by 50% when FES was combined with the LUK-RGO. This was a significant reduction, which was also reflected in the energy consumption measurements shown in table 2. Walking between parallel bars with a standard RGO gave a PCI of 3.1 beats/m. After ten sessions of training with a LUK-RGO, the PCI was reduced by 34% to 2.03 beats/m, and with the LUK-RGO and FES combined it was reduced by 56% to 1.36 beats/m. At this stage he moved on to walking with a rollator. After a further twelve sessions of training, the PCI was 2.47 beats/m with a conventional RGO. However, this was reduced by 12% to 2.17 beats/m with the LUK-RGO on its own, and by 36% to 1.58 beats/m with the hybrid LUK-RGO and FES system.

TRAINING SESSIONS	PCI		
	RGO	LUK-RGO	LUK-RGO and FES
10 sessions between parallel bars	3.1	2.03	1.36
3 further sessions with rollator	2.47	2.26	2.04
12 further sessions with rollator	2.47	2.17	1.58

Table 2. Performance Cost Index (PCI) for patient 'A' with the RGO on its own, with the LUK-RGO or with the LUK-RGO and FES. Each session involved 2.5 hours of training. PCI values are in beats/metre.

7 Discussion

The significant reductions observed in both peak forces on the arms and PCI, when using the LUK-RGO and FES in comparison with a conventional RGO, confirmed our hypothesis that allowing a knee flexing gait would reduce the energy requirement of upright mobility. A similar gait can also be achieved without an orthosis by using a surface FES system such as the **Parastep** produced by Sigmedics Inc. (Winchester *et al.*, 1994) The same subject, patient (A) was also assessed after a further two months of lower limb muscle conditioning and training with 'The Parastep System'. This system used a microprocessor controlled, six channel stimulator with twin surface electrodes positioned on the skin over the gluteus maximus, the quadricepts and peroneal nerve of both lower legs. As with our system, the latter elicited a flexion withdrawal response at the beginning of the swing phase, followed by quadricepts stimulation to extend the leg again prior to heel strike. A key difference compared with our LUK-RGO and FES system is that quadricepts stimulation is maintained throughout the stance phase of the contralateral leg to prevent collapse of the knee under body weight.

The quadricepts and hamstring muscles of patient A had been fully conditioned by FES over a previous five year period. Nevertheless, after a further two months of conditioning and training with the Parastep system (Supplier: Sigmedics Inc., Northfield, Illinois, U.S.A.), we found that he could only walk 20 metres before his knees started to give way due to muscle fatigue. By comparison, his quadricepts showed no signs of fatigue after walking over 1000 metres with the LUK-RGO and FES system. This was because the orthosis supported any moments tending to bend the knee.

The progress of the patient was slow during the early stages of training with the LUK-RGO. This was because he found it difficult to ensure that the orthotic knee joint was fully locked at heel strike. This could be overcome by dipping the upper body forwards against the chest strap to cause the knee to extend against ground contact at the heel. However, the resulting gait then became ungainly. His performance was considerably improved when FES was added to the orthotic system, provided quadriceps stimulation was maintained to just beyond heel strike.

The positive nature of these clinical results has encouraged us to extend the study to a larger number of spinal cord injured patients.

References

Douglas, R., Larson, P.F., D'Ambrosia, R.D., and McCall, R.E. (1983) The LSU reciprocating gait orthosis. *Orthopaedics,* **6:** 834-838.

Edwards, J. and Bataweel, A.B. (1993) A joint for a lower limb orthosis UK Patent Application No. 9315090. 21 July.

Hirokawa, S., Grimm, M. LeT., Solomonow, M., Baratta, R.V., Shoji, H., and D'Ambrosia, R.D. (1990) Energy consumption in paraplegic ambulation using the reciprocating gait orthosis and electric stimulation of the thigh muscles. *Arch. Phys. Med. Rehabil.,* **71.**

Isakov, E., Douglas, R., and Berns, P. (1992) Ambulation using the reciprocating gait orthosis and functional electrical stimulation. *Paraplegia,* **30:** 239-245.

MacGregor, J. (1979) The objective measurement of physical performance with long term ambulatory physiological surveillance equipment (LAPSE). In: F.D. Stott, E.B. Raftery and L. Goulding (eds.) *Proceedings of 3rd International Symposium on Ambulatory Monitoring,* pp. 29-39.

MacGregor, J. (1981) The evaluation of patient performance using long term ambulatory monitoring technique in domiciliary environment. *Physiotherapy,* **67:** 30-33.

Ralston, H.J. (1965) Effects of immobilisation of various body segments on energy cost of human locomotion. *Proc. 2nd I.E.A. Conf.,* Dortmund, 19674. [Supplement to] Ergonomics, p. 53.

Solomonow, M., Baratta, R., Hirokawa, S., Rightor, N., Walker, W., Beaudette P., Shoji, H., and D'Ambrosia, R. (1989) The RGO Generation II: Muscle stimulation powered orthosis as a practical walking system for thoracic paraplegics. *Orthopaedics,* **12:** 1309-1315.

Sykes, L., Edwards, J., Powell, E., and Ross, E.S.R. (1995) Reciprocating Gait Orthosis: Long term usage patterns. *Archives of Physical Medicine and Rehabilitation,* **76:** 779-783.

Winchester, P., Carollo, J.J., and Habasevich, R. (1994) Physiologic costs of reciprocal gait in FES assisted walking. *Paraplegia,* **32:** 680-686.

Whittle, M. and Cochrane, G. (1988) A comparative trial of the Hip Guidance Orthosis and the Reciprocating Gait Orthosis. Nuffield Orthopaedic Centre, Oxford, England, Department of Health and Social Security: 1-54.

Chapter 8

Clinical Applications of Surface FES for Motor Functions

Multichannel Electrical Stimulation in Hemiparetic Patients

S. Hesse, M. Maležič, K.-H. Mauritz
Department of Neurological Rehabilitation,
Freie Universität Berlin, Berlin, Germany

1 Introduction

Since the first reports on the stimulation of the peroneal nerve in hemiparetic patients (Liberson et al.,1961), single-channel stimulators have become common in daily routine. Multichannel surface stimulation of gait in hemiparetic patients has been so far restricted to research laboratories. After reports on simultaneous stimulation of N. peroneus, knee flexors and plantar flexors to support swing phase in the early seventies (Kralj et al.,1971) 6-channel stimulators were designed for the stimulation of the knee extensors, hip abductors, and hip extensors during the stance phase (Trnkoczy et al.,1978). Percutaneous and implantable systems followed later only in single cases (Marsolais et al.,1990).

Single channel stimulation of hemiplegic hand opening followed a decade after the first reports on FES (Rebersek and Vodovnik,1973). Stimulation of hand opening, elbow extension and in a single cases shoulder abduction was introduced shortly after (Merletti et al.,1975). Percutaneous stimulation of finger and wrist muscles was restricted to tetraparetic patients (Peckham et al.,1980).

Despite proved advantages (Alfieri, 1982; Bogataj et al.,1989; Malezic et al.,1987), clinical applicability of the multichannel stimulation of hemiparetic patients was hampered by complicated, research oriented devices and by physical, cognitive and communication impairments of stimulated patients. Therefore an FES program has been installed for in-patients with a temporary stimulation fitted to individual needs and supervised by experienced therapists. This program included the restoration of standing and weight-shift, gait and arm function.

1 Standing and Weight Shift

Requirements for normal walking are posture and balance (Nutt et al., 1993). Regular physiotherpy includes training of standing and weight-shift. Standing and weight-shift of the hemiparetic patient are hampered proximally by weak pelvic alignment and knee instability. Three muscle groups: gluteus maximus, quadriceps and hamstring muscles, were stimulated (surface 4x6cm electrodes) by trains of biphasic pulses (20Hz, 0.2ms, 50-90mA) from Stratec Biocy-8 stimulator.

Eleven non-ambulatory hemiparetic patients (age 39-64; 8 males, 3 females; 5 right, 6 left hemiparesis, mean stroke interval 127 days) stood with the feet at 30 degrees and toes 30cm apart on two triaxial Kistler force plates. The patients then shifted their weight onto the paretic leg without leaning to the non-affected side. The following parameters normalized by the body weight were assessed during the trials without stimulation, with the optimal stimulation and 5 minutes after it:

- vertical ground reaction forces to the affected and non-affected limb before the weight shift (standing symmetry),
- slope during the transient phase as % of body weight per second (weight shift),
- maximum force to the affected leg after the weight-shift.

Three phases were distinguished during the weight-shift:

1. initial weight shift to the non-affected lower limb to generate momentum for the shift to the affected side,
2. transient phase in which the weight was shifted to the affected side and
3. stabilisation phase, in which the maximum ground reaction force was achieved.

Mean values averaged over three trials showed that during the stimulation the patients stood with 11.4% more weight on the affected limb (paired t-test: $p=0.009$), shifted their weight 50.8% faster to the affected limb ($p=0.004$), while the maximum force increased for 5% (not significant).

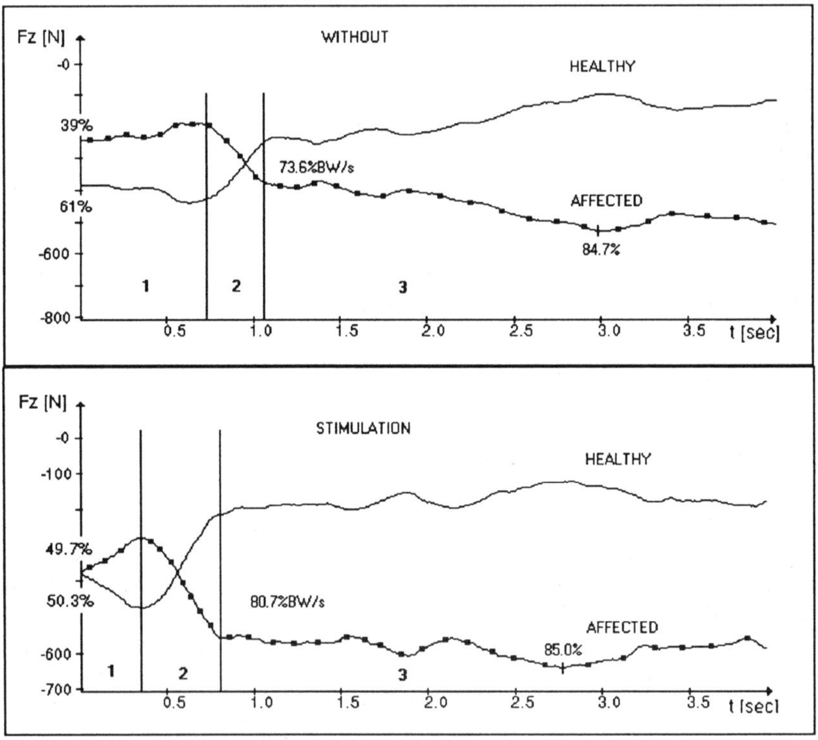

Fig. 1. Standing and weight-shift without and with stimulation. 1,2,3: Momentum generating, transient and stabilization phase.

After the stimulation they stood with 8% more weight on the affected limb (n.s.), the weight-shift was 23% faster (p=0.047) and their maximum loading of the affected limb was 7% higher (p=0.007). Without stimulation the weight distribution was 35% versus 65% BW, corresponding to the literature (Dettmann et al.,1987). The three phases of generating the momentum, weight-shift and stabilisation were clearly expressed in less affected patients, while the first one was less explicit in the severely affected ones, where the last phase also displayed more oscillations.

The stimulation stabilized the pelvis and knee, enabling better standing symmetry and faster weight-shift. A carry-over effect (faster and higher loading) was observed after the stimulation. FES of standing and weight-shift could be administered in addition to regular physical therapy, in particular with severely affected patients, who require a considerable physical effort from the therapists.

3 Gait

Immediate and therapeutic effects of an individually tailored multichannel stimulation of the patients' gait (Bogataj et al.,1989; Malezic et al.,1987a, 1987b) were studied with the help of time parameters and symmetry. Number of stimulating channels were not set in advance, but together with parameters of the stimulation fitted to personal needs of each patient, i.e. a rigid paradigm was avoided in favour of an individually tailored simple stimulation. The selection of stimulation sites was based on a qualitative gait analysis.

Two to three programmable IJS dual channel stimulators (Malezic et al.,1992) were connected together to one stimulating unit for stimulation of more than 2 muscle groups. Foot-switches synchronised the stimulation with the phases of gait. The stride phases were averaged during the sessions for follow-up of the treatment. Trains of biphasic pulses (25Hz, 0.15-0.35ms, 10-50mA) were applied in kinesiologicaly appropriate sequences by surface electrodes: round 2.5cm active felt pad cathode and 2x8cm anode to the peroneal nerve, 5x8cm felt pad electrodes to the quadriceps, hamstrings and gluteus maximus, 2x15cm felt pad electrodes to gluteus medius and minimus muscles and 5x13cm self adhesive PALS electrodes to the supraspinatus, deltoideus and triceps brachii muscles.

3.1 Examples

In one of the patients (59, male, right hemiparesis, ischemic stroke left a. cerebri media, onset 14 weeks) the peroneal nerve was stimulated during the swing to clear the foot and during the loading to prevent the foot slap. The quadriceps muscle was stimulated in the terminal swing to provide a selective knee extension and during the first part of stance to enable a safe weight acceptance. The hamstring muscles were stimulated together with the quardriceps during the first part of stance to stabilize the knee and prevent its hyperextension and then in the pre-swing and initial swing to support the knee flexion. The gluteus maximus muscle was stimulated throughout the stance phase to assist the hip extension.

In another patient (47, male, right hemiparesis, ischemic stroke left a. cerebri media, onset 33 weeks) the peroneal nerve was stimulated during the swing and loading as in the first patient. The gluteus maximus muscle was stimulated by one channel and both the gluteus medius and minimus muscles by another one throughout the stance phase. Additionally a severe shoulder depression with consecutive trunk shortening on the affected side was present. Thus a combined shoulder-arm stimulation with one large electrode on the supraspinatus and part of trapezius muscles and another on the deltoideus and long head of the triceps brachii muscles was introduced to elevate the shoulder and to enable the arm swing.

In the next patient (40, male, left hemiparesis, ischemic stroke right a. cerebri media, onset 17 weeks) the peroneal nerve was stimulated during the swing and loading phases. The quadriceps muscle was stimulated from the terminal swing to mid-stance phase for a controlled knee motion and weight acceptance. The hamstring muscles were stimulated together with the quadriceps muscle in the first part of stance to prevent the knee hyperextension and in the initial swing phase to support the foot clearance. As this patient also suffered from a shoulder depression and lack of arm-swing, the combined shoulder-arm stimulation was applied too.

The treatment included 25 stimulation sessions from 15 minutes at the beginning to an hour at the end besides the regular physiotherapy. The patients were not encouraged to walk faster or long distances, but the correct gait pattern was stressed throughout the sessions. Mean gait velocity, stride length, cadence and stair climbing velocity were assessed together with clinical analysis of the gait pattern, hierarchical Rivermead motor assessment score designed for hemiparetic patients and Ashworth spasticity scale before, in the middle and at the end of treatment. To illustrate direct effects of the gait stimulation, vertical ground reaction forces were recorded by the Infotronic force shoe system with and without the stimulation.

All patients improved functionally: 33% in gait velocity, 5% in cadence, 26% in stride length and 18% in stair climbing when walking with the self adopted speed. During the fastest possible gait the mean improvements reached 33% in the gait velocity, 13% in cadence and 17% in stride length. The initial contact and foot clearance changed to a functional level in all three patients. In patient No. 1 the knee became stabilized, whereas the lack of hip extension was not alleviated by the treatment. In patient No. 2 the trunk was erected and the pelvic alignment was stabilized enabling a better hip extension during the stance phase. Patient No. 3 could control his knee better, avoiding the hyperextension. His shoulder and trunk position improved too. The Rivermead score raised for 19.5% and the Ashworth scale showed a reduced spasticity for 11%. The mean stance-to-swing ratio of the affected side improved from 0.49 to 0.95 and the stance symmetry from 0.62 to 0.97 in a uniform increase.

Mean vertical ground reaction forces and trajectories of the center of pressure under both feet are shown in Figure 2 for the patient No. 3 without and with the stimulation. Note a 140N increase of the mean force in the midstance with 200N lesser standard deviation, better gait dynamics reflected in the loading and push-off peaks.

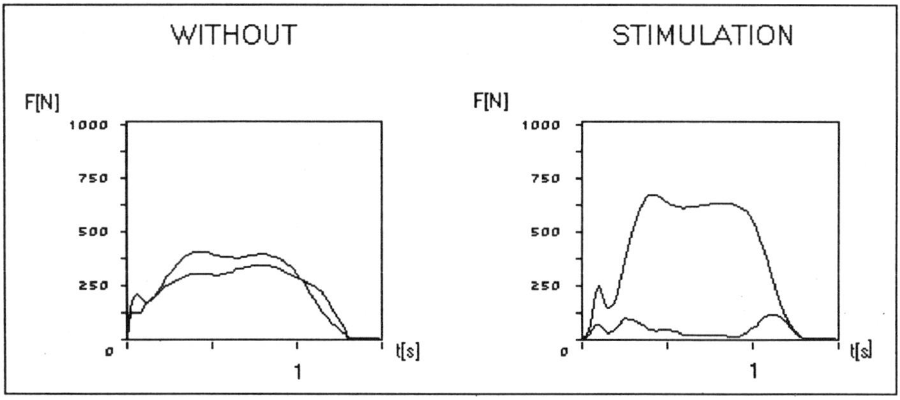

Fig. 2. Vertical force diagram (mean, SD) without and with stimulation.

In conclusion the patients improved functionally and the gait pattern was partly restored as documented by clinical analysis and the symmetry ratios. Besides gait, other motor functions improved (Rivermead Score) and spasticity was reduced (Ashworth Scale).

The stimulation algorithm was not firm but individually fitted with regard to sequences, stimulation sites and their number. Stimulation unit, consisted of the available IJS devices, proved to be a viable solution for daily clinical use. Besides known stimulation sites the shoulder-arm stimulation with the direct and indirect effects was introduced. The latter was a sustained trunk erection, providing a stable trunk and pelvic alignment.

4 Arm Function

Deltoideus, supraspinatus and part of trapezius muscle were stimulated for the shoulder abduction by 13x5cm self-adhesive PALS electrodes, triceps brachii muscle for the elbow extension by 10x4cm sponge electrodes, while 10x4cm neutral and 3x3cm active sponge electrode were applied to the wrist, finger and thumb extensor muscles. Patients simultaneously stimulated the three muscle groups by pressing a button. Stratec BIOCY-8 multichannel stimulator delivered 20Hz, 0.3ms biphasic current pulses with the amplitudes adjusted to strong but still confortable limb segment movements.

After positive results of a feasibility study in 4 patients, an A-B-A single-case design study with two hemiparetic patients (male, 58 and 56 years, right and left hemiparesis, stroke interval 12 and 17 weeks) was conducted by Cybex elbow extension/flexion torque measurements. The affected and non-affected sides were measured. Additionally the Rivermead score, Ashworth scale and Motricity Index were recorded weekly.

One patient could only protract the shoulder while lying, the second patient was able to hold the extended arm in elevation and beginning flexion and extension movements of the elbow were visible while lying. During the A-phases (8 days) with measurements every second day the patients received regular physiotherpy. In the B-phase the FES treatment of 30 minutes per day was added 25 times with weekly measurements.

The Cybex data, normalized by the non-affected side, showed a large variability in both patients, particularly for the extension torques. The mean values of the extension (flexion) torques improved for 37% (23%) during the B-phase and remained stable during the next A-phase in one patient. In the other patient the extension (flexion) torques improved for 30% (11%) during the B-phase. Extension decreased for 11% and flexion for 68% in the second A-phase. The Motricity Index of the paretic arm increased from 40 to 45 (29 to 53), the Rivermead score from 3 to 6 (1 to 3), while the mean Ashworth score increased from 0.7 to 1.2 and remained stable in the second patient.

The program has not been continued. The stimulation itself raised initially rather high expectations in the patients who were disappointed on its outcome at the end of treatment. The first patient developed shoulder pain resulting in moderately increased spasticity. Besides the patients remained passive during this method.

References

Alfieri V. (1982) Electrical treatment of spasticity; reflex tonic activity in hemiplegic patients and selected specific electrostimulation. Scand J Rehabil Med 14, 177-182.

Bogataj, U., Gros, N., Malezic, M., Kelih, B., Kljajic, M., and Acimovic, R. (1989) Restoration of gait during two to three weeks of therapy with multichannel electrical stimulation. Phys Ther 69, 319-327.

Dettmann, M. A., Linder, M. T., and Sepic S. B. (1987) Relationships among walking performance, postural stability and functional assessments of the hemiplegic patient. Am J Phys Med 66, 77-90.

Kralj, A., Trnkoczy, A., and Acimovic, R. (1971) Improvement of locomotion in hemiplegic patients with multichannel stimulation. In Proceedings of the Conference of Human Locomotor Engineering, Sussex, England, 60-68.

Liberson, W. T., Holmquest, H. J., Scott, H., and Dow, M. (1961) Functional electrotherapy: stimulation of the peroneal nerve synchronized with the swing phase of gait of hemiparetic patients. Arch Phys Med Rehabil 2, 101-107.

Malezic, M., Kljajic, M., Acimovic-Janezic, R., Gros, N., Krajnik, J., and Stanic, U. (1987a) Therapeutic effects of multisite electric stimulation of gait in motor-disabled patients. Arch Phys Med Rehabil 68, 553-560.

Malezic, M., Bogataj, U., Gros, N., Kelih, B., Kljajic, M., Acimovic, R. (1987b) Evaluation of gait with multichannel electrical stimulation. Orthopedics 10, 769-772.

Malezic, M., Bogataj, U., Gros, N., Decman, I., Vrtacnik, P., Kljajic, M., and Acimovic-Janezic, R. (1992) Application of a programmable dual-channel adaptive electrical system for the control and analysis of gait. J Rehab Res & Develop 29, 41-53.

Marsolais, E. B., Kobetic, R., Barnicle, K., and Jacobs, J. (1990) FNS application for restoring function in stroke and head-injury patients. J Clin Eng 15, 489-496.

Merletti, R., Acimovic, R., Grobelnik, S., and Cvilak, G. (1975) Electrophysiological orthosis for the upper extremity in hemiplegia: feasibility study. Arch Phys Med Rehabil 56/12, 507-513.

Peckham, P. H., Marsolais, E. B., Mortimer, J. T. (1980) Restoration of key grip and release in a C6 tetraplegic patient through functional electrical stimulation. J Hand Surg 5, 462-469.

Rebersek, S. and Vodovnik, L. (1973) Proportionally controlled functional electrical stimulation of hand. Arch Phys Med Rehabil 54/8, 378-382.

Trnkoczy, A., Stanic, U., and Malezic, M. (1978) Present state and prospects in design of multichannel FES stimulators for gait correction in paretic patients. TIT J Life Sci 8, 17-27.

Extended reference list due to ongoing research:

Malezic, M., Hesse, S., Schewe, H., and Mauritz, K.-H. (1994) Restoration of standing, weight-shift and gait by multichannel electrical stimulation in hemiparetic patients. Int J Rehab Res 17, 169-179.

Malezic, M., and Hesse, S. (1995) Restoration of gait by functional electrical stimulation in paraplegic patients - modified programme of treatment. Paraplegia 33, 126-131.

Hesse, S., Bertelt, C., Jahnke, M. T., Schaffrin, A., Baake, P., Malezic, M., and Mauritz, K.H. (1995) Treadmill training with partial body weight support as compared to physiotherapy in non-ambulatory hemiparetic patients. Stroke 26, 976-981.

Hesse, S., Malezic, M., Schaffrin, A., and Mauritz, K.H. (1995) Restoration of gait by a combined treadmill training and multichannel electrical stimulation in non-ambulatory hemiparetic patients. Scand J Rehab Med 27, 199-205.

Multi-Channel FES Therapy in Rehabilitation of Gait in Stroke Patients

U. Bogataj[1], N. Gros[2], M. Kljajić[1,3], R. Aćimović-Janežič[2]
[1] J. Stefan Institute, Ljubljana, Slovenia
[2]Institute of Republic Slovenia for Rehabilitation, Ljubljana, Slovenia
[3]School of Organisational Science, University of Maribor, Kranj, Slovenia

Abstract - Established gait rehabilitation in severely involved hemiplegic patients requires substantial effort. Preliminary studies indicated the beneficial effects of using multi-channel functional electrical stimulation (MFES) for gait relearning. In this study, a new method of gait rehabilitation for non-ambulatory hemiplegic patients by means of MFES, as an adjunct to conventional therapy, was introduced. The results of the method's application were evaluated by comparing it with conventional therapeutic methods. The proposed rehabilitation method was tested on a group of 20 hemiplegic patients. Each subject participated three weeks in either of the compared therapeutic methods and was randomly assigned to one of two groups with a reversed sequence of treatments. The effects of each treatment were evaluated by measurements of temporal-distance variables, and by assessment of physical status of each patient according to the Fugl-Meyer evaluation scale. The statistical analysis showed improved performance of the patients during MFES therapy combined with conventional therapy compared with conventional therapy alone. The superiority of the presented therapeutic method was mainly attributed to the enhanced motor learning accomplished by application of MFES.

1 Introduction

In patients with hemiplegia the gait pattern is often destroyed due to the damage caused by cerebrovascular accident (CVA) in the central nervous system (CNS). In mild cases the damage is not extensive, which usually enables patients to start with gait training immediately after stabilising their medical condition. After finishing a rehabilitation program some anomalies in gait may remain in some patients. The situation is quite different in patients with severe involvement. These patients are bedridden for a prolonged period of time. Muscle weakness due to inactivity and disturbed muscle control are usually accompanied by a balance problem, disturbances in proprioception, contractures in joints, poor understanding, aphasia, emotional lability, etc. (Anderson 1982). In such cases the re-learning of gait is very difficult and long-lasting. The patient must learn to stand, perform independent straight standing, shifting weight from one leg to another and maintain balance. Muscles must be strengthened by physical exercises or FES. At the same time the patient must regain confidence in the ability to use the affected side. In many cases synergistic movement patterns develop (flexor or extensor), which additionally disturb coordinated movement (Brunström 1970). The transition from standing to coordinated ambulation, therefore, represents quite an effort for the patient as well as for the therapist.

Recent kinesilogical studies and clinical assessments showed that surface MFES of the six main muscle groups of the affected limb can modify pathologic gait, improve correction of gait anomalies, accelerate rehabilitation and enhance the endurance of the patient (Malezic et al 1987, Bogataj et al 1989). Despite the good results, surface MFES was never routinely used as an orthotic aid in hemiplegic patients. The main reason is that patients are unable to position up to six pairs of electrodes. Therapeutic use of MFES produced effects which are quite substantial during therapy and tend to fade away during a period of 6-12 months after the end of therapy. On the other hand, the status of the patients is not significantly better compared to the non-stimulated control group (Malezic 1987). These are probably the reasons why there are currently no reports on the routine use of MFES in rehabilitation of gait in hemiplegic patients. Lately Marsolais et al (1990) reported the use of MFES for gait in hemiplegic patients. These researchers, however, are working on the development and application of implantable systems designed not for therapy, but for orthotic use. The same group reported also beneficial results in a single case follow-up of therapeutic application of MFES system with intramuscular electrodes (Jacobs-Daly et al 1993)

Patients treated in previous studies were ambulatory patients where the main reason for MFES application was to correct the pathological gait pattern (Malezic et al 1987, Bogataj et al 1989, Marsolais et al 1990, Jacobs-Daly 1993). The rapid and good correction of gait anomalies in those patients raised the question, concerning how MFES would perform in the initiation of gait pattern in severely involved hemiplegic patients. A pilot study was therefore carried out (Bogataj et al 1989). It showed that MFES can help to establish an initial gait pattern and improve weight bearing in non-ambulatory patients. However, it showed no comparative value of the method to existing therapeutic programs.

The purpose of this study was to show the real value of MFES therapy in the rehabilitation of gait in severely involved hemiplegic patients compared to existing generally accepted methods and techniques.

2 Methods

2.1 Experimental design

Each subject participated for half the time in the experimental and for half the time in a control procedure. To avoid a problem of the bias produced by sequencing procedures, the patients who participated in the study were randomly assigned to two groups with reversed sequences of therapies. This design provides a method for controlling individual differences among subjects. A relatively more complex statistical analysis, however, is required to obtain valid results with such a design (Krishnaiah 1980). Each subject was monitored following the same methodology through the period of 6 weeks, participating for 3 weeks in each therapeutic program.

2.2 Subjects

Twenty severely involved hemiplegic patients due to CVA participated in the study. They were randomly assigned to two groups of 10 subjects each. One group started with conventional therapy and continued with MFES therapy, and the other group had the reversed sequence of therapies.

Candidates were selected on the basis of neurological, internist, physiatric and psychological examinations. Subjects were assigned to our program on the basis of the following indications and contra-indications:

- The cardiovascular system of the patient had to be in such condition that exertion during therapy or measurement should not represent any hazard to the patient's health;
- The physical status and motor functions, especially in the lower extremities of the patient, had to be in such condition that enabled the patient to stand independently or with the aid of a therapist. Only patients who required the substantial support of one or two therapists to ambulate were included;
- The patient's perceptual and intellectual abilities had to be preserved;
- Sufficient functional response or at least muscle contraction with indicated movement in the corresponding joint should be obtained by FES;
- Patients with extreme reflex activities, hypersensitivity, pains, lower motor neurone lesions, changes to the skin in the area of stimulation and in bone-joint structures (contractures, deformations, etc.), and subjects who refused application of FES were excluded;
- Each patient who passed the described conditions was included in the study only on the basis of his or her informed consent to participate.

The subjects in group 1 (5 male and 5 female) started with conventional therapy and continued with MFES. The 2 left and 8 right hemiplegic patients in this group ranged in age from 38 to 73 years ($\overline{X}$=53.4, SD=11.5) and in mean time between CVA and start of therapy from 53 to 273 days ($\overline{X}$=116, SD=66). The subjects in group 2 (6 male and 4 female) started with MFES and continued with conventional therapy. The 9 left and 1 right hemiplegic patients in this group ranged in age from 43 to 75 years ($\overline{X}$=59.1, SD=9) and in time between CVA and start of therapy from 27 to 227 days ($\overline{X}$=104, SD=62). The t-test showed no difference between the groups in these two variables. Table 1 shows some basic data about the subjects. In all subjects the pre-CVA side of dominance was the right side.

2.3 Conventional therapy

According to the nature and extension of affection, hemiplegia is a very complex condition and therefore an adequately compound rehabilitation program is required. Specialists from different areas (a physician, orthopaedist, internist, neurologist, physical therapist, occupational therapist, psychologist, speech therapist, etc.) must work in a coordinated manner to cover the whole spectrum of a patient's affection. Although all these areas are closely interconnected, we will restrict ourselves to the physiotherapy of gait, so as not to exceed the boundaries of this study.

Subject	Age	Gender	Side of paresis.	T_d [d]	D_i [m]	D_f [m]
Group 1 (started with conventional therapy and continued with MFES)						
1	39	M	R	218	183	600 (7)
2	43	M	R	75	180	400
3	53	F	L	53	109	600 (4)
4	60	M	R	59	42	165
5	73	F	R	129	160	270
6	38	M	R	91	198	600 (13)
7	67	F	R	77	17	186
8	51	F	R	149	33	195
9	57	M	R	76	253	447
10	53	F	L	273	26	212
Mean	Age ± SD			T_d ± SD		
	53.4 ± 11.5 years			116 ± 66 days		
Group 2 (started with MFES and continued with conventional therapy)						
11	63	F	L	125	90	450
12	58	M	L	48	25	215
13	54	M	R	102	90	600 (15)
14	58	F	L	139	72	161
15	67	M	L	116	97	600 (7)
16	43	M	L	51	53	270
17	50	F	L	154	92	350
18	75	F	L	227	60	102
19	59	M	L	27	90	212
20	64	M	L	46	42	209
Mean	Age ± SD			T_d ± SD		
	59.1 ± 9 years			104 ± 62 days		

Table 1: Basic data about subjects participating in study. T_d = time elapsed between accident and start of our program. D_i = initial distance walked by patient on the first day of MFES therapy. D_f- final distance walked by patient on the last day of MFES therapy. If the patient reached the upper limit of 600 m the number of therapy sessions, when accomplished for the first time, is included in parentheses. D_i and D_f data are not available for conventional therapy.

Before an adequate program of therapy could be prescribed the patient's status was assessed and his or her past medical history, history of the present state, social history and communication were evaluated. The assessment of the patient's status comprised information about the patient's functional level (muscle tone, range of motion, coordination, sensation/perception, voluntary control and activities in changing the positions) with special emphasis on gait evaluation.

The patient's functional abilities were the basis for his or her treatment. There was no general pattern of therapy which would apply to all patients. Each patient received the therapy adapted to his or her deficiencies and needs. The same therapist worked with the individual patient through the whole program of conventional treatment. In general, the conventional treatment consisted of a passive and active approach.

With the passive approach we wanted to reduce spasticity, increase or preserve the range of motion in the joints, and enhance sensory input. In order to accomplish that, icing, heating and brushing was applied, and the patient was placed in different positions (sitting, verticalisation on a tilt-table, etc.).

With the purpose of normalising the postural tonus and facilitating activities in order to achieve functional movement, the emphasis was on the following active methods: Bobath technique (Bobath 1971), proprioceptive neuromuscular facilitation (Brunström 1970, Bobath 1971, Fay 1954) and biofeedback exercises (Mulder et al 1986). The decision of which therapeutic approach or their combination was to be used, has been made by the patient's therapist according to his or her professional training, experience and status of the patient. In all patients different kinds of audio-visual biofeedback devices, (from mirrors to EMG biofeedback devices) were used. When the patient reached conditions for gait, he or she started gait training using a passive ankle-foot orthosis or knee-ankle-foot orthosis.

The whole therapy program was conducted at the Institute of the Republic Slovenia for Rehabilitation in Ljubljana, Slovenia. All of the participating subjects were hospitalised in the center for at least the duration of our program (approximately 6 weeks).

2.4 MFES therapy

Surface electrical stimulation was applied on the peroneal nerve for ankle dorsiflexion, the soleus muscle for ankle plantar flexion, the hamstring muscles for knee flexion, the quadriceps muscle for knee extension, the gluteus maximus muscle for hip extension and stabilisation of the pelvis during stance, and optionally the triceps brachii muscle for reciprocal arm swing during the swing phase of ipsilateral leg. The stimulation sites were determined with cyclic stimulation before commencing the therapy. With the patient in a seated or prone position one pair of electrodes were shifted along each muscle or muscle group selected for stimulation until an optimal response was obtained. When determined, the sites were marked on the skin with non-conductive, semi-permanent ink. Amplitudes were raised until the functional response was satisfactory, or up to the level where the patient still felt comfortable with the sensation, if the functional response was unsatisfactory. Stimulation of the triceps brachii muscle was applied in patients with spastic arm if no pain was present with the purpose of relieving the muscle tonus and reducing shoulder subluxation (Rebersek et al 1982).

The following day, when commencing with gait, the amplitudes of the stimulating pulses were set to about 80% of the previously determined value because muscle response on FES in a standing position is different than in a seated or lying position. An excessive stimulation on all channels at the beginning could disturb the patient instead of providing assistance. All of the patients started gait using a crutch. The first steps were begun with the stimulation of the peroneal nerve, and after several steps, other channels were gradually switched on. The therapist accompanying the patient, supporting him or her on the affected side, induced correct weight shifting from one leg to the other, helped perform a step by rotating the pelvis, and orally provided some other essential instructions. In patients with disturbances in coordination another therapist assisted the patient in shifting and loading the crutch. Gradually, according to the progress of the particular patient crutch assistance was reduced and gait support diminished. The MFES therapy session generally lasted from 30 minutes to 1 hour, including the application of electrodes.

In MFES therapy the same therapist worked with all patients. In all MFES sessions an engineer was also present to handle the stimulator according to the instructions of the therapist, because the therapist was engaged in guiding and supporting the patient and could not handle the stimulator as well. The engineer was also needed in the event of some technical problems.

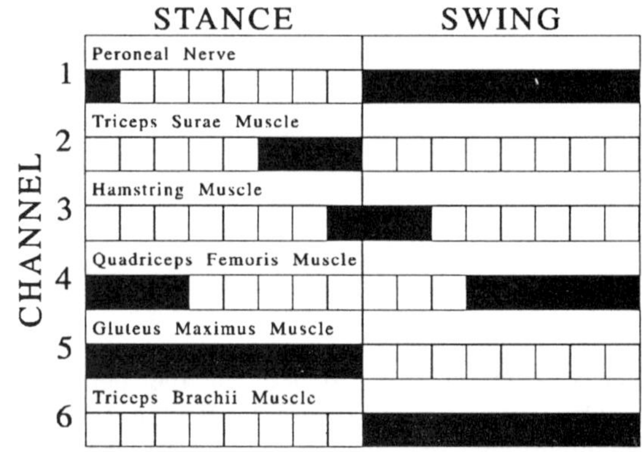

Fig. 1. Initial pattern of stimulation sequences. Stance and swing phases are each divided into eight equal time segments, which are represented by squares. Black squares represent stimulation on, and white squares represent stimulation off in the corresponding time segment of the stride phase.

An individualized stimulation sequence was determined for each patient, starting with a general initial pattern (Fig. 1) and modifying it during the first couple of stimulation sessions. Modification of a stimulation sequence consisted of prolonging, shortening and shifting the stimulation cycle with regard to the gait cycle. A trial-and-error approach based on previous experience was used for the correction of stimulation sequences until an optimum correction of anomalies was achieved. This optimum was usually achieved during the first two or three sessions. The stimulation sequence, was in some cases, modified once more later during the therapy if the patient developed some new gait anomaly (e.g. knee hyperextension).

During the MFES therapy period the "conventional" gait therapy described above was replaced by MFES assisted gait therapy or training. In our study, all patients continued to attend their other prescribed programs. Each patient participated in one therapy session per day (MFES or conventional therapy), five times a week. No therapy sessions were conducted on Saturdays and Sundays so that the patient could rest and go home for the weekend.

The patients walked on a 100 m walkway. At the beginning they covered a short distance, repeating it after a rest period. The initial distance depended on the subject's ability to avoid overexertion, or it was determined by the subject's physician. In the course of treatment the distance was gradually increased. The subjects, however, were instructed not to ambulate more than 600 m per session because the patient had to save some strength to participate in other rehabilitation programs. The distances that each patient covered on the first and on the last day of MFES treatment are listed in the right two columns of Table 1.

2.5 Instrumentation

The stimulator used in MFES therapy in this study contained six independent, galvanically separated channels with intermittent rectangular monophasic stimulation pulses (Pirnat et al 1981). The selected stimulating sequence on each channel was triggered optionally by a left or right foot-switch. Each foot-switch consisted of three switches connected in parallel, mounted into an insole and positioned one under the heel, one under the head of the first and one under the head of the fifth metatarsal. The amplitude of stimulation pulses was set between 0-120V in each channel separately, while frequency and pulse duration were preset internally to 30 Hz and 200 μs for all channels and were not varied. The maximum stimulating current was limited to 50 mA. No modulation of amplitude and pulse duration was used at the onset and end of the stimulation sequence. Stimulation timing during one gait cycle (the stimulation sequence) was timed for each channel using 16 switches, 8 for the stance phase and 8 for the swing phase. Each switch represented one eighth of the stance or swing phase. When the switch was on, stimulation occurred during the corresponding time interval of the stride phase. The durations of stimulation sequences were automatically adjusted to the walking rate of the patient by a microprocessor incorporated in the stimulator, permitting a stride time of up to seven seconds. The duration of stance and swing phases for both legs separately were extrapolated according to the durations of the last four phases, which were measured according to the signals from the foot-switches.

We used 5x9 cm self-adhesive electrodes or 5x8 cm felt pad electrodes for the stimulation of larger muscles and 5x5 cm electrodes for smaller muscles. We used 2.5 cm gauze button electrodes for peroneal nerve stimulation. The felt pad and button electrodes are soaked with tap water and fixed in position with elastic bandage.

At the beginning, at switch-over and at the end of the therapy period, the patient's gait speed, stride length and stride time was measured. The general physical status of the patient was also evaluated according to the Fugl-Meyer evaluation score. Stride length, time and speed were measured by a potentiometer with a wheel and fishing line (Bajd et al 1981).

The measurements described are mostly aimed at measuring time-distance variables during gait, but they tell little about the general condition of the patient. Therefore, additional subjective evaluation of the patient's physical performance was performed. A Fugl-Meyer evaluation system was selected (Fugl-Meyer et al 1975) to evaluate motor function, balance, several sensation qualities and joint function in hemiplegic patients. The test was performed in all subjects and evaluations by the same therapist. The result is a cumulative numeric score (range=0-226 points). The test evaluates the affected side and is divided into several parts: upper extremity, lower extremity, balance, sensation, and passive range of motion and pain.

2.6 Statistical procedures

The effects of compared therapies were evaluated according to the following measured variables: the results of mean gait speed, mean stride length, mean gait cadence and the Fugl-Meyer test. Each subject was measured three times: at the beginning of therapy, at switch-over and at the end of therapy. According to the selected experimental model a multivariate analysis of variance (MANOVA) of results was performed (Cochran et al 1957). Three factors were evaluated in the design: order of treatment (conventional/MFES, MFES/conventional), side of impairment (left, right), and performance of the patient (first, second, third). This lead to a $2 \times 2 \times 3$ MANOVA with the first two factors being between subjects and the last being a within subjects (repeated measures) factor. The performance of the patient was determined by set of four variables: gait speed, stride length, gait cadence and Fugl-Meyer score. The Wilks multivariate tests of significance involving performance within-subject effect for main effect of the performance, for the order of treatment $\times$ performance interaction and for order of treatment $\times$ side of impairment $\times$ performance interaction are presented. The side of impairment $\times$ performance interaction is not presented, because it gives no meaningful information concerning the particular experiment.

Source	Value	Exact F	DF_h	DF_e	p
Performance	0.094	7.234	8.00	6.00	0.013
Order × performance	0.094	7.244	8.00	6.00	0.013
Order × side × performance	0.301	1.696	8.00	6.00	0.268

Table 2. MANOVA of patients' performance determined by four measured parameters (gait speed, stride length, gait cadence, Fugl-Meyer score). DF_h=hypothetical degree of freedom. DF_e=error degree of freedom. p=probability established by Wilks multivariate tests of significance.

3 Results

Table 2 shows the results of MANOVA for four measures (gait speed, stride length, gait cadence and Fugl-Meyer test score) represented as performance. It can be seen that there is a significant main effect for performance ($p = 0.013$). The interaction between order of therapy and performance shows a significant impact of $p = 0.013$. Mean values of all individual measures that compose performance show, that during the therapy applied first, the improvement is greater compared to the improvement in the therapy applied second. The mean improvements during therapy with MFES were greater compared to the mean improvements during conventional therapy. These results show that MFES therapy combined with traditional therapy is more successful than conventional therapy alone. In an experiment such as this, with a relatively small number of subjects, there is the possibility that a distribution of subjects may bias one of the tested methods. In the experiment described, that happened for the distribution of subjects according to their side of affection. This parameter was not controlled by the protocol for assigning subjects to different groups. One group had 9 left and 1 right hemiplegic patient and the other group had 2 left and 8 right hemiplegic patients. To determine whether the affected side influenced the outcome of therapy, side of impairment was included as a factor in MANOVA. No effect could be shown in order of treatment × side of affection × performance interaction ($p > 0.1$). The side of affection did not appear to play significant role in the outcome of the study.

	T	L	V
FM	0.53 (0.02)	0.57 (0.01)	0.59 (0.01)

Table 3. Correlation coefficients between FM - Fugl-Meyer score, T - stride time, L - stride length, and V - gait speed.

	Age	T_p
FM	-0.29 (0.21)	-0.19 (0.43)
T	-0.17 (0.47)	0.004 (0.99)
L	-0.28 (0.26)	-0.13 (0.61)
V	-0.18 (0.46)	-0.15 (0.56)

Table 4. Correlation coefficients between the measured variables (FM - Fugl-Meyer score, T - stride time, L - stride length, V - gait velocity) and AGE - age of subjects, and T_p - time between onset of CVA and beginning of therapy.

Since the Fugl-Meyer test (FM) is designed to evaluate the integral physical status of the patient, we were also interested if it could be replaced by the measurement of T (mean stride time), L (mean stride length) or V (mean gait speed) or vice versa. Therefore, correlation coefficients between gait parameters (T, L, V) and FM were calculated. Table 3 presents the coefficients with their standard deviations (in parentheses). A relatively poor correlation could be found between the Fugl-Meyer score and T, L and V. This means that, although, these measures all show and backup the same general result, we can not use e. g. gait velocity for representation of patient's general status. Besides the described correlation coefficients, a couple more were calculated. We were interested in whether the measured parameters are correlated to the age of subjects (AGE) and to the time elapsed between the onset of CVA and the beginning of our program (T_p). As shown in Table 4, there is almost no correlation between those parameters. In most cases the coefficients are negative, which means better improvement at lower AGE and lower T_p, but the correlation is very poor. Other authors found a high correlation of improvement during rehabilitation with age and T_p (Andrews et al 1981, Katz et al 1966, Cassavan et al 1976) The inconsistency of our results with previous findings can be attributed to the fact that our group is relatively small and does not include a representative sample for the whole hemiplegic population.

4 Discussion

Conventional physiotherapeutic methods use different kinds of exercises to prepare the patient to bridge the gap between standing and gait. In our case, by using MFES, we enabled the patient to start gait without any special pre-training right at the beginning of therapy. The results of such an approach or the long-term effects are easy to assess or measure. There are two parameters which show the summation of effects of MFES therapy. The first one is independent gait. If the patient accomplishes independent gait as he or she continues to perform it, then the effect of the therapy is permanent. The second parameter is the duration of therapy. It is impossible to claim for any patient who participated in the study that he or she would not have been able to manage independent gait if MFES was not applied. However, according to the course of therapy, we clearly see that the progress during MFES therapy combined with traditional therapy was better than during conventional therapy. That means the patients need much less time in MFES therapy combined with traditional therapy to achieve the same state as they would with conventional therapy alone, i.e. rehabilitation time is shorter, patients return to their normal environment sooner and, last but not the least, rehabilitation costs are reduced.

In no case should MFES therapy be regarded as an autonomous therapeutic method. It can form only a part of an integral rehabilitation program. Excluding a patient from his whole program because of therapy with MFES would be unacceptable even from the ethical point of view. The patients, therefore, continued to attended all of their other normal therapeutic programs. A reduction of their intensity might have been allowed in order not to overexert the patient.

When we are looking for an explanation as to why MFES therapy is more successful than conventional therapies, we can see that MFES activates on two levels: direct and indirect. The direct effects are: functional movement as a result of FES induced muscle contraction, corrected synergistic movements, better coordination of extremities, better security and self-confidence of the patient and immediate start with gait at the onset of therapy. The indirect effects could be: improved and richer sensory feedback information to the CNS, possible enhancement of CNS plasticity, better and faster motor learning, and high motivation to participate in the program. All the direct effects enable the patient to walk and, by doing so, the rich influx of sensory information to the CNS is at least partially restored. It is known that sensory information is required for motor learning. If the patient wants to regain the volitional control of movement, a motor program or compensatory program must be established and, therefore, the motor system should be reorganized. It is presumed that useful motor activity is recognised as successful in higher centers in CNS and then somehow transferred back to lower centres (Brooks 1983). Learning, therefore, depends on previous experiences, sensations and movement. The ongoing communication between the motor and sensory system enhances learning. The feedback information is of crucial importance for learning as well as for the stimulation of CNS plasticity. The environment of a healthy subject is rich with sensations, while the abilities of perception in hemiplegic patients could be very limited. Therefore, we tried to use every possibility to improve the sensory inflow. This could be of great importance especially in patients with affected speech or understanding. Most of the conventional methods are based on verbal teaching and directing the patient's activities. If this communication channel is interrupted or damaged the efficiency of the method is much lower. MFES therapy also uses other channels which supplement or replace verbal communication.

Motivation is a vital factor in rehabilitation. The depression which could be regarded as opposite to motivation is highly correlated to the rehabilitation rate (Mayo et al 1991). The motivation of the patients in MFES therapy was quite evident. Every patient would like to get up and walk the way they used to, therefore, the immediate commencement with gait turned out to be very important for them and great eagerness to walk was observed.

Of course, there are also some limitations regarding MFES therapy. The stimulator used in the study was heavy and relatively large so that it sometimes additionally burdened the patient, who carried it on his/her back. In the most severe cases, another person had to carry the stimulator behind the patient. The daily application of electrodes is sometimes complicated and long-lasting. The staff involved in the application of MFES have to be highly trained and well experienced to perform the program. These limitations are more or less related to technology and can be considerably reduced in the future by employing high technology and a user-friendly stimulator design.

5 Conclusion

The study presented shows that an aggressive approach to gait relearning in severely involved hemiplegic patients by means of MFES offers the patient rapid progress in gait training, improved correction of gait anomalies, and a shorter period in which to reach independent gait. The MFES method is, however, in no case a comprehensive rehabilitation program; it serves only as a supplement to all existing therapeutic methods currently used in everyday practice. The target population comprises severely involved hemiplegic patients who are unable to walk independently or with an attendant. The method described should help those patients to progress faster and easier through the period from getting out of bed to independent gait or the point when they can continue rehabilitation of gait using simpler FES devices or various passive orthoses.

The experimental design, where each subject serves as his/her own control, turned out to be very effective. The number of participating subjects was reduced to 20, and despite the large heterogeneousness of the hemiplegic population, highly significant statistical results were obtained.

References

Anderson, T. P. (1982) Rehabilitation of patients with completed stroke. In Kottke FJ., Stillwell GK., Lehmann JF. (eds.), *Krusen's book of physical medicine and rehabilitation*, 3rd edition, W.B. Saunders Co., Philadelphia, pp. 583-603.

Brunnström, S. (1970) Movement therapy in hemiplegia, Harper & Row Publishers, New York.

Malezic, M., Kljajic, M., Acimovic R., et al. (1987) Therapeutic Effects of Multisite Electrical Stimulation of Gait in Motor-disabled Patients. *Arch Phys Med Rehab*, **68**, 553-560.

Bogataj, U., Gros, N., Malezic, M., et al. (1989) Restoration of gait during two to three weeks of therapy with multichannel electrical stimulation. *Phys Ther*, **69**, 319-327.

Marsolais, E. M., Kobetic, R., Barnicle, K., and Jacobs J. (1990) FNS application for restoring function in stroke and head-injury patients. *J of Clinical Engineering*, **15**, 489-496.

Jacobs-Daly, J., Barnicle, K., Kobetic, R., and Marsolais, E. B. (1993) Electrically induced gait changes post stroke, using an FNS system with intramuscular electrodes and multiple channels. *J Neuro Rehab*, **7**, 17-25.

Krishnaiah, P. R. (1980) Analysis of variance. Elsevier Science Publishers, New York.

Bobath, B. (1971) Adult hemiplegia evaluation and treatment. William Clowers & Sons Limited, London, Great Britain.

Fay, T. (1954) The use of pathological and unlocking reflexes in the rehabilitation of spastics, *Am J Phys Med*, **33**, 347-352.

Mulder, T., Hulstijn W., and van der Meer J. (1986) EMG feedback and the restoration of motor control. *Am J Phys Med*, **65**, 173-188.

Rebersek, S., Gros, N., Valencic, V. (1982) Functional electrical stimulation of arm swing during walking of hemiplegic patients. *World Congr. on Physics and Biomed. Eng.*, Hamburg, Gremany, 12.35.

Pirnat, P. and Trnkoczy, A. (1981) Further technical improvements of multichannel FES using microprocessor control. In Proc *7th Int. Symp. on External Control of Human Extremities*, Dubrovnik, Yugoslavia, pp. 317-326.

Bajd, T. and Kralj, L. (1980) Simple kinematic gait measurements. *J Biomed Eng*, **2**, 129-132.

Fugl-Meyer, A. R., Jääskö, L., Leyman, I., et al. (1975) The post stroke patient: A method for evaluation of physical performance. *Scand J Rehab Med*, **7**, 13-31.

Cochran, W. G., and Cox, G. M.(1957) Experimental designs. 2nd ed., John Weiley & Sons.

Katz, S., Ford, A. B., Chinn, A. B., and Newill, V. A. (1966) Prognosis after strokes. Part II: Long term course of 159 patients. *Medicine* (Balt.), **45**, 236-246.

Cassavan, A., Ross, A. L., Dyer, P. R., and Zane, L. (1976) Lateralisation in stroke syndrome. A factor in ambulation. *Arch Phys Med Rehab*, **57**, 583-587.

Brooks, V. B. (1983) Motor control: How posture and movements are governed. *Phys Ther*, **63**, 664-674.

Mayo, N. E., Korner-Bitensky, N. A., and Becker, R. (1991) Recovery time of independent function post-stroke. *Am J Phys Med Rehab*, **70**, 5-12.

Restoration of Gait by FES in Stroke and Spinal Cord Injury Patients

M. Maležič, S. Hesse, K. H. Mauritz
Klinik Berlin, Dept. of Neurological Rehabilitation, Free University Berlin, Germany

Abstract - Restoration of gait by functional electrical stimulation was updated in chronic non-ambulatory hemiparetic patients and in clinically complete paraplegic patients. In 6 hemiparetic patients, individually fitted multichannel stimulation of the lower, trunk and upper limb muscles, motor driven treadmill and body weight support induced functional gait without associated mass synergies in 3 to 6 weeks. Improvements of functional ambulation category, Rivermead Score, Motricity Index, stride length, cadence and gait velocity were recorded together with corrected gait pattern. The approach showed advantages when compared to regular physiotherapy and might restore gait in non-candidates for independent ambulation. Electrical stimulation of standing and gait in clinically complete paraplegic patients was modified in the course of treatment and in stimulation parameters. By substituting cyclic muscle strengthening by an active standing, 4 patients with T3 to T11 lesions started walking in 10 to 17 days. Stimulation of the quadriceps muscle and peroneal nerve by 16 and 60Hz respectively, reduced the fatigue and improved the flexor response.

1 Introduction

The aim of this study was to introduce recently modified techniques of restoration of gait by functional electrical stimulation (FES) both in chronic non-ambulatory hemiparetic patients and in clinically complete paraplegic patients. In the hemiparetic patients an intensive therapeutic treatment was conceptualized in order to initiate their gait and to reestablish the correct pattern within three to six weeks. In the paraplegic patients however, a permanent use of FES was applied.

It has been shown recently that a motor driven treadmill with partial body weight support and enforced stepping movements could effectively restore gait in spinal cord injury patients with various degrees of spastic paresis within 1.5 to several months (Wernig and Müller, 1992). It was efficient in single ambulatory hemiparetic patients without (Waagfjörd *et al.*, 1990) and with partial body weight support (Gregor *et al.*, 1992), as well as in 9 barely- or non-ambulatory hemiparetic patients (Hesse *et al.*, 1994).

It had also been shown before that five- to six channel electrical stimulation of the main lower extremity muscle groups, synchronized with the phases of stride, could successfully initiate the gait pattern and antigravity support in hemiparetic patients after stroke and brain injury. When applied in kinesiologicaly correct sequences it could restore their gait faster and further than conventional physiotherapeutic techniques within a couple of weeks. Eventually it could provide an independent ambulation with or even without a cane or crutch in severely affected hemiparetic patients, who would otherwise remain wheelchair bound (Malezic *et al.*, 1987; Bogataj *et al.*, 1989).

Therefore the multichannel FES and treadmill with partial body weight support were applied together for the restoration of gait in severely affected non-ambulatory hemiparetic patients. A combination of interactive stepping and externally induced muscle activation was expected to render potentiated effects of both methods. Additionally, by stabilization of the trunk, gait pattern could be restored without associated mass synergies (Davies, 1990), relieving also strenuous support of the therapist.

Clinically complete spinal cord injury patients were treated by a well established four channel surface electrical stimulation method for restoration of standing and walking (Kralj and Bajd, 1989). Both quadriceps muscles were stimulated for standing, while stepping was induced by the stimulation of combined ankle dorsiflexion and flexor withdrawal response at the peroneal nerve. Alternating stimulation between the quadriceps muscle and peroneal nerve on both lower limbs was controlled with manual switches by patients themselves.

According to the established method, the patients had been treated by a muscle strengthening program with a cyclic stimulation of the quadriceps muscle while lying preceding the electrically induced standing. The strengthening might have lasted weeks or even months before reaching standing ability of several minutes required for initiation of stimulated gait (Kralj and Bajd, 1989; Cybulski *et al.*, 1984). The stimulation frequency of 20Hz had been regarded optimal for both stimulation sites in all phases of the treatment. The modified method presented in this paper approached the time course of treatment and the stimulation parameters differently in order to substitute the preparatory period and improve responses to the stimulation.

2 Methods

2.1 Hemiparetic Patients

Six non-ambulatory male hemiparetic patients with the age from 30 to 71 years have completed the treatment so far. They were 3 right and 3 left side hemiparetic patients from 10 weeks to 6 years after stroke (4 subjects), tumor surgery (1 subject) and brain injury (1 subject). Two of the patients suffered from a neglect syndrome (Brain, 1941), one was hemianopic, one had Wallenberg syndrome with remained ataxia, one was globally aphasic, while the patient with brain injury had an additional incomplete T11-12 spinal cord lesion. They were all severely affected and were not able to walk in spite of previous conventional comprehensive rehabilitation program.

Similar treadmill system as described previously was used (Barbeau *et al.*, 1987). The patients walked suspended by a modified tandem parachute harness over a motor driven treadmill. The body weight support was set at approximately 30% by a spring scale and system of pulleys at the beginning and was gradually reduced to 5% during the first two weeks of the treatment. The spring scale with a rather long range of motion also dampened sudden loading during the stance phases of affected limb. The treadmill speed was chosen according to measurements of the free level gait and daily adjusted to abilities and preferences of the patients.

Multichannel electrical stimulation of the affected lower limb, trunk and upper limb muscles was applied by surface felt pad or self adhesive polymer electrodes. Two to three programmable dual channel stimulators (Malezic *et al.*, 1992) were connected together, forming so a four-to six channel stimulation unit. It provided a selection of the stimulation within 8 stance and 8 swing phase increments for every channel. Stimulator's microprocessor continuously adapted the duration of selected stimulation sequences to patient's gait cadence and synchronized them within the swing and stance phases respectively. Triple foot switches under both heels, lateral and medial metatarsals measured the phases of stride. Number of strides, average swing, stance and stride times for both legs were extracted from the stimulators together with their standard deviations and stance symmetry (affected versus nonaffected stance ratio) for a follow-up after each stimulation session.

Rectangular biphasic constant current pulses with the duration of 0.1 to 0.5ms and frequency of 20 to 30Hz were adjusted up to 50mA for strong but painless muscular contractions. Number of stimulation channels, electrode sites and sequences of the stimulation within the gait cycle were fitted to individual needs of the patients. A rather rigid stimulation paradigm, as used previously (Bogataj *et al.*, 1989; Malezic *et al.*, 1987), was tried to be avoided in favor of a simple, clinically viable application. Less intervention for the same effect was one of the main criteria there. Three to six stimulation channels were applied for the correction of gait deficiencies, as assessed by clinical gait analysis (Perry, 1992).

Quadriceps muscle was stimulated for knee extension in the terminal swing and first part of the stance phase in all six patients. Wet, 8 x 5cm bipolar felt pad electrodes were placed over the muscle bellies with the distal cathode placed more medially and proximal anode more laterally. Peroneal nerve was stimulated for dorsal flexion and moderate eversion during the swing and initial stance phase in five patient. Monopolar electrode set with a 10 x 2.5cm anode and 2.5cm round cathode on a single Velcro band was used. In one patient, who could not tolerate the peroneal nerve stimulation, the 8 x 5cm bipolar electrodes were placed over tibialis anterior, extensor hallucis and extensor digitorum longus muscles, covering also a part of peroneus longus and brevis muscles. Gluteus maximus muscle was stimulated for hip extension throughout the stance phase by the

8 x 5cm bipolar electrodes five times, in one of the four patients bilaterally. Gluteus medius and minimus muscles were similarly stimulated for the hip abduction in four patients. A combined shoulder/arm stimulation was applied during the swing of ipsilateral leg in four patients and abdominal muscles were stimulated during the stance phase of affected leg twice.

The combined shoulder/arm stimulation was performed by bipolar 13 x 5cm self adhesive polymer electrodes, one over supraspinatus and part of trapezius muscles and another slanting downwards from the lower part of deltoid muscle over the lateral head of triceps brachii muscle. The stimulation was introduced for simultaneous abduction and elevation of the shoulder, its retroversion and extension of the elbow. It should provide a release of associated spastic pattern of arm flexion during gait (Davies, 1990) when present, correction of the depressed shoulder and a reactive reciprocal arm swing during the following swing of contralateral leg. In addition, a sustained trunk erection was expected by a compensatory reflex activation of the lumbar erector spinae muscles (Ertiken and Ertekin, 1981 and 1982) that should stabilize the trunk and align the pelvis, both considered as integral parts of physiological gait (Davies, 1990).

Instead of separate stimulation of the knee extensors and flexors for a good weight acceptance and prevention of the knee hyperextension in the first part of stance phase, adding also separate stimulation of the hip extensors and/or hip abductors during the stance phase when necessary, a stimulation of the abdominal muscles was introduced in two patients. Instead of previous three to four stimulation channels a single one, with lower of the bipolar 13 x 5cm self adhesive electrodes over both rectus abdominis muscles under the navel and the upper one extending from the rectus abdominis to the external abdominal oblique muscle on the affected side above the navel, was applied for a protraction of the pelvis during the stance phase.

The treatment included 13 to 33 daily treadmill/stimulation sessions from 10 minutes at the beginning to something more than half an hour at the end of treatment, depending on physical and psychical condition of the patients. The patients found walking on the treadmill tiresome after that period, probably both from physical (walking with reduced inertia) and psychological reasons (monotony). They were also not encouraged to walk faster or "long distances", but the correct gait pattern was stressed throughout the sessions. Besides verbal support the patients were helped manually at the beginning of the treatment by a skilled physiotherapist. The help included stabilization of the trunk, its alignment, initiation of the swing or placement of the foot when necessary The stimulation parameters were also readjusted with changes of gait pattern during the course of treatment.

First four patients received the treadmill/stimulation treatment besides their conventional physiotherapy. They were clinically tested and their gait was measured at the beginning, in the middle and at the end of treatment. In the last two patients a single case research approach B-A-B study was applied with 15 treadmill/stimulation treatments (B phase), 15 days of comprehensive neurodevelopmental (Bobath, 1978) physiotherapeutic program (A phase) and again 15 days of the treadmill/stimulation. They were clinically tested once and their gait was measured twice every five days of the weekly sessions.

The clinical tests included functional ambulation category assessment, hierarchical Rivermead motor assessment score designed for hemiparetic patients, motricity index and modified Ashworth spasticity scale (Wade, 1992). The same two independent physiotherapists tested the patients throughout the treatment. Mean gait velocity, stride length, and cadence were assessed together with ground reaction forces before, in the middle and at the end of treatment. Infotronic CDG system with a RAM recording unit and overshoe slippers, containing 8 sensors each, was used for measurements of the vertical ground reaction forces and time parameters of gait. The velocity, stride length, cadence and ground reaction forces were recorded at self adopted speed.

The stance and swing phase duration and symmetry statistics during the stimulation were recorded by the stimulators themselves daily after each session. To illustrate direct effects of the stimulation, the ground reaction forces were recorded with and without the stimulation in the last patient.

2.2 Paraplegic Patients

Four male paraplegic patients with the age from 24 to 38 years have been treated so far. They were all clinically complete with the lesions at T3, T4, T6 and T11 spinal cord levels after car accidents dating back from 16 months to 16 years. Two of them were in-patients and had two FES sessions a day, while the other two out-patients came for one daily session during the first month of treatment. The patients had practiced passive standing attached to a standing board, two of them had also used knee-ankle-foot ortheses before the FES program.

Two commercially available IJS ALT-2 dual channel stimulators were used for the alternating stimulation of quadriceps muscle and peroneal nerve on both sides. Bipolar 8 x 5cm felt pad electrodes were used for the quadriceps muscle, while the peroneal nerve was stimulated by a 2.5cm round active electrode, using the distal quadriceps electrode as a neutral one. In two patients the 2.5cm electrodes were replaced by 1cm round ones in order to stimulate the nerve by lower amplitudes more selectively.

The stimulation program excluded any preceding cyclic stimulation in a lying or sitting position. Instead, the patients started standing by the bilateral quadriceps muscle stimulation at the very beginning. They first used a standing frame with handles and elbow support and switched to a rolling walker before starting electrically stimulated stepping. One of the patients combined the walker with elbow crutches at the later stage of rehabilitation.

At the beginning, constant current charge balanced stimulation pulses (up to 150mA, 0.25ms) with the 20Hz frequency were used for both stimulation sites. As the flexor response was diminished after several months of the stimulation, higher amplitudes were required, stimulating not only the peroneal but also the tibial nerve in vicinity. The hip and knee flexion were accompanied by a plantar flexion, which prevailed over the dorsal flexion in the ankle due to the stronger triceps surae muscles. Functional flexor response was impeded by the diminished foot clearance. Therefore, higher stimulation frequencies were investigated for elicitation of the flexor response together with the smaller electrodes.

Medelec Mystro MS 92 electrophysiologic system was used for that purpose. Surface EMG responses of the tibialis anterior, soleus, biceps femoris and rectus femoris muscles were recorded by IVM Ag-AgCl electrodes attached 2.5cm apart over the muscle bellies. The responses were stimulated by the electrodes and sites as used for the stimulation during gait. Besides 20Hz, frequencies of 50Hz and 100Hz with amplitudes adjusted for a functionally optimal response were tested with the patient in a supine position. The response itself was measured in the sagittal plane during the stimulation while standing. Reflective markers were attached to the hip, knee and ankle joint axes, heel and toes. Selspot II 3D motion analysis system with two cameras was employed for recording of the stimulated flexor response in the lower limb at different frequencies.

3 Results

3.1 Hemiparetic patients

Clinical tests showed an improvement of walking ability in all the patients. Results of the assessment of functional ambulation category, Rivermead motor assessment score for the leg and trunk and motricity index for the affected leg are presented in table 1.

Pat	FAC				RLT				MIL			
	S	B	A	E	S	B	A	E	S	B	A	E
1	0			3	2			4	34			43
2	2			5	3			5	34			45
3	2			3	5			6	43			43
4	1			2	6			7	34			62
5	1	2	2	4	5	6	8	8	33	54	54	54
6	0	1	1	3	2	3	4	5	24	34	24	24

Table 1. Clinical tests. Pat: patient, FAC: functional ambulation category, RLT: Rivermead score for the affected leg and trunk, MIL: motricity index for the affected leg, S: start, B: treadmill/stimulation, A: physiotherapy, E: end

The functional ambulation category, observing required assistance of the therapist, improved in average for 233%. It increased from the initial 0 (unable to walk / 2 patients), 1 (continuous support / 2 patients) and 2 (intermittent support / 2 patients) to final 2 (1 patient), 3 (stand by /3 patients), 4 (independent, level ground / 1 patient) and maximum possible 5 (independent / 1 patient). The Rivermead score, assessing maneuvers of the leg and trunk while lying and standing, improved somewhat less: in average for 52%, from 3.8 to 5.8 of maximum possible 10 points. Average improvement of the motricity index, assessing volitional ankle, knee and hip flexions while sitting, reached 34%, from mean 34 to 45 points out of possible 100. In the last two patients, assessed in the B-A-B study, the functional ambulation category improved only during the treadmill/stimulation phases, the Rivermead score improved throughout the treatment, while the motricity index levelled after the first treadmill/stimulation phase.

Improvement of the Rivermead score for general functions, such as transfer from bed to wheelchair, from sitting to standing etc., was moderate (32%) and independent of the treatment. Motricity index of the affected hand did in average not progress and Ashworth spasticity scale remained stable regardless of the treatment.

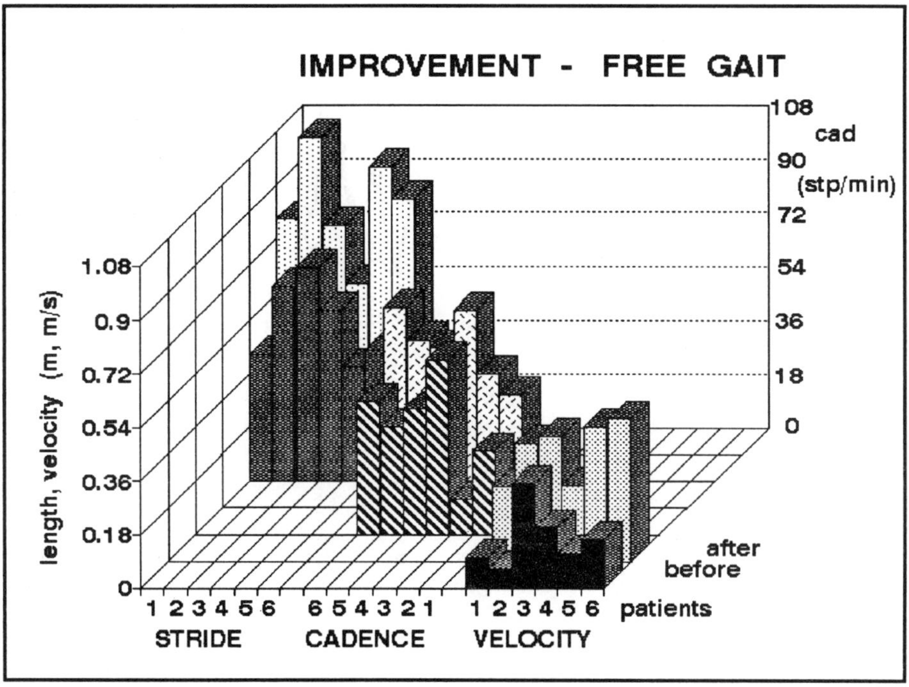

Fig. 1. Improvements in the 6 hemiparetic patients during level gait without stimulation.

Mean stride length, cadence and velocity, assessed together with the ground reaction forces before and after the treatment, are displayed in figure 1. They improved in all the patients, with the exception of stride length, which remained the same in patient No. 4. Average improvements reached 66% in stride length, 76% in cadence and 196% in gait velocity. The improvements substantially increased during the first treadmill/stimulation phase in the patient No. 5: stride length 126%, cadence 55%, velocity 247%, and levelled-up during the subsequent physiotherapy and treadmill/stimulation phases to final 149%, 56% and 281% respectively. With the levelling-up of the stride length, cadence and gait velocity during the physiotherapy and second treadmill/stimulation phases, symmetries of the stance, swing, step and double support durations improved further during the last treadmill/stimulation phase in this patient, all eventually approaching 90%. In patient No. 6, a considerable improvement (stride length 65%, cadence 8.4%, velocity 79%) was followed by a moderate further change during the physiotherapy (+17%, +11.2%, -1%) and again by an increase to the final 98%, 40% and 176% respectively. Improvements of the cadence reached their peaks in the middle of second treadmill/stimulation phase in both patients and of the velocity in the last one.

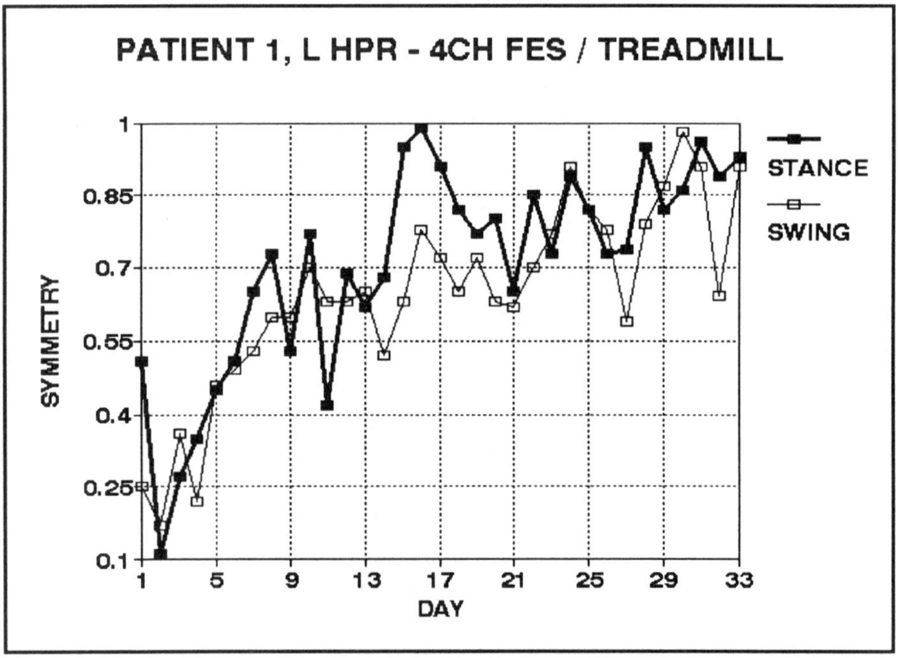

Fig. 2. Stance and swing time symmetry in the left hemiparetic patient No. 1 during the 4-channel stimulation on the treadmill.

The stance and swing phase duration and symmetry statistics during the stimulation, recorded daily after each session, showed a decrease of average stance and swing times on both sides. Stance to swing ratio improved especially on the affected side, the same as the stance and swing symmetry ratios between the affected and non-affected lower limb. As seen in figure 2, the stance and swing duration symmetries of patient No. 1, very low at the beginning of therapy, increased consistently and reached almost one at the end of treatment.

3.2 Paraplegic Patients

All 4 patients tolerated the modified training program with immediate standing well. There were no cardiovascular or orthopedic problems. As presented in figure 3, they stood from 1.5 to 10 minutes in the standing-frame during the first session. They reached 25 to 40 minutes of standing in 10 to 17 days and the next day the FES-walking program was initiated. Drop of the standing time during the preparatory period in the second patient (T4 lesion) in figure 3 was due to a high temperature for 2 days, which delayed the beginning of FES walking. One day drops of the standing duration in the third and fourth patient were caused by a switch from the standing frame to rolling walker before the start of FES gait.

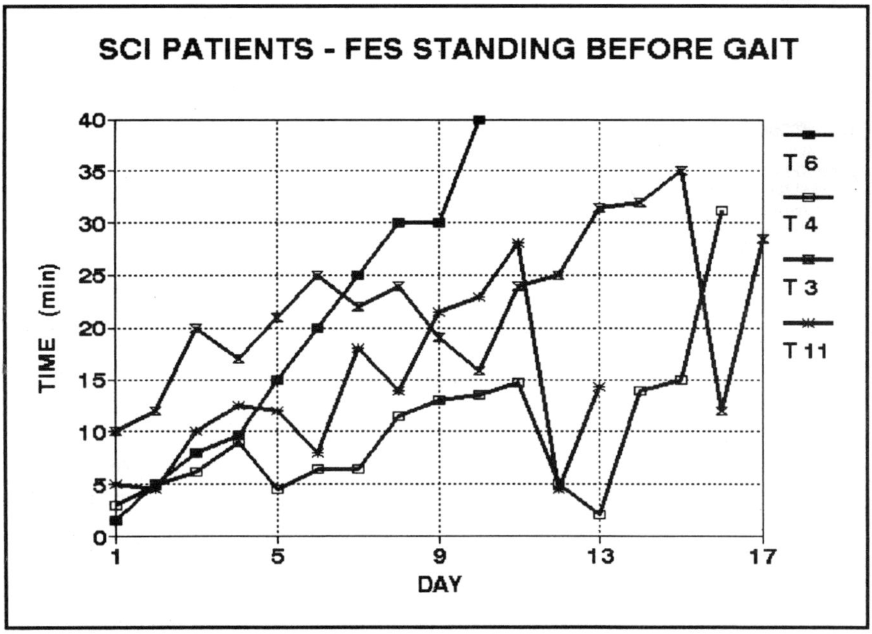

Fig. 3. Standing of the 4 paraplegic patients by FES before the stimulated gait.

The first patient (T6) started walking for 30 minutes in the first day (figure 4), reached 45 minutes in five days and over one hour in 10 days. The second patient started walking for 3 minutes and reached 30 minutes in eight days. The third patient started walking with 12 minutes, dropped to 4 minutes the next day and reached 20 minutes in eight days. The fourth patient started with 3 minutes and reached 30 minutes in ten days. The patients walked very slowly at the beginning, covering only short distances. Their walking speed gradually increased and reached a functional level much later. Only the first patient has been able to cover long distances and walk for a couple of hours so far. Presently he also walks with crutches and climbs stairs.

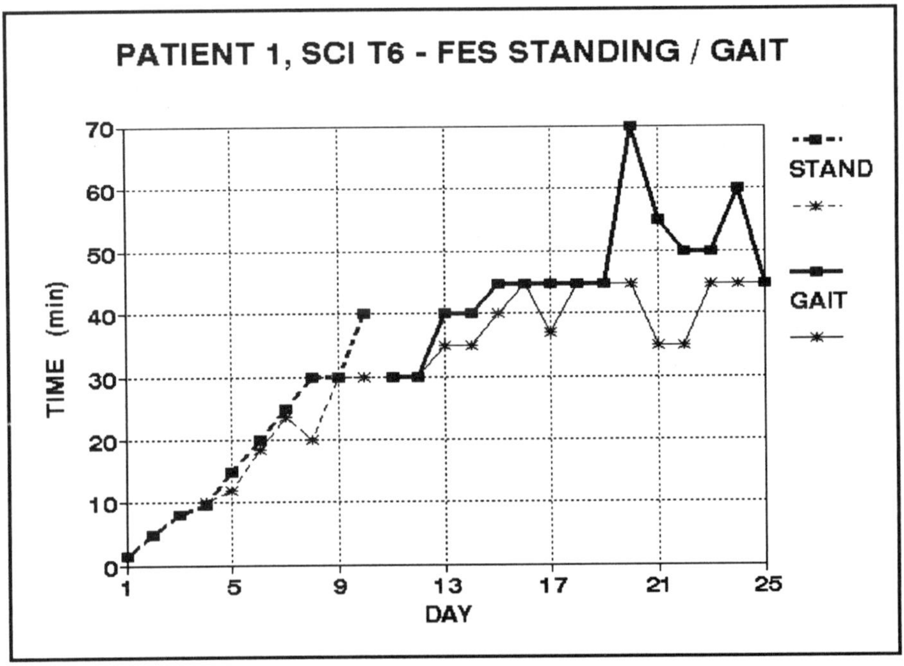

Fig. 4. FES standing and gait of the paraplegic patient No. 1 (T6 lesion) during the first 25 days.

The others perform FES standing and gait for exercise purposes with a reduction of spasticity, improved muscles, appearance and self-esteem. The second patient, whose lower limbs had been exceedingly cold before the FES-program, benefited from a better thermoregulation. He could abandon wool underwear and heating in bed during the summer. In the fourth patient dysaesthesias at the level of lesion were diminished. A urinary infection with the need for antibiotic treatment occurred only once over a period of several months in one patient.

In the first (T6), second (T4) and fourth patient (T11) a diminution of the flexor response was observed after several months of the stimulation. Therefore a higher stimulation frequency was successfully applied. The effect of higher stimulation frequency for the flexor response is illustrated in figure 5. Selspot II stick-figures display better flexions of all three lower limb joints in the sagittal plane at 50Hz when compared to 20Hz. The corresponding EMG recordings revealed better ratio among the flexor response of the tibialis anterior, soleus, biceps and rectus femoris muscles. At 50Hz the area and peak-to-peak amplitude of the tibialis anterior and biceps femoris muscles remained similar whereas the values of the soleus and rectus femoris muscles decreased. A diminished ankle dorsal flexion with good knee- and hip flexions were recorded at 100Hz.

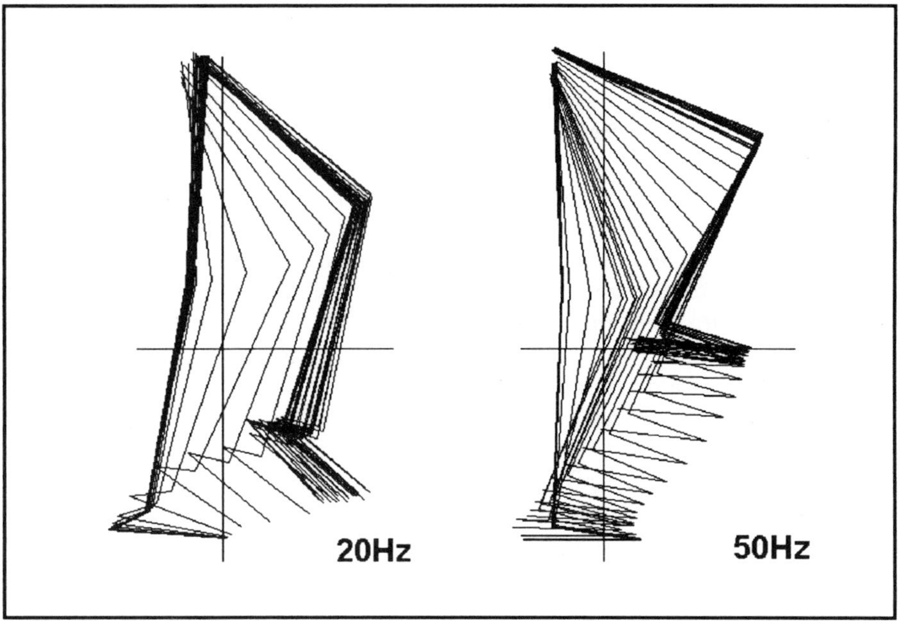

Fig. 5. Effect of the stimulation frequency on the flexor response.

4 Discussion

4.1 Hemiparetic Patients

The treadmill with partial body weight support combined with the multichannel electrical stimulation was expected to render potentiated results of both methods. By stabilization of the trunk and reduction of the load, missing equilibrium reflexes were substituted. Enforced stepping movements, together with externally activated major lower limb and trunk muscles, enabled the execution of complex gait instead of only its single elements. Physiotherapists, relieved of strenuous manual support, could better concentrate on patient's gait. The gait pattern was additionally induced and restored by the multichannel electrical stimulation of the lower middle and upper body segments. Its methods have been updated during the still going-on study.

The introduced shoulder/arm stimulation compensated for a lack of abduction, elevation, and retroversion of the shoulder, as well as for an extension of the elbow, providing a release of associated spastic pattern of arm flexion during gait (Davies, 1990), correction of the depressed shoulder and a reactive reciprocal arm swing during the following swing of contralateral leg at the same time. Besides, it was found previously that single electrical stimuli, applied to the brachial plexus at the Erb's point, caused compensatory reflex activation of the ipsilateral and more strongly of the contralateral lumbar erector spinae muscles within 100ms while standing (Ertekin and Ertekin, 1981). Size of the response was increased in patients with spastic hemiparesis as compared with normal subjects (Ertekin and Ertekin, 1982). By the shoulder/arm stimulation, as described in this paper, a sustained contraction of the paraspinal muscles with erection of the trunk was also achieved by a train of 20 to 30Hz pulses.

The problem of poor weight acceptance, followed by the knee hyperextension with associated ankle plantar flexion, insufficient hip extension and abduction often originate in weak or inactive lower abdominal muscles, as the pelvis is not tilted up in the front (Davies, 1990). Instead of previous three to four stimulation channels, used for the stimulation of knee extensors and flexors together with the hip extensors and/or hip abductors, a single one on the abdominal muscles corrected the above deficiencies in two patients. By tilting the pelvis forward, it was also stabilized together with the correction of an excessive lordosis in one of the patients.

The studied severely affected patients had been previously treated by a comprehensive neurodevelopmental rehabilitation program (Bobath, 1978) without regaining walking ability. Their time after disease onset excluded major influence of spontaneous recovery. They all could walk after the treadmill/stimulation program with at least an intermittent support in one patient, while three needed a stand-by verbal support and two were independent. Patient No. 4, who gained only one functional ambulation category level, suffered from ataxia due to an additional Wallenberg syndrome.

With the substantial improvement of walking ability, Rivermead score, not related to gait and only partly to posture, did not improve to such extent and the motricity index, performed while sitting, even less. This indicated a significance of the task-oriented training for restoration of gait. Improvement of the walking ability only during the treadmill/stimulation phases in the last two patients, with unspecific improvement of the Rivermead score and levelling of the motricity index in the first treadmill/stimulation phase, additionally support this indication. With unchanged Ashworth spasticity scale, the role of tone-inhibiting maneuvers, prevailing in the neurodevelopmental technique, might also be questionable.

Velocity, cadence and stride length improved uniformly in all the patients. The improvements exceeded 60% in all three parameters, while the mean velocity, as the final intent of mobility, increased even three times. Two patients, included in the B-A-B study, showed a marked increase of the stride length, cadence and velocity during the first phase. Later the parameters levelled-up in one patient, while after a delay during the physiotherapy phase they increased further in the second treadmill/stimulation phase. In spite of plateau of the parameters after the first B phase in the patient No. 5, symmetries of the stance, swing, step and double support additionally improved further during the second B phase, all eventually approaching normal values. After reaching functional stride length, cadence and gait velocity levels, the gait pattern thus improved further by the treadmill/stimulation treatment. Moreover, its value was pointed out by the increase, delay and again increase of the values during the three phases in the patient No. 6.

The treadmill/stimulation therapy could play an important role in the restoration of gait in hemiparetic patients, who had not been able to achieve an independent ambulation through conventional physiotherapeutic techniques. Only in stroke patients, one third of them do not regain their gait ability at least in the first three months with meager prospects for further improvement (Wade *et al.*, 1987). The new approach could successfully be applied as an intensive initial treatment of these patients. They could later follow less demanding rehabilitation methods in- or outside clinical environment.

4.2 Paraplegic Patients

Currently used FES methods for standing and walking of spinal cord injury patients include also an initial strengthening program of the antigravity muscles. Cyclic stimulation of the quadriceps muscles at isotonic conditions in a lying patient might last several months before sufficient knee joint torques of around 50Nm for the beginning of standing and walking are achieved (Kralj and Bajd, 1989). The average re strengthening time was found to be approximately 1 month, but there was a considerable variability (Cybulski *et al.*, 1984). In a recent report on incomplete spinal cord injury patients, the inferior isotonic strengthening was replaced by a progressive resisted quadriceps conditioning with weights attached at the ankle (Granat *et al.*, 1993) which lasted 6 months and was completed by all the patients.

On the other hand, it was demonstrated in chronic nonambulatory hemiparetic patients that an immediate walking with FES could provide their gait without support of accompanying therapist in two to three weeks (Malezic *et al.*, 1987; Bogataj *et al.*, 1989). With sometimes much better preserved lower limb muscles due to spasticity and complete support of the upper limbs in paraplegic patients, the immediate standing without previous tedious conditioning was found rational. The active approach as an alternative challenged both research and patient part of the team. Possible hazards due to disuse bone demineralization in the paraplegic patients were reduced by the fact that they had performed passive standing and even braced walking before the FES program. In the heaviest patient (84kg), long bones of the lower limbs were additionally examined by X-ray.

Standing by the help of electrical stimulation itself appeared to be much more efficient muscle strengthening exercise than cyclic conditioning with the patient lying. During the latter, the patients had not been participating actively from obvious reasons; sometimes they were reading or even sleeping. By the stimulated standing however, the quadriceps muscles were strengthened isometrically with an active participation of the patient, including the remained trunk and whole upper extremity muscles, postural reflexes and acquaintance with the new body position.

The acquaintance correlated with a feeling of security and ability of the patient. Its importance was clearly demonstrated during the switch from standing in the frame to standing with the walker in the last two patients. The ability of uninterrupted standing was reduced to 34% in the third patient and even to 14% in the fourth one during the first day with walker. The standing time already increased from 14% to 36% in the fourth patient during the afternoon session of the same day. During the second day with the rolling walker it returned to 80% and 50% respectively in both patients and the next day they started walking.

Habituation of the flexion reflex with prolonged electrical stimulation had been reported in spinal cord injury patients both in basic (Dimitrijevic and Nathan, 1970 and 1971) and clinical reports (Jaeger and Kralj, 1983; Nicol *et al.,* 1991). During neurophysiological studies of the flexion reflex in spinal cord injury patients 500 to 1000Hz (Hagbarth, 1960) or 2000Hz stimulation (Dimitrijevic and Nathan, 1970 and 1971) had been applied. Clinical reports on FES, however, sticked to the 20Hz not only for the stimulation of quadriceps muscle but also for the flexor response. While the low frequency is perfectly justified for the antigravity muscles in order to reduce fatigue, the reason for its application in the flexor response is not obvious.

The present work showed that an increased frequency rendered better flexor response. As the reflex response was combined with direct stimulation of the ankle dorsal flexion, the frequency of 60Hz was finally chosen. It also offered a viable solution for small portable stimulators. For this reason and from the aspect of fatigue, the frequency for the quadriceps muscle was reduced to 16Hz, which still provided a tetanic contraction.

5 Acknowledgements

The study was supported by a Grant No. 91.050.1 of the Wilhelm Sander - Stiftung. The authors are also indebted to Ms. Antje Schaffrin and Ms. Daniela Lücke for their contribution in the study.

References

Barbeau, H., Wainberg, W., and Finch, L. (1987) Description and application of a system for locomotor rehabilitation. Med Biol Eng Comput, 25 341-344.

Bobath, B. (1978) Adult Hemiplegia; Evaluation and Treatment. Heinemann, London.

Bogataj, U., Gros, N., Malezic, M., Kelih, B., Kljajic, M., and Acimovic, R. (1989) Restoration of gait during two to three weeks of therapy with multichannel electrical stimulation. Phys Ther, 69 319-327.

Brain, W. (1941) Visual disorientation with special reference to lesions of the right cerebral hemisphere. Brain, 64 244272.

Cybulski, G. R., Penn, R. D., and Jaeger, R. J. (1984) Lower extremity functional neuromuscular stimulation in cases of spinal cord injury. Neurosurgery 15 132-146.

Davies, P. M. (1990) Right in the Middle; Selective Trunk Activity in the Treatment of Adult Hemiplegia. Springer-Verlag, Berlin, Heidelberg, New York, London, Paris, Tokyo, Hong Kong.

Dimitrijevic, M. R. and Nathan, P. W. (1970) Studies of spasticity in man: 4. changes in flexion reflex with repetitive cutaneous stimulation in spinal man. Brain, 93 743-768.

Dimitrijevic, M. R. and Nathan, P. W. (1971) Studies of spasticity in man: 5. dishabituation of the flexion reflex in spinal man. Brain, 94 77-90.

Ertekin, N. and Ertekin, C. (1981) Erector spinae muscle responses while standing. J Neurol Neurosurg Psychiatry, 44 73-78.

Ertikin, N., and Ertekin, C. (1982) Reflex erector spinal responses in disorders of the central nervous system. Acta Neural Scand, 66 690-696.

Granat, M. H., Ferguson, A. C. B., Andrews, B.J., and Delargy, M. (1993) The role of functional electrical stimulation in the rehabilitation of patients with incomplete spinal cord injury - observed benefits during gait studies. Paraplegia, 31 207-215.

Gregor, R. J., Dobkin, B., and Fowler, E.G. (1992) Interaction between motion analysis lab and physical therapy. Proceedings of the European Symposium on Clinical Gait Analysis, Zurich, Switzerland, 99-103.

Hagbarth, K. E. (1960) Spinal withdrawal reflexes in human lower limbs. J Neurol Neurosurg Psychiatry, 23 222-227.

Hesse, S., Bertelt, C., Schaffrin, A., Malezic, M., and Mauritz, K. H. (1994) Restoration of gait in non-ambulatory hemiparetic patients by treadmill training with partial body weight support. Arch Phys Med Rehabil, submitted.

Jaeger, R. J. and Kralj, A. (1983) Studies in functional electrical stimulation for standing and forward progression. Proc 6th Annual Conference on Rehabilitation Engineering, San Diego, California, RESNA, Bethesda, 75-77.

Kralj, A. and Bajd, T. (1989) Functional electrical stimulation: standing and walking after spinal cord injury. CRC Press, Inc., Boca Raton, Florida.

Malezic, M., Bogataj, U., Gros, N., Kelih, B., Kljajic, M., and Acimovic, R. (1987) Evaluation of gait with multichannel electrical stimulation. Orthopedics, 10 769-772.

Malezic, M., Kljajic, M., Acimovic-Janezic, R., Gros, N., Krajnik, J., and Stanic, U. (1987) Therapeutic effects of multisite electric stimulation of gait in motor-disabled patients. Arch Phys Med Rehabil, 68 553-560.

Malezic, M., Bogataj, U., Gros, N., Decman, I., Vrtacnik, P., Kljajic, M., and Acimovic-Janezic, R. (1992) Application of a programmable dual-channel adaptive electrical system for the control and analysis of gait. J Rehab Res & Develop, 29 41-53.

Nicol, D. J., Granat, M.H., Baxendale, R.H., and Andrews B. J. (1991) Dishabituation of the flexion reflex in spinal man. J Physiol.

Perry, J. (1992) Gait Analysis; Normal and Pathological Function. Slack Inc., Thorofare, New Jersey.

Waagfjörd, J., Levangle, P. K., and Certo, C. M. E. (1990) Effects of treadmill training on gait in a hemiparetic patient. Phys Ther, 70 549-560.

Wade, D. T. (1992) Measurement in neurological rehabilitation. Oxford University Press, Oxford, New York, Tokyo.

Wade, D. T., Wood, V. A., Heller, A., Maggs, J., and Hewer, R. L. (1987) Walking after stroke. Scand J Rehab Med,19: 25-30.

Wernig, A. and Müller, S. (1992) Laufband locomotion with body weight support improved walking in persons with severe spinal cord injuries. Paraplegia, 1992 30 229-238.

Long Term Electrically Induced Cycling in SCI. A Pilot Study

T. Mohr[1,2], P. Tornøe[2], F. Biering-Sørensen[3], J. Pødenphant[2], J. Andersen[4], A. Wagner[5], H. Galbo[1] and M. Kjær[2]
[1]Dept. of Med. Physiology, University of Copenhagen, Panum Institute, DK
[2]Copenhagen Muscle Research Centre, Department of Internal Medicine, DK
[3]Centre for Spinal Cord Injured, Neuroscience Centre, Copenhagen, DK
[4]August Krogh Institute, University of Copenhagen, DK
[5]Dept. of Neuroradiology, National University Hospital, Copenhagen, DK

Abstract - The aim of the present study was to evaluate the long term effects of electrically induced bicycling performed by spinal cord injured subjects. The stimulation was applied via a closed loop controlled stimulator, using the REGYS rehabilitation system. Subjects were scheduled to train for a period of one year, training three times a week for 30 minutes.

Pre- and post training evaluation was done. Parameters thought to be influenced by level of physical activity were measured before and after different periods of training.

The whole body exercise performance was evaluated by measurement of maximal oxygen uptake rate and cardiac performance by echo cardiography and isotope scintigraphy of the myocardium. Pulmonale status was evaluated by measuring diffusion capacities and by functional tests. Muscle and bone adaptation to training was evaluated by histochemistry, single fibre types determination, enzyme activity and MR images of the thigh. Furthermore, bone mineral content of the lower limb was measured and blood lipid status as well as coagulation parameters were determined.

After 6 months of training in three subjects, an increase in maximal oxygen uptake rate and in muscle mass of the thigh was found. In addition a shift in muscle fibres of the trained muscles towards fibres with higher oxidative capacity was seen. Bone mineral content of the proximal tibia was increased at one-year of training. At this preliminary state, we conclude that this training is of potential value in preventing inactivity related secondary problems in spinal cord injured persons.

1 Introduction

Spinal cord injury (SCI) is not only a problem due to the various paralysis of the body, but serious secondary problems are related to the physical inactive lifestyle of the SCI individuals. In the years postinjury these individuals usually develop a variety of degenerative changes associated with inactivity. These changes are previously described to include cardiovascular deconditioning, decreased pulmonary function, muscular atrophy including decreased muscle volume, decreased enzyme activity and fibre type transformation towards glycolytic type II fibres (Cowell et al.1986; Biering-Sorensen et al.1991; Davis 1993; Bauman et al.1992b; Bauman et al.1992a). When lack of sensibility is present, muscle atrophy together with decreased muscle blood flow is the major course to pressure sores. Furthermore postinjury changes also involve increased levels of blood lipids, increased coagulability and osteoporosis of the lower extremities in spinal cord injured individuals (Biering-Sorensen et al.1990; Ragnarsson et al.1981; Winther et al.1992; Biering-Sorensen et al.1988).

It has previously been described that functional electrical stimulation has a beneficial effect on some of the inactivity-related parameters (Ragnarsson et al.1988; Ragnarsson 1986). However, most literature on the topic only concerns evaluation of the effects of training by means of FES after relatively short term use and our aim was to establish whether these effects are increased when the training period was prolonged. Some of the parameters shows no change in previous studies, and we wanted to investigate if the lack of change was due to the short period of training that has been used in previous studies (Leeds et al.1990; Rodgers et al.1991; Petrofsky et al.1992; Garland et al.1992; Faghri et al.1992).

2 Materials and Methods

Three individuals with SCI participated in a one year pilot program of functional electrical stimulation (FES) of their paralysed leg muscles. They had all complete loss of motor functions below the level of lesion, but one had some sensibility, yet not enough to make the stimulation intolerable.

To gain benefits from the training, the aim was to train three times a week, 30 minutes each training bout.

Each training bout was carried out in the unit for spinal cord injured and supervised by a physiotherapist. The SCI subjects were placed in a sitting position, fastened with a belt around the hips, on the computer-controlled functional electrical stimulation exercise ergometer (REGYS I Clinical Rehabilitation System, Therapeutic Technology Inc., Tampa, USA) (Petrofsky et al.1984b; Petrofsky et al.1984a). The system was comprised of three subsystems: a lower extremity ergometer (Monark ergometer), a stimulus control unit and a reclinable patient chair. The stimulus control unit was a computer controlling and monitoring the electrical stimulation according to prescribed parameters (see below) entered into a microprocessor by a remote control keyboard. Before exercise, surface electrodes were placed over motor neuron end-plates (motor points) of the quadriceps, hamstrings and gluteal muscle groups of both legs. Three electrodes (two active and one reference) were applied over each muscle group. Each electrode was coated with a buffered electrode gel that provides a conductive interface between the electrode and the skin. Six separate channels for sequential surface muscle stimulation were used during ergometry with a computer-controlled closed loop system. Each channel supplies monophasic rectangular pulses lasting 350 microseconds and delivered at 30 Hz to each of the two active electrodes over a given muscle. Stimulation intensities ranged from preset threshold levels determined for each individual muscle group to elicit a palpable contraction (18-40 mA (range)) up to a maximum of 130 mA. An ergometer power output, based upon prior studies, was chosen to enable subjects to work 20-30 min. A pedal position sensor, allowing continuous calculation of velocity, was used by the computer to control the instantaneous stimulus amplitude required for each of the six muscle groups to result in a smooth motion and a constant cranking frequency of 50 revolutions per min. Fatigue was defined to occur when revolutions per minute decreased below 35 in the face of maximal stimulation intensity (130 mA). Stimulation was automatically stopped at fatigue.

During the training a complete diary was kept, including biking time and workload.

Before each subject was included in the training program, pre-training evaluation was done, and this evaluation was repeated after specific periods of training.

Echo cardiography and isotope myocardial scintigraphy was performed, pulmonale function was measured by diffusion capacity and inspiratory and expiratory peak pressure, an evaluation of bone mineral density in the lower limbs was done by using dual photon absorptiometry. Cross section area of the thigh muscles was determined by magnetic resonance imaging (MRI). On muscle biopsies taken from the lateral vastus muscle, histochemical staining for different fibre types was performed, myosin heavy chain (MHC) isoforms from single fibres were determined in a one-dimensional SDS-Page system and enzymatic measurements were done.

Furthermore, blood samples for lipid status and coagulation parameters were performed. After 6 weeks of habituation to the electrically induced exercise, peak oxygen uptake was measured using a Jaeger-oxyscreen during maximal biking effort.

3 RESULTS

Initially the capability of each subject was of great interindividual variance (Fig.1). One subject was almost immediately able to bike for 30 minutes, whereas the other two only could carry out the exercise for a few minutes training per session. Although it has been the general recommendation for FES bicycling that subjects who were not able to bicycle for 30 minutes after 3 months would never be able to do so later - one of the subjects in our study did increase his exercise capacity in the period of 5 to 7 months and reached the 30 minutes at that point (Ragnarsson et al.1988).

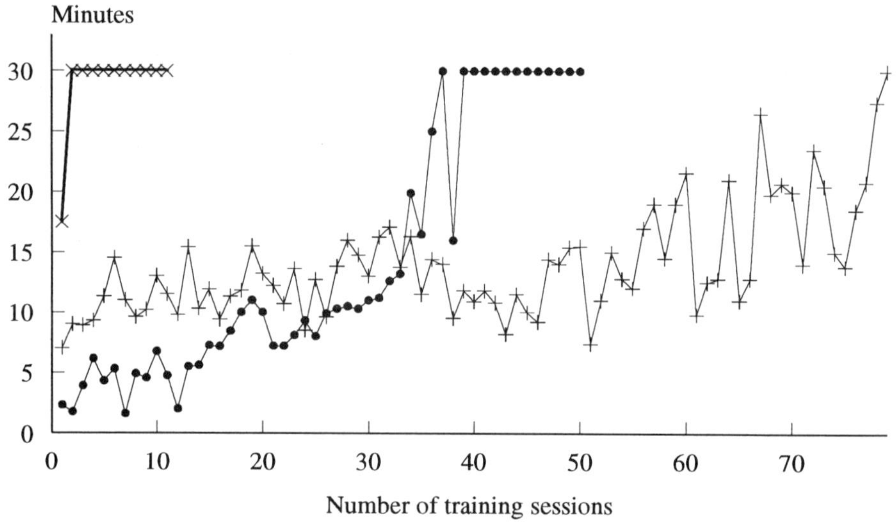

Fig. 1. Progression of the training. • Pt 1 , + Pt 2 and x Pt 3

After 6 weeks of habituation to FES, maximal oxygen uptake rate was 1.08 ± 0.20 l O_2/min (mean and SE). In response to intensive training maximal oxygen uptake increased by 53 % ($p<0.01$).(Fig.2).

A great increase in muscle mass was found on MR images of the thigh, both on the quadriceps and the hamstring muscles. As an example is shown the MR image of a cross section of the thigh before and after 6 months of training (Fig.3).

Biopsies of the lateral vastus muscle in the pretraining state indicated disuse of the muscle in the spinal cord injured subjects, with thin round muscle fibres imbedded in connective and fatty tissue. As a response to training, the muscle structure almost normalised after a period of 6 months (Fig.4).

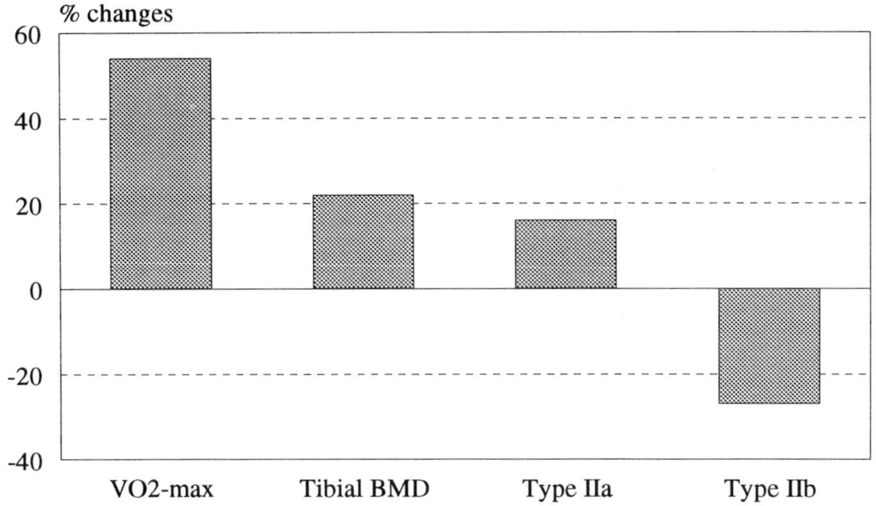

Fig. 2. Overview of the changes.

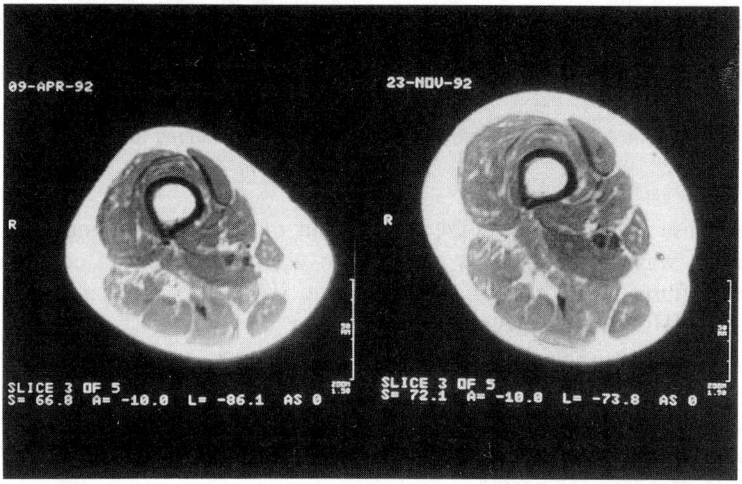

Fig.3. MRI cross sectional image of Pt 1, before and after 6 months of training.

Prior to training the proportion of fibres containing a co-expression of MHC isoforms IIA/IIB was dominating (42%). Fibres with only MHC isoform IIA were 30% and with only MHC isoform IIB were 28%.Fibres containing MHC isoform I were undetectable.

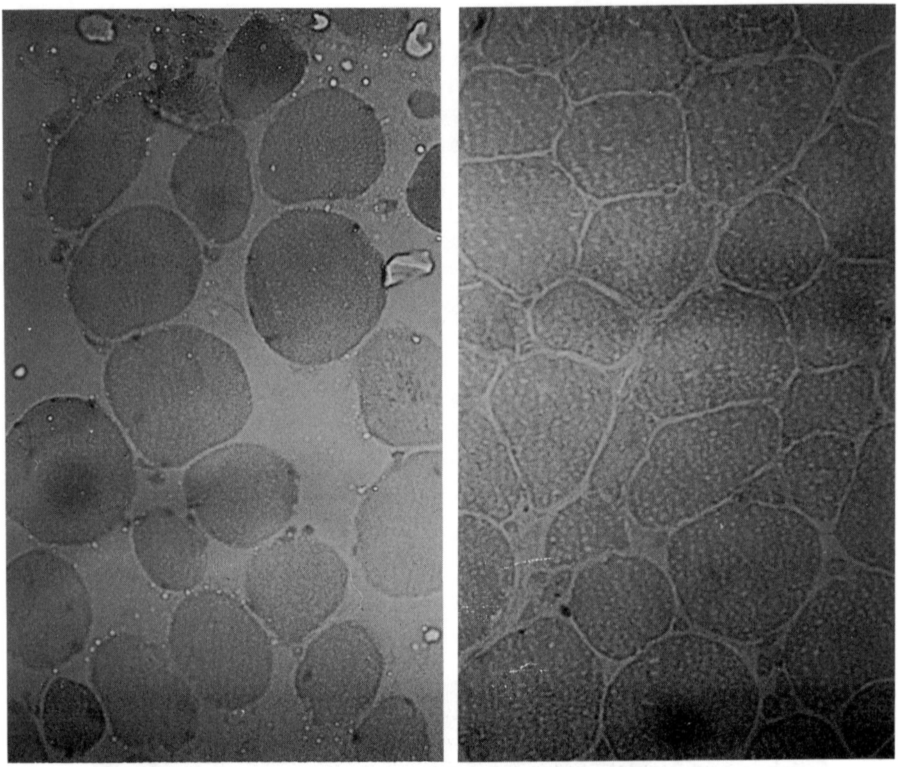

Fig.4. Micro photo-before and after 6 months of training in pt. 2.

In response to training, a total abolishment of fibres containing only MHC isoform IIB was observed. This observation was followed by a corresponding increase in fibres co-expressing MHC isoform IIA/IIB to 55%, and those only expressing MHC isoform IIA (42%).

In response to one year of training total bone mass (TBM) was not significantly changed, but leg bone mass increased by 15%. Bone mineral density (BMD) of lumbar spine (L2-L4) and the hip region was unchanged in response to training, whereas BMD in the proximal tibia increased by 22 ∀ 9 % after a one year training period.

4 Discussion

Functional electrical stimulation is not only a mean to gain control of impaired functions of paralysed muscles, but also a very valuable therapeutic tool to prevent secondary complications to SCI. Long term training with electrically induced bicycling in spinal cord injured individuals results in benefits as seen in able bodied subjects when they are subjected to similar amounts of training (Åstrand et al.1986).

Increased whole body aerobic capacity enhanced the disabled subjects everyday activity performance.

The increasing muscular volume of the stimulated muscles as well as the normalised muscle structure and fibre type composition can be important in relation to pressure sores of the gluteal region. The average cost of pressure sores are usually enormous, and if this can be decreased by using regular FES training, the equipment will save itэs own cost in a limited period of time (Yarkony et al.1992; Levine et al.1990; Barbenel et al.1992; Mawson et al.1993a; Mawson et al.1993b).

The osteoporosis following spinal cord injury is not described reversed due to FES training in previously studies (Leeds et al.1990; Rodgers et al.1991). Therefore it is interesting that we have found an increase in tibial mineral content by more than 20 %. The change seen in our study indicates a very slow training adaptation of the bone metabolism but indicate that non-weight bearing activity of a certain duration and intensity can reverse the osteoporosis in spinal cord injured subjects. This increased leg bone mass and bone mineral density in the proximal tibia might prevent following complications associated with osteoporosis (Biering-Sorensen et al.1990).

Conclusively, this study indicates that long term physical training of paralysed leg muscles with FES can reverse local muscle atrophy, local bone mineral loss and the cardiovascular deconditioning often seen in SCI, and thus increase the well-being and health of the spinal cord injured population, leading to a place for this kind of training in the everyday life of the spinal cord injured person.

5 Acknowledgements

This study was supported by grants from Danish Medical Research Council (J.nr. SSF 12-9360), The NOVO Foundation, The Hamilton Foundation and P. Carl Petersens Foundation; Danish Hospital Foundation for Medical Research (Region of Copenhagen, The Faroe Islands and Greenland); The Danish Heart Foundation; The Foundation of J. and O. Madsen and The Danish Medical Association Research Found.

References

Åstrand, P. O and Rodahl, K. (1986) Textbook of work physiology. 3rd ed. New York: McGraw-Hill Book Company;

Barbenel, J. C and Paul, J. P. (1992) Bioengineering developments for paraplegic patients. Paraplegia 30:61-4.

Bauman, W. A., Spungen, A.M., Raza, M., Rothstein, J., Zhang, R. L., Zhong, Y. G., Tsuruta, M., Shahidi, R., Pierson, R. N., Jr., and Wang, J., et al. (1992a) Coronary artery disease: metabolic risk factors and latent disease in individuals with paraplegia. Mount Sinai Journal of Medicine 59:163-8.

Bauman, W. A., Spungen, A. M., Zhong, Y. G., Rothstein, J. L., Petry, C., and Gordon, S. K. (1992b) Depressed serum high density lipoprotein cholesterol levels in veterans with spinal cord injury. Paraplegia 30:697-703.

Biering-Sorensen, F., Bohr, H., and Schaadt, O. (1988) Bone mineral content of the lumbar spine and lower extremities years after spinal cord lesion. Paraplegia 26:293-301.

Biering-Sorensen, F., Bohr, H. H, and Schaadt, O. P. (1990) Longitudinal study of bone mineral content in the lumbar spine, the forearm and the lower extremities after spinal cord injury. Eur J Clin Invest 20:330-5.

Biering-Sorensen, F., Lehmann Knudsen, J., Schmidt, A., Bundgaard, A., and Christensen, I. (1991) Effect of respiratory training with a mouth-nose-mask in tetraplegics. Paraplegia 29:113-9.

Cowell, L. L, Squires, W. G., and Raven, P. B. (1986) Benefits of aerobic exercise for the paraplegic: a brief review. Med Sci Sports Exerc 18:501-8.

Davis, G. M. (1993) Exercise capacity of individuals with paraplegia. Med Sci Sports Exerc 25:423-32.

Faghri, P. D., Glaser, R. M., and Figoni, S. F. (1992) Functional electrical stimulation leg cycle ergometer exercise: training effects on cardiorespiratory responses of spinal cord injured subjects at rest and during submaximal exercise. Archives of Physical Medicine & Rehabilitation 73:1085-93.

Garland, D. E., Stewart, C. A., Adkins, R. H., Hu, S. S., Rosen, C., Liotta, F. J., and Weinstein, D.A. (1992) Osteoporosis after spinal cord injury. Journal of Orthopaedic Research 10:371-8.

Leeds, E. M., Klose, K. J., Ganz, W., Serafini, A., and Green, B. A. (1990) Bone mineral density after bicycle ergometry training. Archives of Physical Medicine & Rehabilitation 71:207-9.

Levine, S. P., Kett, R. L., Gross, M. D., Wilson, B. A., Cederna, P. S., and Juni, J. E. (1990) Blood flow in the gluteus maximus of seated individuals during electrical muscle stimulation. Archives of Physical Medicine & Rehabilitation 71:682-6.

Mawson, A. R., Siddiqui, F. H., Connolly, B. J., Sharp, C. J., Stewart, G. W., Summer, W. R., and Biundo, J. J., Jr. (1993a) Effect of high voltage pulsed galvanic stimulation on sacral transcutaneous oxygen tension levels in the spinal cord injured. Paraplegia 31:311-9.

Mawson, A. R., Siddiqui, F. H., Connolly, B. J., Sharp, C. J., Summer, W. R., and Biundo, J. J., Jr. (1993b) Sacral transcutaneous oxygen tension levels in the spinal cord injured: risk factors for pressure ulcers? Archives of Physical Medicine & Rehabilita tion 74:745-51.

Petrofsky, J. S., Heaton, H. H., and Phillips, C. A. (1984a) Leg exerciser for training of paralysed muscle by closed-loop control. Medical & Biological Engineering & Computing 22:298-303.

Petrofsky, J. S. and Phillips, C. A. (1984b) The use of functional electrical stimulation for rehabilitation of spinal cord injured patients. Central Nervous System Trauma 1:57-74.

Petrofsky, J. S. and Stacy, R. (1992) The effect of training on endurance and the cardiovascular responses of individuals with paraplegia during dynamic exercise induced by functional electrical stimulation. European Journal of Applied Physiology & Occupational Physiology 64:487-92.

Ragnarsson, K. T. and Sell, G. H. (1981) Lower extremity fractures after spinal cord injury: a retrospective study. Archives of Physical Medicine & Rehabilitation 62:418-23.

Ragnarsson, K. T. (1986) Spinal cord injury: old problems, new approaches. Bulletin of the New York Academy of Medicine 62:174-81.

Ragnarsson, K. T., Pollack, S. F., O'Daniel, W., Jr., Edgar, R., Petrofsky, J. S., and Nash, M. S. (1988) Clinical evaluation of computerized functional electrical stimulation after spinal cord injury: a multicenter pilot study. Archives of Physical Medicine & Rehabilitation 69:672-7.

Rodgers, M. M., Glaser, R. M., Figoni, S. F., Hooker, S. P., Ezenwa, B. N., Collins, S. R., Mathews, T., Suryaprasad, A. G., and Gupta, S. C. (1991) Musculoskeletal responses of spinal cord injured individuals to functional neuromuscular stimulation-induced knee extension exercise training. Journal of Rehabilitation Research & Development 28:19-26.

Winther, K., Gleerup, G., Snorrason, K., and Biering-Sorensen, F. (1992) Platelet Function and Fibrinolytic Activity in Cervical Spinal Cord Injured Patients. Thromb Res 65:469-74.

Yarkony, G. M., Roth, E. J., Cybulski, G. R., and Jaeger, R. J. (1992) Neuromuscular stimulation in spinal cord injury. II: Prevention of secondary complications. Archives of Physical Medicine & Rehabilitation 73:195-200.

Preliminary Results of Muscle Strength, Endurance and Metabolism in the Wrist Extensors of Tetraplegics Following 12 Weeks of Electrically Induced Training

A. Hartkopp[1], S.D.R. Harridge[2], M. Mizuno[3], A. Ratkevicius[3],
H. Gregersen[1], E. Hagen[1], M. Kjær[2], B. Quistorff[3], F. Biering-Sørensen[1]
[1]Centre for Spinal Cord Injured, Neuroscience Centre
[2]Muscle Research Centre, National University Hospital, Copenhagen
[3]NMR Center, Department of Medical Biochemistry and Genetics
The Panum Institute, University of Copenhagen, Denmark

Abstract - Spinal cord injury will, below the level of lesion, cause a muscle to atrophy and reduce its oxidative capacity. Electrical stimulation may reverse these changes. However, it remains uncertain what parameters constitute the optimal conditioning protocol for muscles. The aim of the present study is to evaluate two different protocols (strength and endurance) on partially paralysed wrist extensor muscles in $C_{5/6}$ tetraplegics. This preliminary presentation includes results from the first four participants who have completed the study. Before and after a training period of 12 weeks, muscle strength, fatigue resistance and muscle metabolism, through phosphorus magnetic resonance spectroscopy (^{31}P-MRS), were evaluated. Both of the endurance trained subjects showed an increase in fatigue resistance, while one of the strength trained subjects showed an increase in maximal wrist extensor torque production, as well as an increase in fatigue resistance. In the three tetraplegics who were able to complete the ^{31}P-MRS-evaluation, the anaerobic ATP-production rates were found to be decreased by approximately 40% after training, indicating a lower energy cost for muscle contraction. Furthermore, a faster resynthesis of PCr during aerobic recovery was observed after training, suggesting an increase in oxidative potential.

1 Introduction

Paralysis, as a result of central or peripheral neuro-trauma, has a profound effect on the properties of skeletal muscle (Grimby et al. 1976, Martin et al. 1992, Pette and Staron 1990, Round et al. 1993). A period of prolonged paralysis has been shown to result in muscle fibre atrophy and to increase the proportion of type IIB, at the expense of type I fibres. Furthermore, a decrease in mitochondrial enzyme activity and a decrease in capillary density are related to the decrease in oxidative capacity.

Electrical stimulation of paralysed muscle has been able to reverse some of the effects of disuse (Andersen et al. 1995, Grimby et al. 1976, Pette and Vrbova 1992, Stein et al. 1992). However, despite the widespread use of electrical stimulation for conditioning in man, the optimal stimulation protocols for conditioning specific muscles remains uncertain (Bremner et al. 1992, Gordon and Mao 1994, Rabischong and Ohanna 1992, Stein et al. 1992, Yarkony et al. 1990).

Increasing the strength and endurance of paretic/paralysed muscles may allow functional stimulation to aid in the quality of life, for example in the restoration of a key grip, or grasp in tetraplegics. However, the methods known to improve muscle strength i.e. a low number of repetitions generating high muscle forces, differ from those known to improve muscle endurance, where low intensity contractions performed over a longer period of time are required.

The present study aimed to evaluate the effects of 12 weeks of electrically evoked strength or endurance training on the contractile and metabolic (studied using ^{31}P-MRS) properties of the wrist extensor muscles in tetraplegics with paresis of the forearms i.e. $C_{5/6}$ spinal cord lesions. The training was performed at home and both protocols involved dynamic loaded contractions in which the wrist joint moved throughout the whole range of motion. This presentation gives preliminary results from this study.

2 Methods

2.1 Participants

In total 12 tetraplegics (3 women and 9 men) with spinal cord injuries at the level of $C_{5/6}$ have been selected for the study. Details of the four subjects included in this preliminary presentation are given in Table 1. The patients had chronically complete transections of the spinal cord.

Table 1. Data of the participants.

Partici-pants $C_{5/6\ SCI}$	Year of Birth	Gen-der	Year of in-jury	Cause of injury	Occupation	Wrist function before*	Stimulation protocol
KGN	1965	M	1984	traffic	unemployed	1	endurance
KN	1965	F	1993	traffic	unemployed	2	endurance
HS	1964	F	1981	trampoline	unemployed	3	strength
AP	1959	M	1991	traffic	unemployed	4	strength

* Voluntary muscle function assessed on a scale from 0-5

The subjects were fully informed about the nature and possible risks of the experiment before they gave oral and written consent to participate in the study, which was approved by the Local Ethics Committee.

2.2 Training equipment

2.2.1 Stimulator

An ordinary pocket battery TENS stimulator (Asah Medico 2020, Denmark) was custom made to satisfy the required stimulation parameters and to be easy to use. The stimulator delivered a constant current (0-60 mA) biphasic square wave pulses (150-350 μs), which could be controlled with respect to stimulus frequency and timing.

2.2.2 Resistance orthosis instrument

In order to provide a resistance over the whole range of movement, a training orthosis instrument was specially developed. It consisted of a stable platform on which to rest the forearm. This was linked to a moveable bar placed over the back of the hand. The axis of rotation between the stationary and the moveable part of the orthosis was aligned with the axis of the wrist joint. Simple adjustable springs were connected to the moveable bar to provide the resistance (2.0 - 14.7 N). The whole training orthosis was placed on a adjustable photo-arm (143 Magic arm, Italy), which enabled the best ergonomic training position to be found for the participants, who trained whilst sat in their wheel chairs.

2.3 Stimulation protocols

The conditioning took place for 30 minutes per day, 6 times per week for 12 weeks. The participants trained at home with minimal assistance from their personal helper. Both protocols indvolved dynamic loaded contractions, in which the wrist joint moved throughout the whole range of motion. Following pre-training measurements a strength or endurance training protocol was followed with six subjects being randomly assigned to each group.

2.3.1 Strength training

For this training regimen the stimulation frequency used was 30 Hz (pulse width 250 μs), with the current chosen so as to elicit large muscle forces. During the 12 week period the stimulation and recovery times were fixed to 5 s on/20 s off

(Table 2). The resistance was chosen, so that at the end of the training session the wrist could just move through the range of motion (starting - ~40° below horizontal to full extension). Every 3 weeks the loading was evaluated and the stimulating current adjusted accordingly.

2.3.2 Endurance training

For the endurance training, the muscle was stimulated at a lower frequency of 15 Hz (250μs pulse width), with the current chosen so that repeated contractions could be performed. The adjustable resistance was chosen in such a way that the range of motion of the wrist at the end of the training session was - ~40° below horizontal (starting position) to maximal extension. The stimulation frequency of 15 Hz resulted in lower forces than that at 30 Hz. Every 3 weeks the current and resistance were evaluated and adjusted. The stimulation and recovery times were changed according to Table 2. Although the total protocol time was 30 min the effective excercise duration was increased from 20 to 50% of the protocol time.

Table 2. The stimulation protocol.

	0-3 weeks	3-6 weeks	6-9 weeks	9-12 weeks
Strength-training, 30 Hz 5 s on/ 20 s off	max force	max force	max force	max force
Endurance-training 15 Hz 50 % of maximum force	5/20 (s) on/off time	5/10 (s) on/off time	7,5/10 (s) on/off time	5/5 (s) on/off time

2.4 Evaluation of contractile properties

Strength and endurance were measured in a purpose built isometric dynamometer. The forearm was placed on a stable platform connected to a rotation bar, placed at an angle of 20°, which was attached to a strain gauge (Tedea - 300). The signal was amplified (Nobel Elektronik BKI-5, Sweden, Gould, USA) and fed to an analogue to digital converter (Cambridge Electronic Design 1401,UK) connected to a PC which sampled the data at 2kHz. Muscle force was expressed in the form of torque (Nm) around the wrist joint. Careful placement of the forearm in the ergometer ensured that the axis of rotation of the wrist was aligned with the axis of rotation of the bar connected to the strain gauge. The length of the lever arm was 5 cm. Detailed photographs were taken and anthropometric measurements made of each experiment to ensure that the position of the arm in the ergometer and the stimulating electrodes could be reproduced after training.

Stimulating electrodes in the form of silicon rubber pads (3.5 x 4.5 cm) were placed over the extensor carpi radialis longus and brevis muscle bellies (-) ~7 cm proximal to the axis of rotation in the wrist (+). The muscle was stimulated using positive square wave pulses (pulse width of 100 μs), delivered from a constant current stimulator (Digitimer DS7, UK), controlled by an external timer (Duvoisin et al. 1987).

To determine maximal tetanic force, 2 s contractions at 50 Hz (P_{o50}) were evoked where the current was increased in steps of 5 or 10 mA over one minute intervals from a below threshold current until no further increases in torque were observed. The same procedure was also performed at 30 (P_{o30}) and 15 Hz (P_{o15}).

Following a 5 minutes rest, an endurance test was performed where the muscle was stimulated for 0.3 s at 30 Hz at repeated every second for two minutes at the current which gave a maximal torque response. A fatigue index (FI) was calculated as the ratio of the mean torque generated by the last three contractions divided by the mean generated by the first three contractions.

2.5 Evaluation of muscle metabolism

This was performed using non-invasive phosphorus magnetic resonance spectroscopy (^{31}P-MRS).

2.5.1 ^{31}P-MRS.

A spectrometer (Vivispec, Otsauka Electronics) and an 80-cm-long 2.9-T horizontal superconducting magnet with a 26-cm bore (Magnex Scientific) was used. A 4-cm-diameter two-turn surface coil was placed over the wrist extensor muscles centered at a point corresponding to one-third the distance between the olecranon and the styloid process. Thus, the coil was expected to cover the extensor carpi radialis longus, brevis and also portions of the brachioradialis and extensor digitorum and digitorum minimi muscles. Small portions of the supinator and extensor carpi ulnaris muscles may also have been within the detection volume of the coil.

^{31}P spectra were obtained at 49.83 MHz by single 90° pulse-excitations with pulse-power and -width optimized by the height of the phosphorcreatine, (PCr) peak. Data were collected in 2K points over 205 ms at 5 s of interpulse intervals. Each spectrum consisted of 4 FID's, thus providing 20 s time resolution.

2.5.2 Spectral analysis

After application of an exponential line broadening of 5 Hz to each spectrum, muscle pH was calculated according to Taylor et al. 1983, using the chemical shift value at the maximum heights of inorganic phosphorus (P_i) and PCr resonances.

The peak areas of P_i, PCr, and β-ATP were measured by a curve-fitting program of the Vivospec spectrometer software (Otsuka electronics Inc, USA), assuming Lorentzian line shape. The peak areas were corrected for partial saturation, (Mizuno et al. 1994). The resting ratio of PCr/P_i and PCr/ATP as well as muscle pH were determined in a spectrum summed over 6 min.

The anaerobic ATP turnover rate during electrical stimulation was calculated as described by Kemp et al. (1994). The rate was calculated from a spectrum averaging the last minute before electrical stimulation and during one minute of ischaemic recovery.

In this calculation the PCr concentration at rest was assumed to be 18.6 mmol x kg^{-1} w.w (Bangsbo et al. 1993). The kinetics of PCr resynthesis during recovery was evaluated by fitting data to a monoexponential function applying least square regression. The half time ($t_{1/2}$) for recovery of PCr was calculated from the fitted curve. For this evaluation 20 s spectra obtained during recovery were used.

2.5.3 ^{31}P-MRS exercise protocol

A modified non-magnetic forearm ergometer, connected to a strain gauge was used. This has been described elsewhere (Quistorff et al. 1990). The participants lay supine on a stretcher with the testing arm used for training in the magnet. The elbow joint was stretched and extensor carpi radialis muscles were centered over the surface coil. The strain gauge of the ergometer was connected to an amplifier. The amplified signal was recorded on a strip chart recorder and was also digitized at a sampling rate of 1 kHz by a 12-bit A-D converter and subsequently stored on disk in an AT 486-66 computer. Muscle force was expressed as torque (Nm) around the wrist joint.

The muscles were activated by monophasic positive square wave pulses (pulse width 200 μs) delivered from a constant current stimulator (DISA, Denmark). Stimulation was carried out with self-sticky electrodes (4 cm diameter)(Biodan, Denmark). These were placed as described in the strength measurements. To improve the signal to noise ratio in the MR spectra the wires were wound together in a coil and placed sagittally in the magnet.

To determine maximal tetanic force, 1 sec contractions at 50 Hz, were evoked the current being increased in steps of 2.5 to 5 mA in one minute intervals until no further increases in torque were observed. The maximal current was then used to stimulate the muscle for 40 s at a frequency of 10 Hz . The force developed was equivalent to approximately 40-50 % of maximal tetanic force at 50 Hz.

MR spectra were aquired during 6 min of rest, during 40 s of 10 Hz stimulation, and during a further 5 min 20 s of recovery. A tourniquet placed around the upper arm, was inflated up to a pressure of 280 mmHg after 1 min of rest and released 1 min after the end of electrical stimulation, which thus gave 1 min of ischaemic recovery.

Total isometric 'work' (Nm x s) over the 40 s period was calculated by measuring torque every second. The results were corrected for shifts in baseline.

3 Results and Discussion

3.1 Preliminary results and comments on dynamometer evaluation

Table 3. Pre and post training contractile data for participant KN

Endurance protocol	Wrist extensor function (0-5)	P_{o15} (Nm)	P_{o30} (Nm)	P_{o50} (Nm)	FI
Control arm, pre-	2	0.42	0.46	0.50	0.39
Control arm, post-	-	0.37	0.41	0.46	0.35
Training arm, pre-	2+	0.73	0.90	1.03	0.47
Training arm, post-	-	0.88	1.01	1.04	0.80

After training KN showed a marked (70%) improvement in fatigue resistance (FI). She also reported that following training she was able to grasp and hold objects for a longer period of time.

Table 4 Pre and post training contractile data for participant KGN

Endurance protocol	Wrist extensor function (0-5)	P_{o15} (Nm)	P_{o30} (Nm)	P_{o50} (Nm)	FI
Control arm, pre-	2	1.14	2.03	2.19	0.62
Control arm, post-	-	1.08	1.59	1.92	0.42
Training arm, pre-	1	0.97	1.30	1.44	0.23
Training arm, post-	-	1.27	1.39	1.79	0.53

During the training KGN became ill and was in bed for 9 days. During this time she performed no training and also exhibited a minor loss of weight. A clear (130 %) improvement in fatigue resistance was nevertheless observed after training. However, no improvements in daily function were reported.

Table 5 Pre and post training contractile data for participant AP

Strength protocol	Wrist extensor function (0-5)	P_{o15} (Nm)	P_{o30} (Nm)	P_{o50} (Nm)	FI
Control arm, pre-	4	0.82	2.51	2.57	0.73
Control arm, post-	-	0.40	1.79	2.51	0.58
Training arm, pre-	4	-	2.34	2.52	0.65
Training arm, post-	-	0.51	2.03	2.63	0.60

AP exhibited the best voluntary wrist extensor function and highest stimulated torques of the four subjects tested. He suffered, however, from a high number of spasms which interfered with some of the contractile measurements. Post-training this participant reported that he could now hold and drink a filled bottle of beer!

Table 6 Pre and post training contractile data for participant HS

Strength protocol	Wrist extensor function (0-5)	P_{o15} (Nm)	P_{o30} (Nm)	P_{o50} (Nm)	FI
Control arm, pre-	3	0.25	0.46	0.62	0.28
Control arm, post-	-	0.23	0.39	0.56	0.39
Training arm, pre-t	3	0.29	0.41	0.42	0.36
Training arm, post-	-	0.41	0.59	0.65	0.68

HS showed an increase in torque production at all stimulus frequencies and also showed an increase (89%) in fatigue resistance.

3.1.1 Summary

Voluntary wrist extensor function and the maximal electrically stimulated wrist extensor torque showed a large inter-subject variation. With only a small number of subjects tested so far it is not possible to come to any firm conclusions regarding the effects of the specific training protocols. However, of note is the fact that the two endurance trained subjects showed a marked improvement in fatigue resistance after training. This was also observed in one of the strength trained subjects, who also showed a notable increase in strength at each of the three stimulus frequencies. No major changes were observed in either strength, or endurance, in the second strength trained subject. This may be partly due to the higher number of spasms experienced by this subject, in other words his wrist extensor muscles may have been in a relatively greater state of adaptation before training, and thus his capacity for training adaptation was relatively small.

3.2 Preliminary results and comments on the ^{31}P-MRS data

3.2.1 Resting conditions

Table 7. Resting data

Participants $C_{5/6}$SCI	PCr/P_i		PCr/ATP		Muscle pH	
	pre	post	pre	post	pre	post
AP	8.6	9.5	5.7	7.0	7.02	7.05
HS	8.8	7.6	5.2	5.0	7.15	7.07
KGN	18.5	16.2	3.9	2.7	7.03	7.08

Based on these 3 participants no changes in the resting values of ^{31}P-MRS determined PCr/P_i, PCr/ATP or muscle pH were observed. This result suggests that concentrations of PCr and ATP were unchanged in response to the training. This has also been reported to be the case following training in normal individuals (Kent-Braun et al. 1990). The resting PCr/P_i and PCr/ATP ratios and muscle pH are higher in Type II than in Type I muscles in both animal (Meyer et al. 1985) and human skeletal muscle (Boicelli et al. 1989, Kuno et al. 1991). The data would suggest that no shifts in the major fibre-types have occurred in response to this type and duration of training. However, the possibility of a transformation from Type IIB to Type IIA cannot be ruled out.

3.2.2 Anaerobic end-stimulation conditions

Table 8 End of stimulation data

Partici-pants $C_{5/6}$ SCI	PCr break-down (mmol x kg^{-1} w.w.)		pH		ATP from PCr break-down (mmol x kg^{-1} w.w. x min^{-1})		ATP from Glycolysis (mmol x kg^{-1} w.w. x min^{-1})		Total ATP turnover (mmol x kg^{-1} w.w. x min^{-1})	
	pre	post	pre	post	pre	post	pre	post	pre	post
AP	12.2	10.3	6.74	6.81	18.5	15.6	51.4	41.0	69.9	56.6
HS	13.2	11.3	6.70	6.78	20.0	17.1	62.7	41.8	82.6	58.9
KGN	5.5	5.3	6.71	6.75	8.4	8.0	43.6	31.2	51.9	39.2

w.w: wet weight

The total 'work' performed during 40 s of stimulation improved in all three subjects. The relative increases in work for AP, HS and KGN were 21%, 52%, 48%, respectively

After training the breakdown of PCr, and thereby corresponding decrease in ATP production from PCr breakdown, in response to electrical stimulation was less in all three subjects amounting to 19%, 17% and 5% in AP, HS and KGN respectively. The muscle pH at the end of stimulation was also higher after training, indicating a lower production of lactate. A 25%, 50% and 40% lower rate of glycolytic ATP production was also observed in post-training in AP, HS, and KGN respectively.

Even when the increase in the total amount of work done in the post-training test is not considered, the energy cost during electrical stimulation expressed as total anaerobic ATP turnover rate was 19% (AP), 29% (HS) and 24% (KGN) lower as compared to the pre-training status.

3.2.3 Aerobic recovery

Table 9 $t_{1/2}$ for recovery of PCr.

$t_{1/2}$ for recovery of PCr	pre-training	post-training
AP	(2 min 49 s)	49 s
HS	47 s	29 s
KGN	28 s	18 s

All 3 participants showed a faster $t_{1/2}$ for recovery of PCr in the post-training condition. The longest $t_{1/2}$ observed in AP at pre-training may be explained by the fact that this individual had many spasms during the recovery phase, particularly before training, thereby delaying PCr resynthesis. It has been shown that the resynthesis of PCr after exercise requires ATP produced through mitochondrial oxidative phosphorylation (Quistorff et al. 1993). Thus, the faster PCr resynthesis may reflect an increased oxidative potential of the wrist extensor muscles after training.

3.2.4 Summary

A comparison of anaerobic ATP production rate before and after training indicates a large decrease in energy cost during muscle contraction as a result of training among these participants. The faster resynthesis of PCr during aerobic recovery observed in the post-training condition probably reflects an increase in oxidative potential of the muscle.

References

Andersen, J.L., Mohr, T., Biering-Sørensen, F., Galbo, H., and Kjær, M. (1995) Myosin heavy chain isoform transformation in single fibres from m. vastus lateralis in spinal cord injured individuals: Effects of long term functional electrical stimulation (FES). *Pflügers Arch* (In press)

Bangsbo, J., Johansen, L., Quistorff, B., and Saltin, B. (1993) NMR analytic biochemical evaluation of CrP and nucleotides in the human calf during muscle contraction. *J Appl Physiol* **74**: 2034-2039.

Boicelli, C.A., Baldassarri, A.M., Borsetto, C., and Conconi, F. (1989) An approach to non-invasive fiber type determination by NMR. *Int J Sports Med* **10**: 53-54.

Bremner, L.A., Sloan, K.E., Day, R.E., Scull, E.R., and Ackland, T. (1992) A clinical exercise system for paraplegics using functional electrical stimulation. *Paraplegia* **30**: 647-655.

Duvoisin, M.R., Reed, H.E., Doerr, D.F., Dudley, G.A., and Buchanan, P. (1988)A newly developed EMS unit. *IEEE Trans Biomedical Engineering* **10**:677-678.

Gordon, T., and Mao, J. (1994) Muscle atrophy and procedures for training after spinal cord injury. *Physical Therapy*, **74**: 50-60.

Grimby, G., Broberg, C., Krotkiewska, I., and Krotkiewski, M. (1976) Muscle fiber composition in patients with traumatic cord lesion. *Scand J Rehab Med* **8**: 37-42.

Kemp, G.J., Thompson, C.H., Barnes, P.R.J., and Radda, G.K. (1994) Comparisons of ATP Turnover in Human Muscle During Ischaemic and Aerobic Exercise Using 31P Magnetic Resonance spectroscopy. *Magn Reson Med*, **31**: 248-258.

Kent-Braun, J.A., McCully, K.K., and Chance, B. (1990) Metabolic effects of training in humans: a ^{31}P-MRS study. *J Appl Physiol*, **69**: 1165-1170.

Kuno, S., Akisada, M., Anno, I., Niitsu, M., Itai, Y., and Katsuta, S. (1994) Heterogeneity of Muscle Energetics in Human Muscle Fiber Type Using ^{31}PNuclear Magnetic Resonance. *Clin J Sport Med*, **1**(4): 247-250.

Martin, T.P., Stein, R.B., Hoeppner, P.H., and Reid, D.C. (1992) Influence of electrical stimulation on the morphological and metabolic properties of paralyzed muscle. *J Appl Physiol*, **72**: 1401-1406.

Meyer, R.A., Brown, T.R., and Kushmerick, M.J. (1985) Phosphorus nuclear magnetic resonance of fast- and slow-twitch muscle. *Am J Physiol*, **248** Cell Physiol 17: C279-C287.

Mizuno, M., Horn, A, Secher, N., and Quistorff, B. (1994) Exercise-induced ^{31} P-NMR metabolic response of human wrist flexor muscles during partial neuromuscular blockade. *Am J Physiol*, **267**: R408-R414.

Mizuno, M., Secher, N.H., and Quistorff, B. (1994) ^{31} P-NMR spectroscopy, rsEMG, and histochemical fiber types of human wrist flexor muscles.*J. Physiol.***76**: 531-538.

Pette, D., and Staron, R.S. (1990) Cellular and molecular diversities of mammalian skeletal muscle fibres. *Revs Physiol Biochem, Pharm* **116**: 1-76.

Pette D.,and Vrbova G. (1985) Neural control of phenotypic expression in mammalian muscle fibers. *Muscle Nerve* **8**: 676-689.

Quistorff, B., Johansen, L., and Sahlin, K. (1993) Absence of phosphocreatine resynthesis in human calf muscle during ischaemic recovery. *Biochem J,* **291**: 681-686.

Quistorff, B., Nielsen, S., Thomsen, C., Jensen, K.E., and Henriksen, O. (1990) A simple calf muscle ergometer for use in a standard whole-body MR scanner. *Magn Reson Med,* **13**: 444-449.

Rabischong, E., and Ohanna, F. (1992) Effects of functional electrical stimulation (FES) on evoked muscular output in paraplegic quadriceps muscle. *Paraplegia,* **30**: 467-473.

Round, J.M., Barr, F.M., Moffat, B., and Jones, D.A. (1993) Fibre areas and histochemical fibre types in the quadriceps muscle of paraplegic subjects. *J Neurol Sci,* **116**: 207-211.

Stein, R.B., Gordon, T., Jefferson, J., Sharfenberger, A., Yang, J.F., Dezepetnek, J.T., and Belanger, M. (1992) Optimal Stimulation of Paralyzed Muscle After Human Spinal Cord Injury. *J Appl Physiol,* **72**: 1393-1400.

Taylor, D.J., Bore, P.J., Styles, P., Gadian, D.G., and Radda, G.K. (1983) Bioenergetics of intact human muscle. A ^{31}-P nuclear magnetic resonance study. *Mol Biol Med,* **1**: 77-94.

Yarkony, G.M., Jaeger, R.J., Roth, E., Kralj, A.R., and Quintern, J. (1990) Functional neuromuscular stimulation for standing after spinal cord injury. *Arch Phys Med Rehab,* **71**: 201-206.

Chapter 9

Implanted Systems and Neuroprosthetics for Autonomic Functions

Biomechanical Basis of the Choice of the Stimulated Muscles for CALIES Program

P. Rabischong
INSERM U103, Appareil Moteur et Handicap, Montpellier, France

Abstract - CALIES (Computer Aided Locomotion by Implanted Electrical Stimulation) is an European project, with the goal to implant an electronic box in spinal cord injured patients to restore motor function by means of electrical stimulation applied on muscles and nerves. According to the complexity of gait patterns and the normal activation of more than fifty muscles for each lower limb, it is necesarry to make an appropiate choice in order to allow implanted patients to stand up and to deambulate in an elegant manner. After a description of the three major functional systems of the lower limbs - the hip motor, the knee length controller, and the foot propulser - the choice of the four muscle groups to be stimulated (iliopsoas, glutei, quadriceps, and hamstrings) is justified, allowing to control hip and knee motion.

1 The Lower Limb "Mobile Functional Units"

Each functional group of joints and muscles of the lower limbs has specific role in posture and locomotion. Obviously, they are not working separately and their coordination is assumed by motor nervous system, which commands all muscles, on a proportional mode, due to the variable recruitment of motor units and which controls the achievement of a particular task by processing many inputs coming from muscles, tendons, articular capsule, ligaments and skin, in a closed loop regulation system. It's particularly important, in this manner, to emphasize on the importance of cutaneous inputs, playing a crucial role for the identification of position and movements of the different segments in three dimensions, thanks to the goniometric information coming from the skin deformation around joints. Obviously, in paraplegic patients with complete section of spinal cord, the lower limbs are in "virtual reality", what we called asomatognosia, due to loss of cutaneous inputs. Anyway, it's possible to identify in a simplified manner three functional systems in lower limbs:

1.1 The walking motor: the hip complex

Gait is a cyclic activity generated by a scissor movement of lower limbs with pendular and stance phases in an unstable mode, requiring a very complex dynamic stabilisation. The propulsion phase is achieved by the active contraction of two muscular groups: the **iliopsoas muscle**, which has a mono-articular component fixed on the medial part of the iliac bone and a poly-articular component fixed to the lumbar spine, from T12 to L5 (Fig.1) and the **rectus femoris** (Fig. 2), the poly-articular part of the quadriceps which also generates the extension of the knee. The ballistic movement of the leg has to be controlled, just before the heel strike by a cocontraction **quadriceps/harmstrings**, which guarantee the fixation of the knee during stance phase as well as the extension of the lower limb. In fact, the intermediate part of the cerebellum is responsible for the appropriate control of antagonists muscles to give a braking effect, explaining the natural smoothness of human movements. The **gluteus maximus**, which is a very powerful extensor of the tight is not playing a great role in this sequence when walking in horizontal ground. However, his action is particularly important for standing up, climbing stairs or walking on a slope.

In addition to the propulsion action during the pendular phase, a lateral stabilisation of the trunk during stance phase is achieved by the couple **gluteus medius and minimus** (Fig. 3). Those two muscles are doing an horizontal internal rotation of the pelvis (pelvic step) as well as a lateral fixation of the trunk on the hip joint. Paralysis or weakness of gluteus medius imposes the use of a crutch in order to stabilise the trunk during stance phase. In fact, many other muscles are also acting on pelvis to stabilize it during gait, like oblique abdominal muscles and erector spinae.

1.2 The length controller: the knee complex

The knee joint is one of the most difficult joints to replace, due to its biomechanical conception. It is normally responsible for a movement of flexion-extension, allowing the lower limb to shorten, during the pendular phase of the gait and for all the motor tasks like climbing stairs, sitting on a chair, etc. However, knee joint is also located between the three degrees-of-freedom hip joint and the suropodal cardan joint, which is in contact with the ground. A similar problem exists in upper limb between hand and shoulder. In this case, the pronosupination mechanism can easily absorb the torsion stresses, explaining why the elbow joint can achieve flexion-extension by the way of a one degree of freedom joint, representing really a rigid hinge articulation. In the lower limb, such a pronosupination system does not exist and the torsion stresses have to be absorbed by the knee itself. That could explain why two ingenious systems exist:

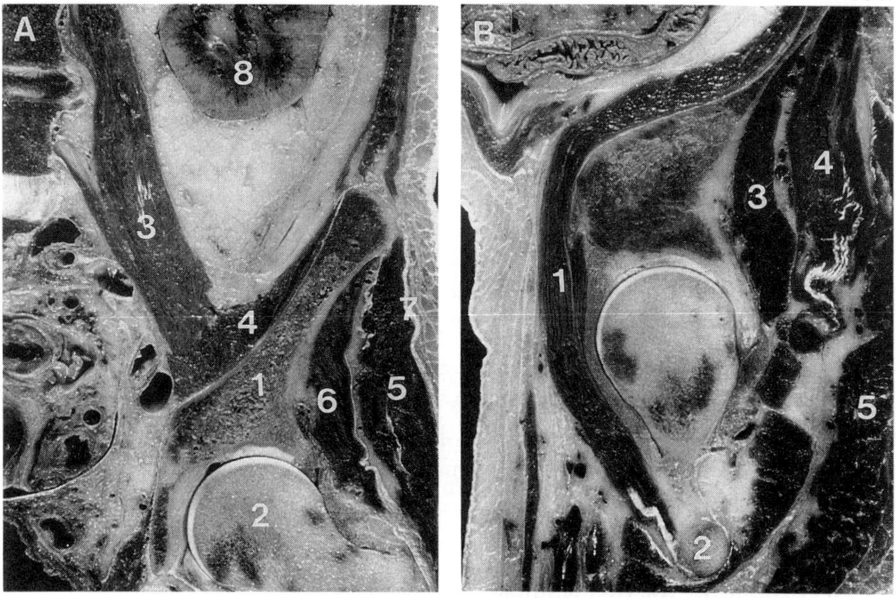

Fig. 1. Cross sections of abdominal cavity. **A:** coronal section showing: 1- Iliac bone. 2- Femur head. 3- Psoas muscle. 4- Iliac muscle. 5- Gluteus medius. 6- Gluteus minimus. 7- Iliotibial tract. 8- Kidney. **B:** Sagittal section of hip joint: 1- Iliopsoas muscle. 2- Little trochanter. 3- Gluteus minimus. 4- Gluteus medius. 5- Gluteus maximus

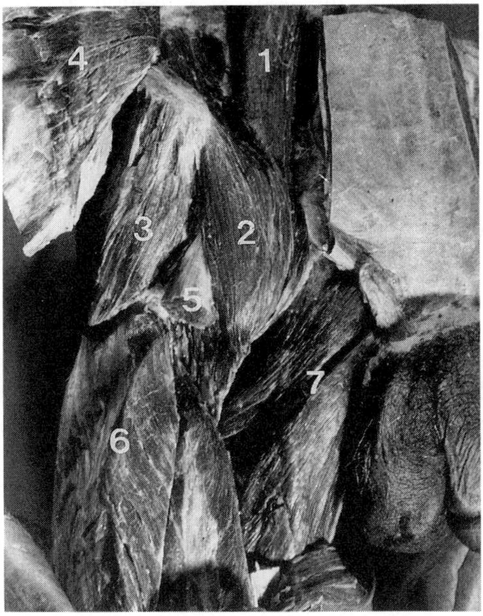

Fig. 2. Anterior aspect of right hip joint: 1- Psoas muscle. 2- Iliac muscle. 3- Gluteus medius. 4- Abdominal wall muscles. 5- Rectus femoris. 6- Vastus lateralis. 7- Adductor

- The first one is the "cam effect", due to the particular geometry of the condyle with a spiral projection of the center of rotation, which generates a full blockage of the knee during extension and a loose state during flexion with a possible axial rotation of the leg of roughly 15°.
- The second one is the oblique axis of all the lateral ligaments of the knee which are crossed each other (lateral, anterior and posterior cruciate, medial), representing a very effective torsion protection. In fact, an overnormal torque of rotation, like for instance in ski traumatology, can generate a painful distension of those ligaments.

On the other hand, no bony locking system exists in knee joint, explaining the progressive recurvatum, in case of lack of harmstrings contraction. Therefore those muscles are fixed on both sides of the knee (lateral with the biceps and medial with semitendinous and semimembraneous) allowing active axial rotation of the leg during knee flexion.

1.3 The propulsor: the foot complex

The foot has many interesting features in his conception. Without going in details, it's important to understand, at least, four systems:

- *The suropodal cardan joint:* two separate degrees of freedom are needed to link leg and foot, to allow the body stabilisation along two axis: antero-posterior (ankle joint) and lateral (subtalar joint). That is particularly important for bipodal and monopodal posture.
- *The two foot triangles:* the posterior is devoted to the stabilisation and the shorter anterior one to the propulsion. Both are hyperstatic systems.
- *The propulsion foot lever:* activated by the very powerful triceps muscle, having monoarticular and polyarticular components fixed on the calcar, the posterior triangle of the foot can be lifted up, generating propulsion forces. The five tarso-metatarsal joints are aligned along a curved line, allowing propulsion in any direction. Therefore, those forces are needed to walk in rough terrain or slopes, but not to walk in horizontal ground, explaining why a patient without ankle activation can walk in this condition using only the hip motor.
- *The multipieces "breaking up conception"* of the foot, in which many pieces of bones linked together by ligaments allow microdeformations of the structure and increase considerably the mechanical resistance of the whole. That explains, in fact, why this complex viscoelastic system is so difficult to be analysed mechanically, if conceived as rigid bodies, like in conventional mechanics.

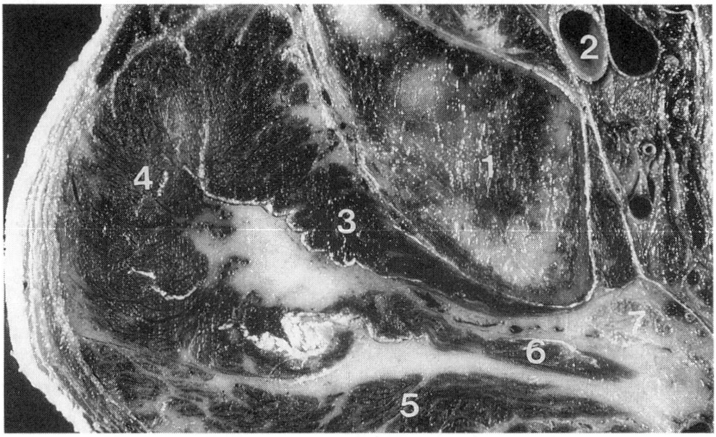

Fig. 3. Axial section of the left hip joint (superior aspect): 1- Acetabulum roof. 2- Iliac artery. 3- Gluteus minimus. 4- Gluteus medius. 5- Gluteus maximus. 6- Musculus piriformis. 7- Ischiatic nerve.

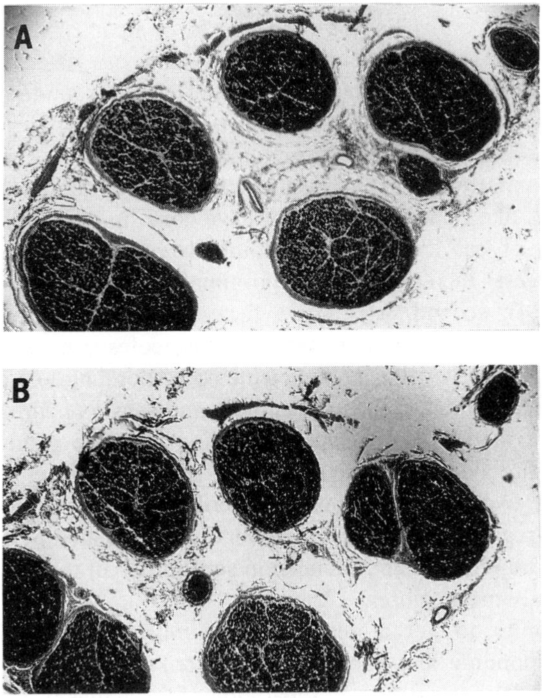

Fig. 4. Histological section with myelin impregnation of ulnar nerve in men. 7 cm are between A and B, showing the formation of new fascicules (superior right and inferior left).

In conclusion of this paragraph, it appears that, in order to reproduce an elegant walking which is one of the main goals of CALIES, it is absolutely needed to take into consideration the main muscles responsible for the smoothness of the gait. Hip and knee control are basically crucial. Ankle can be passively controlled by an orthotic device, if the functional program provided for the patient wants only to allow standing up / sitting down and deambulation on horizontal ground.

2 The CALIES FES Program

The CALIES package is made by a 24 channels implant, cables and connectors, electrodes, external antenna and portable programmer, activated by the patient on a push button mode. Two kinds of implantable FES electrodes are available. The first type is fixed on the aponeurosis of a muscle, as close as possible at the penetration point of the muscular nerve. It is a patch of 1 cm diameter which contains a platinum electrode in the centre. This kind of electrode has to be used for muscles in which the nerve is deeply penetrating, making the surgical approach difficult and invasive. The second type is represented by neural electrodes, made by a cuff placed around a nerve or a part of nerve.

Therefore the need for a selective stimulation can take advantage of the internal organisation of peripheral nerves. They are surrounded by a connective tissue called **epineurium** and the different types of fibres: motor, sensitive and vegetative are grouped in fascicules or bundles, isolated by a strong connective tissue called **perineurium**. This fasciculation of nerves has been studied by different authors, like Sunderland and we have done, in our lab, some research on the distribution of fascicules. Three points have to be noted: first, it is a progressive process increasing from proximal to distal part the number of fascicules (Fig. 4); second, it is not a fuzzy process and even if some distal exchanges of fibres exist, the organisation of fascicules is made in relation to the final distribution of nerves; third, a fascicule corresponding to a muscle is always composed by motor fibres, alpha and gamma, and sensitive fibres Ia and Ib from muscular spindles and Golgi organs, explaining why the suture of a muscular nerve gives less functional result than suture of sensitive nerve, made only by one way fibres. Only two exceptions can be described: the vocal cord, for which the tension regulation generating the sound diversity is regulated by ear and the facial muscles, which are regulated by facial skin sensibility. In those two cases, nerves are containing only motor fibres.

In fact, in order to get a very selective muscular activation, stimulating fascicules corresponding to a particular target looks the best approach. However the neurolysis made surgically to do separation of fascicules is not a complete safe procedure, but according to the fact that, as shown in Fig. 5, blood supply of nervous fibres is included within fascicules and nerves, a competent surgeon can do that, under the microscope, without too much bleeding and consequently too much risk of fibrosis. An endoscopic approach of those nerves in mechanically quiet area will also be able to prevent an hyperfibrosis around electrodes.

Finally, according to what we discussed previously, the list of muscles which will be stimulated for the first set of implantation will be as follows:

MUSCLES	ELECTRODES
Ilio-psoas	Epimysial
Gluteus maximus	Epimysial
Gluteus medius	Epimysial
Gluteus minimus	Epimysial
Quadriceps	Neural on femoral nerve (Fig. 6)
Hamstrings	Neural on ischiatic nerve (Fig. 7)

Before surgical implantation, it has been decided, among the CALIES group, that the patient has to be trained using external FES by means of cutaneous electrodes in order to reinforce muscle power and to decrease fatigue, which is the most difficult problem to solve stimulating paraplegic muscles. It is also a question to use assisted deambulation with external FES only or combined with orthotic braces in an hybrid mode. Anyway, the main advantage expected from implanted FES will be to stimulate muscles which are not possible to be stimulated by skin electrodes like iliopsoas and to get better proportionality and coordination, even if the recruitment curve of neural or epimysial electrodes is steep, with a nonlinearity.

3 Conclusion

In conclusion, the choice of the muscle which will be stimulated in CALIES program has been done according to the need of a good control of hip and knee movement, in order to allow the selected patients to walk in an elegant manner, using crutches to guarantee a good stabilisation. Therefore, the final success of CALIES is mainly based on the common work of the three teams of CALIES: Rehabilitation, chaired by Dr. K. R. Krishnan, Surgical, coordinated by Prof. J. Haase and Technical, managed by Prof. A. Pedotti. It is really a European challenge.

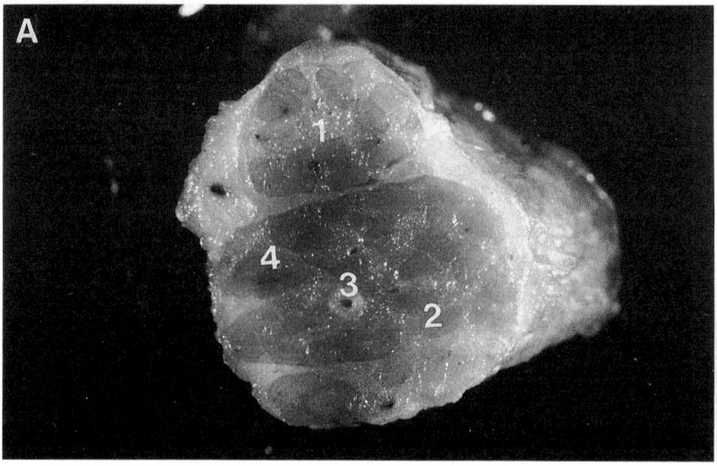

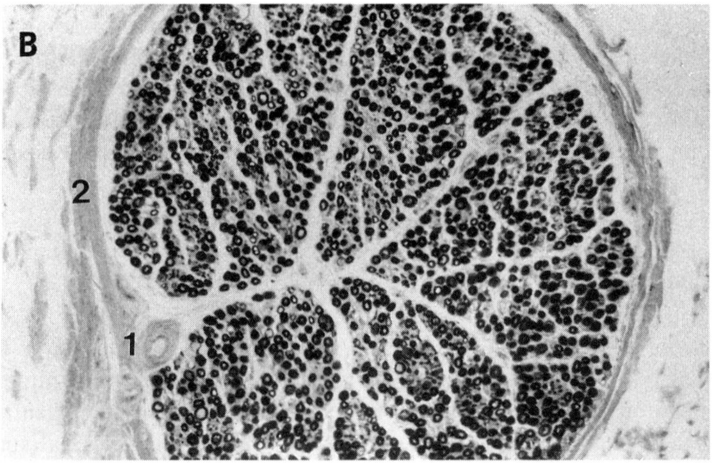

Fig. 5. Internal structure of human nerve. **A:** cross section of human ischiatic nerve showing: 1- Medial ischiatic nerve. 2- Lateral. 3- Internal artery. 4- Fascicules which have to be defined as anatomical or surgical (group of anatomical fascicules which can be isolated by surgical neurolysis). **B:** histological section of a fascicule in human nerve, with myelin impregnation. The black circles are myelin sheaths with a variable diameter corresponding to motor and sensitive fibres: 1- Fascicular artery. 2- Perineural sheath.

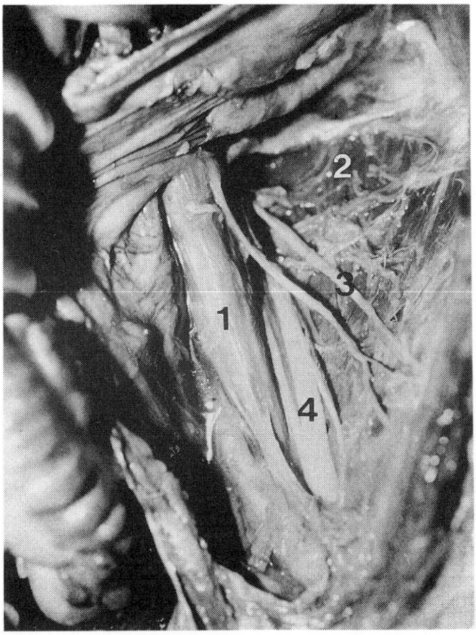

Fig. 6. Dissection of the left retroperitoneal space of abdominal cavity: 1- Psoas muscle. 2- Iliac muscle. 3- Abdominal wall cutaneous nerves. 4- Femoral nerve.

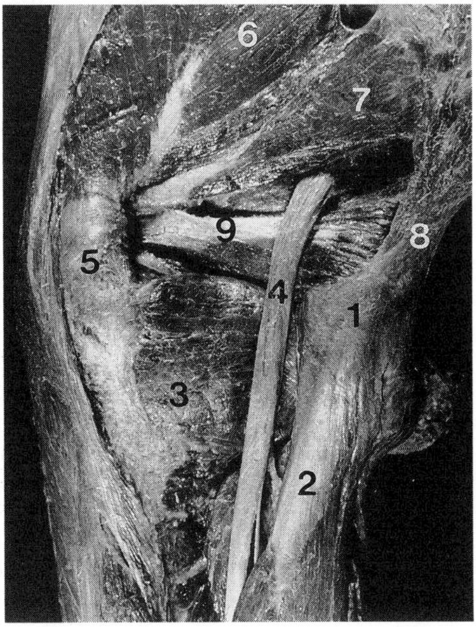

Fig. 7. Dissection of a left gluteal area after resection of the gluteus maximus: 1- Ischion. 2- Hamstrings. 3- Quadratus femoris muscle. 4- Ischiatic nerve. 5- Great trochanter. 6- Gluteus medius. 7- Piriformis muscle. 8- Sacrotuberal ligament. 9- Medial obturatorius muscle

References

Brown, M. D., Jones, R., and Frearson, N. (1989) Effects of activity on the contractile characteristics of developing skeletal muscle. In: *Neuromuscular Stimulation, Basic Concepts and Clinical Application* (Rose FC, Jones R, Vrbova G, eds.) Comprehensive Neurologic Rehabilitation, vol 3, 37-56.

Burke, R. E. (1981) Motors units: anatomy, physiology, and functional organization. In: Brooks VB, ed, *Handbook of Physiology, The Nervous System II*, Bethesda, MD: American Physiological Society, **2**: 345-422.

Edwards, R. H. T. (1981) Weakness and fatigue of skeletal muscles. In: *Advanced Medicine 18* (Sarner M, ed). RCP London Pitman Medical, London, 100-119.

Henneman, E. and Mendell, L. M. (1981) Functional organization of motoneuron pool and its inputs. In: Brooks VB ed., *Handbook of Physiology, The Nervous System II*. Bethesda, MD: American Physiological Society, 2: 423-507.

Rabischong, E., Ohanna, F., and Gilbert, B. (1990) Paraplegic Standing with FNS. A clinical application of a closed loop control. In: Annual Meeting of the International Medical Society of Paraplegia, Ramat Gan, Israël.

Rabischong, E. and Guiraud, D. (1993) Determination of fatigue in the electrically stimulated quadriceps muscle and relative effect of ischaemia. In: *Journal of Biomedical Engineering*, vol.15, November, 443-450.

Woloszko, J., Graille, J., Rabischong, E., and Rabischong, P. (1987) Closed loop control of knee during standing with FNS. In: Proceedings of the 9th Conference of the IEEE Engineering in Medicine and Biology Society, Boston.

Dual Channel Implantable Stimulator System for Selective Stimulation of Ankle Dorsal Flexors and Evertors

M. Tomsic[1], U. Bogataj[1], U. Stanič[1], M. Kljajić[2], R. Aćimović[3], F. Gider[1]
[1]Department of Automatics, Biocybernetics and Robotics, Jozef Stefan Institute, University of Ljubljana, Ljubljana, Slovenia
[2]Faculty of Organisational Sciences, University of Maribor, Maribor, Slovenia
[3]Institute of the Republic of Slovenia for Rehabilitation, Ljubljana, Slovenia

Abstract - A novel dual channel implantable stimulator system has been developed. The purpose of the stimulator is to achieve selective activation of muscles by stimulating peripheral motor nerves selectively and obtain a functional movement in certain applications. We intend to use the stimulator mainly as a peroneal brace with selective stimulation of the peroneal nerve for selective activation of ankle dorsal flexors and evertors. The stimulator comprises an implantable receiver and an external transmitter providing power and stimulus information for the receiver. The stimulator is small, low cost and potentially useful for various applications. Animal implantation experiments are in progress in order to measure different parameters and to test selective activation of the muscles, technology of our system in vivo (reliability, functionality, repeatability) and to make histological examinations. Some preliminary results are presented.

1 Introduction

Many surface as well as implantable functional electrical stimulation devices for the control of paralysed muscles have been developed since the widely known first published Liberson's idea of using a functional electrical stimulation (Liberson et al. 1961). Among them the stimulators used as orthotic devices for correction of the foot drop in hemiplegic patients have been the most popular devices. A great advance in technology has been made through decades of development of stimulators (Vodovnik et al. 1981). Various electronic devices for permanent total implantation have been made since the first implantable cardiac pacemaker. However, implantable functional electrical stimulators for the control of paralysed extremities are by far not as successful as cardiac pacemakers. Only a few stimulators have been used for human implantation. Such devices are open-loop control systems usually because of some problems and limitations regarding the use of closed-loop control systems (Stanic et al. 1974). In spite of this fact, good results have been achieved with implantable peroneal nerve stimulators in Ljubljana. Research and experiences of a single channel implantable stimulator and some successful human implantations (Kljajic et al. 1992, Rozman et al. 1994) resulted in development of different dual channel devices (Holsheimer et al. 1993, Talonen et al. 1983), and further in development of multichannel devices (Keith et al. 1989, Lanmüller et al. 1994, Strojnik et al. 1993) where more precise and complex movement is achieved by activation of more paralysed muscles. Experiences and results from clinical rehabilitation of gait using surface electrical stimulation systems (Malezic et al. 1992) contributed to the design and development of implantable systems. Dual channel implantable stimulator has been used for many years with different aims (Jeglic 1972).

2 Methods

The presented implantable system is an open-loop control system with no sensors and no feedback signals except a heel switch giving the information about the position of the leg. We tried to develop simple, small, low cost device with minimum number of channels for designated application. What can be done with two channels? One idea was to improve the push-off phase of the gait with the second channel (Jeglic 1972). Our idea is to get reliable, functional and useful selective activation of the nerve fibres using two channels with variable impulse parameters.

2.1 Purpose

The purpose of our dual channel implantable FES system is to provide neuromuscular control in two muscles and thus accomplish better correction of gait. The main aim is reliable selective stimulation of the common peroneal nerve. Thus it would be possible to control ankle dorsiflexion and eversion respectively and achieve more normal gait pattern. The system could be equally used in some other applications. Our approach is to solve problems consequently. In this phase of development we try to apply dual channel stimulator to solve the electrode positioning problem in single channel implant where excessive eversion of the foot usually dominated dorsal flexion (Kljajic et al. 1992).

2.2 Description of the system

Our system consists of three main parts: an implantable receiver (implant) with three electrodes, a small microcontroller based external programmable control unit with a transmitting antenna and a portable programmer/stride analyser (Figure 1). The microcontroller is a Motorola M68HC11 with internal memory. An asynchronous serial communications interface is used for communication between the programmer and the control unit. One heel switch is used to synchronise the stimulation with gait cycle. The antenna of the control unit transmits the operating power for the implant and all stimulus parameters. The control unit is simple for use: it has four keys to select the amplitude of the stimulation impulses, one switch for power on and a LED indicator. All other adjustable parameters of the impulses can be set by means of the programmer.

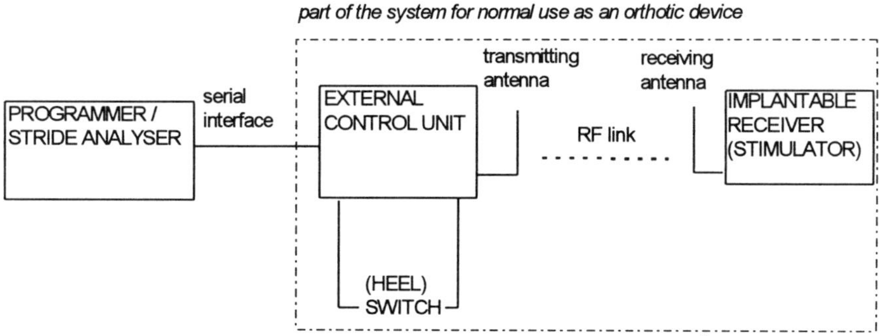

Fig.1. Block diagram of the complete system

In addition an auxiliary stimulator with auxiliary stimulating electrodes has been developed as an implantation tool. By changing software in the control unit different stimulation sequences can be obtained.

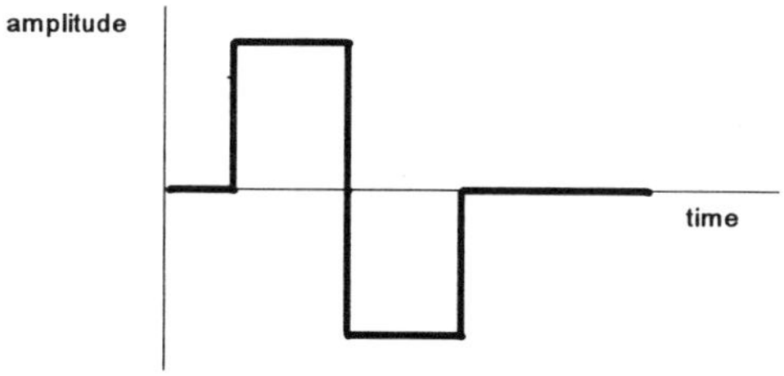

Fig.2. Stimulation impulse

2.3 Stimulation impulses

Trains of rectangular biphasic constant current stimulation impulses with adjustable net charge flow can be triggered by internal timer or synchronised with gait cycle using one heel switch. Figure 2 shows the shape of the impulses used for the stimulation. The output stage of the implant gives the constant current impulses up to the load impedance of 1000 Ohm. The delay between the positive and negative part of the impulse is zero. Stimulus parameters ranges were chosen according to effects of using different stimulus parameters on recruitment of nerve fibres (Gorman et al. 1983). Impulse parameters are collected in Table 1.

impulse parameter	from	to
amplitude (current)	**0**	**10 mA**
impulse width (positive part)	**80 μs**	**500 μs**
impulse width (negative part)	**80 μs**	**500 μs**
frequency	**10 Hz**	**60 Hz**
intermittent stimulation (cycle)	**2 s**	**12s**

Table 1. Adjustable stimulation impulse parameters

The impulse of the second channel is delayed after the impulse of the first channel because of the encoding and the modulation of the transmitted signal.

2.4 Implant description

Figure 3 displays the implantable stimulator with electrodes. The stimulator is made of biocompatible materials. The encapsulation procedures against the depredations of body fluid have been known for long time (Donaldson 1976). The implant was designed according to different criterion: anatomical, surgical, functional and dimensional.

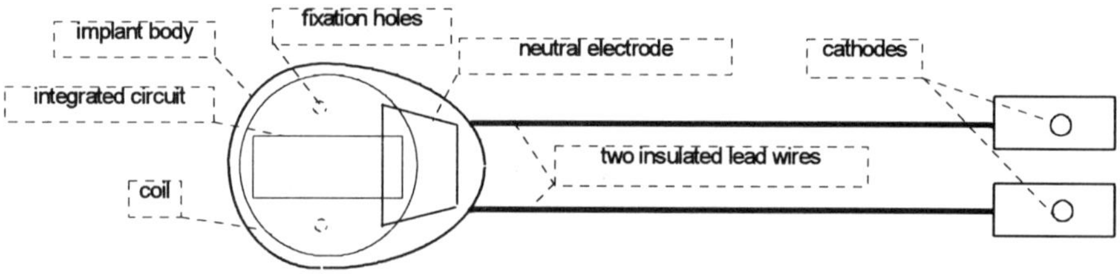

Fig.3. Scheme of the implantable stimulator (implant)

A body of the implant contains the receiving antenna (coil), a hybrid integrated circuit and electrode connectors. Necessary high overall efficiency and good displacement tolerance of radio frequency transcutaneous link lead the design of resonant coupled coils which are used as transmitting antenna and receiving antenna (Donaldson et al. 1983). The dimensions of the implant body are: 29mm x 24mm x 5mm. A neutral electrode (anode) is mounted and fixed on the one side of the implant body. Two stimulating electrodes are connected to the body by means of biomedical wires (stainless steel). They are disc-shaped and imbedded in the silicon fixation sheets. Peripheral nerve electrodes for selective activation of muscles (McNeal et al. 1985) and monopolar excitation technique is used for selective stimulation of superficial peripheral nerve trunk regions (Sweeney et al. 1990). Recruitment of nerve fibres is more stable for intrafascicular electrodes than for extraneural electrodes (Veltink et al. 1989). However, we use extraneural electrodes to avoid any damage to nerves. The complete electronic circuit of the implant is integrated into a 14 pin dual in-line ceramic-metal package. The main part of the electronic circuit is realised as a novel custom designed chip. Only the receiving antenna (coil) and electrode lead wires are connected to the integrated circuit.

3 Results

The system passed preliminary testing and experiments in vitro. Long-term test has been carried out to determine the stability of the materials used in the implant and the operational stability, reliability and durability of the implant. The biphasic charge density for electrodes is much smaller than maximum allowable for the geometric areas of the electrodes and is in the safe charge injection range for the stimulation of the nerve tissue (Brummer et al. 1977).

Two systems have been implanted in two experimental animals. A special implantation procedure of the stimulating electrodes has been used to get optimal functional response. Electrophysiological and biomechanical measurements are done during periodical experiments. Goniometers, EMG recorders, dynamometers, special electronic brace for measuring ankle torque, data acquisition systems, X-ray are used. The response dependence on different stimulation impulses and different stimulation parameters is observed and measured. Periodical tests are done to track the operability and the functionality of the systems. All results are recorded by means of data acquisition systems. Both implanted systems are operable. The effects of the tissue encapsulation of the stimulating cathodes and electrode migration can be overcome by changing the stimulus parameters.

4 Discussion

Restoration of the function of paralysed limbs and rehabilitation of various forms of neuromuscular dysfunction is possible by using functional electrical neuromuscular stimulation. Reliable, selective, reproducible force recruitment characteristics with determined electrode-muscle recruitment characteristics can be obtained by developing different approaches to the stimulation. Two channels can assure reliable selective activation of peripheral nerves by using proper stimulating electrodes, correct positioning of the electrodes (which depends on the application), good fixation technique for the implantable part of the system, rest period after the implantation and changing the intensity of the stimulation of each channel. This is only one step in development of the stimulator, which could be widely accepted as a helpful electronic brace. Instead of the open-loop control systems the closed-loop control systems could be used. Sensory nerve signals could be used as a feedback signal in the closed-loop control (Haugland et al. 1994).

Obtaining good results from animal implantation experiments we will be able to extrapolate our experiences to human implantation. Thirty-five hemiparetic patients had single channel peroneal stimulators implanted during the period from 1981 to 1991 in Ljubljana. Large population of hemiplegic patients dominating the field of neurologic rehabilitation is waiting for a simple solution that could restore their gait and return them to the normal life. At the present our main goal is successful human implantation of the dual channel stimulator within the next two years. The dual channel implantable system could be useful also for other applications, for example in hemiparetic patients with persistent improper quadriceps muscle strength that disturb walking. It would demand relatively minor surgical procedure.

References

Brummer, S.B. and Turner, M.J. (1977) Electrochemical considerations for safe electrochemical stimulation of the nervous system with platinum electrodes. IEEE Transactions on Biomedical Engineering, 24: 59-63.

Donaldson, N. de N. and Perkins, T.A. (1983) Analysis of resonant coupled coils in the design of radio frequency transcutaneous links. Medical and Biological Engineering and Computing, 21: 612-627.

Donaldson, P.E.K. (1976) The Encapsulation of Microelectronic Devices for Long-Term Surgical Implantation. IEEE Transactions on Biomedical Engineering, 23: 281-285.

Gorman, P.H. and Mortimer, J.T. (1983) The Effect of Stimulus Parameters on the Recruitment Characteristics of Direct Nerve Stimulation. IEEE Transactions on Biomedical Engineering, 30: 407-414.

Haugland, M.K. and Hoffer, J.A. (1994) Artifact-free sensory nerve signals obtained from cuff electrodes during functional electrical stimulation of nearby muscles. IEEE Transactions on Rehabilitation Engineering, 2: 37-46.

Holsheimer, J., Bultstra, G., Verloop, A.J., van der Aa, H. E., and Hermens, H.J. (1993) Implantable dual channel peroneal nerve stimulator. Proceedings of the Ljubljana FES Conference, Ljubljana, pp. 42-44.

Jeglic, A. (1972) Two channel implant - approach to an orthotic device. Proceedings of the Fourth International Symposium on External Control of Human Extremities, Dubrovnik, pp. 647-656.

Keith, M.W., Peckham, P.H., Thrope, G.B., Stroh, K.C., Smith, B., Buckett, J.R., Kilgore, K.L., and Jatich, J.W. (1989) Implantable functional neuromuscular stimulation in the tetraplegic hand. The Journal of Hand Surgery, 14A: 524-530.

Kljajic, M., Malezic, M., Acimovic, R., Vavken, E., Stanic, U., Pangrsic, B., and Rozman, J. (1992) Gait evaluation in hemiparetic patients using subcutaneous peroneal electrical stimulation, Scand J Rehab Med, 24: 121-126.

Lanmüller, H., Mayr, W., Sauermann, S., Schnetz, G., Thoma, H., and Unger, E. (1994) A fully implantable ECG triggered multichannel nerve stimulator. Basic and Applied Myology, 4(2): 141-145.

Liberson, W.T., Holmquest, H.J., Scot, D., and Dow, M. (1961) Functional Electrotherapy: Stimulation of the peroneal nerve synchronised with the swing phase of the gait of hemiplegic patients. 3rd Int. Con. of Phy. Med., Washington, 1960, Arch. Phys. Med. and Rehab., 42: 101-105.

Malezic, M., Bogataj, U., Gros, N., Decman, I., Vrtacnik, P., Kljajic, M., and Acimovic-Janezic, R. (1992) Application of a programmable dual-channel adaptive electrical stimulation system for the control and analysis of gait. Journal of Rehab. Res. and Devel., 29: 41-53.

McNeal, D.R. and Bowman, B.R. (1985) Selective activation of muscles using peripheral nerve electrodes. Medical and Biological Engineering and Computing, 23: 249-253.

Rozman, J., Acimovic-Janezic, R., Tekavcic, I., Kljajic, M., and Trlep, M. (1994) Implantable stimulator for selective stimulation of the common peroneal nerve: a preliminary report. Journal of Medical Engineering & Technology, 18: 47-53.

Stanic, U. and Trnkoczy, A. (1974) Closed loop positioning of hemiplegic patient's joint by means of functional electrical stimulation. IEEE Transactions on Biomedical Engineering, 21: 365-370.

Strojnik, P., Schulman, J.H., Byers, C.L., and Meadows, P. (1993) PULSAR™ - CLARION™ cochlear stimulator modified for FES application. Proceedings of the Ljubljana FES Conference, Ljubljana, pp. 27-29.

Sweeney, J.D., Ksiensky, D.A., and Mortimer, J.T. (1990) A nerve cuff technique for selective excitation of peripheral nerve trunk regions. IEEE Transactions on Biomededical Engineering, 37: 706-715.

Talonen, P., Malmivuo, J., Baer, G., Markkula, H., and Hakkinen, V. (1983) Transcutaneous, dual channel phrenic nerve stimulator for diaphragm pacing. Medical and Biological Engineering and Computing, 21: 21-30.

Veltink, P.H., van Alste, J. A., and Boom, H.B.K. (1989) Multielectrode intrafascicular and extraneural stimulation. Medical and Biological Engineering and Computing, 27: 19-24.

Vodovnik, L., Bajd, T., Kralj, A., Gracanin, F., and Strojnik, P. (1981) Functional electrical stimulation for control of locomotor systems. CRC Critical Reviews in Bioengineering, Vol. 6/2, pp. 63-131.

Lumbar Anterior Root Stimulator for Lower Limb Control in Paraplegia

D. N. Rushton[1], N. de N. Donaldson[2],
F. M. D. Barr[3], V. J. Harper[4], T. A. Perkins[2], P. N. Taylor[4], A. M. Tromans[4]
[1]The London Hospital Medical College, U.K.
[2]Department of Medical Physics, University College, London, U.K.
[3]RNOH Stanmore, U.K.
[4]Salisbury General Hospital, U.K.

Abstract - We have implanted an intradural array of 12 tripolar electrodes on the anterior roots L2-S2, left and right, at cauda equina level, in a 33 year old woman with a complete T9 cord lesion of 3 years duration. They are driven by an implanted multiplexor stimulator system. All channels give movements, in patterns that might be predicted from the known anatomy of the cauda equina. In particular, L2,3 give hip adduction; L3,4,and 5 give quadriceps femoris; L5, S1,2 give hamstrings; and S1,2 give plantarflexion. L5 gives mixed movements at the ankle. Some thresholds have varied, probably as a result of tissue encapsulation. The moment generated within each degree of freedom of the legs has been measured for each root, using a specially-developed multi-moment measurement apparatus.

1 Introduction

Standing using quadriceps surface electrodes and was first demonstrated in the laboratory over thirty years ago (Kantrowitz, 1963). However, if the system is elaborated to provide other functions by stimulating other muscle groups, applying the electrodes soon becomes too time-consuming. Also, surface stimulation is wasteful of current, good skin-care is essential, and stimulation varies with movements of the limbs. For these reasons, many workers (Brindley et al, 1979; Marsolais and Kobetic, 1986; McNeal and Bowman 1986) concluded that the scope of surface stimulation methods is essentially limited to experimental work, and that to obtain selective and consistent results, the electrode system will need to be implanted. Three types of implanted system have been developed. The first type is percutaneous wires, which are inserted through the skin, and located to the motor point using trial stimulation (Marsolais and Kobetic, 1986). These are easy for a practised operator to insert, and do not require formal surgery. It is possible to add as many wires as are needed; but they break eventually, and require skin-care at the entry-point. The second type is the nerve-cuff electrode, which is inserted around peripheral motor nerves in a formal surgical procedure. Self-wrapping helical electrodes (Naples et al, 1988) are a variant on this type.

The third group is the epimysial type of electrode, which is an implanted disc electrode attached to the muscle surface. In the case of large muscles it is usually placed near the motor point. These require less dissection than the cuff type, but multichannel lower-limb systems still require extensive surgery. Cuff and epimysial electrode types both require implanted cabling in the limb. Up to now, implanted cabling in the lower limb has not been very satisfactory; cable conductor fractures are common. The other problem with peripheral stimulator types is that a multichannel system for paraplegic standing and walking calls for increasingly extensive surgery, in order to access all the required nerves. Implantable microstimulators which will avoid some of these problems are under development, but have not yet reached the stage of starting patient trial. We have developed a new approach to lower limb FNS, which employs 12-channel stimulation of the lumbosacral anterior roots, between L2-S2 inclusive.

2 Methods

The external controller hardware and software, the patient selection procedure, and the 'multi-moment chair', used to measure the responses to root stimulation, are all specially developed for this application.

2.1 Surgery and electrode mounts

Many aspects of the electrode design, cable type, surgical approach and implantation technique are based on the successful and long-proven sacral anterior root stimulator implant ('SARSI'), which is widely used in Europe and elsewhere to restore bladder control in paraplegia (Brindley et al, 1986; Brindley and Rushton, 1990; Brindley, 1994, 1995). The surgical approach requires a laminectomy of L2-L4, and the electrodes are placed intradurally. The electrodes are tripolar, assembled in a book shape with four leaves, with three slots to accommodate three roots, which can be accessed via three separate stimulation channels, in each book. The books resemble those in SARSI in general form, but the dimensions are slightly smaller. They also differ in that the books are separate, rather than being linked to each other. This enables a book to trap three adjacent roots on one side, while the neighbouring book traps three roots on the opposite side. This arrangement leaves more room for untrapped roots to pass, in comparison with linked electrode books placed in the midline. There are far more passing untrapped roots than is the case for SARSI, partly because the implant is higher in the cauda equina, and partly because, unlike SARSI, the associated posterior roots are not sectioned. The implant receiver and cables (but not the electrode mounts) are coated with antibiotic-impregnated silicone rubber, which greatly reduces the chance of infection (Rushton et al, 1989).

2.2 Stimulator implant

The implantable stimulator assembly is shown in Figure 1. It has been described by Donaldson et al (1995). The multiplexor stimulator is designed for root stimulation, with a 5mA stimulus pulse current, and pulse duration which is adjustable between 2 and 910 microseconds, in 256 increments, each of 6%.

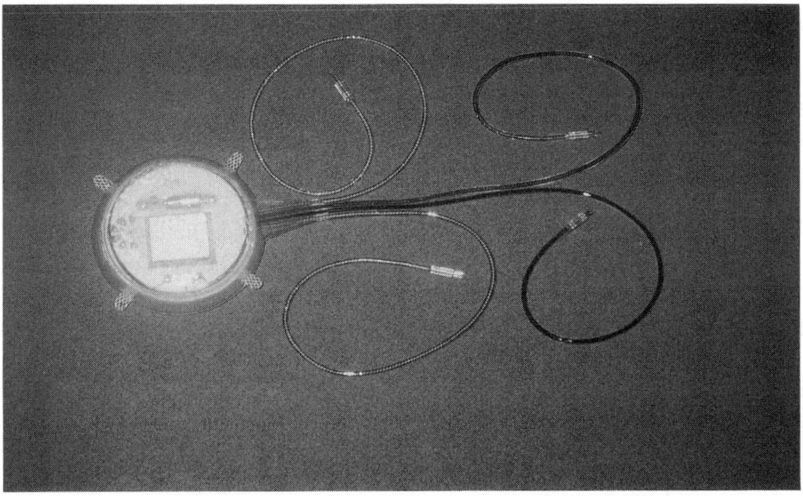

Fig. 1. 12 channel lumbosacral root stimulator implant

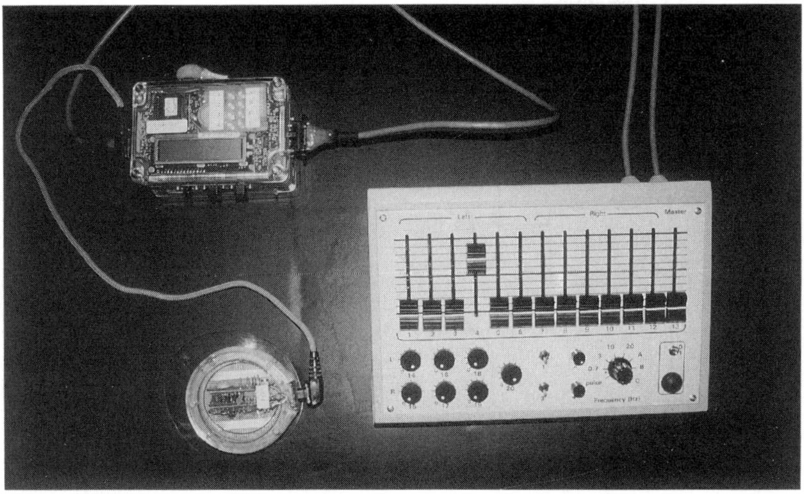

Fig. 2. Portable stimulator, modulator-transmitter and 'slider-box'.

2.3 The Control box

The battery-powered portable control box (Figure 2) is worn on a belt or in a pocket, and is connected to the modulator-transmitter block by a short cable. The modulator-transmitter is glued or taped to the skin in the correct location, and the control box gives a numerical indication of coupling, to assist in location. A moulded location shell attached to the transmitter block helps to maintain the correct location.

2.4 Controlling the Control Box

The control box contains two 68HC11 microprocessors. One of them, the Link Processor, generates the stimulus patterns for the implant, while the other, the Control Processor, executes FES applications programs. In this way, new applications programs can be developed and tested without fear that programming errors might cause inappropriate stimulation commands. The control box can currently be controlled in three different ways (Command Source Options, Figure 3). Programs that have been previously loaded through the RS232 link can be executed by buttons on the box. Alternatively, roots or combinations of roots can be activated by way of a 'slider box' control unit, which is useful in the laboratory as a way of rapidly testing responses. The third method is to download stimulus patterns generated in a PC, again via the RS232 link. These can be for immediate use, or for memorising as a stored program in the control box.

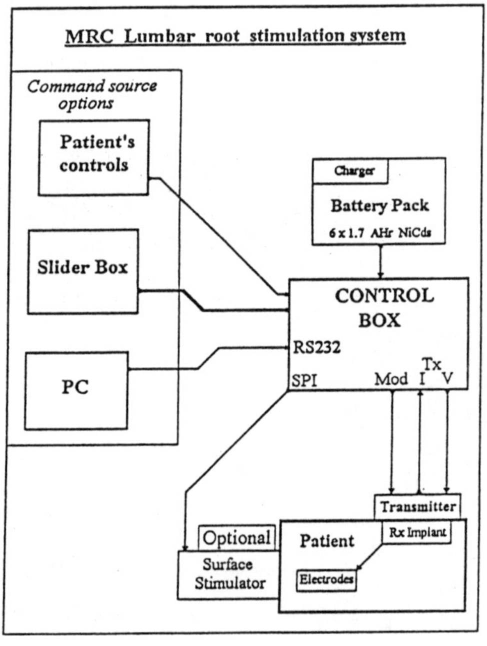

Fig. 3. Block diagram of Control Box and its controls

2.5 Patient

The patient is a woman aged 33 years, with a complete T9 traumatic cord lesion of 3 years duration. She is the first patient to be implanted with this design of system, although an earlier version with a different multiplexer was implanted in 1990, in a man aged 50 years with a complete T6 traumatic cord lesion of 15 years duration (Rushton, 1991). This patient underwent a selection procedure which has been described elsewhere (Barr et al, 1995), and which was designed to ensure that selected patients were physically, psychologically and socially suited, and that their muscles could be adequately trained. This included ratings of neurology, joint mobility, spasticity, muscle strength with surface stimulation, psychological assessments, social support and employment, response to a 12-week muscle training programme, and ability to stand using open-loop and closed-loop control of a surface stimulator system in the laboratory.

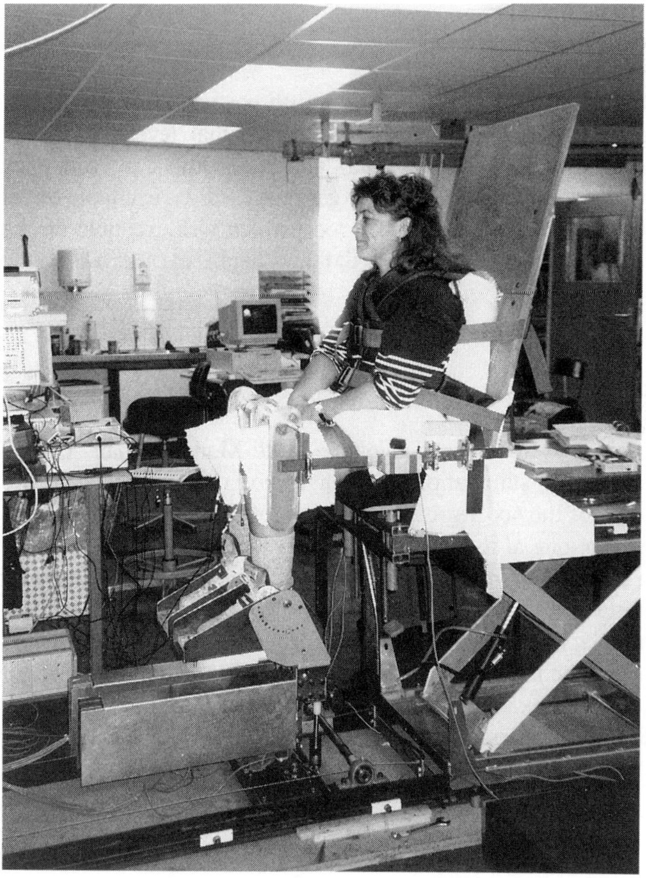

Fig. 4. Patient in the Multi-Moment Chair

2.5 Multi-moment chair

We knew that many motor nerve roots would have complex actions, involving more than one degree of freedom, and often more than one joint, in the lower limb. In order to facilitate the analysis of results, and in order to allow rapid data collection and maximise patient comfort, we therefore developed a 'multi-moment chair' apparatus (Figure 4), which would allow us to measure isometric moments in all the important degrees of freedom in both lower limbs simultaneously (Donaldson et al, 1995). The chair was designed to do this with the lower limbs in a range of postures. The automated stimulation and data collection methods used allow us to collect up to 180 stimulation/response samples in 30 minutes testing. This is the longest practicable uninterrupted testing period, because of the patient's need for pressure relief.

3 Results

3.1 Preliminary testing

Preliminary testing was done starting on the fifth postoperative day. Early tests were designed to record acute-phase threshold and maximal levels, to describe clinical movement responses (Rushton et al, 1995), and to document any root damage. Roots which are damaged accidentally during surgery may still be excitable on the fifth day. One such result was found: the right L2 root, which was excitable on the fifth day, subsequently became inexcitable, and did not begin to recover until the eighth postoperative month.

3.2 Moment measurements

These measurements were obtained using the Multi-Moment Chair. The first task was to map the effects of stimulation of each motor root in terms of the moments generated in each of the six degrees of freedom of the relevant leg (three degrees of freedom at the hip, one at the knee, and two at the ankle). An example of the data obtained from stimulation of roots one at a time is given in Figure 5. Eleven of the 12 roots give substantial stimulation-evoked moments, but in four cases there were superadded time-varying moments, usually in a flexor direction, which appeared to be reflex. These could be minimised by repeat stimulation, but in some cases they could not be eliminated. An example is seen at the right of the upper part of Fig 5, when S2R is stimulated; a transient hip flexor moment appears (downward deflection in the solid trace).

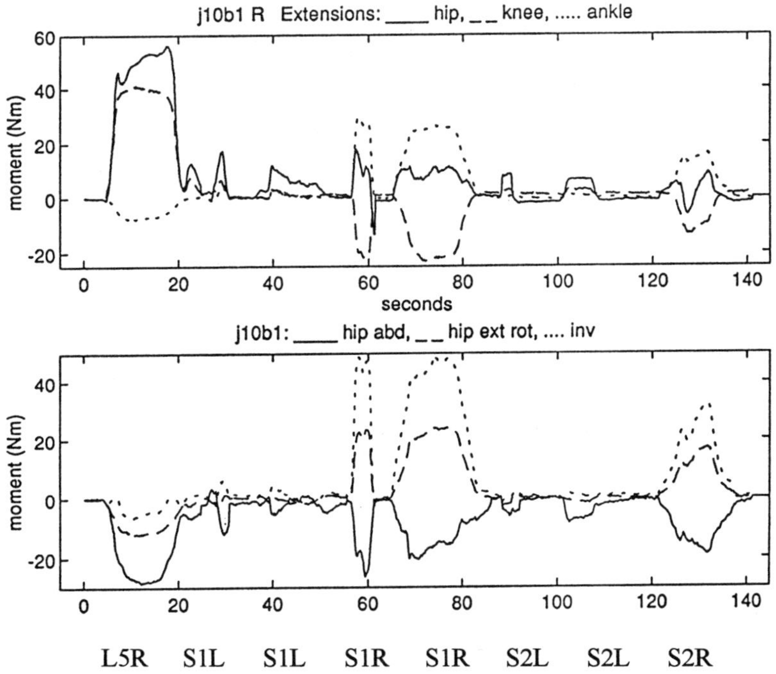

Fig. 5. Sequence of rampup-hold-rampdown stimulation patterns

3.3 Additivity

The moments resulting from stimulation of different roots should in theory not inhibit, occlude or facilitate each other, so that the effects of stimulating two or more roots should be predictable by adding the sets of moments algebraically. However, this prediction needs to be tested, since for practical purposes it is likely that all the most useful stimulation patterns will involve more than one root. The next task therefore was to check that the effects of stimulation of single roots could be added algebraically in the mapping space between the 6 roots and 6 moments. Table 1 shows results for some moments (hip extension, knee extension and hip abduction) and root combinations (L4 and L5). Roots are stimulated separately and together; the combined moments are expressed as a percentage of the sum of the moments obtained when the roots are stimulated separately. In this subject, additivity is always less than complete, and sometimes significantly so. The reasons for this are not yet established.

Test	Root	Stimulus	Hip Ext	Knee Ext	Hip Abd
1	L4	40	-12	11	-12
2	L5	54	-9	21	-11
3	L4 add L5	40, 54	-12	26	-17
4	L5 add L4	54, 40	-14	26	-17
A = (1+2)			-21	32	-23
B = (3+4)/2			-13	26	-17
B/A*100 (%)			62	81	74

Table 1. Additivity of root responses in moment space

3.4 Hyperspace mapping

The multi-moment chair enables us to measure the moments resulting from stimulation of roots, singly or in combination. However, what we actually need is a map or table which will tell us what combination of roots to stimulate, at what strengths, in order to achieve a desired combination of moments for a particular functional purpose. To do this, we need as complete a description as possible of the map relating roots and moments. For each leg there are 6 roots and 6 or 7 degrees of freedom (depending on whether rotation of the foot with the knee flexed is included as a separate degree of freedom). The map, if it exists, is therefore in 6-dimensional hyperspace.

To obtain this data set, for each root we selected three stimulation strengths (just above threshold, mid-range, and just below maximal). We stimulated 3-root samples using different strength combinations, and permuted a large proportion of the whole set of such samples. Samples could be presented at a rate of one every 10 seconds, so that during a thirty minute testing session we could collect 180 mapping data points (Figure 6). Thirty minutes is the duration of a run, because of the need for periodic pressure relief.

The results of these 'hyperspace mapping' experiments showed that the mapping was broadly predictable, and that it was possible to define the 'islands' of interest on the moment side of the map, where the pattern of moments was likely to be useful for standing or stepping. The variations induced by moment changes from one testing session to another were attributable to changes in the pattern of reflex responses, and continuing changes in the strength and state of training of different muscle groups.

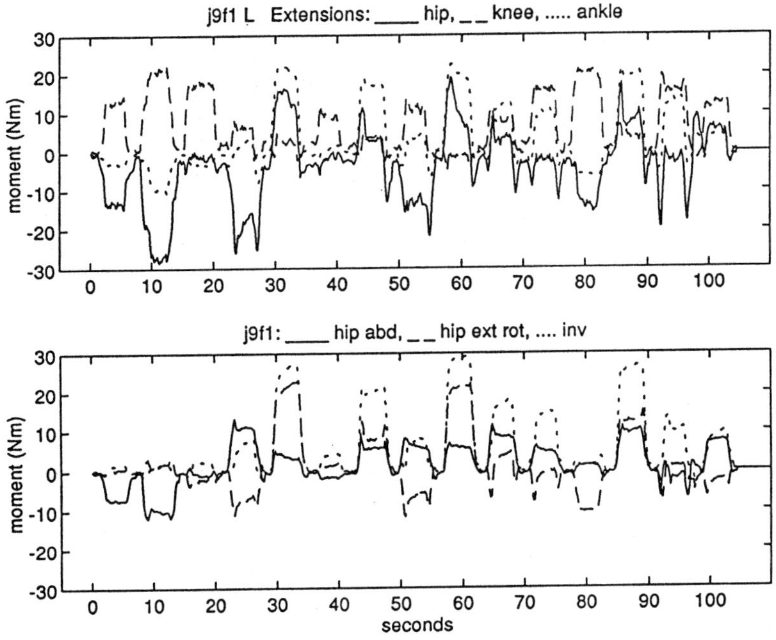

Fig. 6. Fragment of a hyperspace mapping sequence: Different 3-root combinations at different strengths

4 Discussion

The strength and fatigue-resistance of all muscle groups in this patient have continued to improve during the first six postoperative months, in spite of the fact that she trained every day, using surface stimulation, for six months prior to surgery. This is likely to be because root stimulation gives access to the whole motor output, while surface stimulation reaches only part of it. One root (L2, right) has given small moments throughout (except on the day of surgery, and at the first test on the fifth postoperative day), and it is likely that this is attributable to surgical damage. Regeneration began to occur after 9 months, as evidenced by an increasing moment obtained from this root at that time. It is known from experience with the SARSI implantations that spinal roots are sometimes damaged, in spite of every surgical precaution (Brindley and Rushton, 1986), and that after damage of this sort they often regenerate.

Besides training, and the moment mapping experiments reported here, the patient has stood regularly using her implant. The flexion reflexes noted on the moment measurements have also been clinically present on standing, particularly hip flexion and ankle inversion. With continued practice they have progressively diminished, but they are still troublesome.

In this patient, the combinations of lower limb moments that are accessible to root stimulation include those that are essential for standing and stepping. The stimulator control programmes, the multi-moment chair apparatus, and the data collection programmes together enable the rapid collection of large quantities of data. This enables us to make the testing sessions 'friendly' for the patient.

The mapping procedure requires a lot of data (the variables are root, stimulus strength, and posture), but the apparatus and testing software enable us to measure a different root-strength combination, including ramp-up and ramp-down times, and a quiescent interval between each test, at between 4-6 combinations per minute, depending on the parameters used.

5 Acknowledgements

This work was supported by the UK Medical Research Council. We are grateful to our patient for her cheerful cooperation through long hours of testing, and to her husband for his support, and for making significant parts of the apparatus.

References

Barr, F. M. D, Harper, V. J., and Rushton, D. N. et al (1995). Screening and assessment for a lumbosacral anterior root stimulator implant program. In: Proceedings, 5th Vienna International Workshop on Functional Electrostimulation, pp 95-98. Department of Biomedical Engineering and Physics, University of Vienna.

Brindley, G. S. (1994). The first 500 patients with sacral anterior root stimulator implants: general description. Paraplegia, 32: 795-805.

Brindley, G. S. and Rushton, D. N, (1990). Long-term follow-up of patients with sacral anterior root stimulator implants. Paraplegia, 28, 469-475.

Brindley, G. S., Polkey, C. E., and Rushton D. N. (1979). Electrical splinting of the knee in paraplegia. Paraplegia, 16: 428-435.

Brindley, G. S., Polkey, C. E., Rushton, D. N., and Cardozo, L. (1986). Sacral anterior root stimulators for bladder control in paraplegia: the first 50 cases. Journal of Neurology, Neurosurgery and Psychiatry, 49: 1104-1114.

Brindley, G. S. (1995). The sacral anterior root stimulator as a means of managing the bladder in patients with spinal cord lesions. In: Neuroprostheses. Eds GS Brindley and DN Rushton. Baillière Tindall, London.

Donaldson, N. de N., Perkins, T. A., and Worley, A. C. M. (1995). Lumbar root stimulation for restoring leg function. Methods: Stimulator and measurement of muscle actions. In: Proceedings, 5th Vienna International Workshop on Functional Electrostimulation, pp 323-326. Department of Biomedical Engineering and Physics, University of Vienna.

Kantrowitz, A. (1963). Electronic physiologic aids. Report of the Maimonides Hospital of Brooklyn.

Marsolais, E. B. and Kobetic, R. (1986). Implantation techniques and experience with percutaneous intramuscular electrodes in the lower extremities. Rehabilitation Research and Development 23, 1-8.

McNeal, D. R. and Bowman, B. R.(1986). Selective activation of muscles using peripheral nerve electrodes. Medical and Biological Engineering & Computing, 23: 249-253.

Naples, G. G., Mortimer, J. T., Scheiner, A., and Sweeney, J. D.(1988). A spiral cuff electrode for peripheral nerve stimulation. IEEE Transactions, BME-23: 905-916.

Rushton, D. N., Donaldson, N. de N., Barr, F. M. D et al (1995). Lumbar root stimulation for restoring leg function: results in paraplegia. In: Proceedings, 5th Vienna International Workshop on Functional Electrostimulation, pp 39-42. Department of Biomedical Engineering and Physics, University of Vienna.

Rushton, D. N., Brindley, G. S., Polkey, C. E., and Browning, G. V. (1989). Implant infections and antibiotic-impregnated silicone rubber coating. Journal of Neurology Neurosurgery and Psychiatry, 52: 223-229.

Initial Results with a Lumbar/Sacral Anterior Root Stimulator Implant

T. A. Perkins[1], N. de N Donaldson[1], A. C.Worley[1], V.Harper[2], P.Taylor[2]
D.E.Wood[2], D.N.Rushton[3]
[1]University College, London, U.K.
[2]Odstock Hospital, Salisbury, U.K.
[3]Royal London Hospital, London, U.K.

Abstract - Root stimulation responses and effects of training are presented for one female subject with a complete T9 spinal lesion. For standing, lumbar root stimulation stabilises the knees and sacral root stimulation stabilises the hips. The primary clinical aim for the patient to stand under her own control with sufficient stability to take one hand off the balance handles has been attained.

1 Introduction

The companion paper presented at this workshop by D.N.Rushton provides the background to this work. Figure 3 of that paper illustrates the control system used with three possible command sources. The backup option of surface stimulation in conjunction with the implant has not been necessary as the implant is working well.

2 Obtaining Correct Stimulation Levels

2.1 Getting started

Initially stimulation levels were adjusted using the slider box as the command source (see Figure 2 of D. N. Rushton's paper in this volume). Muscle responses were detected both visually and by palpation as in Figure 1 here. Thresholds are easy to obtain this way, the response being either present or not. Judgement of maximal levels by palpation is more subjective. Nevertheless initial estimates of 'maximal' levels for training purposes were set by this method to get training under way as soon as possible (see Figure 2). Thus muscle atrophy due to inactivity following the implantation surgery was largely avoided.

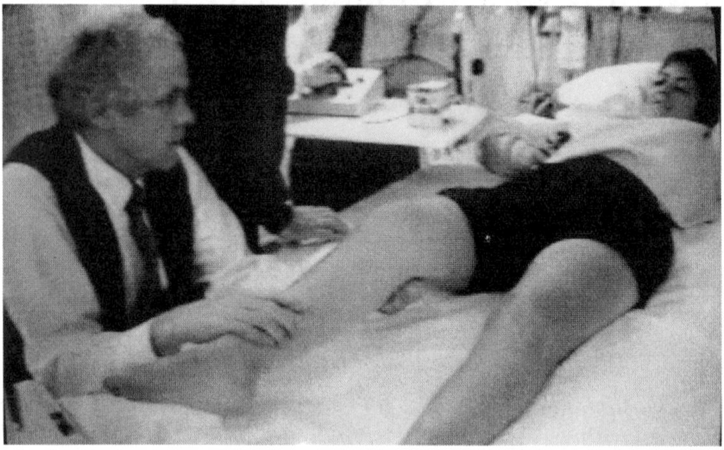

Fig. 1. Still from video presented: palpation of L3R response, 5 days post op.

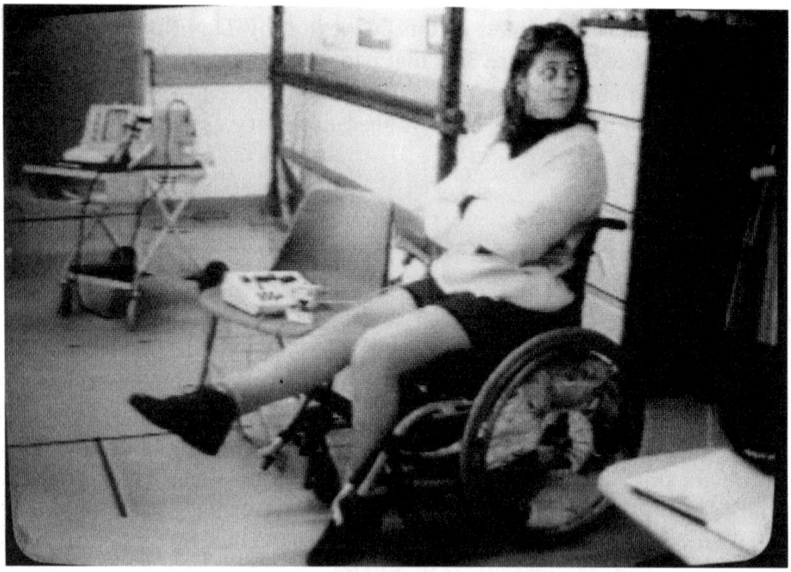

Fig. 2. Still from video presented: initial training using implant, 2 weeks post op.

2.2 Settling of threshold and maximal levels

Thresholds were closely monitored and, as shown in Figures 3, 4, and 5, had largely settled within 3 months of the operation.

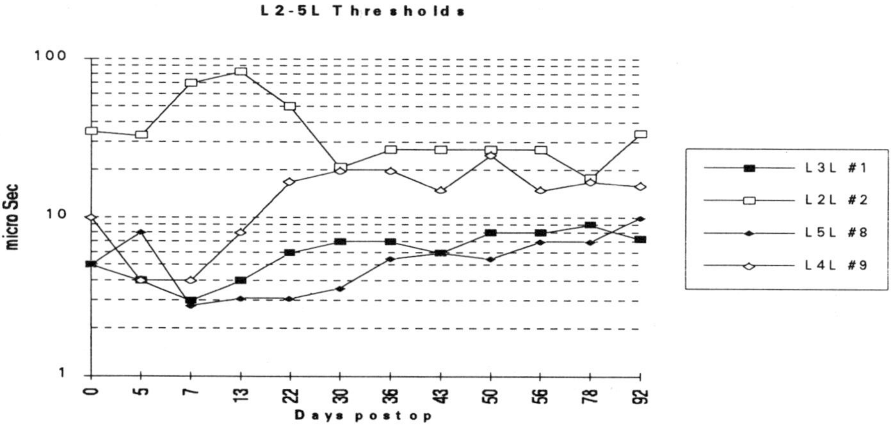

Fig. 3. Left lumbar thresholds: 56 days post op by palpation, then by moment chair

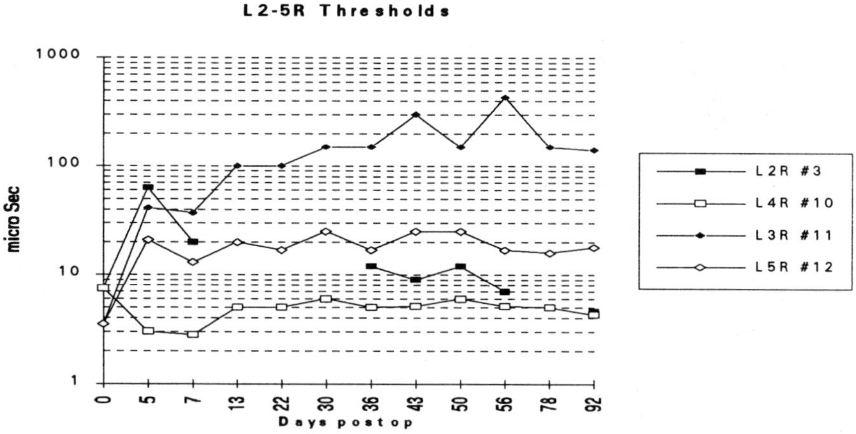

Fig. 4. Right lumbar thresholds: 56 days post op by palpation, then by moment chair

Ten out of the twelve channels have always shown strong responses, the exceptions being L2R and S2L. Initially, L2R gave strong hip adduction but its response faded after a week, returning as a weak hip flexor at five weeks post op (see Figure 4). The response of S2L also disappeared temporarily (see Figure 5) but recovered well after a month. The stimulus current in this implant was fixed at 5 mA. The dynamic range of threshold pulse width at 92 days post op was about 50 fold from ca 4 uS for L4R (in Figure 4) to more than 200 uS for S2L (in Figure 5). The sensitivity difference between the S1 and S2 roots is striking.

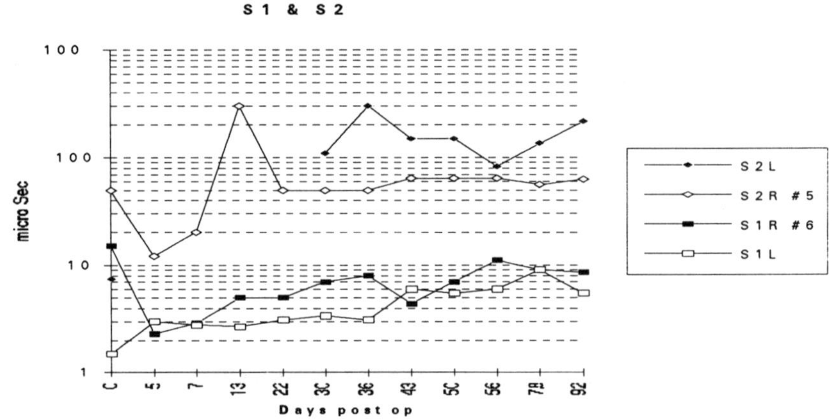

Fig. 5. Sacral root thresholds: 56 days post op by palpation, then by moment chair

Now, over nine months after implantation, L2R and L3R are slightly more sensitive and S2L rather less. The other thresholds remain similar to those at 92 days post op.

2.3 Measuring thresholds and maximals by multi-moment chair

As soon as practicable after the operation, the multi-moment chair was used to measure the responses to root stimulation (see Figure 4 of the companion paper). For threshold and maximal measurement we modulated the stimulation intensity of the test channel with a slow linear ramp up from zero to a target percentage (50% of full scale in the case shown in Figure 6). This linear percentage scale (used for convenience) corresponds to a logarithmic scale of pulse width from a minimum of about 2.5uS to a maximum of 910uS. The stimulation was held at the target level for 5 seconds and then ramped down to zero again. Even for L2R here, the weakest channel, threshold and maximal points can readily be seen. Errors due to timing skew can be cancelled out by taking the average of the results for the upward and downward ramps.

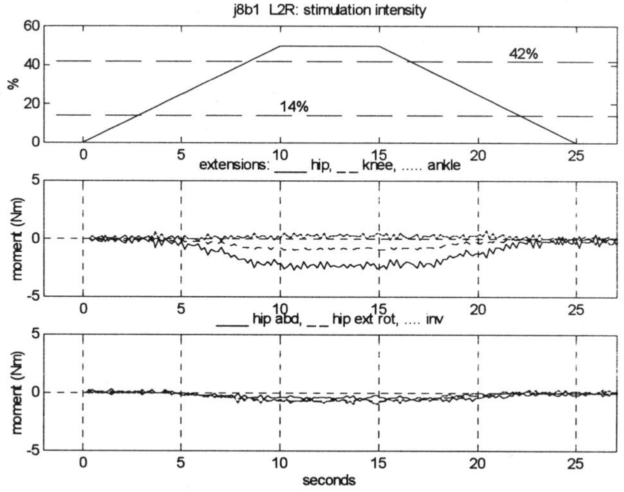

Fig. 6. **Multi-moment chair measurement of hip, knee and ankle moment responses to L2R stimulation up to 50% full scale.**

In Figure 6 the threshold corresponds to 14% full scale stimulation intensity and maximal level to 42%. In Figures 3, 4 and 5 threshold results derived by this method are plotted for the 56th and 92nd post operative days and are in general agreement with results obtained by palpation. While it is quicker to find a threshold by palpation, it is easier to see a maximal level from the multi-moment chair plot.

2.4 Stimulation levels for training

Several adjustments in training stimulation levels were needed to allow for the initial rise in maximals in the first few weeks after the operation. Because of the rising trend in maximals we undoubtedly set the training levels too high for some channels. No further action occurs above maximal stimulation for L2R, so a training stimulation level a little above maximal is not critical in this case. However several of the other roots give more complex (as well as much stronger) responses. Figure 7 shows that L4R has a maximal for knee extension moment at about 40% full scale stimulation. However at higher stimulation intensities hip flexion continues to increase. For standing the desired action is knee extension. There is no point in stimulating above the 40% level in this case, only to gain further unwanted hip flexion for negligible additional knee extension.

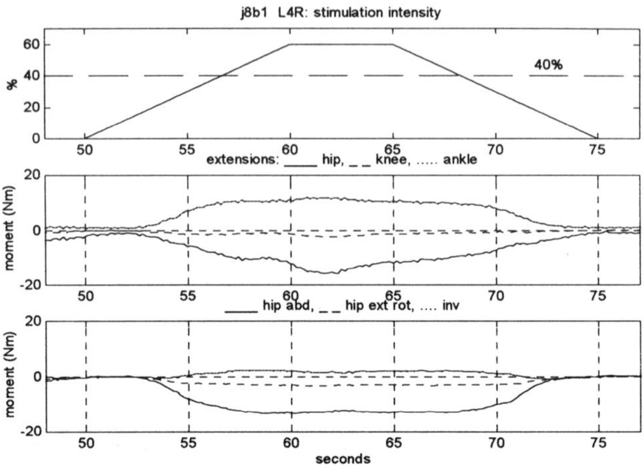

Fig. 7. Multi-moment chair measurement of hip, knee and ankle moment responses to L4R stimulation up to 60% full scale.

As training with the implant continued, muscle strength increased. This was most striking for movements, such as hip flexion and ankle inversion, which had not been obtained during the six months of pre-operative exercise with surface stimulation. Accordingly, as multi-moment chair results became available, the exercise stimulation levels were reduced to the maximal of the desired response for standing so as not to over strengthen the unwanted hip flexion and ankle inversion. From Figure 8 it is clear that L5L can give an unacceptable 30Nm of ankle inversion on its own. With half the patient's body weight supported on one foot, only about 15Nm of inversion renders the ankle unstable. Consequently L5L is now used neither for exercise nor standing.

2.5 Automation of response measurement

Figure 8 is an example of automated measurement using the multi-moment chair. In this case the command source was the same personal computer (PC) that recorded the response data from the chair. The stimulation patterns and timing data were held in a prepared floppy disc text file and read out to the stimulation control box via the RS232 link. After the control box stimulated with one pattern for the specified time, it sent a signal back to inform the PC it was ready for the next pattern. Two plots like that of Figure 8 were needed for the left leg responses for each of the 12 implant channels. Data for the two right leg plots (one is Figure 5 of D.N.Rushton's presentation) was collected at the same time. Thus all 12 single root response measurements could be obtained in a patient-friendly six minutes.

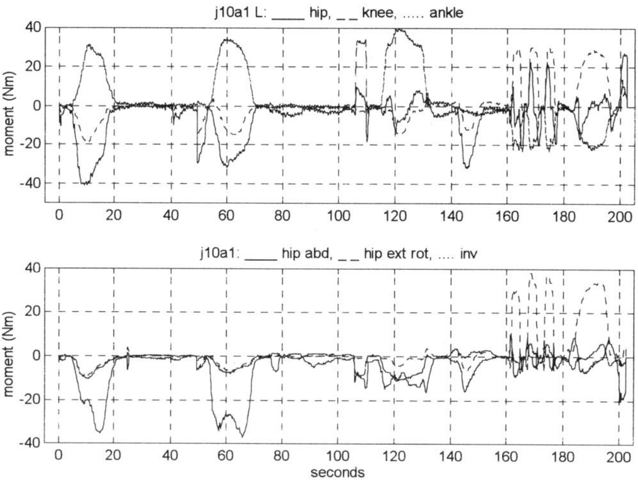

L2L (L2R) L3L (L3R) L4L L4L (L4R) L5R ....

Fig. 8. Left response to single root ramp-up, hold, ramp-down stimulation patterns measured in near extended posture 22/9/ 95

3 The Effect of Posture

The Fig. 8. measurements were carried out with only about 15 degrees of flexion at both hip and knee. In this test the three roots L2L, L3L and L4L all gave strong knee extension, useful to the patient getting up from her wheelchair. However only L4L was sufficiently free of hip flexion to be useful in maintaining standing.

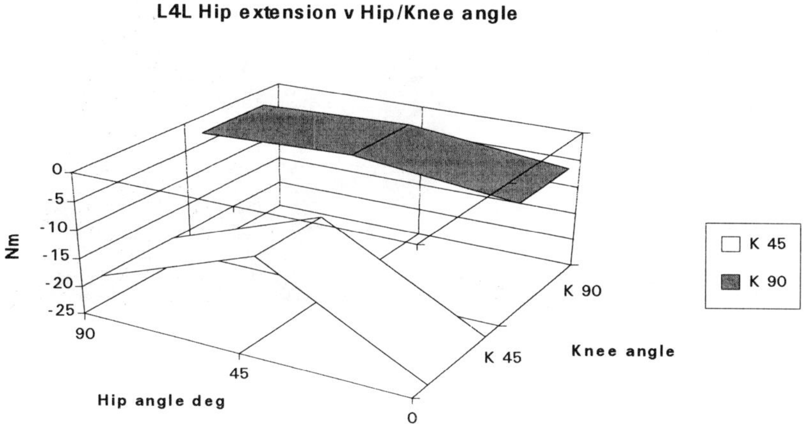

Fig. 9. L4L hip moment response versus hip and knee angle.

Some earlier hip moment measurements at a variety of postures are shown in Figure 9 It is only too obvious that joint angles can very greatly affect joint moments. We have therefore been obliged to use one stimulation pattern for getting up from the wheelchair, while the knees and hips are still somewhat flexed. Then for standing erect we have had to use a different pattern. It also appears that posture in training can influence subsequent stimulation response.

4 Response Adjustment Cycle

For six months prior to the operation, the patient had exercised her quadriceps muscles quite satisfactorily while seated, using a surface stimulator. She found training in her wheelchair convenient. Furthermore, just before the operation, she was able to stand quite erect with the aid of surface stimulation. As seen from Figure 2, the initial training by implant stimulation was also given in a seated posture. Figure 10 shows the patient standing after some months of seated implant training. With the amount of hip flexion shown, there was no chance of her remaining stable after removing one hand off a balance handle.

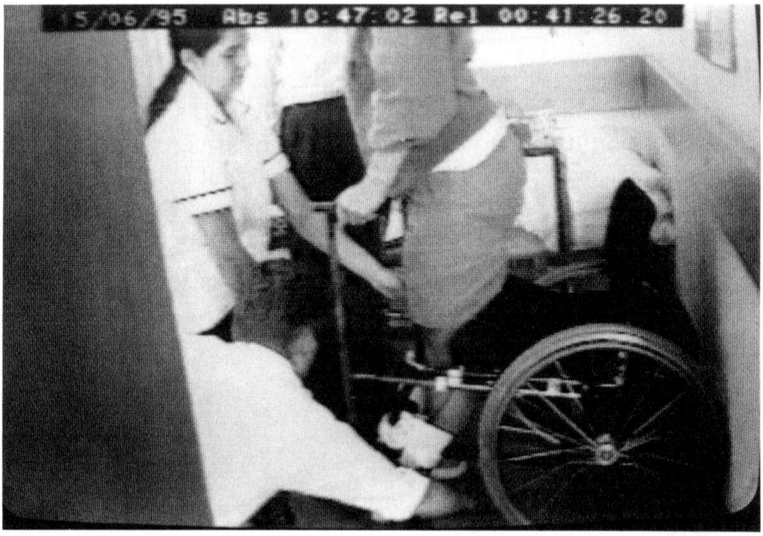

Fig. 10. Early stand with implant stimulation prior to training being optimised.

We concluded that implant driven exercise had to be done in an extended posture, which the patient has now been using for over 4 months. She has accepted training lying on her back. We are yet to persuade her to exercise while lying on her front.

Following the changes both in posture and in the stimulation levels used during training, our volunteer's responses to stimulation have become considerably more stisfactory. Good knee extension is available, with less hip flexion and ankle inversion. As we have continued to monitor responses, so we have been able to adjust the training program further to emphasize the desired actions and reduce the unwanted. With the benefit of experience, we hope to reduce the time taken on this response adjustment cycle by several months for any future patient.

5 Selecting the Best Stimulation Pattern for Standing

Most of the lumbar roots give hip flexion as well as knee extension. The sacral roots give hip extension at the cost of some knee flexion. In table 1 the roots giving the best ratios of moments have their results given in bold type. As S1R was stronger than S2R and gave less ankle inversion, S1R was preferred. Thus the asterisks mark the 4 channel 'best standing' stimulation pattern.

Table. 1. Ratios of hip and knee moment from multi-moment chair results 22/5/95

Side Root Ratio	Left Knee Ext/Hip Flex	 Hip Ext/Knee Flex	Right Knee Ext/Hip Flex	 Hip Ext/Knee Flex
L2	0.30			
L3	0.36		0.67	
L4	0.75*		0.48	
L5	Knee flex + ankle invers. Do not use!		0.75*	
S1		1.33		1.5* less ankle inv
S2		2.0*		1.5 weaker

6 Standing Control Program

Since table 1 was prepared, changes to training have been made (as mentioned in section 4) and lumbar root responses now give better ratios of knee extension to hip flexion. The standing pattern is now incorporated into the simple open loop control program illustrated in the finite state diagram of Figure 11 Each state in this diagram is defined in terms of actions on entry to the state; a target pattern of stimulation to be held for a specified time during the state and the exit conditions to other states. On entry to a state there is a ramp for a specified time in which the previous stimulation pattern is linearly adjusted to the new target stimulation pattern. Other action on entry can include a warning bleep. At present the 'patient's control' command option for the control box consists of two switches mounted on her right balance handle. The 'UP' switch allows her, after a one second pause, to get up smoothly and stand.

Pressing the 'DOWN' button allows her to sit down. As can be seen from Figure 12, she can now stand in a much more relaxed manner than shown in Figure 10, with a more erect posture. She has sufficient stability at knees and hips to take one hand off the balance frame and hold an object (in this case a glass of water) in her free hand.

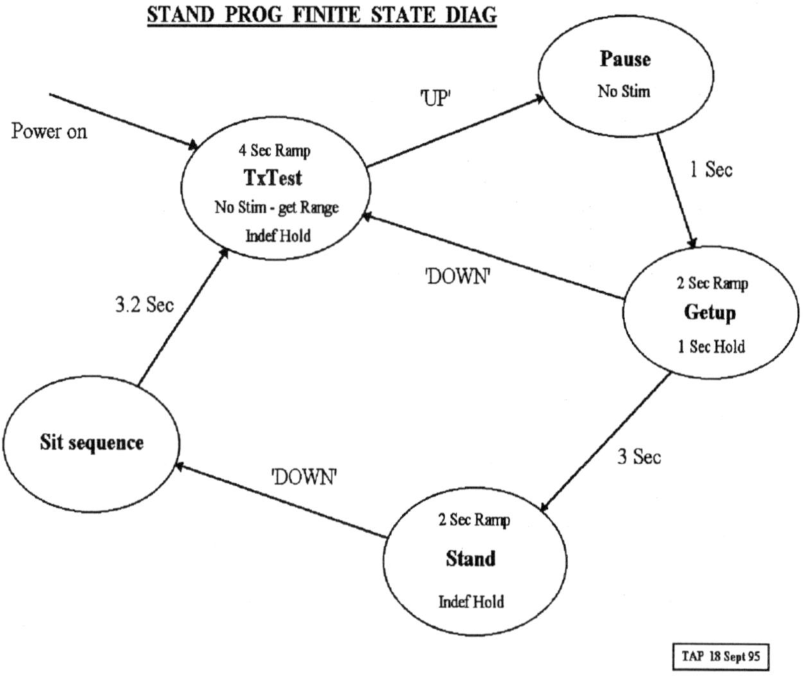

Fig. 11. Standing control program - as used in Figure 12

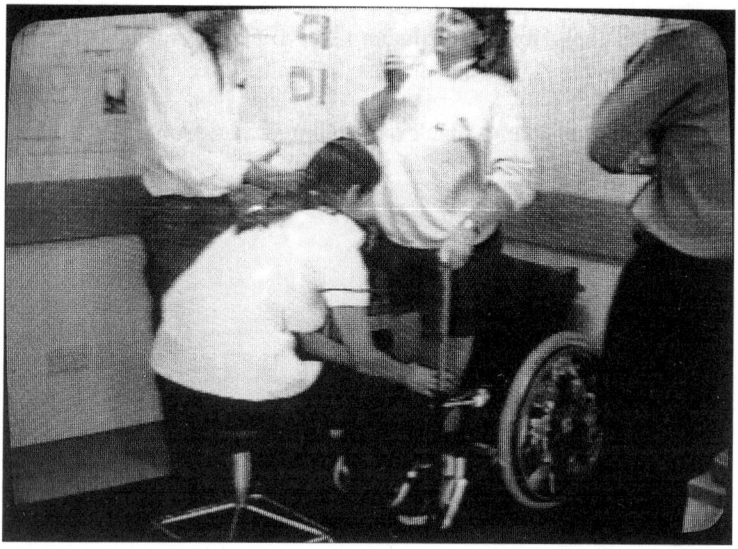

Fig. 12. Standing with implant stimulation after improved training 13/9/95

7 Discussion

The primary clinical target of enabling a paraplegic to stand with sufficient stability to have one hand free to reach for an object has been achieved. Even after neurological stability had been attained, as indicated by the settling of thresholds, we found the muscle responses to stimulation could be modified considerably by alterations to the patient's exercise regime. Because of this plasticity of response, the correct exercise posture and optimised stimulation levels are crucial to obtaining the desired actions from the patient's leg muscles.

8 Acknowledgements

We are grateful to the British Medical Research Council for funding this work and also to the following contributors:

Adler, J.	Stanmore Micro Systems; for power PCB and slider box assembly
Barr, F.	RN Orthopaedic Hospital, Stanmore, for help with patient selection
Chaffey, N.J.	Retired MRC NPU; for peripheral connector PCB assembly
Phillips, G.	FES Research Unit, Stanmore; for lab space and program advice

Shafik, T.	Kingston University student; for processor PCB assembly
Swain, I.	Odstock Hospital, Salisbury; for planning and advice
Tromans, A.	Odstock Hospital, Salisbury; for implant surgery and slider box idea
Wood, G.	University College student; for transmitter and battery assembly

Most of all we would like to thank our volunteer patient for her enthusiasm and tolerance during the many hours of testing.

Augmentation of Pulmonary Ventilation by Electrical Stimulation of Abdominal Muscles

U. Stanič[1], L. Lenart[1], J. Šorli[2], F. Kandare[2], R. Jaeger[3]
[1]Institute J.Stefan, Ljubljana, Slovenia
[2]Institute for Chest Diseases Golnik, Golnik, Slovenia
[3]Pritzker Institute of Medical Engineering, Chicago, IL, USA

Abstract - The possibility of electrical stimulation of the abdominal muscles during ventilation of normal subject was tested. The stimulation was triggered by expiratory airflow at the mouth, what resulted in increased tidal volume. This supports the idea, that similar electrical stimulation can be used in patients on mechanical ventilation. The Elite optical system was preliminary tested for measurement of lung volume.

1 Introduction

Respiration and ventilation are key functions in maintaining human life. Under normal conditions, a person typically takes 12 breaths per minute at rest, the volume of each breath being about 500 ml. Inspiration is brought about by the contraction of the diaphragm, and expiration occurs passively due to the elastic recoil of the chest. In some cases when adequate ventilation does not occure, mechanical ventilation (MV) is considered, Tobin (1984). This typically consists of introducing a fixed volume of air into the lungs under pressure. The expiratory phase occurs passively. The hypothesis of this study is that by electrical stimulation of abdominal muscles the respiratory rate and tidal volume can be changed what can be of some benefit for patients that have to rely on MV.

2 Methods

In this study five neurologically intact male subjects were included. For measurements of lung parameters Oxycon system was used: tidal volume (V_T,ml), frequency of respiration (fR, breaths/minute), minute ventilation (V_E,l/min), respiratory quotient (RQ,dimensionless). The measured data was processed of-line for statistical analysis (SPSS/PCt). Some preliminary tests were made by Elite optical system (BTS,Italy) for measurements of lung volume, but the data are not included in this study.

Large (3 × 8 cm) rectangle self - adhesive surface electrodes were used (PALS, Axelgaard). After some initial experiment by two pairs of electrodes, where several electrode sites were tested, in the present study only one pair of electrodes was used, the upper 6 cm above umbilicus, the lower one 6 cm below the umbilicus.

A custom built microprocessor controlled stimulator was used in the experiments, Sorli (1994). The stimulator was triggered by a flow sensor signal that was set at 15% of peak expiratory flow measured during quiet breathing. The amplitude of stimulation was gradually increased from zero to the value that caused effective contraction of abdominal muscles at tolerable comfort.

Figure 1 showes the experimental site with the subject in supine position with mouth piece and electrodes in place.

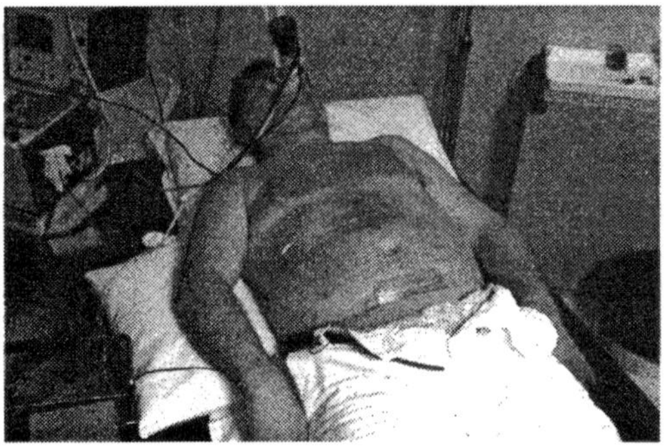

Fig. 1. Position of electrodes

The measurement consisted of four 10 minute periods of breathing: first period of quiet breathing was recorded, then period under the condition of electrical stimulation, followed by second period of quiet breathing, and finally 10 minutes of manually assisted period concluded the experiments. For statistical analysis means and standard deviations were computed for all subjects and for all four conditions.

Out of several parameters of lung function measured by Oxycon system, in Figures 2 and 3 the typical results of tidal volume and respiratory quotient are given for one subject.

3 Results

It was shown by statistical analysis that periods 1 and 3 were similar, but statistically significally different to periods 2 and 4. No difference between this two groups were observed. In average in all subjects tidal volume was increased from approximately 700 ml to 1100 ml in the periods of assisted ventilation. Respiratory rate was on the average 17 breaths/min during 1 and 3 periods of normal respiration, 19.5 during electrically assisted ventilation and 21.6 during mechanically assisted one. Ventilation was approximately 11.5 l/min during normal breathing, increasing to 21 l/min during electrically assisted expiration and 25 l/min during manually assisted expiration. The respiratory quotient was below 1.0 during normal breathing, and above 1.0 during the hyperventilating periods of assisted expiration.

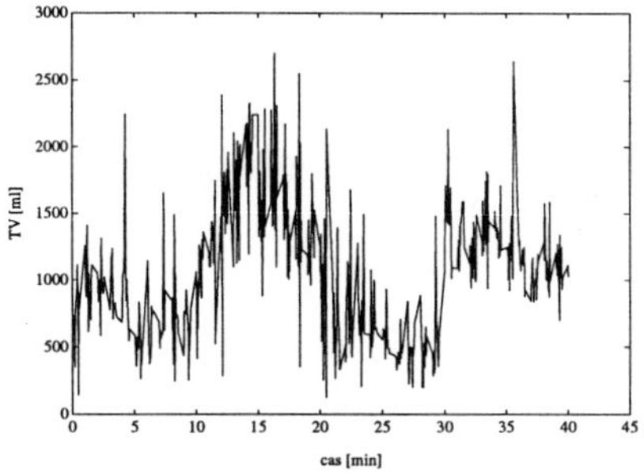

Fig. 2. Tidal volumes

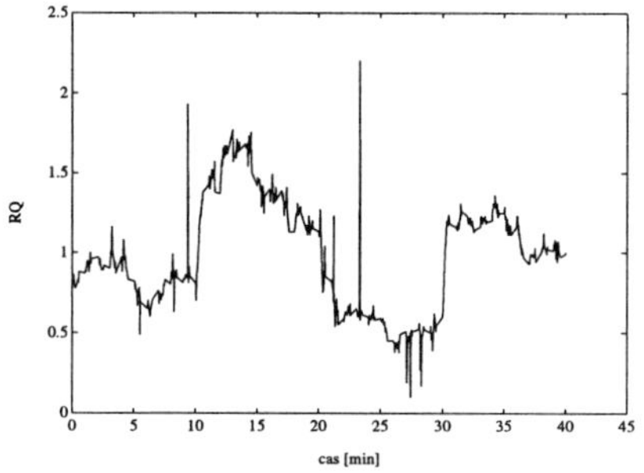

Fig. 3. Respiratory quotient

4 Conclusion and Discussion

In the study it was shown by the experiments on normal subjects that both respiration rate and tidal volume increased during assistance expiration. The subjects reported on more comfortable sensation during periods of electrical stimulation compared to mechanical one. The results offer perhaps some alternative to the elctrical stimulation of the diaphragm, Elefteriades (1992). It is to early to bring any conclusions of possible benefits for the patients now dependant on MV before the experiments are made.

References

Tobin, M. J. (1994) Mechanical Ventilation. J.Medicine,330:1056-61
Sorli, J. (1994) Kandare F. Jaeger R. Stanic U. Ventilatory augmentation using electrical stimulation of abdominal muscles. Proc 16th Ann Int Conf IEEE Eng Med & Bio Soc. Baltimore. Nov 1-6
Elefteriades, J. A., Hogan, J. F., Handler, A. L., Jacob, S., (1994) Long-term Follow-up of Bilateral Pacing of the Diaphragm in Quadriplegia. New England Journal of Medicine, 326:1433-34

Functional Recovery of Respiration: Phrenic Nerve Stimulation

D. Caldiroli[1], C. Carozzi[2], L. Cubattoli[2], G. C. Razionale[2]
[1]Dept. of Anesthesia and Intensive Care - Spinal Cord Injury Center, Sondalo, I
[2]Dept. of Anesthesia and Intensive Care - Spinal Cord Injury Center, Legnano, I

Abstract - Diaphragm Pacing (DP) has proved to be very effective as ventilatory support in patients suffering from chronic respiratory insufficiency caused by organic and functional abnormalities of the brain-stem respiratory center or by inadequate neural conduction as in quadriplegic. The ventilatory response with DP is satisfactory only when the indication to apply it is appropriate. The choice of the device and the implant site is based upon two considerations: the results of the neurophisiological testing and the characteristics of the electrode. The patients we treated were all quadriplegics and are all able to live at home and breathe free of ventilator. Although the complications of electrophrenic ventilation were found to be negligible, it should be emphasized that stimulator failures have occurred and in such cases had to be replaced. Adjusting the electrical parameters allow to obtain good diaphragm contraction under fatigue threshold even during the conditioning period. DP is nevertheless only one step in the rehabilitation program and the success is very closely linked to a careful screening of the candidates.

1 Introduction

For over 200 years physicians have tried to obtain artificial ventilation by phrenic nerve stimulation. The earliest meaningful experiences date back to 1783 when Hufeland applied phrenic stimulation in order to artificially ventilate asphictic newborns (Schechter, 1970). In 1814 Ure demonstrated how it was possible to obtain ventilation in freshly hanged man criminal (Schechter, 1970). In 1872 Duchenne de Boulogne (1872) was the author of a publication entitled "Respiration artificielle par la faradisation des nerfs phreniques" which added scientific meaning to this technique and defined it as the best method to imitate spontaneous breathing. Finally in our century this technique has found an extended area of application. In 1948 Sarnoff (Sarnoff *et al.*, 1948) applied diaphragm pacing as an alternative to mechanical vantilation during a poliomyelitis epidemic. Interest in this technique greatly decreased because for transcutaneous stimulation high voltage was necessary and this cause pain and burns. Another reason for the decrease in the use of DP at this time was the simultaneous development of intermittent positive pressure ventilation (IPPV). In 1964 Glenn (Glenn *et al.*, 1964) developed a method for transcutaneous inductive transmission of electrical energy with the use of an implantable nerve pacemaker. Since 1977 numerous centers apply phrenic stimulation in various pathologies of the nervous system using different types of electrodes and electric current wave forms. The first system for phrenic nerve stimulation was conceived by Glenn (Glenn *et al.,* 1964) and developed (and built) by Avery Laboratories N.Y., U.S.A. in 1960. The external components which comprise the device are an electrical impulse generator, an antenna coil, and a receiver that is in implanted in the subcutaneous tissue of the thorax or abdomen of the patient. The generator produces a series of electrical impulses which can be adjusted to variable settings of frequency, amplitude and intensity. The impulses are conveyed under the form of radio waves (at 1600 mHz) through the antenna coil to the receiver. The receiver converts the radio-waves to an electrical signal that is conveyed by means of an electrode (internal component) to the phrenic nerve. The electrode may be either monopolar or bipolar with the anode integrated in the receiver. Today it is no longer necessary to replace the receiver every 5 years because of batteries with an unlimited life.

The Finnish system Atrostim-Atrotech (Talonen *et al.,* 1985) because of the use of a quadripolar electrode and because of different type of stimulation called "sequential". On every inspiration each pole of the electrode stimulates one of the four quadrants in which the phrenic nerve is theoretically divided, thus reducing the frequency with which each single axon is stimulated, thereby allowing a comprehensive recruitment of a greater number of nerve fibres and motor units that shortens the period of muscular conditioning and limits the onset of muscle fatigue.

The Austrian system introduced by Thoma (Medimplant Biotechnisches Laboratories-Wien) in 1984 requires a complicated micro-surgical technique in order to implant the electrode (Thoma *et al.,* 1989). The device produces a characteristic stimulation called "carousel" which allows 16 electrode combinations during inspiration. From a physiological perspective DP represents a perfect hybrid between spontaneous and mechanical ventilation. In fact its function is to supply a respiratory drive as in mechanical ventilation although it utilized the patients own neuromuscular apparatus to create a negative intrathoracic pressure as spontaneous ventilation does. The indications to implement diaphragm pacing can be summed up as "any clinical condition characterized by chronic respiratory insufficiency caused by a dysfunction of one, or more components of ventilation (functional or organic alterations of brain stem respiratory centers, trauma of the cervical cord located above the emergence of the phrenic nerve)". The evaluation of a correct indication cannot disregard an accurate appraisal of the causes which led to respiratory paralysis. This is accomplished through functional explorations of the respiratory center, the conductivity of the phrenic nerves, diaphragm contractility, thoraco-pulmonary mechanics and the gas exchanges (Show *et al.,* 1980). It is therefore equally important to precisely define which patients would not benefit from the implementation of DP. It is very important to associate the interpretation of the neurophysiological and clinical data (Show *et al.,* 1980) obtained with stimulation tests of the phrenic nerve through percutaneous stimulation at the neck, intravascular stimulation in the thorax (Ishii *et al.,* 1990) or direct stimulation during surgery. The muscle action potential is recorded at the 6th or 7th intercostal space. It is advisable to radioscopically visualize diaphragm movement and measure the excursion even if the neurophysiological values are within normal range (Phrenic Nerve Conduction Time - PNCT < 12 msec. and Amplitude ≥ 0.5 mV. This can be a valuable assistance in the interpretation of uncertain neurophysiological data. The contractile efficiency can be quantifiably expressed by measuring the Pdi (Trandiaphragmatic Pressure) (Bellemare and Bigland-Ritchie, 1984; Aubier *et al.,* 1985; Bellemare and Grassino, 1982) during monolateral or bilateral electrical stimulation with a magnetic stimulator.

2 Methods

We are currently following four patients with DP implant (Table 1). All are males ranging from 18 to 51 years of age. All are tetraplegic with a lesion above C3, caused by traumas to cervical cord. Two patients were involved in auto accidents, one had a diving accident, and the last suffered a complication after a surgical procedure. Three of these patients were submitted to decompressive surgery after the acute event. The time which transpired between the accident causing the lesion, and the stimulator was never less than three months, in order to allow the stabilization of the neurological profile, and to exclude a possible recovery of spontaneous respiratory activity.

Pt.	Age (years)	Lesion level	Cause	Treatment
1	18	C1-C2	Diving	None
2	18	C1-C2	Car accident	Decompression
3	14	C1-C2	Surgical	Decompression
4	51	C2	Car accident	Decompression

Table 1. Patients

The choice of implant site was at the cervical level for three patients and the thoracic level for the fourth. In all cases the implant was carried out bilaterally. This was dictated by the material available and by the results of the functional exploration tests for phrenic conductivity and diaphragm contraction. For the first three cases we utilized American material (Avery-Framingdale,N.Y.) with small monopolar electrodes which necessitate only a minimal surgical exposure of the phrenic nerve. In the fourth case we used a Finnish model (Astrostim Pekka Atrotech Tampere) with a quadripolar cathode for which was necessary to implant the electrode into mediastenum through the thorax. The fundamental difference between the two models lies in the stimulating cathode. In the first three cases the cathode was monopolar whereas in the last case the cathode was quadripolar, which allows the sequential stimulation of each of the four quadrants in which the nerve is theoretically divided, for each respiratory act, thus limiting the electrical damage by reducing the intensity of the current thereby delaying the onset of perineural fibrosis (Table 2). In the final analysis the implant site (thoracic or cervical) was chosen in order to be able to stimulate the greatest possible number of nerve fibres with the maximum recruitment of motor units during inspiration.

Pt.	Time from accident (month)	PNS	Site	Electrode
1	6	Avery	Neck bilat.	Monopolar
2	8	Avery	Neck bilat.	Monopolar
3	3	Avery	Neck bilat.	Monopolar
4	6	Atrotech	Thorax bilat.	Quadripolar sequential

Table 2.

3 Results

There were no side effects noted after the first five years from the implant of the stimulator. In one case simultaneous stimulation of the brachial plexus was produced in relation to hyperextention and rotation of the head thereby bringing the plexus to a more superficial level, this phenomenon was also caused by the high current intensity which was utilized. On the contrary, many technical malfunctions of the external stimulator were recorded. In one case the stimulator (Avery model) had to be replaced twice, whereas in the last patient the stimulator (Atrotech model) had to be replaced once. The defects were caused in the first case by an imperfect adherence of the connections between the antennas, in the second case by electrical dispersion and rapid energy loss, and in the third case by the loss of the capacity to regulate ventilation. Each malfunction resulted in a reduction of diaphragm muscle contraction. Three have not been noted to this date any defects concerning any of the implantable components. Since the time of implant the electrical parameters (current amplitude, respiratory rate, inspiratory time, slope of inspiration and pulse interval) in all patients were modified in relation to the following:

1. modification of the minimum threshold of stimulation necessitating increments in current intensity, thus reaching a plateau after about four months;

2. structural modification of the muscle during the conditioning period (8 months after implant) changing type 2 "rapid contraction" fibres into type 1 "slow contraction" fibres (Salmons *et al.*, 1978; Salmons and Henriksson, 1981);
3. muscle contraction under the fatigue threshold.

All patients were bilaterally stimulated with a current inferior to 3 mA with a frequency below 20 Herz, Ti = 1 sec. (Inspiratory Time) and a respiratory rate < 12 breath\min. These parameters allowed us to obtain a TTdi < 0.15 (Tension Time Index of diaphragm)(Grassino and Clanton, 1991; Bellemare and Grassino, 1982) well underneath the fatigue threshold as well as the harmful level of charge density for nervous tissue (375 mc Coulombs\cm2).

Pt.	PNS	Side effect	Structural Failure
1	Avery	Nine	None
2	Avery	None	nr.2 Changes
3	Avery	Brachial Plexus Stimulation	None
4	Atrotech	None	nr.1 Change

Table 3.

Pt.	Living Home (years)	nr. Hospitalization and Reasons	nr. Respiratory problems
1	6	5,bedsores,gastric bleeding	None
2	4	2,routine control stimulator	1 (pneumonia)
3	3	1,routine control stimulator	None
4	3	2,routine control stimulator	None

Table 4.

The hospital stay for all patients ranged 7-13 months. Since the time that they were released from the hospital and returned to their home only once was readmission into the hospital necessary for respiratory problems, whereas readmission for other causes such as bedsore lesions, and intestinal problems were more numerous. The efficacy of phrenic stimulation is illustrated in table 5. All patients utilize phrenic ventilation all day or night long except for one patient (patient number 3), for whom the indication for the implant was not carefully evaluated. In one case the tracheostomy was closed. It worth to note how two patients implanted still tetraplegic can breathe spontaneously, respectively for over 8 hours and 12 hours a day utilizing accessory respiratory muscles of the neck without great difficulty. It is demonstrated however that DP does not prevent the recovery of spontaneous respiratory activity.

Pt.	Follow-Up	Tracheostomy	DP *	MV **	SB ***
1	6	Yes	24	0	>12
2	4	Closed	24	0	>12
3	4	Yes	2	22	No
4	3	Yes	24	0	No

* = Diaphragm Pacing   ** = Mechanical Ventilation   *** = Spontaneous Brething

Table 5.

4 Conclusion

Undoubtedly DP today has advanced a great deal technologically so as to achieve the desired respiratory response, however success is tightly linked to a careful preoperative selection of candidates, an accurate surgical technique and a competent follow-up. Currently there is still no wide consensus on many aspects of DP and many questions still remain. There are many advantages in DP such as the simplicity of use, the ventilatory pattern similar to normal, the absence of devices of any sort connected to the airway, the possibility to have a normal tone of voice, the absence of complications deriving from mechanical ventilation, and a reacquired increase in mobility, However we must also consider the cost, the incidence of stimulator failure, the necessity to perform tracheostomy in many cases, and the instability of the upper airways caused by obstructive syndromes if and when the tracheostomy is closed, and we must also consider the length of training.

Recent analyses indicate however, a greater acceptance and satisfaction by most of the patients for DP with respect to mechanical ventilation, with a decrease in maintenance cost and assistance.

DP however has to be considered as part of a global rehabilitation program that is also comprehensive of physiokinesitherapy, control of spasticity, accessory respiratory muscle enhancement, psychological assistance and learning of the instruments for environmental control.

References

Aubier, M., Murciano, D., Lecocguic, Y. et al. (1985) Bilateral phrenic stimulation: a simple technique to assess diaphragmatic fatigue in humans. J Appl Physiol; 58: 58-64

Bellemare, F. and Grassino, A. (1982) Evaluation of human diaphragmatic fatigue. J Appl Physiol 1982; 53: 1196-1206

Bellemare, F. and Grassino, A. (1982): Effects of pressure and timing of contraction on human diaphragn fatigue. J Appl Physiol; 53: 1190-1195

Bellemare, F. and Bigland-Ritchie (1984) Assessment of human diaphragm strength and activation using phrenic nerve stimulation. Respiration Physiology; 58: 263-277

Duchenne de Boulogne, G. (1855, 1872) De l'electisation localiseè et de son application à la physiologie et à la therapeutique.Paris, Bailliere II ed. 1855 et III ed. 1872

Glenn, W. W. L., Hageman, J. H., Mauro, A., et al. (1964) Electrical stimulation of excitable tissue by radiofrequency trasmission. Ann Surg; 160: 338

Grassino, A. and Clanton, T. (1991) Respiratory Muscle Fatigue. Seminars Respirat Med 1991;12(4):305-321

Ishii, K., Kurosawa, H., Koyanagi, H. et al. (1990) Effects of bilateral tranvenous diaphragm pacing on hemodynamic function in patients after cardiac operations: experimental and clinical study. J Choroc Cardiovasc Surg; 100: 108-114

Salmons, S., Gale, D. R., and Sreter, F. A. (1978) Ultrastructural aspects of the transformation of muscle fiber by long-term stimulation: changes in Z discs and mithochondria. J Anat; 127: 17-31

Salmons, S. and Henriksson, J. (1981) The adaptive response of the skeletal muscle to increased use. Muscle Nerve; 4: 94-105

Sarnoff, S. J., Hardenberg, E., and Whittenberg, J.L. (1948) Electrophrenic respiration. Am J Physiol; 155: 1-9

Schechter, D. C. (1970) Application of electrotherapy to non cardiac thoracic disorders. Bull N Y Acad Med; 46: 932-951

Show, R. K., Glenn, W. N. L., Hagen, J. F., et al. (1980) Electrophysiological evaluation of phrenic nerve function in candidates for diaphragm pacing. J Neurosurg; 53: 345-354

Talonen, P., Baer, G. A., Huhti, M., and Hakkinen, V. (1985) Control of muscle force by sequential motor unit stimulation of peripheral nerves: J Med Biol Eng Comut 23 (suppl 1): 396-397

Thoma, H., Girsch, W., Holle, J., and Mayr, W. (1989) Technology and long-term application of an epineural electrode. Asaio Trans; 35: 490-494

Modelling and Evaluation of a Nerve Cuff Electrode

D.M. Fitzpatrick[1],L. M. Costa Monteiro[2], R.H. Baxendale[2]
[1]Bioengineering Unit, Strathclyde University, Glasgow, Scotland, U.K.
[2]Institute of Physiology, The University, Glasgow, Scotland, U.K.

Abstract - Urinary incontinence is a major problem. Although it affects a substantial part of the population, in many cases it lacks any adequate conventional solution. One novel approach is to take direct control of the lower urinary tract musculature by electrical stimulation via electrodes on sacral spinal roots. This technique has been successful in some hundreds of cases world-wide but its more widespread acceptance is limited by the unsuitable recruitment characteristics of bipolar stimulating electrodes. This paper describes a new tripolar design for stimulating electrodes. Initial mathematical modelling studies predicted some very attractive features for this design. These predictions have been supported by in vivo testing in isolated nerve trunks and in experimental animals.

1 Introduction

Dysfunction of the control of the urinary bladder presents problems to a significant proportion of the population and unfortunately, conventional treatments are often inadequate to control the problem. Brindley and his co-workers have used electrical stimulation of sacral spinal roots via a bilateral array of electrodes. By judicious selection of roots for stimulation and adjustment of stimulation parameters the bladder can be brought under functional control. This work has met with considerable success in several hundred patients in many countries (Brindley *et al.*, 1982; Sauerwein *et al.*, 1990).

The principal limitation of more widespread application of this approach lies in the recruitment characteristics of the bipolar stimulating electrodes. Bipolar electrodes cause action potentials to propagate in both directions away from the stimulus site. In addition, they excite large axons at lower currents than small axons. The result of these properties are:

1. that volleys travelling orthodromically in afferents can give rise to unwanted reflexes or pain sensations.
2. that large motor axons innervating skeletal muscle and the external urethral sphincter are excited at lower current intensity than the smaller autonomic motor fibres which initiate bladder contraction.

The difficulties associated with 1. can be overcome by performing a dorsal rhizotomy to block afferent transmission and so eliminate possible pain sensations or unwanted reflexes. However, this is a relatively large surgical procedure which may have other unwanted effects.

The difficulties associated with 2. are harder to overcome. In addition to the unfortunate recruitment sequence for motor axons, the skeletal muscles of the sphincter contract faster than the smooth muscle of the bladder wall. The combined effect results in the sphincter closing before the bladder wall contracts. This prevents the bladder emptying and may cause potentially troublesome high pressures in the bladder. This problem can be addressed by adopting complex stimulation strategies but other electrode configurations may offer better solutions which could lead to a more widespread application of the Brindley technique.

We have been concerned with the modelling and testing of the characteristics of a more modern electrode, the preliminary results of which have been reported in recent scientific meetings (Fitzpatrick *et al.,* 1992; Costa Monteiro *et al.,* 1993).

2 Background

This paper describes experiments performed to evaluate a computational model of the properties of a tripolar cuff electrode (TCE) with a cathode placed asymmetrically between two anodes. Details of this design (Fitzpatrick *et al.,* 1991) and other similar designs (Wijkstra *et al.,* 1991; Rijkhoff *et al.,* 1992) have been published elsewhere . The design allows for the excitation of axons at the cathode with differential blocking of the action potentials at the anodes. The two anodal currents are regulated independently to allow for a complete anodal block at one end of the cuff with a controllable differential block at the other end.

The effect of varying the current intensity and the anodal current ratios on axons of different diameters were studied. The model predictions for the TCE are summarised in table 1. Briefly these are:

a. that it is possible to elicit action potentials which are anodally blocked at one end of the cuff but which are allowed to escape from the other end.
b. that it is possible to regulate the intensity of the anodal current at the escape end of the cuff to provide for the selective blocking of large skeletomotor axons whilst allowing the escape of action potentials in the smaller autonomic motor axons.

3 Results

We have begun testing the predicted properties of the triple electrode configuration in experiments performed in vitro and in vivo.

3.1 In Vitro Experiments

In experiments performed in sciatic nerves dissected form recently killed New Zealand white rabbits, electrical activity was recorded simultaneously from both proximal and distal ends of the nerve whilst currents were delivered via the TCE located in the central region of the nerve. The viability of the nerve was confirmed by the presence of

Ratio of anodal currents 0.7:0.3

Fibre	Current mA										
size	**325**	**371**	**410**	**428**	**451**	**454**	**458**	**555**	**600**	**636**	**800**
12	X	X	X	X	X	X	X	X	X	X	X
10		X	X	X	X	X	X	X	X	X	X
8									X	X	X
6										X	X
4											

Ratio of anodal currents 0.8:0.2

12	X	X	X	X	X	X	X	X	X	X	X
10	X	X	X	X	X	X	X	X	X	X	X
8						X	X	X	X	X	X
6										X	X
4											

Ratio of anodal current 0.9:0.1

12					X	X	X	X	X	X	X
10								X	X	X	X
8											X
6											
4											

Table 1: Summary of results of the computational model calculated for a cuff length of 10mm, fibre diameters between 4 and 12 mm and currents between 325 and 800 mA. The duration of the stimulation pulse is 300 ms. Three ratios of current splits are shown. **X** indicates block of action potentials at both ends of the cuff.

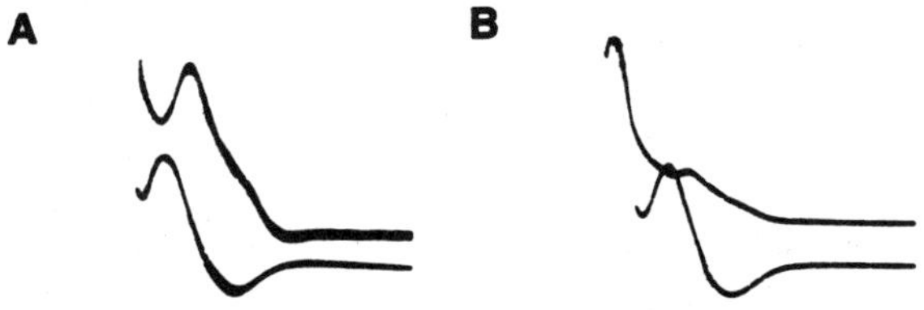

Fig. 1. This figure shows CAPs recorded simultaneously at the ends of an isolated rabbit sciatic nerve during stimulation via an electrode located in the central portion. All records were made from one preparation within a few minutes and at the same gain. Vertical scale bars indicate 1 mV. Horizontal scale bars indicate 1 msec. *A* shows CAPs recorded at both ends during conventional **bipolar** stimulation ie the action potentials escapes in both directions. *B* shows CAPs recorded during **tripolar** stimulation. A CAP is recorded at one end only. At the other end only a small residual CAP has escaped the block.

compound action potentials (CAPs) recorded at either end of the nerve during conventional bipolar stimulation. (figure 1a). When the nerve was stimulated with the tripolar electrode, a CAP was still recorded escaping from one end of the cuff whilst no CAP was seen at the other end of the nerve (figure 1b). These observations confirmed the modelling studies prediction that it is possible to set up unidirectional action potentials.

However, such an experiment provides information about the behaviour of only the larger axons found in the sciatic nerve. For technical reasons it is very difficult to record the CAP associated with the smaller autonomic axons. The recruitment characteristics of the TCE for these smaller fibres was investigated in a second series of experiments.

3.2 In Vivo Experiments

This project was reviewed by the Home Office and awarded Project Licence No PPL60/01193.

Experiments were performed in deeply anaesthetised adult male New Zealand white rabbits with a low lumbar-sacral laminectomy with dorsal rhizotomy to expose the S_1-S_3 ventral roots. The roots were stimulated in turn to identify which roots are most effective in generating contractions in the lower urinary tract. A cannula was positioned in the bladder to record the pressure generated during ventral root stimulation. The frequency and pulsewidth of stimulation were kept constant at 20Hz and 300ms, the current intensity was adjusted to produce activity. Periods of stimulation of 5-30 seconds were used. The TCE was then placed on the ventral roots and electrical stimulation applied to excite or block axonal activity,

During the TCE stimulation any other skeletal muscles innervated by the same sacral root were detected by visual inspection of the hindlimb and tail region. This was used to direct for the insertion of needles for intramuscular electromyography.

The TCE could be used for conventional bipolar stimulation by using the two outer electrodes. Bipolar stimulation produced the expected pattern of results in that whenever the current was intense enough to excite the small autonomic fibres causing bladder contraction there was accompanying activity in the larger skeletomotor axons. Typical results of bipolar sacral root stimulation are shown in figure 2a, b. Fig 2a shows the M wave recorded for a muscle in the perineal region during stimulation sufficiently intense to initiate bladder contractions, fig 2b. When used in the tripolar mode it was possible to set up equally strong bladder contractions, fig 2d, in the complete absence of any skeletal muscle activity, fig 2c.

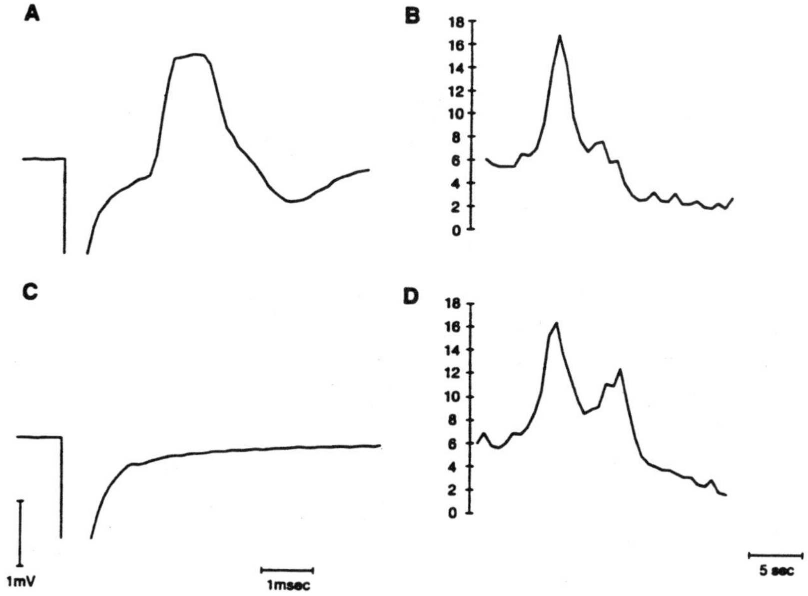

Fig.2. Figures showing the results of sacral root stimulation. *A* and *B* show the results of conventional bipolar stimulation of a single sacral ventral root. Activity is present in both skeletal muscle, *A*, recorded as the averaged EMG as picked up by intramuscular wire electrodes and *B*, the bladder wall, recorded as an increase bladder pressure. Skeletal muscle was always activated at lower current intensities than bladder contractions. This illustrates the expected recruitment sequence (larger axons first) for bipolar electrodes. *C* and *D* show tripolar stimulation of the same root. In this case bladder contractions are not accompanied by any EMG activity. This shows conclusively that the normal recruitment sequence of larger axons first has been reversed to allow selective stimulation of small motor axons.

4 Conclusion

Incontinence and its management is such a major cost to the health service that any prospective advance is potentially of enormous importance. These results show that a preliminary evaluation of the TCE support the modelling study predictions that the TCE offers the prospect of unidirectional excitation of axons and the possibility of exciting the smaller preganglionic motor fibres without concurrent excitation of larger somatic motor fibres. These are very new and exciting observations.

These properties may allow the benefits of the Brindley type FES strategies for restoration of bladder function to be more widely applied since they eliminate the need for a dorsal rhizotomy. The possibility of activation of the bladder musculature without simultaneously increasing the sphincter activity should also lead to better emptying avoiding the problems associated with bladder contraction with simultaneous sphincter contraction leading to very high bladder pressures or the problems associated with retention of urine due to incomplete emptying of the bladder.

References

Costa Monteiro, L. M., Baxendale, R. H., and Fitzpatrick, D. M. (1993) Stimulation of sacral roots for restoration of bladder control. Proc XXXII Congress of the International Union of Physiological Sciences: 89, 96.19P.

Brindley, G. S., Polkey, C. E., and Rushton, D. N. (1982) Sacral anterior root stimulators for bladder control in paraplegia. Paraplegia 20: 365-381.

Fitzpatrick, D. M., Struijk, J. J., and Andrews, B. J. (1991) A nerve cuff design for selective activation and blocking of myelinated nerve fibres. .Proc. IEEE-EMBS, 13 2/5: 906-907. ISBN 0-7803-2016-8.

Fitzpatrick, D. M., Baxendale, R. H., and Costa Monteiro, L. M. (1992) A new design of tripolar electrode for sacral root stimulation. 4th Vienna International Workshop on Functional Electrical Stimulation: ISBN 3-900928-02-9.

Rijkhoff, N. J. M., Holsheimer, J., Koldewijn, E. L., Debruyne, E. L., and Wijkstra (1992). Sacral root stimulation for bladder control: a study by computer modelling. Proc 4th Vienna International Workshop on Functional Electrical Stimulation: 164-167. ISBN 3-900928-02-9.

Sauerwein, D., Ingunza, W., Fisher, J., Madersbacher, H., Polkey, C. E., Brindley, G. S., Colombel, P., and Teddy P. (1990) Extradural implantation of sacral root stimulators. J. Neurol, Neurosurg & Psychiat, 53: 681-684.

Wijkstra, H., Rijkoff, N. J. M, Holsheimer, J. Kerrebroeck, Ph. v., Koldewijn, Boom, H. B. K., and Debruyne, F. M. J. (1991) Selective activation and blocking of sacral nerves: research set-up and. preliminary results. Proc. IEEE-EMBS, 13 2/5: 910-911. ISBN 0-7803-2016-8.

List of Authors

Abello, G. 411
Acimovic-Janezic, R. 541, 603
Alev, K. 67
Alexandrov, A. 3
Alfieri, A. 447
Alfieri, V. 447
Andersen, J. 45, 569
Andersen, O.T. 373
Anogianakis, G. 21
Apostolakis, M. 21
Baardman, G. 163, 171, 201
Bahrami, F. 285
Bajd, T. 293
Barner, T. 301
Barr, F.M.D. 217, 611
Bastings, E. 33
Bataweel, A.O.P. 523
Baxendale, R.H. 115, 429, 647
Bela, E. 21
Beliaeff, M. 179
Biering-Sørensen, F. 373, 569, 579
Boedrich, H. 301
Bogotaj, U. 541, 603
Boom, H.B.K. 155, 163, 201,317
Buss, M. 285
Caldiroli, D. 639
Caulfield, B. 51
Cincera, M. 11
Colombo, G. 41
Condie, D.N. 513
Costa Monteiro, L.M. 647
Daunicht, W.J. 263
De Vries, W. 163
Delwaide, P.J. 33, 393
Dietz, V. 41
Donaldson, N. deN. 217, 611, 623
Dorgan, S.J. 91
Duysens, J. 15
Edwards, J. 483, 523
Fernandez, M. 129
Ferrarin, M. 81, 401, 411,493
Fitzpatrick, D.M. 647
Franken, H.M. 155, 201
Frech, R. 437
Freyberger, F. 301
Frigo, C. 81
Galbo, H. 569
Garrett, M. 51
Gaviria, M. 145
Gider, F. 603
Gilbert, B. 179
Gollee, H. 123
Granat, M.H. 115, 513
Gregersen, H. 579
Gros, N. 541
Guiraud, D. 137, 179
Haase, J. 327
Hagen, E. 579
Hansen, S.D. 373
Harper, V 611,623
Harridge, S.D.R. 579
Hartkopp, A. 579
Haugland, M. 327, 335
Heinze, S. 163, 209
Hermens, H.J. 163, 171, 209
Hesse, S. 533, 553
Hoch, G. 183, 189
Huijing, P.A. 209
Iacuone, P. 81
Ijzerman, M. 163
Jaeger, R. 635
Järva, J. 67
Jarvis, J.C. 123
Jensen, L. 41
Jensen, P.L. 209
Kaasik, P. 67
Kandare, F. 635
Karcnik, T. 293
Keller, M. 183
Keller, T. 275
Kjær, M. 569, 579
Kljajic, M. 541, 603

Koopman, H.F.J.M. 209
Korosec, D. 377
Korze, D. 377
Koutsonicolas, D. 21
Krafczyk, S. 305
Kralj, A. 293
Krauß, P. 183, 189
Kwende, M.M.N. 123
Laczko, J. 305
Lenart, L. 635
Lickel, A. 327, 335
Lozza, A. 33, 393
Maertens de Noordhout, A. 33
Malezic, M. 533, 553
Massion, J. 3, 11
Mauritz, K.-H. 533, 553
Maxwell, D.J. 115, 513
Mayagoitia, R.E. 209
Meier, J.H. 359
Mihelin, M. 129
Mingrino, A. 81
Mizuno, M. 579
Mohr, T. 569
Murray-Smith, D.J. 123
Nene, A.V. 163
Nützel, A. 195
O'Malley, M.J. 91
Osio, M. 401, 411
Pääsuke, M. 67
Paul , J.P. 513
Pedotti, A. 11, 81
Pehme, A. 67
Perkins, T. A. 217, 611, 623
Phillips, G.F. 217
Pødenphant, J. 569
Psaier, E. 95
Puhke, R. 67
Quintern, J. 95, 183, 189,233
255, 281, 301, 305
Quistorff, B. 579
Rabuffetti, M. 493
Rabischong, E. 61, 137, 145, 179
Rabischong, P. 593
Rapisarda, G. 33, 393
Ratkevicius, A. 579
Repetto, J.C. 179
Riener, R. 95, 233, 255
281, 285, 301
Riso, R.R. 345
Rithalia, S.V.S. 483
Rowley, D.I. 513
Rugelj, D. 129
Rupp, R. 195
Rupprecht, S. 255
Rushton, D.N. 611, 623
Rutten, W.L.C. 359
Salmons, S. 123
Schmidt, G. 95, 281, 285, 301
Schultheiss, J. 275
Seene, T. 67
Sinkjær, T. 45, 327
Slot, P.J. 345
Soni, B.M. 469
Sorbi, S. 461
Sorli, J. 635
Sorrentino, G. 461
Sostaric, A. 377
Stallard, J. 503
Stanic, U. 603, 635
Straube, A. 255
Taylor, P. 611, 623
Thorsen, R. 373
Tomsic, M. 603
Tornøe, P. 569
Tromans, A.M. 611
Trontelj, J.V. 129
Umnova, M. 67
Van de Crommert, H. 15
Van Wezel, B.M.H. 15
Veltink, P.H. 155, 163, 201
209, 245, 317
Vernazza, S. 3, 11
Villars, S. 281
Volz, S. 255
Vossius, G. 195, 437
Wagner, A. 569
Weiß, A. 189
Wood, D.E. 623
Worley, A.C. 623
Yang, L. 513
Zazula, D. 377
Zilvold, G. 163